D0849816

BIOMECHANICS
AND EXERCISE
PHYSIOLOGY

BIOMECHANICS AND EXERCISE PHYSIOLOGY

Arthur T. Johnson
University of Maryland
College Park, Maryland

A WILEY-INTERSCIENCE PUBLICATION

JOHN WILEY & SONS, INC.

New York ● Chichester ● Brisbane ● Toronto ● Singapore

Library of Congress Cataloging in Publication Data:

Johnson, Arthur T.
  Biomechanics and exercise physiology / Arthur T. Johnson.
    p.   cm.

  Includes bibliographical references (p.   ) and index.
  ISBN 0-471-85398-4
  1. Exercise—Physiological aspects. 2. Biomechanics. I. Title.

QP301.J57 1991
612′.04—dc20   90-12842
                                      CIP

Printed in the United States of America

10 9 8 7 6 5 4 3 2 1

This book is dedicated to Miss Mary R. Humpton,
high school teacher and advisor at Newfield Central School,
who was much more than a teacher to the class of 1959.

We frequently hear the complaint that as the boundaries of science are widened its cultivators become less of philosophers and more of specialists, each confining himself with increasing exclusiveness to the area with which he is familiar.

—James Clerk Maxwell

Every author has much to explain, and the preface serves as a confessional vehicle. It also provides an opportunity for an author to define the philosophy behind the writing. And it tells the reader what to expect.

So I begin by confessing why I wrote this book. Dr. Ralph Goldman is the cause: he showed me that it is possible to quantitatively predict exercise thermal response. Once I saw that, I was hooked—what became most interesting to me was to see what could be predicted. If all exercise responses could be described in equation form, we could start using these equations in exciting ways—designing optimized equipment, producing more convenient respiratory protective masks and similar products, improving training procedures, and, of course, circumventing the university's Human Subjects Committee by resorting to computer modeling. Teaching of physiology would become more precise, because models contain precise (although not necessarily accurate) information. Gone would be terms like "relatively large," and "dominant," and "acute," and "chronic"; in their places would be glorious equations with numbers and precise definitions. So I started planning this book long ago: gathering information, classifying it, and filing it away for later reference.

But why exercise? Exercise is a natural stressful condition for which the body has been built. Physiology of rest is interesting enough, but look at all the changes, compensations , and feedback loops that are manifested during exercise! Extremely fascinating.

I confess next that this book does not contain all the information about exercise that various experts know should really be included. But I hope one strength of the book is its scope. Although large volumes have appeared on respiratory models, cardiovascular models, and thermal models, not a one addresses all three areas. So start here with an overview, then find more details in other tomes. I have tried to include all pertinent concepts, although not all pertinent embellishment. The scope of this book is so broad that I probably would not yet have attempted it, except that Tom Milhorn, author of *The Application of Control Theory to Physiological Systems*, told me how he began writing his inspiring book "before he knew any better" when he was a graduate student.

I confess, too, that, although I tried to include as much physiology as necessary (and I am reasonably familiar with physiology), I wrote this book as an engineer. I am extremely proud to be an engineer, and engineering has taught me to organize thoughts, concepts, and information. I hope there is a reasonable amount of good in this book for those who are not engineers, as well.

The models I chose to include in this book are not always the most modern. Indeed, I confess to having purposely passed over a number of exacting recent models to include some earlier ones. My reason for this was pedantic: some of the older models, although less detailed, give better overviews of the systems they model. And therein lies the connection with the quote from Maxwell at the beginning of this preface.

My biggest confession concerns units. Oh, what headaches! Every sub-, sub-, subdivision of every specialty uses different units. As an example, consider pressure drop by engineers in inches of water, by industrial hygienists in centimeters of water, by physicians in millimeters of mercury, and by some others in atmospheres; or consider rate of work by power engineers in horsepower, by electrical engineers in watts, by exercise physiologists in kilopond-meters per minute, by industrial hygienists in centimeters of water times liters per second. I talk to all of these, and it means constantly juggling conversion factors in my head. When I began writing this book I started using the prevailing units for each object of scrutiny. It soon became apparent that in this method lay madness. Thus you'll find straight metric units here, and not even International system units, because a joule is called a newton-meter, and a watt, or joule per second, is called a newton-meter per second. To accommodate those readers who talk to people in other specialities, I've included some units in parentheses. Perhaps after seeing the standard set of units used here, you'll appreciate why other units are still used.

I also had a problem with the title of this book: it could have included the words "biomechanics," "ergonomics," "exercise physiology," "labor," or "stress"—all recognizable to a portion of the technical field I wish to address. But what do you do when you're dealing with a multidisciplinary subject? You call it what you will, and hope for the best.

Now that I've confessed, I feel better. I hope it wasn't too painful for you. Maybe the next edition of this book will have a section on your work, and a shorter preface as a result.

Arthur T. Johnson

College Park, Maryland
January 1991

ACKNOWLEDGMENTS

Jupiter has loaded us with a couple of wallets: the one, filled with our own vices, he has placed at our back; the other, heavy with those of others, he has hung before.

—Phaedrus

I am deeply indebted to many for the final production of this book. Thanks to Mrs. Thelma deCheubel for typing the early drafts, thanks to Mr. Lovant Hicks for the excellent drawings, and a special thanks to Cathy, who typed the final draft, counting down each equation in turn and cringing at my split infinitives.

A.T.J.

CONTENTS

1. EXERCISE LIMITATIONS   1

    1.1 Introduction / 1
    1.2 Exercise Intensity and Duration / 2
    1.3 Muscle Metabolism / 7
        1.3.1 Muscle Fiber Structure / 7
        1.3.2 Muscle Energy Sources / 8
        1.3.3 Oxygen Debt / 10
        1.3.4 Maximal Oxygen Uptake / 12
        1.3.5 Anaerobic Threshold / 15
        1.3.6 Oxygen Uptake Kinetics / 19
        1.3.7 A Bioenergetics Model / 21
        1.3.8 Chemical Responses / 24
    1.4 Cardiovascular Exercise Limitation / 24
    1.5 Respiratory Limitation / 26
    1.6 Thermal Limitation / 26
    1.7 Prolonged Exercise / 26
Symbols / 28
References / 28

2. EXERCISE BIOMECHANICS   31

    2.1 Introduction / 31
    2.2 Physics of Movement / 31
        2.2.1 Equilibrium and Stability / 31
        2.2.2 Muscles and Levers / 33
        2.2.3 Energy and Motion / 38
            Translational Motion / 38
            Angular Motion / 43
    2.3 The Energy Cost of Movement / 47
    2.4 Walking and Running / 54
        2.4.1 Basic Analysis / 54
        2.4.2 Optimal Control of Walking / 58
        2.4.3 Experimental Results / 64
    2.5 Carrying Loads / 65
        2.5.1 Load Position / 65
        2.5.2 Lifting and Carrying / 65
        2.5.3 Using Carts / 66
    2.6 Sustained Work / 66

Symbols / 67
References / 69

3. CARDIOVASCULAR RESPONSES   **71**

3.1 Introduction / 71
3.2 Cardiovascular Mechanics / 71
    3.2.1 Blood Characteristics / 72
        Composition / 72
        Oxygen-Carrying Capacity / 72
        Viscosity / 78
    3.2.2 Vascular Characteristics / 81
        Organization / 81
        Resistance / 82
        Very Small Vessels / 84
    3.2.3 Heart Characteristics / 89
        Starling's Law / 90
        Blood Pressure / 91
        Heart Rate / 93
        Cardiac Output / 94
        Energetics / 96
3.3 Cardiovascular Control / 99
    3.3.1 Neural Regulation / 100
        Sensors / 100
        Controller / 101
        Effector Organs / 104
        Reflexes / 105
    3.3.2 Humoral Regulation / 107
    3.3.3 Other Regulatory Effects / 108
    3.3.4 Exercise / 108
    3.3.5 Heat and Cold Stress / 111
3.4 Cardiovascular Mechanical Models / 112
    3.4.1 Robinson's Ventricle Model / 112
    3.4.2 Comprehensive Circulatory System Model / 116
    3.4.3 Vascular System Models / 117
    3.4.4 Optimization Models / 118
    3.4.5 Heart Rate Models / 125
        Transient Response / 125
        Heat Effects / 127
        Comparison Between the Two Heart Rate Models / 131
3.5 Cardiovascular Control Models / 131
    3.5.1 The Heart / 131
        The Ventricles / 131
        The Atria / 138
        Heart Rate Control / 139
        Coronary Blood Flow and Heart Performance / 142
    3.5.2 Systemic and Pulmonary Vessels / 143
        Mechanics / 143
        Vascular Resistance Control / 145
        Control of Capillary Pressure and Blood Volume / 146
        Nonlinear Resistances / 147
    3.5.3 Model Performance / 148

Appendix 3.1 Numerically Solving Differential Equations / 149
Appendix 3.2 Pontryagin Maximum Principle / 151
Appendix 3.3 The Laplace Transform / 153
Symbols / 156
References / 160

4. RESPIRATORY RESPONSES   **166**

4.1 Introduction / 166
4.2 Respiratory Mechanics / 166
    4.2.1 Respiratory Anatomy / 167
          Lungs / 167
          Conducting Airways / 169
          Alveoli / 171
          Pulmonary Circulation / 172
          Respiratory Muscles / 173
    4.2.2 Lung Volumes and Gas Exchange / 174
          Lung Volumes / 175
          Perfusion of the Lung / 177
          Gas Partial Pressures / 179
          Respiratory Exchange Ratio / 183
          Lung Diffusion / 185
          Gas Mixing in the Airways / 189
          Diffusion Capacity / 191
          Blood Gases / 192
          Pulmonary Gas Exchange / 196
    4.2.3 Mechanical Properties / 200
          Respiratory System Models / 200
          Resistance / 203
          Compliance / 214
          Inertance / 218
          Time Constant / 219
          Respiratory Work / 220
4.3 Control of Respiration / 222
    4.3.1 Respiratory Receptors / 224
          Chemoreceptors / 224
          Mechanoreceptors / 230
          Other Inputs / 231
    4.3.2 Respiratory Controller / 231
          Respiratory Rhythm / 231
          Airflow Waveshape / 232
          Control Signals / 238
    4.3.3 Effector Organs / 238
          Respiratory Muscles / 238
          Airway Muscles / 238
          Local Effectors / 239
    4.3.4 Exercise / 239
          Initial Rise / 240
          Transient Increase / 240
          Steady State / 241
          Cessation of Exercise / 250
          Anaerobic Ventilation / 250

Ventilatory Loading / 252
Dyspnea and Second Wind / 254
Optimization of Breathing / 256
Summary of Control Theories / 265

4.4 Respiratory Mechanical Models / 271
    4.4.1 Respiratory Mechanics Models / 271
        Jackson–Milhorn Computer Model / 271
        Expiratory Flow Model / 281
        Ventilation Distribution Model with Nonlinear Components / 286
        Theory of Resistance Load Detection / 291
    4.4.2 Gas Concentration Models / 293
        Concentration Dynamics Model / 293

4.5 Respiratory Control Models / 298
    4.5.1 System Models / 299
        Grodins Model / 300
        Saunders Modification of Grodins Model / 310
        Yamamoto CO_2 Model / 320
    4.5.2 Fujihara Control Model / 330
    4.5.3 Optimization Models / 330
        Yamashiro and Grodins Model / 331
        Hämäläinen Model / 335
    4.5.4 Brief Discussion of Respiratory Control Models / 340
Appendix 4.1 Lagrange Multipliers / 341
Appendix 4.2 Method of Calculus of Variations / 341
Symbols / 344
References / 351

5. THERMAL RESPONSES   **361**

5.1 Introduction / 361
    5.1.1 Passive Heat Loss / 361
    5.1.2 Active Resources / 363
5.2 Thermal Mechanics / 364
    5.2.1 Convection / 364
        Body Surface Area / 366
        Respiratory Convective Heat Loss / 367
    5.2.2 Conduction / 368
        Clothing / 369
        Mean Skin Temperature / 370
    5.2.3 Radiation / 372
        Radiant Heat Transfer Coefficient / 374
        Solar Heat Load / 375
    5.2.4 Evaporation / 381
        Respiratory Evaporation / 384
        Sweating / 385
        Clothing / 385
    5.2.5 Rate of Heat Production / 390
        Basal Metabolic Rate / 390
        Food Ingestion / 393
        Muscular Activity / 394
    5.2.6 Rate of Change of Stored Heat / 401
5.3 Thermoregulation / 403

      5.3.1 Thermoreceptors / 403

      5.3.2 Hypothalamus / 405

      5.3.3 Heat Loss Mechanisms / 409

          Vasodilation / 409

          Sweating / 412

      5.3.4 Heat Maintenance and Generation / 413

          Vascular Responses / 413

          Shivering / 415

          Nonshivering Thermogenesis / 415

      5.3.5 Acclimatization / 416

      5.3.6 Circadian Rhythm / 417

      5.3.7 Exercise and Thermoregulation / 418

   5.4 Thermoregulatory Models / 419

      5.4.1 Cylindrical Models / 419

          Gagge Model / 419

          Wyndham–Atkins Model / 422

      5.4.2 Multicompartment Model / 425

      5.4.3 External Thermoregulation / 433

   5.5. Body Temperature Response / 436

      5.5.1 Equilibrium Temperature / 436

          Metabolic Heat Load / 436

          Radiation and Convection Heat Exchange / 439

          Sweating / 439

          Equilibrium Body Temperature / 440

      5.5.2 Variation of Rectal Temperature with Time / 440

          Changes at Rest Under Heat Stress / 441

          Elevation During Work / 441

          Recovery After Work / 442

          Effect of Acclimatization / 443

      5.5.3 Model Limitations and Performance / 444

Symbols / 446

References / 449

INDEX   **457**

BIOMECHANICS AND EXERCISE PHYSIOLOGY

CHAPTER 1

Exercise Limitations

It would be futile to accomplish with a greater number of things what can be accomplished with fewer
—William of Ockham[1]

1.1 INTRODUCTION

The study of exercise is important to the bioengineer. To understand exercise responses is to understand physiological responses to natural stresses to which the body has become attuned. This understanding can be used to facilitate communication with physiologists, veterinarians, occupational hygienists, or medical personnel on multidisciplinary research, development, or management teams. Familiarity with exercise physiology may be a requirement for the proper design decisions when developing a new bioengineering product. Bioengineers, especially those who have accumulated some experience and reputation in their field, are often requested to evaluate research or management proposals or design reports from their subordinates. A basic understanding of exercise physiology can be an invaluable aid toward making the proper evaluation. Furthermore, there is something to be said for the individual who seeks knowledge of the surrounding world for the sake of global understanding and self-actualization. This is the type of individual who would relish the opportunity to study the material with which this book is filled, and this is the type of individual who will see new ways to describe and formulate physiological information.

Like many exercise physiology texts, this book must deal with a broad scope of material. After all, exercise responses are both all-consuming and highly integrated: most physiological systems, artificially divided and separately studied, become one total supportive mechanism for the performance of the physical stress of exercise.

Unlike many exercise physiology texts, the emphasis here is on quantitative description as much as possible. This means that the book is not intended to be a physiology primer; others will have to be used for introductory purposes. This book is intended to demonstrate the vast amount of physiological material that can be quantitatively predicted. For this reason, some physiological facts are not included here, but the hope is that the equations, models, and tables of numerical values will make up for any omission.

Models play an important part in the engineering world. As Grodins (1981) states:

> [Models]...clarify our thinking about a problem by explicitly identifying and clearly stating every assumption and limitation and...set the stage for a rigorous analysis usually expressed in mathematical language.... They provide a compact, clear, rigorously integrated summary of current conventional wisdom about how some natural system works.... Textbooks in the biological sciences are often swollen with detailed verbal descriptions which do not depart very far from raw

---

[1] This statement, known as Ockham's Razor, or the Principle of Parsimony, is the basis for selecting the simplest possible model to describe a process.

experimental observations. Textbooks of physics, on the contrary, are compact because they contain descriptions of models almost exclusively....

The archival function of models implies that they should also serve a valuable teaching function, as indeed they do in the physical sciences. Dynamic respiratory models, especially in their computerized interactive format, should be very valuable in teaching physiologists, medical students, and physicians the essence of normal and pathological pulmonary physiology....

Finally, models provide a mechanism for rigorously exploring the observable implications of physiological hypotheses and thus can help to design experiments to test them. Investigators must know what a particular hypothesis commits them to in terms of experimental observations before they can test it. In a complex system with many interacting variables which cannot be experimentally isolated, rigorous modeling may be the only way to obtain them. Such predictions may sometimes turn out to be unexpected and counterintuitive. If they survive an exhausting recheck of model formulation and computation, this surprising behavior of models is one of their most valuable attributes in hypothesis testing.[2]

This book emphasizes models, quantitative mathematical models if possible, or conceptual models at the very least. Especially in the last three chapters, several models describing cardiovascular, respiratory, or thermal responses are presented. The physiology sections preceding the models are directed toward presentation of sufficient background to understand the models. First, there are some basic concepts concerning exercise in general that must be introduced and kept in mind in succeeding chapters. These concepts deal with exercise duration and limitations to perpetual performance.

1.2 EXERCISE INTENSITY AND DURATION

Generally, intense exercise can be performed for short times only. The intensity–duration curve for any particular individual plots generally as a hyperbola asymptotically approaching each axis (Figure 1.2.1). Although Figure 1.2.1 was used to describe exercise limitations imposed by respiratory protective masks, the general shape is still valid for exercise of various intensities; it shows that for very high rates of work, very short performance times can be expected.

In an interesting summary article, Riegel (1981) compared world-class athletic performance records for running, race walking, cross-country skiing, roller and speed skating, cycling, freestyle swimming, and man-powered flight. He plotted time against distance on logarithmic scales and found a linear relationship between the times of 210 and 13,800 sec (Figure 1.2.2). Below 180–240 sec, athletic competition includes sprints and other activity involving transient body processes. Above 13,800 sec, competition is rarely, if ever, carried to the limit of endurance. Thus over the linear range of 210–13,800 sec (3.5–230 min), performance time is predicted by the following equation:

$$t = ax^b \tag{1.2.1}$$

where t = endurance time, sec
a = constant, sec/km^b
x = distance, km
b = fatigue factor, dimensionless

The constant a is dependent on the units of measurement and has no particular significance. The exponent b determines the rate at which average speed decreases with distance. Values

---

[2] Cobelli et al. (1984) state that "the principle difficulty attached to the mathematical analysis of physiological and medical systems stems from the mismatch between the complexity of the processes in question and the limited data available from such systems."

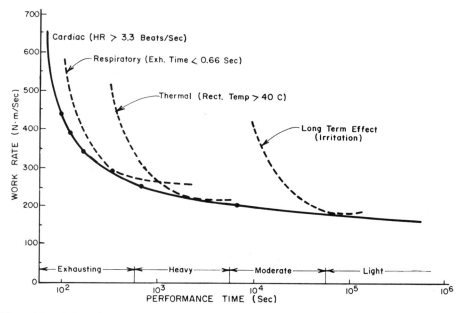

Figure 1.2.1 Schematic representation of performance time while exercising wearing a protective mask. (Adapted and redrawn with permission from Johnson and Cummings, 1975.)

TABLE 1.2.1 Specific Constants and Data for the Endurance Equation

Activity	a^a sec/km^b	(min/km^b)	b^a	Distance Range, km	Time Range, sec	(mm)
Running, men	8,274	(137.9)	1.07732	1.5–42.2	210–7,740	(3.5–129)
Running, men over 40	9,246	(154.1)	1.05352	1.5–42.2	234–7,860	(3.9–131)
Running, men over 50	10,230	(170.5)	1.05374	1.5–42.2	252–8,700	(4.2–145)
Running, men over 60	11,530	(192.2)	1.05603	1.5–42.2	294–10,100	(4.9–168)
Running, men over 70	13,150	(219.2)	1.06370	1.5–42.2	324–11,300	(5.4–189)
Running, women	9,354	(155.9)	1.08283	1.5–42.2	234–8,820	(3.9–147)
Swimming, men	35,770	(596.2)	1.02977	0.4–1.5	234–900	(3.9–15)
Swimming, women	38,080	(634.7)	1.03256	0.4–1.5	246–960	(4.1–16)
Nordic skiing, men	10,210	(170.2)	1.01421	15–50	2,640–6,940	(44–149)
Race walking, men	12,830	(213.9)	1.05379	1.6–50	354–13,300	(5.9–222)
Roller skating, men	5,718	(95.3)	1.13709	3–10	336–1,320	(5.6–22)
Cycling, men	3,654	(60.9)	1.04834	4–100	264–7,680	(4.4–128)
Speed skating, men	4,560	(76.0)	1.06017	3–10	246–900	(4.1–15)
Man-powered flight	11,660	(194.3)	1.10189	1.8–36.2	384–10,100	(6.4–169)

Source: Adapted and used with permission from Riegel, 1981.

[a]Based on records up to November 1, 1979.

for these constants, obtained by a least-squares[3] analysis, are found in Table 1.2.1. World-class runners, men and women, have an identical fatigue factor of 1.08; men and women swimmers share a fatigue factor of 1.03.

[3]This term refers to a standard procedure in statistical regression where the constants are determined such that they minimize the sum of the squares of deviations of the individual data points from the line fitted through them.

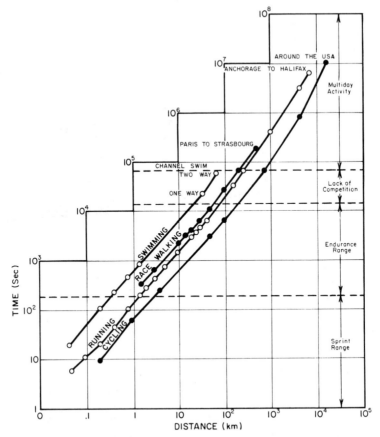

Figure 1.2.2 World records for swimming, race walking, running, and cycling showing the relationship between distance and time. (Redrawn with permission from Riegel, 1981.)

Manipulating the endurance equation gives, for average speed,

$$s = \frac{x^{(1-b)}}{a} \tag{1.2.2}$$

where s = speed, km/sec

These speeds, seen in Figure 1.2.3, are instructive for characterizing individual sports. In cycling, aerodynamic drag is the dominant form of resistance, and cyclists often line up one behind the other, with the lead cyclist breaking the wind for the rest. Speed skaters also operate at high speeds, with their inherent drag, and must also negotiate many turns. Runners are affected by the large forces they must develop or absorb as they overcome the inertia from rapid limb movement. Their bodily centers of gravity rise and fall with each step. Race walkers are not jolted with each step, as runners are, but their body motions must be more contorted and require great stretching effort and use of more of their total musculature. Swimmers compete in a medium that is relatively viscous, which limits their speeds considerably.

Men and women swim and run at the same distances in world-class events. In swimming, women attain speeds of about 94% of those of a man. In running, women achieve about 88% of the speed of men.

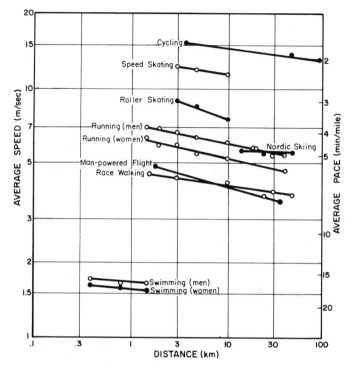

Figure 1.2.3   Speed decreases as distance increases for all world-class activities. Shown here is the average speed from the endurance equation. (Redrawn with permission from Riegel, 1981.)

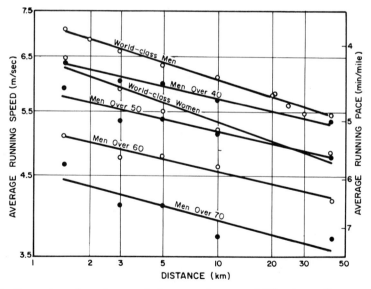

Figure 1.2.4   Comparison of running records for men and women of different ages. Runners provide the greatest amount of data for performance comparison. (Redrawn with permission from Riegel, 1981.)

When comparing running records, age can be seen to decrease average attainable speed (Figure 1.2.4). A septuagenarian can run 70% as fast as a world-class man. The difference with age appears to be greater for the shorter running distances than it does for longer distances. At longer distances, the speed of the fastest 40-year-old is nearly the same as that of a world-class man. It is unclear how much of this is due to relative short-term endurance loss or due to different training or competitive factors with older men. Certainly, older men who hold other jobs cannot spend full time training, nor are they subject to the highest acclaim when winning a race.

Returning to Figure 1.2.1, there are several dashed-line hyperbolas that appear in the plot. This figure suggests that several factors can limit exercise performance. Those shown to be important while exercising wearing a mask are cardiovascular, respiratory, thermal, and long-term effects. Although each of these can contribute to the exercise performance limitation, it is the factor determining shortest time at any particular steady work rate which is the limiting factor in exercise performance. The overall work rate performance time characteristic is the locus of points formed from the individual stress limitations. Approximate time and work rate data have been obtained from published reports, and supporting experimental data appear in Table 1.2.2.

The conceptual framework appearing in Figure 1.2.1 is relative only. Normal individuals not wearing masks probably will not experience a respiratory limitation to exercise. Imposition of heavy clothing may move the thermal stress limitation curve to the left from its position in Figure 1.2.1 such that it dominates the whole figure.

The implications of this hypothetical intensity–duration concept are many. First, the model implies that the various types of stress can be studied independently from one another at appropriate levels of work. Second, any interactions between stresses, if they occur, would be found at work rates and performance times where two component stress limitation curves

TABLE 1.2.2   Subject Data at Their Voluntary End Points for Different Rates of Work

Work Rate, N·m/sec	Performance Time, sec	(min)	Final Heart Rate, beats/sec	(beats/min)	Final Exhalation Time, sec	Final Rectal Temperature, °C
			Subject A			
150	4260	(71.0)	2.93	(176)	0.96	38.83[a]
175	3430	(57.2)	2.83	(170)	0.91	38.50[a]
200	2400	(40.0)	2.93	(176)	0.79	38.66[a]
225	2110	(35.2)	3.13	(188)	0.70	39.00[a]
275	438	(7.3)	2.98	(179)	0.55[a]	38.03
300	240	(4.0)	3.00	(180)	0.50[a]	37.50
325	204	(3.4)	2.93	(176)	0.49[a]	37.50
350	150	(2.5)	3.05	(183)	0.55[a]	37.39
375	144	(2.4)	3.00	(180)	0.50[a]	37.39
400	120	(2.0)	2.93	(176)	0.50[a]	37.61
			Subject R			
200	3660	(61.0)	2.68	(161)	0.842	38.83
250	1560	(26.0)	2.53	(152)	0.913	37.89
350	420	(7.0)	2.72	(163)	0.560[a]	37.36
400	240	(4.0)	2.65	(159)	0.544[a]	36.83

Source: Adapted and used with permission from Johnson, 1976.

[a] Denotes probable limiting measurement.

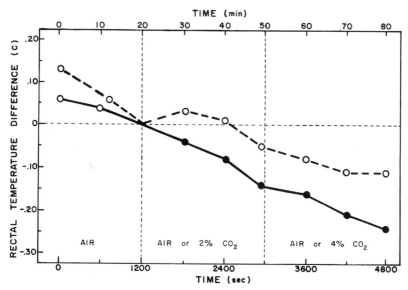

Figure 1.2.5 Differences in rectal temperature of cats with carotid bodies intact when breathing air and carbon dioxide. Reference for the comparison was temperature at the end of the 1200 sec (20 min) period of air breathing. Thereafter, cats were made to breathe either air (open circles) or air and carbon dioxide (closed circles). Other studies with carotid bodies surgically modified showed less carbon dioxide effect on rectal temperature. (Adapted and redrawn with permission from Jennings and Szlyk, 1986.)

intersect on the overall work limitation curve. Thus a cardiovascular–respiratory interaction and a respiratory–thermal interaction could be found, but no cardiovascular–thermal interaction would be expected as long as the respiratory limitation was interposed between them.

There is limited evidence to suggest a respiratory–thermal interaction. Johnson and Berlin (1973) present very tenuous and indirect evidence of this interaction. Jennings and Szlyk (1986) gave a stronger physiological basis to the interaction by demonstrating that the carotid bodies, important in respiratory control (see Section 4.3.1), can also affect temperature regulation (Figure 1.2.5). In their animals they showed that hypoxic stimulation of the carotid bodies suppresses shivering.

Body temperature has been found to have a direct effect on heart rate (Rubin, 1987), and, therefore, a thermal–cardiac interaction might also be expected in some humans. The implications of this intensity–duration concept cannot be drawn too far.

1.3 MUSCLE METABOLISM

Although the previous section suggests many possible limitations to exercise performance, the most widely considered limitation involves the basic energy mechanisms of the muscles themselves. For exercise durations of 0–900 sec (0–15 min), these mechanisms most surely dominate exercise capacity.

1.3.1 Muscle Fiber Structure

Individual muscle fibers have been found to be composed of fibrils (about 1 μm in diameter), which are themselves composed of the protein filaments actin and myosin (White et al., 1959).

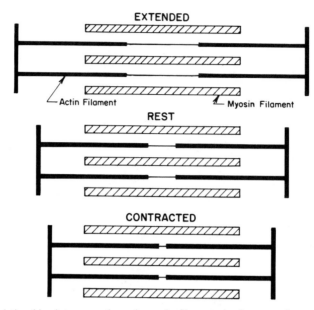

Figure 1.3.1 Relationships between actin and myosin filaments in three muscle conditions. (Redrawn with permission from White et al., 1959.)

These filaments are crosslinked, either directly or indirectly, by chemical bonds (Figure 1.3.1).[4] When muscle contraction occurs, these bonds must be broken and other bonds, which slide the actin filaments along the myosin filaments, must be established. Such a process requires a source of energy which is immediate and can deliver energy over a considerable amount of time.

The force per unit area (also called tension) that a muscle develops varies with the length of the muscle fiber. Tension developed can be measured either during an isometric (or constant-length) contraction or on an unstimulated, passive muscle fiber. Length of the muscle fiber is usually related to resting length. The length–tension relationship between muscles, which affects their efficiencies, is discussed in detail in Section 5.2.5.

Two types of muscle fibers, slow twitch and fast twitch, have been identified. Fast-twitch fibers are primarily those concerned with fine, rapid, precise movement. Slow-twitch fibers are involved in strong, gross, sustained movements (Ganong, 1963). Fast-twitch fibers appear to be more adapted for anaerobic contraction, whereas slow-twitch fibers utilize oxygen better (Kamon, 1981). Therefore, a higher proportion of slow-twitch fibers in a given muscle mass should provide a better aerobic endurance of the muscle.

1.3.2 Muscle Energy Sources

Organic phosphate compounds are the fundamental energy sources for muscle cells. Of particular importance is adenosine triphosphate (ATP).[5] ATP can be hydrolyzed by actomyosin, which affects its physical state. When ATP is hydrolyzed, it forms phosphate plus free energy

---

[4] The muscle can lock (establish stable crosslinking) at any point between 65 and 120% of the resting length (White et al., 1959). A study of mechanisms involved in the process is given by Davis (1986).

[5] Adenosine is an organic nucleic acid adenine linked to ribose (White et al., 1959). When one ring hydroxide is replaced with three phosphate groups (phosphorus and oxygen), the result is adenosine triphosphate. There are two high-energy pyrophosphate bonds in ATP.

plus adenosine diphosphate (ADP). ADP contains one energy-rich bond and can also be used as a muscle energy source. Adenosine monophosphate (AMP), the final product of ATP and ADP hydrolysis, contains no usable energy for muscular contraction. There are severe restrictions on AMP as a phosphate acceptor; it cannot accept phosphate either from anaerobic glycolysis or from oxidative reactions, whch may be one reason why ATP is almost immediately formed from ADP whenever possible.

ATP is used as the energy-rich carrier not only for muscular contraction but also for resting metabolic processes, such as protein formation and osmotic maintenance. For these, there is ample store of ATP within the muscle. ATP formation occurs continually by the oxidation of carbohydrate or acetoacetate (White et al., 1959).

Maximally contracting mammalian muscle uses approximately 1.7×10^{-5} mole of ATP per gram per second (White et al., 1959). However, ATP stores in skeletal muscle tissue amount to 5×10^{-6} mole per gram of tissue, which can meet muscle demands for no more than $\frac{1}{2}$ sec of intense activity.

Initial replenishment of ATP occurs through the transfer of creatine phosphate (also called phosphagen) into creatine, a reaction which is catalyzed by creatine kinase (White et al., 1959). In the resting state, muscle contains four to six times as much creatine phosphate as it does ATP. Phosphocreatine, however, cannot directly affect actomyosin.

Even considering phosphocreatine, the total supply of high-energy phosphate cannot sustain activity for more than a few seconds. Glycogen is a polysaccharide present in muscle tissue in large amounts.[6] When required, glycogen is decomposed into glucose and pyruvic acid. This pyruvic acid, in turn, becomes lactic acid. ATP is formed in this process. All these reactions proceed without oxygen. During intense muscle activity, the oxygen content of blood flowing through muscle tissue can be rapidly depleted (anaerobic conditions).

When sufficient oxygen is available (aerobic conditions), either in muscle tissue or elsewhere, these process are reversed. ATP is reformed from ADP and AMP, creatine phosphate is reformed from creatine and phosphate, and glycogen is reformed from glucose or lactic acid. Energy for these processes is derived from the complete oxidation of carbohydrates, fatty acids, or amino acids to form carbon dioxide and water (Molé, 1983).

Following the manner of Astrand and Rodahl (1970), the foregoing reactions can be summarized by chemical equations:

Anaerobic:

$$ATP \Leftrightarrow ADP + P + \text{free energy} \tag{1.3.1}$$

$$\text{creatine phosphate} + ADP \Leftrightarrow \text{creatine} + ATP \tag{1.3.2}$$

$$\text{glycogen or glucose} + P + ADP \rightarrow \text{lactate} + ATP \tag{1.3.3}$$

Aerobic:

$$\text{glycogen or fatty acids} + P + ADP + O_2 \rightarrow CO_2 + H_2O + ATP \tag{1.3.4}$$

All conditions:

$$2ADP \Leftrightarrow ATP + AMP \tag{1.3.5}$$

Anaerobic and aerobic processes can occur simultaneously in different parts of the body. Lactic acid freely diffuses from muscle cells into interstitial fluid and thence to the blood, where

---

[6]Glycogen has been likened to animal starch. If the amount of energy equivalent to glycogen were present in the form of the simple sugar glucose, the osmotic balance of muscle tissue would be gravely upset.

it is carried to the liver. Most of the lactic acid[7] is resynthesized to glycogen in the liver, at the expense of liver ATP. Liver glycogen is released as blood glucose[8] for utilization by muscle.

If muscular work is at a pace slow enough for sufficient oxygen delivery for aerobic measures to prevail, then the glucose is directly utilized in muscle to generate ATP. If oxygen is not available, then anaerobic processes yield sufficient ATP for muscular action. Because there is a limit to the amount of anaerobic metabolites that can be tolerated by muscle tissue, there is also a limit to the duration of anaerobic metabolism. Oxygen is required to chemically remove these metabolites from the tissue. The greater the concentration of metabolites, the greater is the amount of oxygen required to reform resting levels of glycogen and phosphocreatine.[9] This, in turn, leads to the concept of oxygen debt.

1.3.3 Oxygen Debt

At the cessation of exercise there remains an elevated need for oxygen (Figure 1.3.2). The amount of oxygen utilized after exercise, above normal resting levels, is termed the oxygen debt. As we have discussed, much of this oxygen debt is accumulated by muscle biochemistry. However, there are other contributing factors to oxygen debt: (1) elevated body temperature immediately following exercise increases bodily metabolism in general, which requires more than resting levels of oxygen to service; (2) increased blood epinephrine levels increase general bodily metabolism; (3) increased respiratory and cardiac muscle activity requires oxygen; (4) refilling of body oxygen stores requires excess oxygen; and (5) there is some thermal inefficiency in replenishing muscle chemical stores. Considering only lactic acid oxygen debt, the total amount of oxygen required to return the body to its normal resting state is about double. Viewed the other way, the efficiency of anaerobic processes is about 50% of aerobic processes (Astrand and Rodahl, 1970).

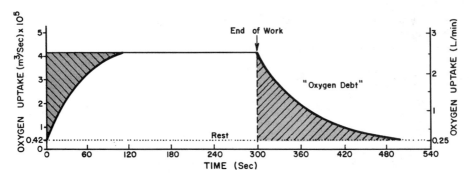

Figure 1.3.2 Oxygen uptake at the beginning of exercise increases gradually until reaching a level high enough to meet demands of the tissues. At the end of exercise, oxygen uptake gradually returns to the resting level as the oxygen debt is filled. (Adapted and redrawn with permission from Astrand and Rodahl, 1970.)

[7] Plasma lactate may play a part in the release of adrenocorticotropic hormone (ACTH) and other hormones associated with mobilization reactions of bodily systems to exercise (Farrell et al., 1983).

[8] There is a very intricate regulation of blood glucose, the complete description of which is outside the purview of this book. Basically, glucose input depends mostly on ingested carbohydrate, which in turn is dependent on hypothalamic and thyroid function. Insulin acts to remove glucose from the blood and produce liver glycogen. Epinephrine and glucagon decrease liver glycogen and increase blood glucose (White et al., 1959).

[9] Also reformed is oxymyoglobin. Muscle tissue contains a protein similar to blood hemoglobin, which also binds to, and stores, oxygen. The major difference between myoglobin and hemoglobin is that the former stores one oxygen atom, whereas the latter stores four oxygen atoms for every hemoglobin molecule in the oxidated state.

This muscular cycle is reflected in the amount of heat generated by the muscles. There is a small amount of resting heat produced by the muscles reflecting basic muscle metabolism; there is an initial heat produced during muscle contraction and relaxation; and there is a heat of recovery during the restoration of the muscle to its preactivated state. Heat of recovery is nearly equal to initial muscle energy expenditure (Mende and Cuervo, 1976).

That muscular activity results in heat as well as useful mechanical work means that muscles are less than 100% efficient. In fact, the large muscles are about 20–30% efficient, about the same as a gasoline engine (Morehouse and Miller, 1967). Efficiency is diminished by excessive loads, excessive rate of work, and fatigue (see Chapter 5).

During heavy work there is a discrepancy between muscular energy demand and aerobic energy available. In Figure 1.3.3 can be seen the relative energy contributions of aerobic fuel utilization and the two anaerobic contributions of anaerobic glycolysis and phosphocreatine utilization. Similar information is available from Table 1.3.1 and Figure 1.3.4. As the level of work decreases, such that performance time increases, the relative contribution of aerobic energy provision increases.

The more a person must rely on anaerobic processes to perform any given task, the greater will be that person's oxygen debt. From Table 1.3.1, an athlete competing in a 60–120 sec (1–2 min) event requires about 167 kN·m (40 kcal) to be repaid as a lactic acid oxygen debt. For each cubic meter (1000 L) of oxygen used, about 20,900 kN·m (5000 kcal) will be delivered, resulting in a lactic acid oxygen debt of 0.008 m^3 (8 L). Reformation of ATP and creatine phosphate requires about 0.001–0.0015 extra cubic meters of oxygen (total thus far of 0.0095 m^3). Assuming the basic efficiency of oxygen repayment is about 50%, an increase in oxygen uptake of about 0.0019–0.0020 m^3 follows the exercise.[10]

With performance times up to 120 sec, anaerobic power dominates aerobic power. At about 120 sec, each is of equal importance. With longer performance time, aerobic power prevails (Figure 1.3.4). Therefore, at performance times below about 120 sec exercise is mostly limited by

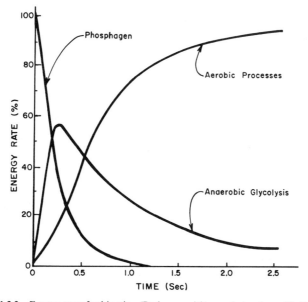

Figure 1.3.3   Energy transfer kinetics. (Redrawn with permission from Molé, 1983.)

---

[10] Blood lactate levels decline more rapidly while exercising during the recovery period than while resting (Stamford et al., 1981).

TABLE 1.3.1 Contributions of Anaerobic (Lactate) Energy Sources to Total Work Requirement[a]

Performance Time, sec	Total Energy			Anaerobic Sources		Aerobic Sources	
	kN·m	(kcal)	kN·m/sec	kN·m	%	kN·m	%
10	121	(29)	12.1	105	85	16.7	15
60	251	(60)	4.18	167	65–70	83.7	30–35
120	376	(90)	3.14	188	50	188	50
240	607	(145)	2.53	188	30	418	70
600	1,190	(285)	1.99	146	10–15	1,050	85–90
1,800	3,050	(730)	1.70	125	5	2,930	95
3,600	5,440	(1,300)	1.51	84.7	2	5,440	98
7,200	10,000	(2,400)	1.39	62.7	1	10,000	99

Source: Adapted and used with permission from Astrand and Rodahl, 1970.

[a] Based on the following assumptions: (1) 20.9 kN·m energy is equivalent to oxygen uptake of 0.001 m³; (2) an individual's maximal aerobic capacity is 188 kN·m; (3) 100% of maximal oxygen uptake can be maintained during 600 sec, 95% during 1800 sec, 85% during 3600 sec, and 80% during 7200 sec.

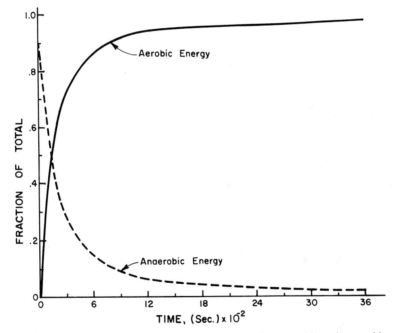

Figure 1.3.4 Relative contributions of total energy requirement from aerobic and anaerobic processes. At 120 sec, both processes are of equal importance. (Adapted and redrawn with permission from Astrand and Rodahl, 1970.)

cellular mechanisms; above 120 sec, up to 3600 sec, performance decrement is more likely to be from systemic causes which interfere with oxygen transport.

1.3.4 Maximal Oxygen Uptake

If an individual exercises while utilizing large muscle groups (so that small muscle fatigue is not a performance factor), performing dynamic, not static work (static work inhibits blood flow), and for a performance time exceeding about 180 sec (so that oxygen can reach steady state before the cessation of exercise), there will be found a rate of oxygen delivery to the muscles which cannot be exceeded. This value is termed the maximal oxygen uptake, or maximal aerobic power for the individual. Maximal oxygen uptake appears at a relatively high work rate (250 N·m/sec in Figure 1.3.5), but not necessarily at the highest attainable work rate, the highest work rate that can be performed for at least 180 sec. Although the rate of work can be increased, the rate at which oxygen is delivered to and used by the body cannot be increased. There is a significant and fast-rising increase in blood lactic acid, indicating that anaerobic metabolism has already begun (Figure 1.3.6).

Below the maximal oxygen uptake, the rate of oxygen use is directly proportional to the rate of work (Figure 1.3.6). The actual rate of oxygen use will depend on the muscle groups used and their relative efficiencies. When maximal oxygen uptake is reached, it too depends on the muscles used and the way in which they are used (Astrand and Rodahl, 1970). As long as exercise is performed in an upright position, and with the legs or arms and legs together, there is no appreciable difference in oxygen uptake (Table 1.3.2) for different kinds of exercise (running, cycling, cross-country skiing, etc.). While supine, however, legs-only exercise gives a maximal oxygen uptake of about 85% of upright maximal oxygen uptake, and swimming (arms plus legs) yields 90%.

The exact mechanism limiting oxygen uptake has been the subject of controversy. Faulkner et al. (1971) suggest that the limiting mechanism is the rate at which blood can be pumped by the heart. With a higher capacity, more oxygen could be delivered to the muscles.

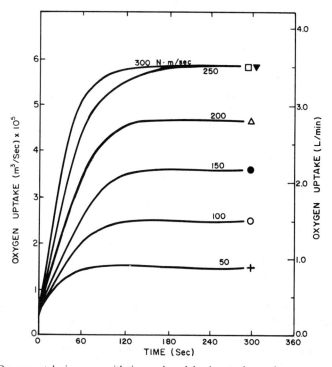

Figure 1.3.5   Oxygen uptake increases with time and work load up to the maximum oxygen consumption. Thereafter, oxygen uptake remains constant and additional required energy is produced by a combination of aerobic and anaerobic processes. Symbols refer to different work levels. (Adapted and redrawn with permission from Astrand and Rodahl, 1970.)

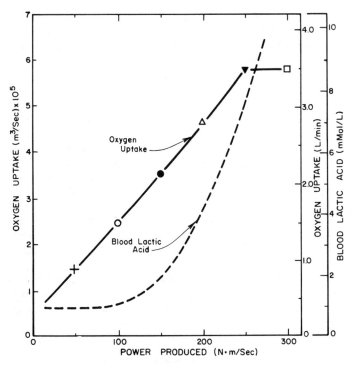

Figure 1.3.6 Steady-state oxygen consumption related to work rate. Oxygen uptake increases linearly with work rate until maximum oxygen uptake is reached. Blood lactic acid begins to rise before maximum oxygen uptake is reached. Symbols refer to work levels in the previous figure. (Adapted and redrawn with permission from Astrand and Rodahl, 1970.)

TABLE 1.3.2   Maximal Oxygen Uptake for Tasks Using Arm and Leg Muscles

	Maximum Oxygen Uptake			
	Women,		Men,	
Age, yr	m^3/sec	$(L/min)^a$	m^3/sec	$(L/min)^a$
20–29	3.57×10^{-5}	(2.14 ± 0.25)	5.27×10^{-5}	(3.16 ± 0.30)
30–39	3.33×10^{-5}	(2.00 ± 0.23)	4.80×10^{-5}	(2.88 ± 0.28)
40–49	3.08×10^{-5}	(1.85 ± 0.25)	4.33×10^{-5}	(2.60 ± 0.25)
50–59	2.75×10^{-5}	$(1.65 + 0.15)$	3.87×10^{-5}	(2.32 ± 0.27)

Source: Adapted and used with permission from Kamon, 1981.

[a] Numbers in parentheses are averages plus or minus 1 standard deviation.

Maximal oxygen uptakes of about $4.2 \times 10^{-5} m^3 O_2/sec$ (2.5 L/min) are typical for young (20–30 years of age) male nonathletes (Astrand and Rodahl, 1970). This figure becomes $6.1 \times 10^{-7} m^3 O_2/kg \cdot sec$ for a typical 68 kg man. Well-trained male athletes possess maximal oxygen uptakes twice as high as this, and untrained women have maximum oxygen uptakes 70% as large. There is a rapid increase in maximum oxygen uptake before the age of 20, with no significant sex difference before the age of 12, and a gradual, nearly linear decline with age after 20, reaching about 70% of the age 20 value at age 65.[11] There is a large individual

[11] Higginbotham et al. (1986) demonstrated that this age-related decline is probably the result of reduced exercise heart rate in older subjects rather than a reduction in stroke volume or peripheral oxygen utilization.

variation, which limits application of these values to particular people. Modern training methods, especially for women, have dramatically altered their relative maximum oxygen uptakes. Active older individuals are likely to possess higher maximum oxygen uptakes than sedentary younger individuals. Since capacity for work depends directly on maximum oxygen uptake, there is a great influence of training on work capacity.

Training increases maximum oxygen uptake and also increases maximum oxygen debt. Muscle metabolism becomes more efficient, and muscle stores of ATP, creatine phosphate, and glycogen increase (Astrand and Rodahl, 1970). Muscle basal metabolism (see Chapter 5) decreases, indicating increased metabolic efficiency (Morehouse and Miller, 1967). Muscle mass increases, the capillary density increases, and myoglobin content increases (Astrand and Rodahl, 1970; Morehouse and Miller, 1967). Heart volume increases dramatically, to the point where it would be considered unhealthy for an untrained individual (see Chapter 3). At the same time, heart rate decreases and blood volume increases. Beyond that, movement efficiency increases due to a learning effect.

Kamon (1981) presented an equation from which can be obtained a relationship between endurance time and the relative work rate, given as a fraction of an individual's maximum oxygen uptake:

$$t_{wd} = 7020 + 7200/f_o \qquad (1.3.6)$$

where t_{wd} = endurance time for dynamic work, sec
  f_o = fraction of maximum oxygen uptake utilized, unitless
Equation 1.3.6 can be used for rhythmic or dynamic work tasks. Static effort occludes flow of blood to the muscles and reduces endurance time (Kamon, 1981):

$$t_{ws} = 34.2/f_o^{2.42} \qquad (1.3.7)$$

where t_{ws} = static effort endurance time, sec

1.3.5 Anaerobic Threshold

The onset of progressive lactic acid accumulation with graded exercise is called the anaerobic threshold (Wasserman et al., 1973). The anaerobic threshold is a benchmark in exercise physiology. Below it, one set of physiological assumptions appears to hold; above it, physiological adjustments are much less simple. The anaerobic threshold occurs at workloads between 50 and 80% of maximal oxygen uptake. Anaerobic threshold for athletes is higher than it is for inactive individuals.

Measured anaerobic threshold has been defined in different ways by different workers. It can be indicated by a threshold level of lactate in the blood (Farrell et al., 1979), increased output of carbon dioxide from the lungs (Sutton and Jones, 1979, Chapter 4), increased rate of respiratory ventilation (linear with work rate below the anaerobic threshold) above the predicted linear value (Davis et al., 1976; Wasserman et al., 1973, Figure 4), an increase in respiratory exchange ratio (rate of carbon dioxide produced divided by rate of oxygen used) above its resting level (Issekutz et al., 1967; Naimark et al., 1964) and various end-tidal gas partial pressure measures (Davis et al., 1976; Martin and Weil, 1979; Wasserman et al., 1973). However, none of these definitions is quite satisfactory; they all suffer from shortcomings of one kind or another. Blood lactate accumulation as a definition suffers from the presence of concurrent lactate removal; therefore, by this definition anaerobic threshold does not accurately reflect the onset of anaerobic metabolism. Rate of exhaled carbon dioxide as a definition suffers from its indirectness and the influence of respiratory anatomical, mechanical, and control factors on carbon dioxide excretion (see Chapter 4). Although ventilation increases above that predicted linearly from work rate, because of the increased acidity of the blood above the anaerobic threshold, this definition is still very indirect and also suffers from the difficulty in estimating just when the relationship of ventilation with work rate becomes nonlinear.[12] Carbon dioxide is excreted at a higher rate above anaerobic threshold than below; thus respiratory exchange ratio should give some information about the threshold, but Wasserman et al. (1973) found the exchange ratio to be among the most insensitive to accurate anaerobic threshold prediction. The various end-tidal gas partial pressure measures are among the most difficult measures to implement.

Skinner and McLellan (1980) provide a succinct description of the events leading to the anaerobic threshold. They indicate that there is not really a single anaerobic threshold, but, instead, there are at least two thresholds and three phases to exercise. In phase I, exercise progresses at a low, but increasing intensity (Figure 1.3.7). Oxygen is extracted from the inspired

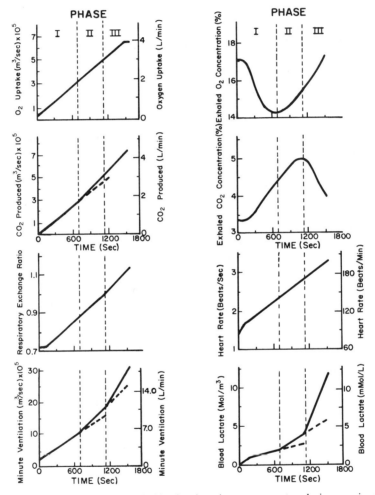

Figure 1.3.7 Concurrent typical changes in blood and respiratory parameters during exercise progressing from rest to maximum. The transitions from phase I to II is called the aerobic threshold and the transition from phase II to III is called the anaerobic threshold. (Adapted and redrawn from Skinner and McLellan, 1980, by permission of the American Alliance for Health, Physical Education, Recreation and Dance.)

[12] In addition, Black et al. (1984) showed that previous exercise raises the anaerobic threshold determined by various ventilatory methods. Scheen et al. (1981) claim that determination of the anaerobic threshold from the hyperventilation threshold is not associated with anaerobic threshold based on lactic acid accumulation.

air, resulting in a lower fraction[13] of oxygen in the expired air. The expired concentration of carbon dioxide increases. There is a linear increase in oxygen intake, ventilation rate, volume of carbon dioxide produced, and heart rate. Respiratory exchange ratio is in the range of 0.7–0.8, indicating normal carbohydrate aerobic metabolism. Little or no lactate is formed in this phase.

As exercise intensity increases to a point between 40 and 60% of maximal oxygen uptake, phase II is reached. Oxygen consumption and heart rate both continue to rise linearly. The rate of lactate accumulation rises and tends to acidify the blood. This acidity is buffered by blood bicarbonate, resulting in an increased evolution of carbon dioxide. The expired fraction of carbon dioxide continues to increase. The respiratory controller attempts to compensate for the increased blood acidity (metabolic acidosis) by stimulating minute ventilation. This increased ventilation contains the acidity increase within close bounds. Because of the excess carbon dioxide produced, respiratory exchange ratio increases, but oxygen, used only to replace ATP, is not removed as much from each breath, so exhaled oxygen fraction increases. The onset of phase II is thus characterized by a nonlinear increase in ventilation and carbon dioxide removal.

As exercise increases further to 60–90% of maximal oxygen uptake, phase III is entered. Heart rate and oxygen uptake increase in linear fashion until maximal oxygen uptake is approached. Blood lactate increases greatly. There is a further increase in minute ventilation and carbon dioxide excreted, but the hyperventilation no longer compensates for the marked rise in lactate. Fractional concentration of carbon dioxide begins to decrease, and oxygen fraction continues to increase. The large increase in respiratory muscle energy expenditure taxes the oxygen-carrying capacity of the blood and leaves less oxygen for use by skeletal muscles. This phase is characterized by a great increase in hyperventilation, which becomes less and less effective in dealing with the effects of blood lactic acid.

Skinner and McLellan (1980) suggested the terms "aerobic threshold" and "anaerobic threshold" to apply to the demarcations between phases I and II and between phases II and III. They suggested blood lactate levels of $2 \, mol/m^3$ (2 mmol/L) and $4 \, mol/m^3$ (4 mmol/L) as quantitative definitions of these two thresholds.

Although others (Kindermann et al., 1979; Ribeiro et al., 1985) usually concurred with these definitions, Schwaberger et al. (1982) indicated that, in individual cases, these empirical definitions are not an adequate description. Lactate values do not account for individual differences in metabolism or for dietary effects (Yoshida, 1984). Schwaberger et al. (1982) thus introduced the concept of "individual anaerobic threshold."

Before reaching the aerobic–anerobic transition, lactate concentration is constant. After the transition, blood lactate concentration increases:

$$c_{LA}(t) = c_{LA}(0) + (\alpha/\eta)P(t)(t - t_0) \qquad (1.3.8)$$

where $c_{LA}(t)$ = blood lactic acid concentration, mol/m^3
$\quad c_{LA}(0)$ = blood lactic acid concentration below the anaerobic transition, mol/m^3
$\quad\quad \alpha$ = proportionality constant, $mol/(N \cdot m^4)$
$\quad P(t)$ = work rate, $N \cdot m/sec$
$\quad\quad \eta$ = mechanical efficiency, dimensionless
$\quad\quad t$ = time, sec
$\quad\quad t_0$ = time at aerobic–anaerobic transition, sec

Since the common procedure for determination of anaerobic threshold uses a stepwise increasing work rate, which can be approximated as a work rate proportional to time,

$$P(t) = kt \qquad (1.3.9)$$

where k = proportionality constant, $N \cdot m/sec^2$

---

[13]See Chapter 4 for a full explanation of these terms.

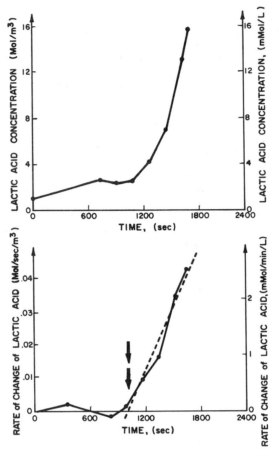

Figure 1.3.8 Method of the determination of the individual anaerobic threshold. (Adapted and redrawn with permission from Schwaberger et al., 1982.)

then

$$c_{LA}(t) = c_{LA}(0) + (\alpha/\eta)kt(t - t_0) \tag{1.3.10}$$

When the rate of lactate production increases above the rate of removal, then the derivative[14] of Equation 1.3.10 will be greater than zero:

$$\frac{dc_{LA}}{dt} = \frac{\alpha}{\eta}k(2t - t_0) > 0 \tag{1.3.11}$$

At this point, Schwaberger et al. (1982) indicate that the individual anaerobic threshold has been reached. Figure 1.3.8 illustrates this concept in an individual subject. In general, Schwaberger et al. found the standard deviations of individual anaerobic threshold values to be much lower than those for aerobic and anaerobic thresholds based on the 2 mol/m³ and 4 mol/m³ definitions.

[14] Equation 1.3.11 differs slightly from the equation presented by Schwaberger et al. (1982) because of an error in their equation.

Individual threshold was indicated at an average blood lactate concentration of 2.87 ± 0.91 mol/m^3; it is claimed to be physiologically well defined and accounts for individual differences in energy metabolism and lactate kinetics. Since Yeh et al. (1983) indicated that anaerobic threshold determination through invasive means (arterial and venous lactate concentrations) is not detectable, and that variability of anaerobic threshold detection by exercise physiologists reviewing ventilatory data is too large for clinical application, more positive definitions, such as the individual threshold, are needed.

1.3.6 Oxygen Uptake Kinetics

Whipp et al. (1981) provided a short mathematical description of oxygen uptake transient changes. Using ramp (linearly increasing) and square wave work rate inputs, they reported that the dynamics of oxygen uptake are linear and of constant first-order (exponential response) both below and above the anaerobic threshold. Therefore, any change in oxygen uptake in response to a step change in work rate is described as

$$\Delta \dot{V}_{O_2}(t) = \Delta \dot{V}_{O_2}(ss)(1 - e^{-t/\tau}) \tag{1.3.12}$$

where $\Delta \dot{V}_{O_2}(t)$ = oxygen uptake change with time, m^3/sec
   $\Delta \dot{V}_{O_2}(ss)$ = difference in oxygen uptake between the old and new steady-state values, m^3/sec
   t = time, sec
   τ = time constant, sec
This means that the general first-order differential equation

$$\tau \frac{d\dot{V}_{O_2}}{dt} + \Delta \dot{V}_{O_2}(t) = \Delta \dot{V}_{O_2}(ss) \tag{1.3.13}$$

governs oxygen uptake dynamics.
   Oxygen deficit, taken as the accumulated difference between oxygen intake and the energy equivalent amount of oxygen actually used, is

$$O_2 D = \Delta \dot{V}_{O_2}(ss) \cdot t - \Delta \dot{V}_{O_2}(ss) \int_c^t (1 - e^{-t/\tau}) \, dt \tag{1.3.14}$$

where $O_2 D$ = oxygen deficit, m^3
When $t \gg \tau$,

$$O_2 D = \tau \Delta \dot{V}_{O_2}(ss) \tag{1.3.15}$$

As previously mentioned, work rate is normally chosen to increase at a constant rate, forcing steady-state oxygen consumption to increase also at a constant rate. Actual oxygen uptake thus becomes

$$\Delta \dot{V}_{O_2}(t) = \Delta \dot{V}_{O_2}(ss)[t - \tau(1 - e^{-t/\tau})] \tag{1.3.16}$$

which, for $t \gg \tau$, reduces to

$$\Delta \dot{V}_{O_2}(t) = \Delta \dot{V}_{O_2}(ss)(t - \tau) \tag{1.3.17}$$

This response is illustrated in Figure 1.3.9.
   Powers et al. (1985) studied the effect of maximum oxygen consumption on time constant of

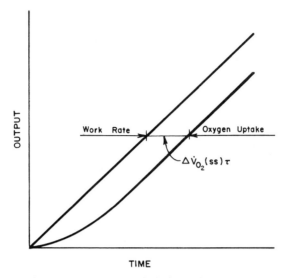

Figure 1.3.9 Oxygen uptake response to progressively increasing exercise work rate. Oxygen uptake would follow the work rate curve except for its exponential time response. With progressively increasing work rate, oxygen uptake always lags behind the ideal value.

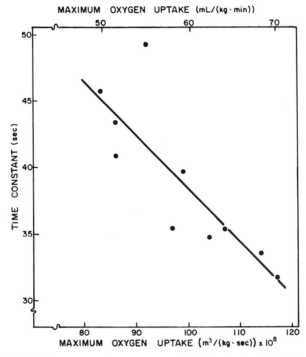

Figure 1.3.10 Relationship between maximum oxygen uptake of trained male athletes and time constant of oxygen uptake. (Data adapted and redrawn with permission from Powers et al., 1985.)

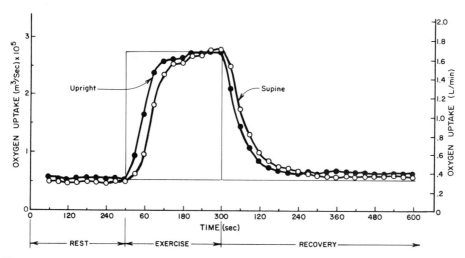

Figure 1.3.11 Rest, exercise, and recovery oxygen uptake for the supine and upright positions. Upright exercise results in faster responses compared to supine. (Adapted and redrawn with permission from Convertino et al., 1984.)

oxygen uptake in 10 highly trained male track athletes with similar training habits. They utilized a modified form of Equation 1.3.12 in characterizing their data:

$$\Delta \dot{V}_{O_2}(t) = \Delta \dot{V}_{O_2}(ss) \left\{ 1 - \exp\left[-\frac{(t - t_d)}{\tau} \right] \right\} \tag{1.3.18}$$

where all terms are as in Equation 1.3.12 except t_d = dead time, sec. Without the inclusion of the dead time, to account for the time when there is no measurable change in oxygen uptake after the beginning of exercise, erroneous values for time constant are calculated.

Powers et al. (1985) found a negative linear relationship between time constant of oxygen uptake and maximum oxygen consumption (Figure 1.3.10). Those individuals with higher maximum oxygen uptake achieve a more rapid oxygen uptake adjustment at the onset of work.

Convertino et al. (1984) presented evidence for an oxygen uptake time constant for supine exercise roughly twice the time constant for upright exercise. This difference contributed significantly to the accumulated oxygen debt. There was no difference in final oxygen uptake between the two exercise modes (Figure 1.3.11).

1.3.7 A Bioenergetics Model

The general scheme of energy utilization by the exercising body was summarized by Margaria (1976) in a three-compartment hydraulic analog. The three compartments (Figure 1.3.12) represent aerobic metabolism, lactic acid formation, and phosphagen breakdown. Energy contributions are modeled by fluid flowing from each hydraulic vessel representing one of the three.

Morton (1985) described the action of this model as follows:

> The fluid in vessel P (representing phosphagen) is directly connected with the outside through the tap T, which regulates the flow, W (total energy expenditure). At rest, with T closed, the upper level of fluid in P is the same as in the communication vessel O (representing the oxidative source). The vessel O is of infinite capacity and is connected through tube R_1. The second communicating vessel L

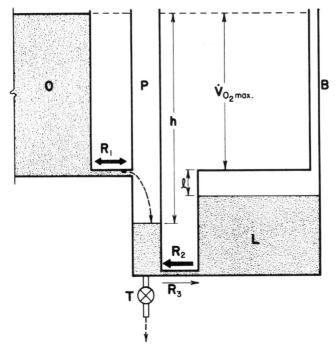

Figure 1.3.12 Hydraulic model representing bioenergetics during exercise. (Adapted and redrawn with permission from Morton, 1985.)

(representing the glycolytic source) is of finite capacity, with upper level the same as the bottom level of vessel O, apart from a very narrow extension tube, B. The fluid in B, corresponding to the resting blood lactic acid, is of very small volume relative to L, and does not contribute to any flows in a measurable amount. L is connected to P through a wider, but one-way tube R_2, and P is connected to L by another, but very much smaller one-way tube, R_3.

If T is partly opened, corresponding to a workload W, the level in P falls, inducing a flow through R_1 (oxygen consumption, $\dot{V}_{O_2}$) in accordance with the difference in levels, h between the two vessels. This induced flow slows the rate at which the level in P falls, and provided W is not too large, an equilibrium will be reached at a level above the inlet R_1. This level in P is below the resting level, and fluid flows continuously from O to P and out through T. If the equilibrium is exactly at the level of R_1, then the oxidative mechanism is at its maximum, denoted $\dot{V}_{O_2 max}$. Once the equilibrium is established, the only energy mechanism contributing is the oxidative; the exercise is purely aerobic, and in theory could continue indefinitely. Prior to equilibrium of course, P has contributed some of its supply, and the empty volume in P above the equilibrium level is known as the alactic oxygen debt.

If T is now closed, i.e. exercise ceases, P will begin to refill through R_1, but at a slower and slower rate as the level in P returns to normal. When it does so, the flow in R_1 ceases and the subject is said to have repaid his oxygen debt during this recovery period.

If T had been widely opened (severe exercise), the initial situation would be as described above, but the level in P would fall below R_1. This happens after about 50% of the fluid in P has been utilized, and the subject is said to have crossed his anaerobic threshold. As soon as this happens, two things occur; the flow in R_1 has reached and continues at its maximum, $\dot{V}_{O_2 max}$, determined only by the height of the vessel O; and a flow through R_2 is induced. This flow is in accordance also with the difference in levels between vessels L and P (the level, I, in L lagging behind the level in P). The flow through R_2 will slow the fall of level in P, but since the flow through R_1 is insufficient and the capacity in L is limited, the levels in both L and P will continue to fall. If exercise is prolonged, L and P will be emptied and the subject will be exhausted!

If T is closed at or before exhaustion, P will again be refilled. Initially it will be filled through R_1 at the maximal rate, and through R_2 until the lag in levels between L and P has been eliminated. This latter flow is the delayed lactic acid formation which occurs after cessation of exercise. Once the levels have been equated, P will fill through R_1, initially at the maximal rate and thereafter at a progressively slower rate as described previously. L will be refilled from P through R_3 at a rate in accordance with the difference in levels between the two. Because R_3 is so small, the level in L will lag behind the level in P; the repayment of this, the lactic oxygen debt is very slow. Finally both P and L are refilled, and the subject is fully recovered.

Morton (1985) analyzed Margaria's model to obtain a mathematical solution. He began by setting the total work rate equal to the sum of flows from the three reservoirs:

$$\beta M = \dot{V}_O - \dot{V}_P - \dot{V}_L \tag{1.3.19}$$

where M = total rate of work, N·m/sec
$\quad \beta$ = conversion of work to volume, m²/N
$\quad V$ = volume, m³
$\quad \dot{V}$ = volume rate of change, m³/sec
and O, P, and L are subscripts denoting the three vessels. $\dot{V}_O$ is the maximal flow from vessel O and corresponds to the maximum oxygen uptake. Also, $\dot{V}_P$ and $\dot{V}_L$ are expected to be negative.

$$\dot{V}_P = A_P \frac{dh}{dt} \tag{1.3.20a}$$

$$\dot{V}_L = A_L = \frac{dl}{dt} \tag{1.3.20b}$$

where A = vessel cross-sectional area, m²
$\quad h$ = height of liquid in vessel P, m
$\quad l$ = height of liquid in vessel L, m
$\quad t$ = time, sec
The flow from vessel L to vessel P is determined by the difference in levels between the two vessels:

$$\dot{V}_L = \dot{M}_{LA}(h - l) \tag{1.3.21}$$

where $\dot{M}_{LA}$ = constant related to maximal rate of lactic acid production, m²
Solving for h and differentiating yields

$$\frac{dh}{dt} = \frac{A_L}{\dot{M}_{LA}} \frac{d^2l}{dt^2} + \frac{dl}{dt} \tag{1.3.22}$$

and substituting into Equation 1.3.19 yields

$$\frac{d^2l}{dt^2} + \frac{\dot{M}_{LA}(A_P + A_L)}{A_P A_L} \frac{dl}{dt} - \frac{\dot{M}_{LA}(\beta M - \dot{V}_O)}{A_P A_L} = 0 \tag{1.3.23}$$

The general solution is

$$l = \frac{-C_1 A_P A_L}{\dot{M}_{LA}(A_P + A_L)} \exp\left[\frac{-\dot{M}_{LA}(A_P + A_L)t}{A_P A_L}\right] + \frac{(\beta M - \dot{V}_O)t}{A_P + A_L} + C_2 \tag{1.3.24}$$

where C_1 and C_2 are constants of integration, values of which are determined from the boundary conditions.

Morton (1985) solved mathematically and numerically for the constants C_1 and C_2 for several conditions. The mathematics is not repeated here because of the specialized nature of the solution, and because Morton asserts that the model is not completely specified and must be modified before further progress can be made. The model as described, however, can give the reader a means to visualize the metabolic processes during exercise.

1.3.8 Chemical Responses

Before turning totally away from the chemical aspects of muscle metabolism and exercise responses, a digression here will be useful to indicate to the reader that bodily responses to exercise are truly complex, highly integrated, and thoroughly redundant. There exists a great chemical response of the body to exercise, much of which is related to the "fight-or-flight" reaction for primitive survival, and much of which is manifested in physical changes. These changes are characterized here and in later chapters. However, it is good to be reminded that their operation depends on a great number of mechanisms.

Hormonal releases occur naturally during exercise (Naveri, 1985). Of these, the most familiar hormones are the catecholamines: epinephrine, norepinephrine, and acetylcholine. These stimulate the nervous system, mobilize free fatty acids, enhance glycogenolysis in liver and skeletal muscle, and stimulate metabolism (Ganong, 1963). They increase the rate and force of heart muscle contraction, either dilate or contract small blood vessels, stimulate breathing, and cause heat to be generated. They work in conjunction with other hormones to produce the effects already discussed as muscle metabolism.

Other hormones, such as ACTH, thyroxin, and glucagon, also enhance exercise responses (Dohm et al., 1985; Farrell et al., 1983; Vanhelder et al., 1985). Endorphins, endogeneous opiates which apparently serve the numerous exercise functions of appetite enhancement, pain suppression, temperature regulation, metabolic control, ventilation control, and blood pressure control (Farrell, 1985; Santiago et al., 1981), have also been found to be released during exercise. Exercise has been shown to produce higher levels of metabolites called prostanoids, with resulting changes in cardiac and platelet behavior (Rauramaa, 1986; Stebbins and Longhurst, 1985). Varying levels of nonexercise hormones, such as those produced during the normal female menstrual cycle, also have been found to influence exercise responses (Berg and Keul, 1981; Bonen et al., 1983). Descriptive models of some of these systems have appeared in the literature (Cobelli and Mari, 1983; Hays, 1984; Salzsieder et al., 1985; Swan, 1982) but are beyond the scope of this book.

1.4 CARDIOVASCULAR EXERCISE LIMITATION

Generally speaking, it is difficult to completely separate cardiovascular exercise limits from metabolic limits. However, there is a limit to the volume rate of blood movement which can be delivered by the heart (see Chapter 3), and additional burdens are placed on the heart when heat production during exercise requires cutaneous vasodilation (see Chapter 5). From Table 1.3.1, we see that exercise durations greater than about 120 sec require at least 50% aerobic metabolism. It is in this region that exercise performance becomes sensitive to blood oxygen delivery. If the cardiovascular system is incapable of delivering sufficient oxygen to the skeletal muscles, then it will not be long before the maximum oxygen debt which the individual can incur will be reached and the individual will be unable to continue. Practically speaking, the cardiovascular limitation to exercise is seen for exercise duration of 120–600 sec, unless there is a respiratory impairment, in which case the cardiovascularly limited exercise duration range is about 120–240 sec. The heart reacts to exercise more rapidly than other bodily systems (Table 1.4.1).

TABLE 1.4.1   Comparison of Response Time Constants for Three Major Systems of the Body

System	Dominant Time Constant, sec	Reference
Heart	30	Fujihara et al., 1973
Respiratory system	45	Fujihara et al., 1973
Oxygen uptake	49	Whipp et al., 1981
Thermal system	3600	Givoni and Goldman, 1972

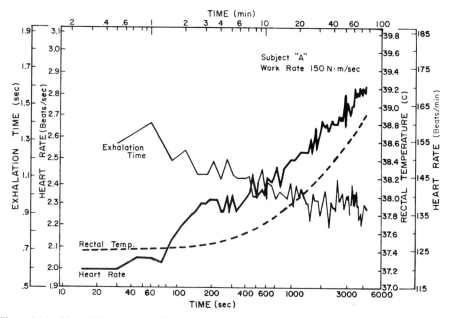

Figure 1.4.1 Plots of three indices of exercise stress on a subject exercising at 150 N·m/sec. Heart rate (cardiovascular stress) responds fastest, with exhalation time (respiratory stress) responding slightly slower and rectal temperature (thermal stress) responding slowest. There are secondary effects of rectal temperature on both heart rate and exhalation time.

Measurements on an exercising subject are seen in Figure 1.4.1 (Johnson, 1976). The work rate was only 150 N·m/sec, which allowed the subject to continue exercising for nearly 6000 sec (100 min). Heart rate moves rapidly to its equilibrium value of about 2.33 beats/sec (140 beats/min). Exhalation time as an indicator of respiratory stress (Johnson and Berlin, 1974; Johnson and Curtis, 1978) decreases somewhat more slowly than heart rate to its equilibrium value near 1.1 sec. Rectal temperature slowly rises from about 37.4°C at the beginning of the session to 38.8°C at the end. After rectal temperature reaches about 37.5°C there is a secondary rise in heart rate, which continues at a rate of about 0.428 beat per second per degree Celsius [25.7 beats/(min·°C)] as long as rectal temperature rises. At about the same time as the start of the secondary rise in heart rate, a fall in exhalation time occurs. If the work rate had been higher, the rise of rectal temperature would have been lower, exhalation time would have tended toward, and be limited at, 0.5 sec, heart rate would have gone quickly to a higher value, and performance time would have been much shorter.[15]

---

[15]Therefore, in designing experimental studies, the work rate and anticipated performance time should be chosen to be sensitive to the particular stress that is the object of the test. An experiment testing heat stress should be designed to last much longer than an experiment testing cardiovascular stress.

1.5   RESPIRATORY LIMITATION

Respiratory adjustments (see Chapter 4) to exercise are slower than cardiovascular adjustments, so that a respiratory limitation, if seen at all, requires a longer time to manifest itself than the cardiovascular limitation. It is generally conceded that for normal, healthy individuals, there is no limit to exercise performance imposed by the respiratory system (Astrand and Rodahl, 1970). However, should the individuals suffer from respiratory function impairment, then there appears to be a definite relationship between exercise performance and respiratory functioning (Johnson and Berlin, 1974; Johnson and Curtis, 1978).[16] In our testing of subjects wearing respiratory protective masks, we have generally seen evidence of respiratory limitation to exercise for constant work rates of duration of about 240–1200 sec.

Martin et al. (1984) found that ventilation levels associated with peak exercise levels approaching maximum oxygen uptake require anaerobic metabolism by the respiratory muscles. This can significantly add to blood lactate levels and presumably reduce the additional amount of oxygen debt utilized by the skeletal muscles in their performance of anaerobic work. This accumulation of blood lactate also probably contributes to overall muscle fatigue.

1.6   THERMAL LIMITATION

It takes a relatively long time for the excess heat generated during exercise to warm the body sufficiently that the individual must either quit exercising or suffer severe discomfort or even death (see Chapter 5). The rate of heat accumulation will depend to a great extent on physiological adjustments during exercise, the rate of exercise, the size of the individual, environmental factors, and clothing worn. Depending on the motivation of the individual, he or she may tolerate severe thermal discomfort before quitting. A usually conservative upper limit on deep body temperature is 39.2°C (102.5°F) before requiring the termination of exercise.[17] It will require at least 600 sec of steady exercise to reach this temperature.[18] The upper range for exercise duration ending in a thermal end point is probably 3600–7200 sec (1–2 h) in moderate environmental conditions.

Physiological mechanisms underlying the reason that hyperthermia limits muscular work are not clearly identified. Obviously, thermal discomfort is a factor determining cessation of exercise. There appears also to be a strong effect of muscle temperature on its metabolism (Kozlowski et al., 1985). Higher muscle temperatures result in decreased levels of ATP and creatine phosphate, more rapid muscle glycogen depletion, and higher levels of muscle lactate and pyruvate (Figure 1.6.1). These effects indicate that higher temperatures reduce the ability of muscles to work.

1.7   PROLONGED EXERCISE

Exercise performed for a prolonged time results in a number of slower and more subtle physiological effects becoming more important for performance. Over a long time, a general

[16] In general, the higher the maximum oxygen uptake of the individual, the smaller the ventilatory response to exercise (Morrison et al., 1983).

[17] One subject who we tested, a physically fit U.S. Marine, had a jump from 39.0°C (102.2°F) to 40.0°C (104°F) rectal temperature in the 600 sec between readings. He was stripped and put into ice water to cool down from this life-threatening temperature. Although we have seen nothing like this rate of rise in other individuals, for this particular individual, 39.2°C was not conservative enough.

[18] To heat up while exercising requires *reducing* the rate of exercise to allow sufficient time for heat to accumulate.

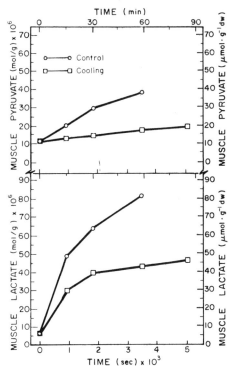

Figure 1.6.1 Muscle contents of pyruvate and lactate in dogs exercising with and without muscle cooling. (Adapted and redrawn with permission from Kozlowski et al., 1985.)

feeling of fatigue may be the reason for quitting, although what constitutes fatigue is not well known. A drop in blood glucose and depletion of muscle glycogen stores appear to be involved (Astrand and Rodahl, 1970). Dehydration due to protracted sweating can be a limiting factor, as can solute balance from loss of salt.

Small irritations produced by clothing or equipment chafing the skin or psychological factors may prove to be the limiting factor to exercise performance. In general, subjects who are kept mentally distracted exercise longer.

A workload of 50% of maximum oxygen uptake is too high for work to last all day. Work lasting this long is usually performed in a steady-state physiological condition.

Fatigue during prolonged exercise has long been thought to be related to depletion of muscle glycogen. The Daedalus human-powered flight from the island of Crete to the Aegean island of Santorini, a distance of 119 km, was expected to last about 21,600 sec (6 h) at a physiological power cost of 900 N·m/sec (Nadel and Bussolari, 1988). Prolonged exercise such as this, without breaks, of course, usually eventually leads to a depletion of muscle glycogen and a concomitant reduction in plasma glucose, followed by a plasma volume reduction (from sweating) and a rise in heart rate (to maintain the required cardiac output despite a reduction in blood volume). Nadel and Bussolari describe their empirical testing of potential Daedalus pilots and the development of a drink to replenish blood glucose, plasma volume, and blood electrolytes. They were successful in avoiding plasma glucose declines over six hours of prolonged bicycle ergometer exercise, and their subjects were able to perform for at least that amount of time. The rest is history: the Daedalus flew the required distance, making it the longest man-powered flight at that time.

SYMBOLS

A	area, m^2
a	constant, sec/km^b
b	fatigue factor, dimensionless
C	constant of integration
c	concentration, mol/m^3
c_{LA}	lactic acid concentration, mol/m^3
$c_{LA}(0)$	initial lactic acid concentration, mol/m^3
f_o	fraction of maximum oxygen uptake utilized during exercise, unitless
h	height, m
k	proportionality constant, $N \cdot m/sec^2$
l	height, m
M	total rate of work, $N \cdot m/sec$
M_{LA}	constant related to maximal ratio of lactic acid production, m^2
O_2D	oxygen deficit, m^3
P	work rate, $N \cdot m/sec$
s	speed, km/sec
t	time, sec
t_{wd}	endurance time for dynamic work, sec
t_{ws}	endurance time for static work, sec
t_d	dead time, sec
V	volume, m^3
$\dot{V}$	volume rate of flow, m^3/sec
$\dot{V}_{O_2}$	oxygen uptake rate, m^3/sec
$\Delta\dot{V}_{O_2}(ss)$	change in steady-state oxygen uptake rate, m^3/sec
x	distance, km
α	proportionality constant, $mol/(N \cdot m^4)$
η	mechanical efficiency, dimensionless
τ	time constant, sec

REFERENCES

Astrand, P.-O., and K. Rodahl. 1970. *Textbook of Work Physiology*. McGraw-Hill, New York.

Berg, A., and J. Keul. 1981. Physiological and Metabolic Responses of Female Athletes During Laboratory and Field Exercise. *Med. Sport*. **14**: 77–96.

Black, A., J. P. Ribeiro, and M. A. Bochese. 1984. Effects of Previous Exercise on the Ventilatory Determination of the Anaerobic Threshold. *Eur. J. Appl. Physiol*. **52**: 315–319.

Bonen, A., F. J. Haynes, W. Watson-Wright, M. M. Sopper, G. N. Pierce, M. P. Low, and T. E. Graham. 1983. Effects of Menstrual Cycle on Metabolic Responses to Exercise. *J. Appl. Physiol*. **55**: 1506–1513.

Cobelli, C., E. R. Carson, L. Finkelstein, and M. S. Leaning. 1984. Validation of Simple and Complex Models in Physiology and Medicine. *Am. J. Physiol*. **246**: R259–R266.

Cobelli, C., and A. Mari. 1983. Validation of Mathematical Models of Complex Endocrine–Metabolic Systems. A Case Study on a Model of Glucose Regulation. *Med. Biol. Eng. Comput*. **21**: 390–399.

Convertino, V. A., D. J. Goldwater, and H. Sandler. 1984. Oxygen Uptake Kinetics of Constant-Load Work: Upright vs. Supine Exercise. *Aviat. Space Environ. Med*. **55**: 501–506.

Davis, J. A., M. H. Frank, B. J. Whipp, and K. Wasserman. 1979. Anaerobic Threshold Alterations Caused by Endurance Training in Middle Aged Men. *J. Appl. Physiol*. **46**: 1039–1049.

Davis, J. A., P. Vodak, J. H. Wilmore, J. Vodak, and P. Kurtz. 1976. Anaerobic Threshold and Maximal Aerobic Power for Three Modes of Exercise. *J. Appl. Physiol*. **4**: 544–550.

Davis, J. S. 1986. A Model for Length-Regulation in Thick Filaments of Vertebrate Skeletal Myosin. *Biophys. J.* **50**: 417–422.

Dohm, G. L., G. J. Kasperek, and H. A. Barakat. 1985. Time Course of Changes in Gluconeogenic Enzyme Activities During Exercise and Recovery. *Am. J. Physiol.* **249**: E6–E11.

Farrell, P. A. 1985. Exercise and Endorphins—Male Responses. *Med. Sci. Sports Exerc.* **17**: 89–93.

Farrell, P. A., T. L. Garthwaite, and A. B. Gustafson. 1983. Plasma Adrenocorticotropin and Cortisol Responses to Submaximal and Exhaustive Exercise. *J. Appl. Physiol.* **55**: 1441–1444.

Farrell, P. A., J. H. Wilmore, E. F. Coyle, and D. L. Costill. 1979. Plasma Lactate Accumulation and Distance Running Performance. *Med. Sci. Sports. Exerc.* **11**: 338–344.

Faulkner, J. A., D. E. Roberts, R. L. Elk, and J. Conway. 1971. Cardiovascular Responses to Submaximum and Maximum Effort Cycling and Running. *J. Appl. Physiol.* **30**: 457–461.

Fujihara, Y., J. Hildebrandt, and J. R. Hildebrandt. 1973. Cardiorespiratory Transients in Exercising Man. *J. Appl. Physiol.* **35**: 68–76.

Ganong, W. F. 1963. *Review of Medical Physiology.* Lange Medical Publications, Los Altos, Calif.

Givoni, B., and R. F. Goldman. 1972. Predicting Rectal Temperature Response to Work, Environment, and Clothing. *J. Appl. Physiology.* **32**: 812–822.

Grodins, F. A. 1981. Models, in *Regulation of Breathing*, T. F. Hornbein, ed. Marcel Dekker, New York, pp. 1313–1351.

Hays, M. T. 1984. Compartmental Models for Human Iodine Metabolism. *Math. Biosci.* **72**: 317–335.

Higginbotham, M. B., K. G. Morris, R. S. Williams, R. E. Coleman, and F. R. Cobb. 1986. Physiologic Basis for the Age-Related Decline in Aerobic Work Capacity. *Am. J. Cardiol.* **57**: 1374–1379.

Issekutz, B., N. C. Birkhead, and K. Rodahl. 1967. Use of Respiratory Quotients in Assessment of Aerobic Work Capacity. *J. Appl. Physiol.* **17**: 47–50.

Jennings, D. B., and P. C. Szlyk. 1986. Carotid Chemoreceptors and the Regulation of Body Temperature, in *Homeostasis and Thermal Stress*, K. Cooper, P. Lomax, E. Schönbaum, and W. L. Veale, ed. Karger, Basel, Switzerland, pp. 30–33.

Johnson, A. T. 1976. The Energetics of Mask Wear. *Am. Ind. Hyg. Assoc. J.* **37**: 479–488.

Johnson, A. T., and H. M. Berlin. 1973. Interactive Effects of Heat Load and Respiratory Stress on Work Performance of Men Wearing CB Protective Equipment. Edgewood Arsenal Technical Report ED-TR-83059, Aberdeen Proving Ground, Md.

Johnson, A. T., and H. M. Berlin. 1974. Exhalation Time Characterizing Exhaustion While Wearing Respiratory Protective Masks. *Am. Ind. Hyg. Assoc. J.* **35**: 463–467.

Johnson, A. T., and E. G. Cummings. 1975. Mask Design Considerations. *Am. Ind. Hyg. Assoc. J.* **36**: 220–228.

Johnson, A. T., and A. V. Curtis. 1978. Minimum Exhalation Time with Age, Sex, and Physical Condition. *Am. Ind. Hyg. Assoc. J.* **39**: 820–824.

Kamon, E. 1981. Aspects of Physiological Factors in Paced Physical Work, in *Machine Pacing and Occupational Stress*, G. Salvendy and M. J. Smith, ed. (Taylor and Francis, London, pp. 107–115.

Kindermann, W., G. Simon, and J. Keul. 1979. The Significance of the Aerobic–Anaerobic Transition for the Determination of Work Load Intensities During Endurance Training. *Eur. J. Appl. Physiol.* **42**: 25–34.

Kozlowski, S., Z. Brzezinska, B. Kruk, H. Kaciuba-Uscilko, J. E. Greenleaf, and K. Nazar. 1985. Exercise Hyperthermia as a Factor Limiting Physical Performance: Temperature Effect on Muscle Metabolism. *J. Appl. Physiol.* **59**: 766–773.

Margaria, R. 1976. *Biomechanics and Energetics of Muscular Exercise*, Oxford University Press, Oxford.

Martin, B. J., H. I. Chen, and M. A. Kolka. 1984. Anaerobic Metabolism of the Respiratory Muscles During Exercise. *Med. Sci. Sports Exerc.* **16**: 82–86.

Martin, B. J., and J. V. Weil. 1979. CO_2 and Exercise Tidal Volume. *J. Appl. Physiol.* **46**: 322–325.

Mende, T. J., and L. Cuervo. 1976. Properties of Excitable and Contractile Tissue, in *Biological Foundations of Biomedical Engineering*, J. Kline, ed. Little, Brown, Boston, pp. 71–99.

Molé, P. A. 1983. Exercise Metabolism, in *Exercise Medicine*, A. A. Bove and D. T. Lowenthal, ed. Academic Press: New York, pp. 43–88.

Morehouse, L. E., and A. T. Miller. 1967. *Physiology of Exercise.* C. V. Mosby, Saint Louis.

Morrison, J. F., S. van Malsen, and T. Noakes. 1983. Evidence for an Inverse Relationship Between the Ventilatory Response to Exercise and the Maximum Whole Body Oxygen Consumption Value. *Eur. J. Appl. Physiol.* **50**: 265–272.

Morton, R. H. 1985. On a Model of Human Bioenergetics. *Eur. J. Appl. Physiol.* **54**: 285–290.

Nadel, E. R., and S. R. Bussolari. 1988. The Daedalus Project: Physiological Problems and Solutions. *Am. Sci.* **76**: 351–360.

Naimark, A., K. Wasserman, and M. McIlroy. 1964. Continuous Measurement of Ventilatory Exchange Ratio During Exercise. *J. Appl. Physiol.* **19**: 644–652.

Naveri, H. 1985. Blood Hormone and Metabolite Levels During Graded Cycle Ergometer Exercise. *Scand. J. Clin. Lab. Invest.* **45**: 599–603.

Powers, S. K., S. Dodd, and R. E. Beadle. 1985. Oxygen Uptake Kinetics in Trained Athletes Differing in $V_{O_{2max}}$. *Eur. J. Appl. Physiol.* **54**: 306–308.

Rauramaa, R. 1986. Physical Activity and Prostanoids, *Acta Med. Scand.*, Suppl. **711**: 137–142.

Ribeiro, J. P., R. A. Fielding, V. Hughes, A. Black, M. A. Bochese, and H. G. Knuttgen. 1985. Heart Rate Break Point May Coincide with the Anaerobic and Not the Aerobic Threshold. *Int. J. Sports Med.* **6**: 220–224.

Riegel, P. A. 1981. Athletic Records and Human Endurance. *Am. Sci.* **68**: 285–290.

Rubin, S. A. 1987. Core Temperature Regulation of Heart Rate During Exercise in Humans. *J. Appl. Physiol.* **62**: 1997–2002.

Salzsieder, E., G. Albrecht, U. Fischer, and E.-J. Freyse. 1985. Kinetic Modeling of the Glucoregulatory System to Improve Insulin Therapy. *IEEE Trans. Biomed. Eng.* **32**: 846–855.

Santiago, T. V., C. Remolina, V. Scoles, and N. H. Edelman. 1981. Endorphins and the Control of Breathing. *N. Engl. J. Med.* **304**: 1190–1195.

Scheen, A., J. Juchmes, and A. Cession-Fossion. 1981. Critical Analysis of the Anaerobic Threshold: During Exercise at Constant Workloads. *Eur. J. Appl. Physiol.* **46**: 367–377.

Schwaberger, G., H. Pessenhofer, and P. Schmid. 1982. Anaerobic Threshold: Physiological Significance and Practical Use, in *Cardiovascular System Dynamics: Models and Measurements*, T. Kenner, R. Busse, and H. Hinghefer-Szalkay, ed. Plenum, New York, pp. 561–567.

Skinner, J. S., and T. H. McLellan. 1980. The Transition from Aerobic to Anaerobic Metabolism. *Res. Q. Exerc. Sport* **51**: 234–248.

Stamford, B. A., A. Weltman, R. Moffatt, and S. Sady. 1981. Exercise Recovery Above and Below Anaerobic Threshold Following Maximal Work. *J. Appl. Physiol.* **51**: 840–844.

Stebbins, C. L., and J. C. Longhurst. 1985. Bradykinin-Induced Chemoreflexes from Skeletal Muscle: Implications for the Exercise Reflex. *J. Appl. Physiol.* **59**: 56–63.

Sutton, J. R., and N. Jones. 1979. Control of Pulmonary Ventilation During Exercise and Mediators in the Blood: CO_2 and Hydrogen Ion. *Med. Sci. Sports* **11**: 198–203.

Swan, G. W. 1982. An Optimal Control Model of Diabetes Mellitus. *Bull. Math. Biol.* **44**: 793–808.

Vanhelder, W. P., M. W. Radomski, R. C. Goode, and K. Casey. 1985. Hormonal and Metabolic Response to Three Types of Exercise of Equal Duration and External Work Output. *Eur. J. Appl. Physiol.* **54**: 337–342.

Wasserman, K., B. J. Whipp, S. N. Koyal, and W. L. Beaver. 1973. Anaerobic Threshold and Respiratory Gas Exchange During Exercise. *J. Appl. Physiol.* **22**: 71–85.

Whipp, B. J., J. A. Davis, F. Torres, and K. Wasserman. 1981. A Test to Determine Parameters of Aerobic Function During Exercise. *J. Appl. Physiol.* **50**: 217–221.

White, A., P. Handler, E.L. Smith, and D. Stetten. 1959. *Principles of Biochemistry*. McGraw-Hill, New York.

Yeh, M. P., R. M. Gardner, T. D. Adams, F. G. Yanowitz, and R. O. Crapo. 1983. "Anaerobic Threshold": Problems of Determination and Validation. *J. Appl. Physiol.* **55**: 1178–1186.

Yoshida, T. 1984. Effect of Dietary Modifications on Lactate Threshold and Onset of Blood Lactate Accumulation during Incremental Exercise. *Eur. J. Appl. Physiol.* **53**: 200–205.

CHAPTER 2

Exercise Biomechanics

Give me a lever long enough, and a prop strong enough, and I can single-handedly move the world.
—Archimedes[1]

2.1 INTRODUCTION

"Mechanics is the branch of physics concerned with the effect of forces on the motion of bodies. It was the first branch of physics that was applied successfully to living systems, primarily to understanding the principles governing the movement of animals" (Davidovits, 1975). In this chapter we are concerned with mechanical approaches to the understanding of exercise, both from a static and from a dynamic viewpoint.

Although the emphasis of this chapter is on walking, running, and moving, there also are treatments of strength, load-carrying, and muscular energy expenditure. The reader should also note that companion material can be found in Chapter 5, Thermal Responses, since an intrinsic part of biomechanical activities is the production of heat.

2.2 PHYSICS OF MOVEMENT

A great deal of understanding of movement can be obtained by consideration of fundamentals. In this section, the human body is reduced to its very simplest form, and simple conclusions result. As realistic complications are added, the analyses must become more complicated as well. However, the conclusions drawn from these involved cases will not necessarily give more insight. Thus we begin simply.

2.2.1 Equilibrium and Stability

Any body, including the human body, is in static equilibrium if the vectorial sum of both the forces and torques acting on the body is zero. Any unbalanced force results in a linear acceleration of body mass, and any unbalanced torque results in a rotational acceleration. Thus for a body to be in static equilibrium,

$$\sum \bar{F} = 0 \qquad (2.2.1a)$$

$$\sum \bar{T} = 0 \qquad (2.2.1b)$$

where $\bar{F}$ = vectorial forces, N
$\bar{T}$ = vectorial torques,[2] N·m

[1] Lever action, torques, and forces form the basis for much of the study of biomechanics.
[2] Usually assumed to be positive for a clockwise rotation.

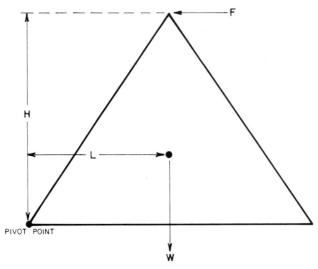

Figure 2.2.1   Body stability. The center of mass must be located over the support for stability. A wider support increases stability. Here, the action of an unbalanced force F tends to topple the body with a torque FH. Acting against this torque is the opposing torque WL. Increasing L increases the resistance to toppling.

TABLE 2.2.1   Fraction of Body Weights for Various Parts of the Body

Body Part	Fraction
Head and neck	0.07
Trunk	0.43
Upper arms	0.07
Forearms and hands	0.06
Thighs	0.23
Lower legs and feet	0.14
	1.00

Source: Used with permission from Davidovits, 1975

The weight of a mass can be considered to be a single force acting through a single point called the center of mass. Body weight acting through its center of mass generally is used to promote stability. That is, body weight can provide the balancing force or torque necessary to maintain stability.

The position of the center of mass with respect to the base of support determines whether the body is stable. A stable body has its center of mass directly over its support base (Figure 2.2.1). The wider the base, the more difficult it is to topple the body. The reason for this is that the lateral distance between the center of mass and the point about which the body would pivot should it topple is located at one side of the base and is increased for a wider base, producing a higher restoring torque.

The center of mass of a human body is located at approximately 56% of a person's height measured from the soles of the feet (Davidovits, 1975) and midway between the person's sides and front-to-back. The center of mass can be made to shift by extending the limbs or by bending the torso (see Table 2.2.1). When carrying an uneven load under one arm, the other arm extends from the body to compensate and shift the center of mass of the body–load combination back over the

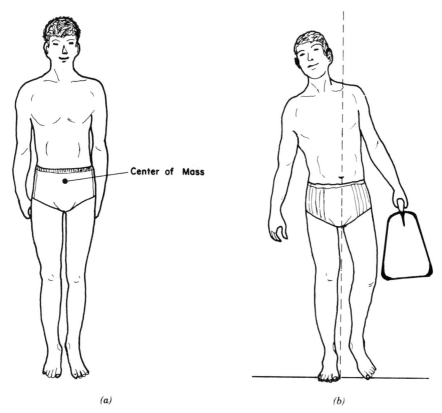

Figure 2.2.2   (*a*) The center of mass of the body is located at about 56% of a person's height and centered over the feet. (*b*) When carrying an uneven load, shifting the position of arms, legs and torso again brings the center of mass over the feet and stability is maintained. (Redrawn with permission from Davidovits, 1975.)

feet. At the same time, the torso bends away from the load and body weight is shifted from the leg nearest the load so that the limb can help maintain stability (Figure 2.2.2).

When performing dynamic exercise, some assistance can be obtained by temporarily forcing the body to become unstable. Running, jumping, and diving are sports where instability must be managed. While wrestling, weight-lifting, and fencing, stability must be maintained. Shifting body position will produce the desired effect.

2.2.2 Muscles and Levers

Skeletal muscles consist of many thousands of parallel fibers, wrapped in a flexible sheath that narrows at both ends into tendons (Davidovits, 1975). The tendons attach the muscles to the bone. Most muscles taper to a single tendon; muscles with two tendons on one end are called biceps and muscles with three tendons are called triceps.

Muscles usually are connected between adjacent movable bones. Their function is to pull the two bones together.

Resting muscle tissue possesses an electrical potential difference across its cell membranes (Figure 2.2.3). This resting transmembrane potential arises as a consequence of the ionic charge distribution on both sides of the membrane (Mende and Cuervo, 1976). Sodium is the chief extracellular cation, and potassium is the most plentiful intracellular cation. Chloride is the main

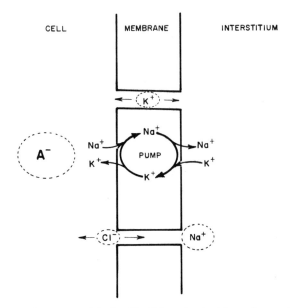

Figure 2.2.3 A transmembrane potential of -90 mV is maintained by active mechanisms that require energy from ATP. Sodium ions are pumped outside and potassium ions are pumped inside the cell membrane. Chloride ions pass freely both ways, but large protein anions cannot escape through the cell membrance.

extracellular anion, whereas relatively large organic acid anions, to which the cellular membrane is impervious, are inside. A source of energy is required to establish and maintain this resting transmembrane potential. Sodium ions that leak inside the cell, due to a concentration difference across the membrane, are actively excluded. The result of this ionic disequilibrium is about a -90 mV potential[3] difference across the membrane.

Whenever a nervous impulse reaches the muscle, a chemical transmitter is released at the site of the conjunction of nerve and muscle, which causes the muscle membrane to become much more pervious to sodium ions. The inrush of sodium actually reverses the resting transmembrane potential, and it momentarily reaches a value of about $+20$ mV ($+30$ mV in neurons). Within about a millisecond, the resting value is reestablished.

This reverse polarization of the transmembrane potential travels from one location of the muscle cell to another, in wavelike fashion. Muscular contraction is triggered by this depolarization wave (see Sections 1.3.1 and 5.2.5).

Since muscles are capable only of contraction, the direction of movement of the bones to which they are attached depends on their points of attachment. In this respect, the joint between the bones acts as a fulcrum, and the muscle acts on a portion of the bone as a force on a lever.

There are three classes of levers, illustrated in Figure 2.2.4 (Davidovits, 1975). In a class 1 lever the fulcrum is located between the applied force and the load. Examples of a class 1 lever are a crowbar and a seesaw. In a class 2 lever the load is between the fulcrum and the force. A wheelbarrow is an example of a class 2 lever. In a class 3 lever, the applied force is between the fulcrum and the load. A pencil writing on a sheet of paper is an example of this class.

Equating the torques caused by the load and the applied force gives

$$Fd_F = Wd_W \tag{2.2.2}$$

---

[3] The transmembrane potential is about -70 mV in nerve cells and -90 mV in skeletal muscle. Intracellular fluid is negative with respect to extracellular fluid.

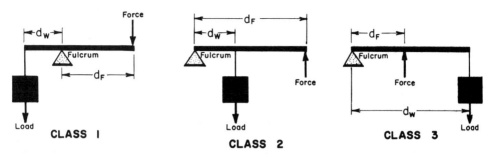

Figure 2.2.4 Three lever classes. The class 2 lever is a very common arrangement for muscles and bones. (Redrawn with permission from Davidovits, 1975.)

from which

$$\frac{F}{W} = \frac{d_W}{d_F}$$ (2.2.3)

where F = applied force, N
$\quad W$ = load, N
$\quad d_F$ = distance from the fulcrum to the point of application of the force, m
$\quad d_W$ = distance from the fulcrum to the point of attachment of the load, m

The applied force will be less than the load if the distance between fulcrum and load is less than the distance between fulcrum and the applied force. Although it may seem to be advantageous to apply a force smaller than the load, this is not the way muscular attachment is built.

Another property of levers is illustrated in Figure 2.2.5. When the load does move, the distance the load moves compared to the distance the force moves is

$$\frac{L_W}{L_F} = \frac{d_W}{d_F}$$ (2.2.4)

where L_W = distance through which the load moves, m
$\quad L_F$ = distance through which the force moves, m

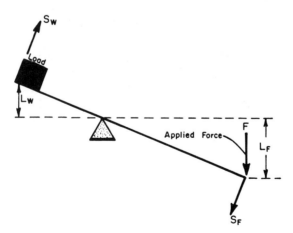

Figure 2.2.5 A class 1 lever showing the relation between distance and speed. (Redrawn with permission from Davidovits, 1975.)

When both distances are divided by time, relative speeds are obtained:

$$\frac{s_W}{s_F} = \frac{d_W}{d_F} \tag{2.2.5}$$

where s_W = speed of load movement, m/sec

s_F = speed of force movement, m/sec

Muscles are capable of generating large forces of about 7×10 N per square meter of cross-sectional area (Davidovits, 1975). They are not capable of moving far, and muscle efficiency decreases as speed of contraction increases (see Sections 3.2.3, 4.2.3, and 5.2.5). Therefore, many limb joints are built as class 3 levers to match the properties of muscle tissue (or vice-versa).

Figure 2.2.6 is a diagram of the upper and lower arm and elbow. The biceps muscle is attached as a class 1 lever. Calculations by Davidovits (1975) indicate that if the angle between the upper and lower arms at the elbow is about 100°, with the lower arm horizontal, then the biceps muscle exerts a force somewhat greater than 10 times the weight supported in the hand. The reaction force that is exerted by the bone of the upper arm (humerus) on the bones of the lower arm (ulna and radius) at the elbow is about 9.5 times the supported weight.

The force exerted on the joint can be significant. At the hip joint (Figure 2.2.7) the reaction force is nearly 2.5 times the weight of the person. Limping shifts the center of mass of the body more directly above the hip joint and decreases the force to about 1.25 times the body weight. This is a significant reduction in force and demonstrates why persons with injured hips limp the way they do.

Maximal expected torques that can be developed at the joints depend on several factors. First

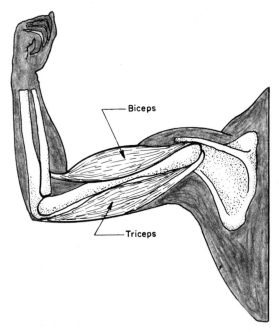

Figure 2.2.6   The muscles and bones of the elbow. The biceps muscle is attached as a class 3 lever and the triceps muscle is attached as a class 1 lever. (Redrawn with permission from Davidovits, 1975.)

of these is the distribution of fast-twitch and slow-twitch muscle fibers in muscles of the joint (see Section 1.3.1; Kamon, 1981). Second of these is the work history of the muscles, where muscles composed largely of fast-twitch fibers can produce larger torques than muscles composed mostly of slow-twitch fibers at all speeds of contraction before muscle exhaustion. After muscle exhaustion, maximal torques are the same for the two muscle types (Kamon, 1981). Age and sex also influence maximum torque. Some of these torques are summarized in Table 2.2.2. In general, women seem to be 60% as strong as men (Kamon and Goldfuss, 1978).

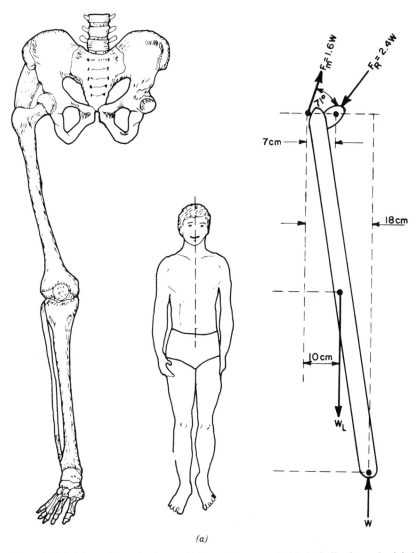

(a)

Figure 2.2.7 The hip joint and reaction forces. (*a*) Normal posture, the hip including leg and pelvic bones, and a lever representation. Weight of the individual is designated W and the weight of the leg, W_L. Muscle force F_m is 1.6 times the body weight and the hip joint reaction force is 2.4 times the body weight. (*b*) Limping decreases the magnitude of both muscle force and hip reaction force on the limping side. (Redrawn with permission from Davidovits, 1975.)

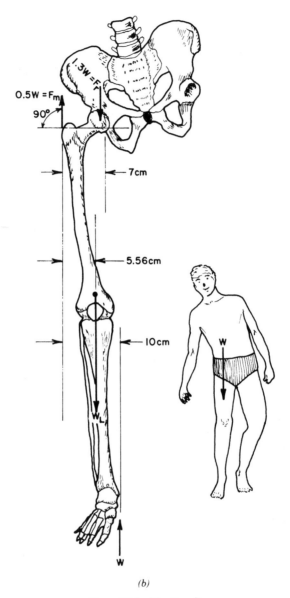

(b)

Figure 2.2.7 *(Continued)*

2.2.3 Energy and Motion

From a general viewpoint, body motion can be considered to be composed of translational motion and rotational motion.

Translational Motion. Translational motion is characterized by identical velocity and acceleration for all parts of the body. To accelerate a body requires an unbalanced force according to the

TABLE 2.2.2 Expected Maximal Torques[a] Around Joints Flexed at Different Angles for Average men and Women Below 40 Years of Age

Joint Action	Sex	Joint Angle		
		45°	90°	135°
Shoulder flexion	Male	67	68	47
	Female	29	30	21
Elbow flexion	Male	52	85	60
	Female	24	43	23
Back extension	Male	—	240	—
	Female	—	130	—
Knee extension	Male	135	196	174
	Female	93	130	136
Foot plantar flexion	Male	110	127	101
	Female	83	111	108

Source: Used with permission from Kamon, 1981

[a] All torque values in N·m

familiar Newton's second law:

$$F = \frac{d(mv)}{dt} = m\frac{dv}{dt} = ma \tag{2.2.6}$$

where mv = translational momentum of a body, kg·m/sec
  m = body mass, kg
  v = body velocity, m/sec
  F = force, N
  t = time, sec
  a = acceleration, m/sec^2
A body that is subjected to uniform acceleration for a time t will reach a speed[4]

$$s = s_0 + at \tag{2.2.7}$$

where s = speed, m/sec
  s_0 = initial speed, m/sec
Integration of Equation 2.2.7 will give distance traveled over that time:

$$L = \int_0^t s\,dt = \int_0^t (s_0 + at)\,dt = s_0 t + \frac{at^2}{2} \tag{2.2.8}$$

where L = distance traveled, m
  Energy is defined as the capacity of a body to do work. Kinetic energy is the result of motion and potential energy is the result of position. For calculation of energy, a force times the distance through which it acts is required:

$$E = FL \tag{2.2.9}$$

where E = energy, N·m

---

[4] The difference between velocity and speed is that the former is a vector quantity (includes a direction and a magnitude) whereas the latter is a scalar quantity (magnitude only).

For kinetic energy, assuming zero initial velocity and uniform acceleration,

$$F = ma \tag{2.2.10a}$$

$$L = \frac{at^2}{2} \tag{2.2.10b}$$

$$v = at \tag{2.2.10c}$$

$$E = (ma)\left(\frac{at^2}{2}\right) = \frac{m}{2}(at)^2 = \frac{mv^2}{2} \tag{2.2.10d}$$

For potential energy within a constant gravitational field,

$$F = mg \tag{2.2.11a}$$

$$L = h \tag{2.2.11b}$$

$$E = mgh \tag{2.2.11c}$$

where h = height above a reference plane, m
$\quad g$ = acceleration due to gravity, 9.80 m/sec^2

Vertical jumps begin from a crouch (Figure 2.2.8). The legs push against the bottom surface until the feet leave the surface, and the body continues to rise until decelerated to zero velocity by gravity. The maximum height of the jump is the point when velocity reaches zero. Energy performed by the legs to raise the body from the crouch (kinetic energy) is translated into potential energy in the process of the jump. From a conservation of energy perspective,

$$Fc = W(c + h) \tag{2.2.12}$$

where F = force produced by the legs, N
$\quad W$ = body weight, N
$\quad c$ = depth of the crouch, m
$\quad h$ = height of the jump, m

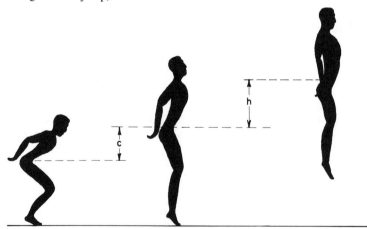

Figure 2.2.8 Vertical jump. Crouching before the jump gives the legs opportunity to develop more jumping energy than if the jump began from a standing position. (Redrawn with permission from Davidovits, 1975.)

Therefore,

$$h = \frac{(F - W)c}{W} \qquad (2.2.13)$$

Experimental measurements have shown that the force produced by the legs is roughly twice the body weight (Davidovits, 1975). Thus

$$h = c \qquad (2.2.14)$$

For an average person, the depth of the crouch is about 60 cm. The height of the jump is also about 60 cm.

A much greater height ought to be attained by beginning the jump from a running start. Horizontal kinetic energy can be converted into vertical potential energy, thus forming the basis for an estimate of the height of the jump:

$$mgh = \tfrac{1}{2}mv^2 \qquad (2.2.15a)$$

$$h = \frac{v^2}{2g} \qquad (2.2.15b)$$

Added to this estimate should be a considerable fraction of the 60 cm previously estimated as the height boost that can be produced in a final pushoff by the legs just before jumping. Also, note that the center of mass of the body is about a meter above the feet, and that by repositioning the body during the high jump to a more nearly horizontal plane (with a net external energy cost of very little because, as the lower body is being raised, the upper body is lowered), a higher level can be cleared. We must subtract from our estimate a very small amount of translational kinetic energy which cannot be converted into potential energy because it is needed to jump over the bar. Therefore,

$$h = \frac{v^2}{2g} + 1.4 \qquad (2.2.15c)$$

The short-distance running speed of a good high jumper is about 8.2 m/sec (Davidovits, 1975). The estimate of height thus becomes 4.8 m.

This estimate for the high jump is about twice the high jump record. Furthermore, the pole vault recorded is near 6.0 m. These facts demonstrate that the efficiency of transforming translational kinetic energy into potential energy is much higher with the aid of a pole than with the unaided foot.

If the vertical jump is performed in a weaker gravitational system, such as on the moon, a greater height can be attained. However, the additional height is not proportional to the decrease in weight. Because of the gravitational system, the maximum force produced by the legs does not change, nor does the depth of the crouch change. Return to Equation 2.2.13:

$$\frac{h_m}{h} = \frac{(F - W_m)}{(F - W)}\frac{W}{W_m} = \frac{(2W - W_m)}{(2W - W)}\frac{W}{W_m} \qquad (2.2.16)$$

where h_m = height of jump on the moon, m
$\quad W_m$ = weight of person on the moon, N

With one-sixth of the earth's gravity, the moon causes a person to weigh one-sixth what he would on the earth ($W/W_m = 6$). Therefore, a person who jumps 60 cm on the earth will jump 6.6 m on the moon.

Energy considerations can also be used to calculate the height of a jump that will produce bone fracture. When assuming bone to be an elastic material, the energy stored in this elastic material is

$$E = \tfrac{1}{2} K (\Delta L)^2 \tag{2.2.17}$$

where K = spring constant, N/m

$\quad \Delta L$ = change in length from resting length, m

The spring constant is a property of an elastic material (analogous to a spring) which relates force required to compress the spring to the compression distance:

$$F = K \Delta L \tag{2.2.18}$$

Stress is defined as the force in a material divided by the cross-sectional area:

$$\sigma = F/A \tag{2.2.19}$$

where σ = stress, N/m^2

$\quad F$ = force, N

$\quad A$ = cross-sectional area, m^2

and strain is defined as the amount of compression or stretch divided by the original length:

$$\varepsilon = \Delta L/L \tag{2.2.20}$$

where ε = strain, m/m

$\quad L$ = original material length, m

$\quad \Delta L$ = change in length, m

The ratio of stress to strain, called Young's modulus (also called modulus of elasticity or elastic modulus), is usually assumed to be constant[5] and has been measured for many materials:

$$Y = \frac{\sigma}{\varepsilon} \tag{2.2.21}$$

where Y = Young's modulus, N/m^2

Young's modulus for bone in compression is 1.4×10^{10} N/m^2 (Davidovits, 1975).

Also measured is the maximum compressive stress that can be resisted without rupture. For bone, this value is 10^8 N/m^2 (Davidovits, 1975).

Combining Equations 2.2.18 through 2.2.21,

$$K = \frac{F}{\Delta L} = \frac{F/A}{\Delta L/A} = \frac{\sigma A}{\Delta L} = \frac{\sigma A/L}{\varepsilon} = \frac{YA}{L} \tag{2.2.22}$$

At the maximum compressive stress,

$$Y = \frac{\sigma_{max}}{\varepsilon} = \frac{\sigma_{max}}{\Delta L/L} \tag{2.2.23a}$$

---

[5] For many biological materials, the ratio of stress to strain is not truly constant, usually becoming lower at higher rates of strain. In this case, Young's modulus is often measured as the slope of the chord joining the origin to a point on the curve with a particular strain.

and

$$\Delta L = \frac{\sigma_{max} L}{Y} \qquad (2.2.23b)$$

where σ_{max} = maximum breaking stress, N/m^2

An energy balance can now be written for the leg bones in compression. The energy input is the body weight times the height of the fall. Energy stored in the bone is given by Equation 2.2.17:

$$Wh = \tfrac{1}{2} K(\Delta L)^2 = \frac{AL\sigma_{max}^2}{2Y} \qquad (2.2.24a)$$

$$h = \frac{AL\sigma_{max}^2}{2YW} \qquad (2.2.24b)$$

where h = height of the fall, m
A = total cross-sectional area of the bones of the legs, m^2
L = length of the leg bones, m
W = body weight, N
σ_{max} = maximum breaking stress, N/m^2

Taking the combined length of the leg bones at about 90 cm and the combined area of the bones in both legs at about 12 cm^2, and assuming an average 686 N body weight (70 kg mass), the allowable height of the jump is 56 cm. Obviously, jump heights greater than 56 cm are safely made. But this does point to the fact that a great deal of energy is dissipated in bone joints and in the redistribution of fall energy on landing.

Not only do the joints aid in protecting the bones from breaking, but they also possess an amazing amount of lubrication, which keeps them from destruction. Since the center of mass is not directly above the hip joint, the force exerted by the bones on the joints is about 2.4 times the body weight (see Figure 2.2.7a). The joint slides about 3 cm (0.03 m) inside the socket during each step. The friction force acting through this distance is the coefficient of friction times the exerted force, or $2.4 \cdot \mu \cdot W$. The energy expanded during each step is

$$E = FL = (2.4W)(\mu)(0.03) \qquad (2.2.25)$$

where μ = friction coefficient, dimensionless

Without lubrication, the coefficient of friction would be about 0.3 and the energy to be dissipated during each step of a 686 N man would be nearly 15 N·m; the joint would be destroyed. As it is, the joint is well lubricated and has a coefficient of friction of only 0.003, reducing friction heat and wear to negligible values.

Angular Motion. Any object moving along a curved path at a constant angular velocity is subject to a centrifugal force:

$$F_c = \frac{mv^2}{r} = \frac{Wv^2}{gr} \qquad (2.2.26)$$

where F_c = centrifugal force, N
m = body mass, kg

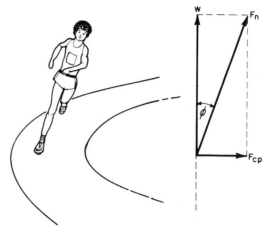

Figure 2.2.9 Runner on a curved track and a representation of the forces acting on the foot of the runner. (Redrawn with permission from Davidovits, 1975.)

v = velocity[6] of the body tangential to the curve of the path taken by the body, m/sec
r = radius of curvature, m
W = body weight, N
g = acceleration due to gravity, 9.8 m/sec²

This centrifugal force component must be balanced by a force of equal magnitude and opposite direction, called the centripetal force, in order that the body does not slide radially outward from the curve. Centripetal force may be supplied by friction:

$$F_{cp} = \mu W = \frac{Wv^2}{gr} \tag{2.2.27}$$

where F_{cp} = centripetal force, N
μ = coefficient of friction, dimensionless

or it may be supplied on a banked curve by the component of force acting toward the center of the curve (Figure 2.2.9):

$$F_{cp} = F_n \sin \phi = \frac{Wv^2}{gr} \tag{2.2.28}$$

where F_n = force normal to the surface of the banked curve, N
ϕ = angle of the curve with respect to the horizontal, rad

Since the vertical component of F_n must support the weight of the body,

$$F_n \cos \phi = W \tag{2.2.29a}$$

$$F_n = \frac{\cos \phi}{W} \tag{2.2.29b}$$

[6]The linear distance traversed in angular motion is

$$D = r\theta$$

where D = distance, m
r = radius of curvature, m
θ = angle of the curve traversed, rad

Dividing both sides of the equation by time gives

$$\frac{D}{t} = v = r\frac{\theta}{t} = r\omega$$

where ω = angular velocity, rad/sec.

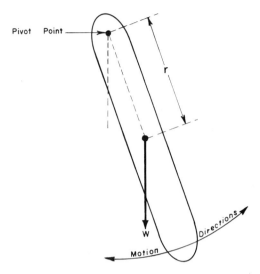

Figure 2.2.10 Diagram of a physical pendulum. (Redrawn with permission from Davidovits, 1975.)

Then, without friction,

$$\tan \phi = \frac{\sin \phi}{\cos \phi} = \frac{v^2}{gr} \tag{2.2.30}$$

The only way that any given banking angle can support various running speeds is by friction to supply the otherwise unbalanced centrifugal force.

A runner rounding a curve, as in Figure 2.2.9, naturally leans into the curve. The reason for this is that the resultant force F_n will pass through the center of mass of the body only if the runner leans inward. If not, there will be an unbalanced torque acting on the body which tends to topple the runner outward. The angle of the lean is the same as calculated by Equation 2.2.30. For the speed of 6.7 m/sec (a 4 min mile) on a 15 m radius track, $\phi = 0.30$ rad (17°). Notice that body weight does not influence this angle. Also to be noted is the fact that the banking on running tracks must be tailored to the speeds expected to be run on them.

For simplistic analysis of walking, consider the legs as pendulums. However, simple pendulums, with all the weight concentrated at the ends, are not a good representation of the legs. The physical pendulum is more realistic because its weight is distributed along its length (Figure 2.2.10).

The period of oscillation for a physical pendulum (Davidovits, 1975) is

$$T = 2\pi \sqrt{\frac{I}{Wr}} \tag{2.2.31}$$

where T = period of oscillation, sec
    I = moment of inertia, N·m·sec^2
    r = distance from pivot point to center of mass, m
    W = weight of the pendulum, N
and

$$I = \frac{WL^2}{3g} \tag{2.2.32}$$

where L = length of the pendulum, m

g = acceleration of gravity, 9.8 m/sec^2

if the center of mass of a leg can be assumed to be at half its length, then

$$T = 2\pi \sqrt{\frac{2}{3}\frac{L}{g}} \qquad (2.2.33)$$

For a 90 cm long leg, the period is 1.6 sec (Davidovits, 1975). If each walking step is regarded as a half-swing (the time of the pendulum to swing forward), then the time for each step is $T/2$. This is the most effortless walk; walking faster or slower requires additional muscular exertion and is more tiring.

Walking speed is proportional to the number of steps in a given time, and the size of each step is proportional to the length of the leg. Therefore,

$$s \propto \frac{L}{T} \qquad (2.2.34a)$$

where s = walking speed, m/sec

But, from Equation 2.2.33,

$$T \propto \sqrt{L} \qquad (2.2.34b)$$

Therefore,

$$s \propto \frac{L}{\sqrt{L}} = \sqrt{L} \qquad (2.2.34c)$$

Thus the speed of walking in a natural stride increases as the square root of the length of the walker's legs. Similarly, the natural walking speeds of smaller animals is slower than those of larger animals.

The situation for running, however, is different. When running, the torque is produced mostly by the muscles instead of gravity. Assume that the length of the leg muscles is proportional to the length of the leg, the cross-sectional area of the muscles is proportional to the length squared, and the mass of the leg is proportional to length cubed[7]:

$$L_m \propto L \qquad (2.2.35a)$$

$$A_m \propto L^2 \qquad (2.2.35b)$$

$$m \propto L^3 \qquad (2.2.35c)$$

where L_m = muscle length, m

A_m = muscle area, m^2

m = leg mass, kg

Maximum muscle force is proportional to the area of the muscle. Maximum muscle torque is proportional to the product of the maximum force times the length of the leg:

$$T_{\max} \propto F_m L \propto L^3 \qquad (2.2.36)$$

[7]Leg mass proportional to length cubed implies that body mass is proportional to its length cubed. Although we like to think this is true, a least squares regression of ideal body weights, as published by the American Heart Association, with height for medium-frame men, gives a dependence of mass on height to the 1.4 power.

where T_{max} = maximum muscle torque, N·m

$\quad\quad F_m$ = maximum muscle force, N

The period of oscillation for a physical pendulum with application of an external torque (Davidovits, 1975) is

$$T = 2\pi \sqrt{\frac{I}{T}} \tag{2.2.37}$$

With the mass of the leg proportional to L^3, the moment of inertia becomes proportional to L^5. Therefore, the period of oscillation becomes

$$T \propto \sqrt{\frac{L^5}{L^3}} = L \tag{2.2.38}$$

Running speed is still proportional to the product of the number of steps per unit time and the length of each step. Therefore,

$$s \propto \frac{L}{T} \propto \frac{L}{L} = 1 \tag{2.2.39}$$

This indicates that the maximum speed of running is independent of leg size. A fox, for instance, can run at about the same speed as a horse (Davidovits, 1975).

This simple analysis, which we will see later needs considerable modification to reflect reality, can be used to give an estimate of the energy expended during running. The legs are assumed to pivot only at the hips and reach their maximum angular velocity as the feet swing past the vertical position. Rotational kinetic energy at this point (Davidovits, 1975) is

$$E_r = 1/2\, I\, \omega^2 \tag{2.2.40}$$

where E_r = rotational kinetic energy, N·m

$\quad\quad \omega$ = angular velocity, rad/sec

and this energy is assumed to be supplied by the leg muscles during each running step. The angular velocity can be calculated (Davidovits, 1975) from

$$\omega = \frac{s_{max}}{L} \tag{2.2.41}$$

where s_{max} = leg speed with the leg in the vertical position, m/sec

$\quad\quad\quad$ = speed of running

Energy calculated using Equation 2.2.40 must be divided by muscular efficiency (about 20%) to obtain total energy expenditure. Using some very simplifying assumptions, Davidovits (1975) calculated the energy of running for a 70 kg person with 90 cm long legs with 90 cm step lengths to be 100 kN·m (24 kcal) when running 1.6 km (1 mile) in 360 sec (6 min). This compares to a value of 1352 N·m/sec (19.4 kcal/min) energy expenditure from Table 2.3.1. The conclusion of this exercise is that there is a good deal more to calculating the energy of running than given in this simple example.

2.3 THE ENERGY COST OF MOVEMENT

We all know that various types of movement require different energy levels. From the data of Table 2.3.1 we can see that the energy contained in a large apple can be expended by 19 min of

TABLE 2.3.1 Calorie–Activity Table: Energy Equivalents of Food Calories, Expressed in Minutes of Physical Activity

Food	Energy, kN·m (kcal)		Activity				
			Walking[a]	Riding Bicycle[b]	Swimming[c]	Running[d]	Reclining[e]
Apple, large	423	(101)	19	12	9	5	78
Bacon, 2 strips	402	(96)	18	12	9	5	74
Banana, small	368	(88)	17	11	8	4	68
Beans, green, 1 c	113	(27)	5	3	2	1	21
Beer, 1 glass	477	(114)	22	14	10	6	88
Bread and butter	327	(78)	15	10	7	4	60
Cake, two-layer, 1/12	1490	(356)	68	43	32	18	274
Carbonated beverage, 1 glass	444	(106)	20	13	9	5	82
Carrot, raw	176	(42)	8	5	4	2	32
Cereal, dry, 1/2 c, with milk and sugar	837	(200)	38	24	18	10	154
Cheese cheddar 1 oz	465	(111)	21	14	10	6	85
Cheese, cottage, 1 tbsp	113	(27)	5	3	2	1	21
Chicken, fried, 1/2 breast	971	(232)	45	28	21	12	178
Chicken, TV dinner	2270	(542)	104	66	48	28	417
Cookie, chocolate chip	213	(51)	10	6	5	3	39
Cookie, plain	63	(15)	3	2	1	1	12
Doughnut	632	(151)	29	18	13	8	116
Egg, boiled	322	(77)	15	9	7	4	59
Egg, fried	460	(110)	21	13	10	6	85
French dressing, 1 tbsp	247	(59)	11	7	5	3	45
Gelatin, with cream	490	(117)	23	14	10	6	90
Halibut steak, 1/4 lb	858	(205)	39	25	18	11	158
Ham, 2 slices	699	(167)	32	20	15	9	128
Ice cream, 1/6 qt	808	(193)	37	24	17	10	148
Ice cream soda	1070	(255)	49	31	23	13	196

Food		Walking[a]	Riding bicycle[b]	Swimming[c]	Running[d]	Reclining[e]
Ice milk, 1/6 qt	603 (144)	28	18	13	7	111
Malted milk shake	2100 (502)	97	61	45	26	386
Mayonnaise, 1 tbsp	385 (92)	18	11	8	5	71
Milk, 1 glass	695 (166)	32	20	15	9	128
Milk, skim, 1 glass	335 (81)	16	10	7	4	62
Milk shake	1760 (421)	81	51	38	22	324
Orange, medium	285 (68)	13	8	6	4	52
Orange juice, 1 glass	502 (120)	23	15	11	6	92
Pancake with syrup	519 (124)	24	15	11	6	95
Peach, medium	193 (46)	9	6	4	2	35
Peas, green, 1/2 c	234 (56)	11	7	5	3	43
Pie, apple, 1/6	1580 (377)	73	46	34	19	290
Pie, raisin, 1/6	1830 (437)	84	53	39	23	336
Pizza, cheese, 1/8	753 (180)	35	22	16	9	138
Pork chop, loin	1310 (314)	60	38	28	16	242
Potato chips, 1 serving	452 (108)	21	13	10	6	83
Sandwiches						
Club	2470 (590)	113	72	53	30	454
Hamburger	1460 (350)	67	43	31	18	269
Roast beef with gravy	1800 (430)	83	52	38	22	331
Tuna fish salad	1160 (278)	53	34	25	14	214
Sherbet, 1/6 qt	741 (177)	34	22	16	9	136
Shrimp, French fried	753 (180)	35	22	16	9	138
Spaghetti, 1 serving	1660 (396)	76	48	35	20	305
Steak, T-bone	984 (235)	45	29	21	12	181
Strawberry shortcake	1670 (400)	77	49	36	21	308

[a] Energy cost of walking for 686 N (70 kg) individual = 363 N·m/sec (5.2 kcal/min) at 1.56 m/sec (3.51 mi/hr).
[b] Energy cost of riding bicycle = 572 N·m/sec (8.2 kcal/min).
[c] Energy cost of swimming = 781 N·m/sec (11.2 kcal/min).
[d] Energy cost of running = 1353 N·m/sec (19.4 kcal/min).
[e] Energy cost of reclining = 90.7 N·m/sec (1.3 kcal/min).

walking, 12 min of cycling, 9 min of swimming, 5 min of running, and by 78 min of reclining. This indicates that running is the most energy-intensive exercise among the five. However, with that same energy expenditure, a walker will cover a distance of about 1.8 km, the cyclist will cover a distance of about 4.8 km, the swimmer will go only 360 m, the runner will travel 2.0 km, and the recliner will not travel at all. Clearly, there is a huge difference between the energy expended on these different tasks. Why this should be so is the topic of this discussion.

The case of the cyclist is most interesting. The cyclist encumbers himself with the extra weight of the apparatus, but he obviously, gains a great deal by being able to travel substantially farther on the same amount of energy compared to walking or running (which have nearly equal distances). We previously noted the special case of swimming (Section 1.2) and the additional energy required to overcome viscous drag on the body. Returning to the case of bicycling, what is it about the bicycle that makes locomotion with it so highly efficient?

Tucker (1975) considered this and other forms of movement. In his article he proposed, as an index of the cost of transport,

$$CT = P_i/sW \qquad (2.3.1)$$

where CT = cost of transport, dimensionless
P_i = input power, N·m/sec
s = speed of movement, m/sec
W = body weight, N

The cost of transport really involves the rate of energy usage moving at an appropriate speed. Because there may be substantial differences in body weight between animals to be compared,[8] the cost of transport includes the weight factor. The result is a dimensionless quantity that can be used to compare different modes of exercise.

The cost of transport for a given animal will vary with speed. If the animal does not move, the cost of transport will be infinite because speed is zero, but a small amount of maintenance energy (see Section 5.2.5) is still supplied. At very rapid speeds, the energy cost is very high due to friction and inertia of various body parts. In Section 2.2.3 we saw that walking and running speeds could be related to the natural periods of pendulums. Faster speeds require the use of additional forcing energy. Thus at very high speeds, as at low speeds, the cost of transport becomes very high. In between, there will be a minimum power expenditure at some point.

The cost of transport will also achieve a minimum, but generally at a higher speed than the power expenditure minimum. For a constant animal weight, the minimum cost of transport will be determined by the ratio of P_i/s, which is equivalent to determining the minimum graphically as the point at which a line through the origin of a graph for P_i and s is tangent to the power curve. Figure 2.3.1 shows this minimum for flight of a budgie (budgerigar parrot).

In Figure 2.3.2 are plotted minimum costs of transport for a variety of runners, fliers, swimmers, and other forms of human locomotion. Over 12 orders of magnitude of body mass are represented, and minimum costs of transport vary widely.

The data in Figure 2.3.2 cluster along three general lines of classification: swimmers, fliers, and walkers (or runners), with the minimum costs of transport for swimmers less than those for fliers and for fliers less than those for walkers. Walking, therefore, is a comparatively inefficient way of moving about.

Cycling has a minimum cost of transport about one-fourth that of walking,[9] which is why a cyclist is willing to assume the burden of the extra weight of the bicycle. Human swimmers, on the other hand, have a minimum cost of transport nearly six times that of human walkers. Many cars

---

[8]Or the body weight of a given animal may change substantially over a short time. Some migrating birds use up to 25% of their body weight as fuel between feeding periods (Tucker, 1975).

[9]A 686 N man (mass of 70 kg) achieves his minimum cost of transport while walking at about 1.75 m/sec (3.85 mi/hr). The metabolic cost of walking at this speed is 452 N·m/sec and his cost of transport is 0.376. By comparison, he expends 1122 N·m/sec while jogging at 3.5 m/sec (7.7 mi/hr) and his cost of transport is 0.467.

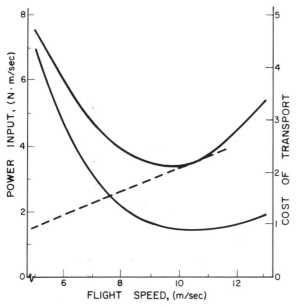

Figure 2.3.1   The cost of transport (upper curve) and power input (lower curve) for a 0.35 kg parrot in level flight. There is a minimum power input at a speed between 10 and 11 m/sec. The minimum cost of transport is found at the point of tangency of the curve and the dashed line. (Redrawn with permission from Tucker, 1975.)

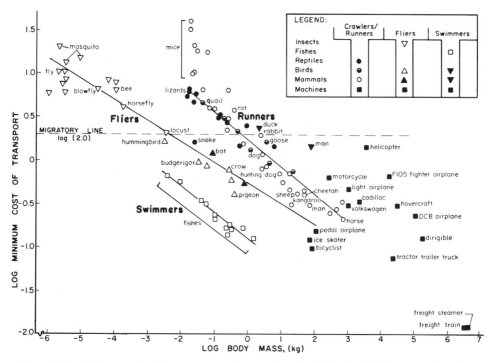

Figure 2.3.2   Minimum costs of transport for various species, which fall naturally into groups depending on their types of locomotion. (Redrawn with permission from Tucker, 1975.)

and airplanes have costs of transport worse than walking animals of equivalent mass, but tractor trailer trucks are nearly as efficient as walking animals of equivalent mass (if they existed!).

A sparrow possesses a mass and metabolic rate equivalent to a mouse but flies nearly 10 times faster than the mouse runs. The sparrow's minimum cost of transport is about 10 times less than that for a mouse.

Tucker (1975) observed that smaller terrestrial animals almost never migrate, but smaller birds often do. Only larger mammal species, such as caribou, bison, and large antelopes, migrate. Figure 2.3.2 shows a horizontal line at a cost of transport of 2.0. Animals with lower costs of transport have usually been observed as migratory species, whereas animals above the line have not. Apparently the costs of transport are too high for migration if they are above 2.0.[10]

The statement of muscular efficiency, at least for the larger muscles, being about 20%, is made several times in this book (Sections 1.3, 2.2, 3.2.3, 4.2.3, 5.2.5). However, considering an act of movement as a whole, mean muscular efficiency often is much lower than this and may approach zero. Such is the case with walking on a level surface.

Muscle power is used, in general, for three purposes: (1) to support the body weight, (2) to overcome aerodynamic drag, and (3) to perform mechanical work. Total input power equals muscle power plus power diverted for nonmuscular purposes:

$$P_i - P_{nm} = \frac{P_{spt} + P_d + P_w}{\eta} \qquad (2.3.2)$$

where P_i = input power, N·m/sec
P_{nm} = nonmuscular power, N·m/sec
P_{spt} = power to support body weight, N·m/sec
P_d = power to overcome drag, N·m/sec
P_w = power to perform external mechanical work, N·m/sec
η = muscular efficiency, dimensionless

Rearranging Equation 2.3.2 to obtain mean muscular efficiency:

$$\eta = \frac{P_{spt} + P_d + P_w}{P_i - P_{nm}} \qquad (2.3.3)$$

For walkers or runners, the power required to support the body weight is very small. So is aerodynamic drag. Since a walker or runner on the level does not raise his body weight,[11] external work is zero. Therefore, mean muscular efficiency for walking and running approaches zero.

Birds do not have the same efficiencies while flying. They must support their body weights with their wing muscles; going faster, they have higher amounts of aerodynamic drag; and they perform external work when they move their wings through the air. Their mean muscular efficiencies are close to 20%.

Why should mean muscular efficiency of walking be so low, and what happens to the input energy? While walking, the center of mass of the body is continually moving up and down. The muscles actively perform external work to raise the body weight, but they cannot recover the potential enenrgy when the center of mass falls. Instead, the muscles act against the body weight by decelerating it. When muscles shorten and produce a force during shortening, they produce external work; when muscles stretch but produce a force against an externally applied force, they

---

[10]Notice that helicopters and F105 fighter planes could migrate, should they be so inclined.
[11]We are talking here about raising or lowering body weight over the entire walking or running cycle. During the cycle, however, body weight does rise and fall considerably.

produce negative external work (work is done on the muscle; see Section 5.2).[12] This stretching of active muscles, attempting to shorten but not producing enough force of their own to overcome the externally applied force, occurs during the decelerating phase of walking. Part of the walking time is spent by muscles producing external work, and part of the walking time is spent by work being done on the muscles. The former is characterized by a positive muscular efficiency and the latter by a negative muscular efficiency. Mean muscular efficiency for the entire act is about zero.[13]

If there were some way of storing mechanical energy at the appropriate points in the walking cycle, it could be recovered to aid in performing other work and muscular efficiency would rise. One way of doing this would be to store energy in an elastic medium. But humans have not developed a very effective elastic medium in the course of their evolution and thus cannot use this mechanism.[14] The energy which is not stored becomes useless heat.

There are other ways of handling the excess of external mechanical energy without elastically storing it. One alternative is to prevent the stretching of active muscles by converting the downward velocity component of the body's center of mass into an upward component later in the walking cycle. This mechanism applies a force to the center of mass at right angles to its direction of motion. When the force is at right angles to the displacement, the muscles that supply the force can neither do work nor have work done on them. The velocity is changed at no expense to muscular work.

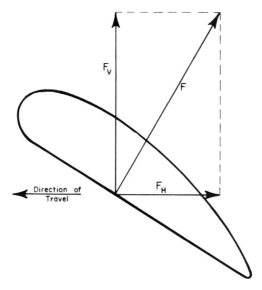

Figure 2.3.3   A wing converts horizontal movement into vertical lift. Here the net force F acting on the wing is decomposed into a horizontal F_H and vertical F_V component.

---

[12]Kinesiology is the study of human movement, and biomechanics is the subdiscipline that relates to neuromusculoskeletal aspects of that movement (Winter, 1983). Kinesiologists usually use the term "concentric" contraction for muscles shortening while producing positive external work. They use the term "eccentric" contraction for muscles shortening and producing negative muscular work.

[13]Alexander (1984) compares the changes in energy and speed during walking and running to alternately braking and accelerating while driving a car. The average speed can be held to the same value as during steady driving, but the use of energy in the form of gasoline is much greater this way. The difference lies in the greater dissipation of energy as heat while braking and accelerating, and the resulting efficiency is very low.

[14]This is true for the case of walking. For running, however, there is a considerable amount of elastic energy storage (see Section 2.4).

An example of this is the pole used by the pole vaulter. The vaulter runs at a high speed and thrusts the pole into a box in the ground. As long as the pole is not exactly horizontal, a component is developed in the pole which is perpendicular to the direction of running. This component lifts the vaulter without a vertical component of muscular work required.

A wing also performs this function. A wing is usually thin and tilted (Figure 2.3.3). The tilt enables a vertical force component to be developed from horizontal movement. With wings, the flying animal can change the downward motion of its center of mass into a forward motion without stretching elastic structures or active muscles. Tucker (1975) provides a dramatic example of the benefits of developing this perpendicular force. He considers the results of dropping a pigeon and a rat from a high place. The pigeon merely extends its wings and the perpendicular force changes its motion from vertical to horizontal. The rat, however, must absorb all the developed kinetic energy at the bottom of the fall by stretching elastic structures and active muscles, probably with extremely damaging effect.

Active muscle stretching can also be prevented by precluding the vertical movement of the center of mass of the body. Many fishes achieve this end by balancing the force of gravity with the buoyancy of their swim bladders. Millipedes, with their large number of legs, can support their centers of mass at all times. The extreme of this strategy leads to the wheel. The wheels of a bicycle stabilize the position of the rider's center of mass, and even pedaling while standing up does not result in the stretching of active muscles because when the center of mass falls the motion is translated into horizontal movement. By using external machinery humans can achieve the muscular efficiencies that swimming and flying animals naturally accomplish.

2.4   WALKING AND RUNNING

Moving about by walking and running has been the object of much study. In this section we proceed from the simplest of biomechanical energetic models to theories about control of these processes to experimental correlations of data.

2.4.1   Basic Analysis

Walking is a natural movement in which at least one foot is on the ground at all times (Figure 2.4.1).[15] Because each foot touches the ground for slightly more than half the time, there are stages when both feet are simultaneously on the ground (Alexander, 1984). While stepping, the leg remains nearly straight, and, the position of the center of mass of the body is therefore highest when the leg is vertical and the body passes over the supporting foot. Contrarily, the body is lowest when both feet are touching the ground.

Running is a different mode of locomotion in which each foot is on the ground less than half the time (Figure 2.4.2). There are stages of running during which neither foot is on the ground. The runner travels in a series of leaps, with the center of mass of the body at its highest in midleap. Its lowest point occurs when the trunk passes over the supporting foot, and the supporting leg is bent at this stage. Walking and running are therefore characterized by many dissimilarities, with the major resemblance between the two being forward motion propelled by the legs.

The transition between walking and running occurs at fairly predictable speed of about 2.5 m/sec (6 mi/hr) for normal-sized adults (Alexander, 1984). Why this should be so can be shown easily by a simple model of walking.

As illustrated by Figure 2.4.3, the walker sets a foot on the ground ahead of himself and, while keeping the leg straight, propels himself forward with a speed v. His hip joint thus moves along an arc of a circle centered on the foot. For purposes of this simple model, the legs will be considered to be sufficiently light that their masses can be ignored compared to the trunk, and therefore the

---

[15]Except for race walking, where, it has been found, there is a very short time during which neither foot has ground contact.

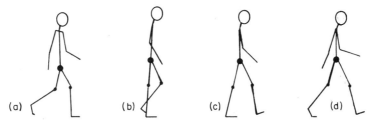

Figure 2.4.1 Four successive stages of a walking stride. In the first stage the trailing foot leaves the ground and the front foot applies a braking force. In the second stage the trailing foot is brought forward off the ground and the supporting foot applies a vertical force. In the third stage the trailing foot provides an acceleration force. In the last stage, both feet are on the ground, with the trailing foot pushing forward and the front foot pushing backward.

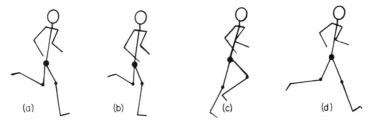

Figure 2.4.2 Four stages of running. Braking and pushing forces are exerted by the feet much as in walking, but much of the otherwise lost energy is stored between the first two stages in the form of elastic strain in the tendons. This energy is then released between the second and fourth stages. During the last stage, no feet are touching the ground; therefore, the opposing forces generated by the feet during the last stage of walking are not present.

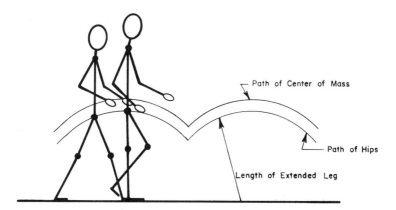

Figure 2.4.3 While walking, the center of mass of the body rises and falls along an arc with a radius depending on the length of the leg. (Adapted and redrawn with permission from Alexander, 1984.)

body center of mass will occupy a fixed position on the trunk. Hence the center of mass will move along an arc of the same radius as that of the hip joint.

Centripetal force can be calculated from Equation 2.2.26:

$$F_c = \frac{mv^2}{r} \qquad (2.2.26)$$

where F_c = centripetal force, N
    m = body mass, kg
    v = tangential velocity, m/sec
    r = arc radius, m

A point moving with speed v along an arc of a circle will have an acceleration toward the center of the circle:

$$\frac{F}{m} = a = \frac{v^2}{r} \tag{2.4.1}$$

where a = acceleration, m/sec^2

When the center of mass is at its highest, this acceleration will be directed vertically downward. Since the walker cannot pull himself downward, his vertical acceleration is limited to the free fall acceleration of gravity:

$$\frac{v^2}{r} \leqslant g \tag{2.4.2a}$$

or

$$v \leqslant \sqrt{gr} \tag{2.4.2b}$$

where g = gravitational acceleration, 9.8 m/sec^2

With a typical leg length of 0.9 m, maximum walking speed is about 3 m/sec, close to the observed 2.5 m/sec in adults. Children, who have shorter legs than adults, break into running at lower forward speeds. These results confirm the analysis resulting in Equation 2.2.34c.

Race walkers exceed this maximum speed, however, traveling about 4 m/sec (Figure 2.4.4). The trick that makes high walking speeds possible is to bend the lower part of the back during walking, thus sticking the pelvis out and lowering the center of mass of the body relative to the hip joint. The center of mass no longer moves in arcs of radius equal to the length of the legs, but in arcs of larger radius. There is less rising and falling, and higher speeds are possible.[16]

More detailed analysis of walking has shown that the simplified approach given previously may be misleading. McMahon (1984) summarizes six movements during walking which modify the gait:

1. *Compass gait.* This is the basic walk characterized by flexions and extensions of the hips and illustrated in Figure 2.4.3. The legs remain stiff and straight.

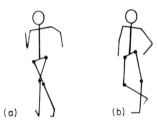

(a)   (b)

Figure 2.4.4 During race walking the center of mass of the body is kept lower than in ordinary walking by the bending of the back and the tilting of the hips. Because the center of mass rises less, higher speeds are possible compared to ordinary walking.

[16] It has also been reported that women expend less energy than men walking at the same speed. Presumably this is because of shorter steps taken by women, with consequent smaller fluctuation of vertical height of the pelvis (Booyens and Keatinge, 1957)

2. *Pelvic rotation.* The pelvis rotates around a vertical axis through the center of the body. The amplitude of this rotation is about $\pm 3°$ during normal walking speeds and increases at high speeds. The effect of this motion is to increase the effective length of the leg, producing a longer stride and increasing the radius of the arcs of the hip, giving a flatter, smoother movement.

3. *Pelvic tilt.* The pelvis tilts so that the hip on the side with the swinging leg falls lower than the hip on the opposite side. The effect of this movement is to make the trajectory arcs still flatter.

4. *Stance leg knee flexion.* By bending the knee of the leg supporting the weight, the arc is made flatter yet.

5. *Plantar flexion of the stance ankle.* The sole, or plantar surface of the foot, moves down and and ankle of the stance leg flexes just before the toe lifts from the ground. A result of this is that the leg muscles can produce the forces necessary to swing the leg forward during the next phase, but it also results in an effective lengthening of the stance leg during the portion of the arc when the hip is falling. The hip thus falls less than it would without this movement.

6. *Lateral displacement of the pelvis.* The body rocks from side to side during walking, with a lifting of the swing leg.

These motions make walking a much more complex process than the simplified models to this point would suggest. The result of these motions is that walking, although still energy inefficient, is not as inefficient as it would be without them.

Results of calculations of expended power made from respiratory gas measurements are seen in Figure 2.4.5. We have already discussed cycling relative to running, and it is not surprising to see that cyclists expend less energy at any given speed than do runners. Power required for

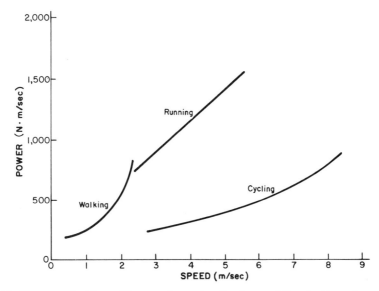

Figure 2.4.5 Power required for walking, running, and cycling by an adult male. Curves for walking and running intersect at about 2.3 m/sec and show that walking is more efficient below the intersection and running is more efficient above. Cycling is more efficient because, presumably, the body does not rise and fall as much as with walking and running. (Redrawn with permission from Alexander, 1984).

walking begins at a low value at low speeds (we would expect there to be a minimum in the curve, based the discussion of Section 2.2.3) and rises rapidly to moderate power levels at higher speeds.

Running power begins at moderate levels and rises less slowly than walking at yet higher speeds. An intersection of the walking and running curves occurs at about 2.5 m/sec. If walking is continued beyond this speed, there will be a higher expenditure of energy than if the person switched to running. Similarly, if running is begun before 2.5 m/sec, a higher amount of energy will be expended than if the person walked. It appears that the switch from walking to running occurs because of energy considerations. There is a gradual shift in the walking gait to maintain an optimal energy expenditure (Alexander, 1984) until the abrupt changeover to running to again maintain an optimal energy expenditure.

Human running uses less energy than might be expected because of elastic energy storage. Between the first and second stages of a running stride (Figure 2.4.2) the body is both slowing and falling, simultaneously losing kinetic and potential energy (Alexander, 1984). This energy must be restored between the third and fourth stages. If the energy lost was not stored somewhere, the metabolic energy required from the muscles would be about 1.8 times the actual energy consumption for slow running and 3.0 times the actual consumption for fast running (Alexander, 1984).

Energy is stored by elastic deformation of the muscles and tendons. Muscles may be stretched about 3% of their length before they yield and the energy cannot be recovered elastically. Tendons can stretch about 6% before breaking (Alexander, 1984). Although elastic energy can be stored in each of these, the tendons are probably the most important structures for energy storage. The ligaments and tendons in the soles of the feet and the Achilles tendon are likely the most important site of energy storage during each running step (Alexander, 1984).

Quadripedal animals have one mode of locomotion, besides walking and running, that humans do not: they gallop at high speed. Galloping involves bending movements of the back which briefly store leg kinetic energy fluctuations as elastic energy, contributing to overall efficiency (Alexander, 1988). These animals appear to have two transitional power points, one from walking to running or trotting and another from running to galloping.

2.4.2 Optimal Control of Walking

Walking has long been recognized as one bodily function that appears to have some built-in optimization operating (see also Sections 3.4.3 and 4.3.4). Walking, for instance, appears to occur at a speed that minimizes the rate of energy expenditure of the body. This can be simply shown from the empirical observation that power consumption of walking, as measured by oxygen consumption, depends on walking speed (Dean, 1965; Milsum, 1966):

$$\dot{E} = a + bs^2 \tag{2.4.3}$$

where $\dot{E}$ = rate of energy usage (or power), N·m/sec
a,b = constants, N·m/sec and N·sec/m
s = walking speed, m/sec
Average power per unit speed is

$$\dot{E}/s = a/s + bs \tag{2.4.4}$$

This represents an average power with two components, one linearly increasing and one hyperbolically decreasing (Figure 2.4.6). Minimum average power can be found by taking the derivative of $\dot{E}/s$ and setting the derivative equal to zero:

$$\frac{d}{ds}(\dot{E}/s) = \frac{-a}{s^2} + b = 0 \tag{2.4.5}$$

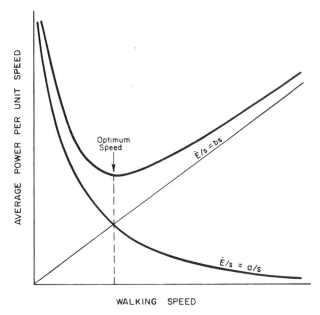

Figure 2.4.6 Walking appears to occur at a speed very close to the optimum based on average power consumption. Two components of average power, one increasing with speed and the other decreasing with speed, make possible a minimum average power.

$$s = \sqrt{a/b} \qquad (2.4.6)$$

where s = optimum speed, m/sec

Biochemical models describing walking and running are necessarily complex, not conceptually but parametrically. As noted by Winter (1983), model inputs of muscle electromyographic signals are many for relatively simple movements. Similarly, model outputs of body segment motions, each with 3 degrees of freedom and 15 variables of forces and moments, can soon become overwhelming. It is no wonder, then, that most modelers have greatly oversimplified, constrained, or limited conditions for their models in order to deal with these problems (Onyshko and Winter, 1980; Siegler et al., 1982).

All this is not necessarily bad, however. Depending on the use of the model, a simplified artificial model may be preferred to a complex realistic model. This preference is especially true if the model is to be used to impart understanding of general patterns rather than to diagnostically treat individual malfunctions. Biomechanical models, used to identify causes of abnormal gait patterns or to improve competitive running performance, are necessarily very complex models. Since the objective for including models in this book is to aid general understanding through mathematical description (see Section 1.1), models chosen for inclusion are of the general or simplistic type.

There are many reasons for developing biomechanical models of walking and running. Pierrynowski and Morrison (1985a,b) developed theirs to predict muscular forces; Williams and Cavanagh (1983) and Morton (1985) developed theirs to predict power output during running; Greene's model (1985) has applications to sports; Dul and Johnson (1985) developed a descriptive kinematic model of the ankle; and Hatze and Venter (1981) used their models to investigate the effects of constraints on computational efficiency. Reviews by King (1984) and Winter (1983) summarize many recent modeling attempts.

The one model chosen to be highlighted here uses stepping motion as the object of the model and includes control aspects as well as mechanical descriptions (Flashner et al., 1987). In this model is postulated a hypothetical, but nevertheless plausible, hierarchical structure of stepping control.

The hierarchy of control, diagramed in Figure 2.4.7, includes both open- and closed-loop components. In general, Flashner et al. postulated a system that normally determines, based on previous experience, the trajectory of a step to be taken. This is used as an open-loop procedure during stepping. Only when the controller determines that the trajectory is not proceeding as planned does it take corrective action.

For instance, if an object stands in the way of the step, the leg and foot must move in such a way as to clear the object. Presumably the individual, over the years, has learned how to optimally perform this task. The trajectory that has been stored from previous trials is then used to program hip, leg, and foot motion. The action is quick and sure as long as nothing unexpected happens. The controller samples sensors in the leg to determine if the intended trajectory is being achieved. This sampling may occur at a slower or faster rate, depending on the needs of the controller.

If conditions are found to be not as anticipated (for instance, if heavier shoes are worn or the object moves), feedback control is used to correct the intended action (for instance, muscle forces are increased or activity times are changed). Since feedback control is slower than feedforward control, and feedback control does not effectively use past experience (at least control with constant coefficients, or nonadaptive control), feedback is used only when required.

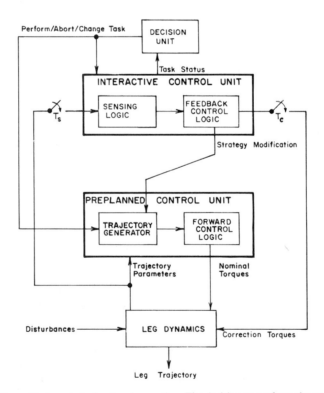

Figure 2.4.7 Hierarchical control of a stepping motion. The decision to perform the motion results in a trial trajectory given to the leg. Sampled data from the leg are sent to the interactive control unit, where it is determined whether or not to send correction torques to the leg to overcome unforseen disturbances. (Adapted from Flashner et al., 1987.)

The highest level of control decides about task performance: to step or not to step, to change task strategy for feedforward or feedback control units. The interactive control unit is activated only when corrections to the preplanned movement are needed. This is the site of feedback control.

At a lower level comes the preplanned control unit, wherein are stored optimal trajectories parameterized by relevant variables of motion such as step height, step length, and step duration (or, more likely, muscle forces and durations).

The leg dynamics level includes both sensing and activation. Its outputs are used by both the feedforward and feedback control units, and it receives input information from both control units.

During learning the interactive control unit is constantly active. The preplanned control unit determines a candidate trajectory. Joint angles and control torques are calculated and sent to the leg dynamics unit. Some performance criterion is calculated and stored. Over the course of the learning period the task is repeated many times with different candidate trajectories. Each of these yields a different value for the performance index. The trajectory with the most desirable (usually the maximum or minimum) cost or performance index is the trajectory that is remembered.

Performance criteria[17] for the task may include any number of aspects. Minimizing time, energy, peak force, or any combination of these is a possible performance criterion. In addition, there are constraints, such as limits to the force of contact with the ground, velocities, and accelerations. These must be included in the model formulation.

Figure 2.4.8 is a diagram of the dynamic leg model. The leg starts in position 1, fully extended. As it moves to position 2 in midswing the hip and knee are bent. Flashner et al. consider ankle bending only when the foot touches the ground. Hip height decreases but the foot is raised to clear the object. Upon landing, the foot again raises the hip and both hip and knee ankles return to their initial values.

Flashner et al. considered cycloidal velocity profiles for hip and knee joints:

$$\dot{\theta}_H = C_1(\omega - \omega \cos \omega t) \tag{2.4.7a}$$

$$\dot{\theta}_K = C_2(\omega - \omega \cos \omega t) \tag{2.4.7b}$$

where $\dot{\theta}_H$ = time rate of change of hip angle, rad/sec
$\dot{\theta}_K$ = time rate of change of knee angle, rad/sec
ω, C_1, C_2 = constant parameters whose values are
chosen to match experimental data, rad/sec

Cycloids have the advantage that their first and second time derivatives vanish at the beginning ($\omega t = 0$) and end ($\omega t = 2\pi$) of the cycle. Experimental evidence suggests that the smooth transition from a stationary state to a moving state and back again requires both velocity and acceleration to be zero. Cycloids also introduce no more new parameters than do sines or cosines, and, once hip motion is specified, all other angles, positions, velocities, and accelerations are determined.

Kinematic equations can be derived for all segments of the model. Flashner et al. presented these for the foot:

$$X_F = X_H + L_{TH} \sin \theta_H - L_{SH} \sin \Theta \tag{2.4.8a}$$

$$Y_F = Y_H - L_{TH} \sin \theta_H - L_{SH} \cos \Theta \tag{2.4.8b}$$

$$\dot{X}_F = \dot{X}_H + L_{TH}\dot{\theta}_H \cos \theta_H - L_{SH} \dot{\Theta} \cos \Theta \tag{2.4.9a}$$

---

[17]Mathematically expressed as a "cost function" or "objective function." See Section 4.3.4.

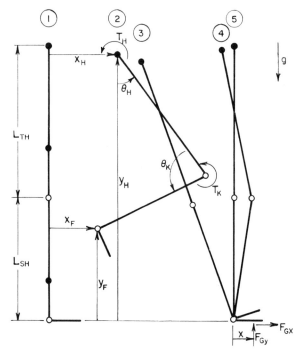

Figure 2.4.8 Schematic representation of the leg dynamic model. Foot and leg motion is not constrained during the swing phase, but once the foot is planted upon landing, leg motion is no longer totally free. Stages represented are (1) begin swing, (2) midswing, (3) begin landing, (4) midlanding, and (5) end landing. (Adapted and redrawn with permission from Flashner et al., 1987.)

$$\dot{Y}_F = \dot{Y}_H + L_{TH}\dot{\theta}_H \cos\theta_H - L_{SH}\dot{\Theta}\sin\Theta \qquad (2.4.9b)$$

$$\ddot{X}_F = \ddot{X}_H - L_{TH}\dot{\theta}_H^2 \sin\theta_H + L_{TH}\ddot{\theta}_H \cos\theta_H + L_{SH}\dot{\Theta}^2\sin\Theta - L_{SH}\ddot{\Theta}\cos\Theta \qquad (2.4.10a)$$

$$\ddot{Y}_F = \ddot{Y}_H + L_{TH}\dot{\theta}_H^2 \cos\theta_H + L_{TH}\ddot{\theta}_H \sin\theta_H - L_{SH}\dot{\Theta}^2\cos\Theta - L_{SH}\ddot{\Theta}\sin\Theta \qquad (2.4.10b)$$

where X_F, Y_F = position coordinates of the foot in a fixed frame of reference, m
$\dot{X}_F, \dot{Y}_F$ = velocity components of foot, m
$\ddot{X}_F, \ddot{Y}_F$ = acceleration components of foot, m
L_{TH} = length of the thigh measured from hip joint to knee joint, m
L_{SH} = length of the shank measured from knee joint to ankle, m
θ_H = hip angle, rad

and

$$\Theta = \theta_H + \theta_K \qquad (2.4.11)$$

where θ_K = knee angle, rad
Notice that Equations 2.4.9a,b and 2.4.10a,b are obtained from Equations 2.4.8a,b by simple derivatives.

Flashner et al. also present inverse kinematic equations, that is, equations to predict hip and knee angles and their derivatives from foot position. The reader is referred to Flashner et al. (1987) for these equations.

Model dynamic equations are derived using the Lagrangian method.[18] In generalized form, dynamic equations related to system energy are

$$\frac{d}{dt}\left(\frac{\partial \mathscr{L}}{\partial \dot{q}_i}\right) - \frac{\partial \mathscr{L}}{\partial q_i} = Q_i + C_i \qquad (2.4.12)$$

where $\mathscr{L}$ = system Lagrangian
= difference between system kinetic energy and system potential energy, N·m
q_i = generalized coordinates, m or rad
Q_i = generalized forces, N or N·m
C_i = constraints, N or N·m
For Flashner et al.'s model, the coordinate vector is

$$q = [q_1 q_2 q_3 q_4]^T = [X_H Y_H \theta_H \theta_K]^T \qquad (2.4.13)$$

and the force vector is

$$Q = [Q_1 Q_2 Q_3 Q_4]^T = [F_{HX} F_{HY} T_H T_K]^T \qquad (2.4.14)$$

where F_{HX}, F_{HY} = force components acting on the hip, N
T_H, T_K = torques acting at hip and knee joints, N·m
The constraint vector is

$$C = J(q)\lambda \qquad (2.4.15)$$

where $J(q)$ = Jacobian matrix[19] that relates the Cartesian coordinates of mass centers to generalized coordinates q_i
λ = vector of length to be determined by the system of constraints
During the swing phase of stepping there are no constraints on the motion of the leg. During the landing phase of stepping the motion of the foot is constrained by the surface of the ground. Flashner et al. introduce these constraints by

$$\begin{aligned} X_F &= 0 \\ Y_F &= 0 \end{aligned} \qquad (2.4.16)$$

These conditions were used to derive equations of motion for the swing and landing phases.

Flashner et al. (1987) fitted their equations to experimental data as seen in Figure 2.4.9. It can be seen from the figure that the agreement is quite close. Because these data were used as the basis for model calibration, the fit would be expected to be very good as long as the model had general validity.[20] The conclusion which can be reached, therefore, is that the model has sufficient capacity to reproduce reality in very limited circumstances. Whether the model is a good description of the actual control of stepping and whether the model is a good predictor of other data to which it has not been calibrated have yet to be determined.

---

[18] Any system of equations which must be solved subject to certain constraints is a candidate for Lagrange's method. Constraints are introduced into the equation set using a series of parameters called Lagrange multipliers. See Appendix 4.1.
[19] The Jacobian matrix contains elements each of which is a partial derivative of a coordinate in one system with respect to a coordinate in another system. All such elements $\partial x_i/\partial q_i$ are included.
[20] Flashner et al. (1987) show closer agreement to their data when the cycloidal motion of the hip is modified using fitting techniques.

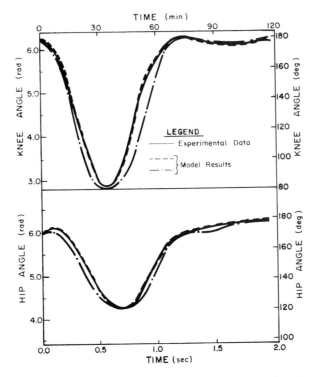

Figure 2.4.9 Comparison of experimental data (solid line) with model results using a cycloidal input (dashed and dashed-dotted lines). (Adapted and redrawn with permission from Flashner et al., 1987).

2.4.3 Experimental Results

Bassett et al. (1985) measured the oxygen cost of running, comparing overground and treadmill running. They found no statistical difference between these two types of running, either on a level surface or on a 5% uphill grade. Level running gave regression lines as follows for treadmill:

$$\dot{V}_{O_2} = 2.22m(10^{-7}s - 10^{-8}), \qquad s \leqslant 4.77 \, \text{m/sec} \tag{2.4.17}$$

and for overland running:

$$\dot{V}_{O_2} = 2.02m \, [10^{-7}s + (2.65 \times 10^{-8})], \qquad s \leqslant 4.77 \, \text{m/sec} \tag{2.4.18}$$

where $\dot{V}_{O_2}$ = oxygen consumption, m^3/sec
m = body mass, kg
s = running speed, m/sec
They also reported that the additional oxygen cost caused by air resistance is

$$\Delta \dot{V}_{O_2} = 3.3 \times 10^{-11}s^3 \tag{2.4.19}$$

where $\Delta \dot{V}_{O_2}$ = additional oxygen cost to overcome air resistance, m^3/sec
Measurements of additional metabolic energy used by a runner to overcome air resistance vary widely—from 2% (Bassett et al., 1985) to 16% (Ward-Smith, 1984).

2.5 CARRYING LOADS

Load carrying is an important aspect of manual labor and of certain sports such as weight lifting. Load carrying has been the subject of a great deal of study by exercise physiologists and ergonomicists, and it has even been quantified to a large extent (see Section 5.5). Yet there are quite a few different ways of carrying loads, and quantitative description of these has not been fully completed.

2.5.1 Load Position

Load position has an important effect on the amount of energy required to carry the load. Body weight, for example, is carried with metabolic cost usually less than externally carried loads, since it is reasonably well distributed and its center of mass passes through the center of mass of the body. Light loads carried on the hands, on the head, and high on the back are carried with almost no additional energy penalty except for the weight itself (Table 2.5.1). Heavy loads on the feet and hands, however, pose a muscular burden out of proportion to weight carried (Martin, 1985; Soule and Goldman, 1969)

2.5.2 Lifting and Carrying

Lifting of loads requires an initial isometric muscular contraction to overcome inertia and set the postural muscles followed by a dynamic muscular contraction as the load is moved. The major part of the lift, when it occurs on the job, is composed of dynamic contraction. Pytel and Kamon (1981) studied workers to determine if a simple predictor test could be devised for maximum lifting capacity of an individual. Such a test would be useful in industrial situations. By measuring the dynamic lifting strength of the combined back and arm muscles and comparing this to voluntary maximum acceptable loads lifted, they were able to obtain this simple equation with an r^2 (statistical coefficient of determination) of 0.941:

$$F_m = 295 + 0.66F_{dls} - 148S_x \qquad (2.5.1)$$

where F_m = maximum load to be lifted repetitively, N

F_{dls} = peak force developed during dynamic lifting strength test, N

S_x = sex indicator, 1 for men and 2 for women, dimensionless

TABLE 2.5.1 Relative Energy Cost for Carrying Loads in Different Positions at Different Speeds

Condition	Speed, m/sec		
	67	80	93
No load	1.0	1.0	1.0
Hands, 39 N (4 kg) each	1.0	1.3	1.9
Hands, 69 N (7 kg) each	2.0	1.8	1.8
Head, 137 N (14 kg)	1.3	1.0	1.3
Feet, 59 N (6 kg) each	4.2	5.8	6.2
No load, actual energy cost[a]			
$10^8 \cdot [m^3 \ O_2/sec]/N$ body wt	1.79	2.18	2.62
([mL O_2/min]/kg body mass)	(10.5)	(12.8)	(15.4)

Source: Data from Soule and Goldman, 1969.

[a]Wyndam et al. (1963) give a regression equation relating oxygen consumption to work rate of $\dot{V}_{O_2} = 6.535 \times 10^{-6} + 2.557 \times 10^{-7} \dot{W}$ where $\dot{V}_{O_2}$ = oxygen consumption, m^3/sec, and $\dot{W}$ = work rate, N·m/sec (original values of equation coefficients are 0.3921 L/min and 3.467×10^{-4} L/ft·lb). The range of applicability of this equation is not known, however, since data were originally obtained from 88 Bantu tribesmen.

Average values for F_{dls} were 379 N for women and 601 N for men. Maximum dynamic loads were 250 N for women and 544 N for men. Further observations on steelworkers exhibited much more data scattering and much less satisfactory regression equations (Kamon et al., 1982). Goldman (1978) reviewed the field of load lifting and Freivalds et al. (1984) produced a biomechanical model of the load lifting task.

Givoni and Goldman (1971) proposed an empirical equation to predict metabolic energy cost of walking at any given speed and grade while carrying a load. In developing this equation they used data from many different sources but found excellent agreement between data and calculations. They proceeded to provide corrections for load placement (as already discussed), carrying very heavy loads (very heavy loads are carried less efficiently), effect of terrain (higher metabolic costs are involved for rougher walking surface), and running (below a critical speed which depends on external load and grade, running is less efficient than walking). A more thorough presentation of this material can be found in Section 5.5.1, and the reader is referred there.

2.5.3   Using Carts

Using handcarts to carry the load has been found to be much easier than carrying the same load by backpacking. Haisman et al. (1972) tested four commercially available handcarts and found that on a treadmill and on a level asphalt surface a 500 N (50 kg) load required a range of 480–551 N·m/sec to pull while walking. The predicted cost of walking alone was about 446 N·m/sec. The difference between these two was the additional power required to transport the load. Taken a different way, about 800 N·m/sec would have been required to transport the same load on the back.

The same advantage does not appear to hold with rough terrain. Haisman and Goldman (1974) loaded a cart with various weights carefully balanced in the cart. On a blacktop surface little difference was found in metabolic rate of the subject whether he was carrying a 200 N (20 kg) load on his back or 200, 600, or 1000 N loads in a handcart. On a dirt road or dry grass terrain, however, metabolic cost increased up to 50% for the 1000 N load in the cart compared to a 200 N load carried by pack. Although the metabolic cost advantage of carrying loads in a cart is not nearly as great over rough terrain as it is over a smooth surface, carts still make possible transporting loads that would not be possible to carry by hand.

2.6   SUSTAINED WORK

The capacity to perform physical work depends on age, gender, and muscle fiber composition (Kamon, 1981). The demands which any given task make on the body can therefore best be studied by standardizing, or normalizing, to maximal body capacity. For dynamic work efforts it is usually maximum oxygen uptake which is considered to be a measure of maximum capacity (see Section 1.3.4). For static work efforts the maximum muscle force or torque that can be developed by the muscles is useful as a measure of maximum capacity. Thus work can be sustained for periods of time depending on the type (static or dynamic) of work and the fraction of maximum oxygen uptake (dynamic work) or maximum voluntary contraction (static work).

Kamon (1981) gives the maximum time to exhaustion for dynamic work as

$$t_{exh} = 7200\left(\frac{\dot{V}_{O_2max}}{\dot{V}_{O_2}}\right) - 7020 \tag{2.6.1}$$

where t_{exh} = time to exhaustion for sustained dynamic work, sec
$\quad\dot{V}_{O_2}$ = oxygen uptake, m^3/sec
$\quad\dot{V}_{O_2max}$ = maximum oxygen uptake, m^3/sec

Maximum oxygen uptake values may be found in Table 1.3.2. Kamon recommends working periods of $t_{exh}/3$ for sustained industrial work involving moving tasks.

Recovery time is generally exponentially related to work intensity. Kamon (1981) suggests that a recovery time of twice the working time is sufficient to replenish ATP in the muscles.

Steady-state (or sustained) dynamic submaximal work at rates above 50% of $\dot{V}_{O_2max}$ is accompanied by lactic acid production (see Section 1.3). Durations of resting periods for work rates above 50% $\dot{V}_{O_2max}$ should be based on the rate at which lactic acid appears in the blood and the rate at which it disappears. Lactic acid appearance in the blood peaks about 240–300 sec (4–5 min) after muscular exercise ceases, and its elimination rate is linear at about 0.05 mg % /sec (Kamon, 1981). From these, Kamon makes the following recommendation for rest times when working above 50% $\dot{V}_{O_2max}$:

$$t_{rest} = 528 \ln\left[\left(\frac{\dot{V}_{O_2}}{\dot{V}_{O_2max}}\right) - 0.5\right] + 1476 \tag{2.6.2}$$

where t_{rest} = resting time, sec

Static work can be sustained for a period of time related to maximal voluntary contraction (Kamon, 1981):

$$t_{exh} = 11.40\left(\frac{MT_{max}}{MT}\right)^{2.42} \tag{2.6.3}$$

where t_{exh} = time to exhaustion for sustained static work, sec

$\quad$ MT = muscle torque, N·m

$\quad$ MT_{max} = maximal muscle torque, N·m

Values for maximal muscle torque may be found in Table 2.2.2.

Rest times for static work are recommended by Kamon (1981):

$$t_{rest} = 1080\left(\frac{t}{t_{exh}}\right)^{1.4}\left(\frac{MT}{MT_{max}} - 0.15\right)^{0.5} \tag{2.6.4}$$

where t = time of sustained contraction, sec

$\quad$ t_{exh} = time calculated from Equation 2.6.3, sec

SYMBOLS

A	area, m^2
a	acceleration, m/sec^2
a	constant, N·m/sec
b	constant, N·sec/m
CT	cost of transport, dimensionless
C_i	constraints, N or N·m
c	depth of crouch, m
c_1, c_2	constants, rad/sec
D	distance, m
d_F	distance from the fulcrum to the point of application of a force, m
d_W	distance from the fulcrum to the point of attachment of the load, m
E	energy, N·m
E_r	rotational energy, N·m
$\dot{E}$	power, N·m/sec

F	force, N
F_c	centrifugal force, N
F_{cp}	centripetal force, N
F_{dls}	dynamic lifting peak force, N
F_{HX}	force at hip in horizontal direction, N
F_{HY}	force at hip in vertical direction, N
F_m	maximum force, N
F_n	normal force, N
g	acceleration due to gravity, 9.8 m/sec^2
h	height, m
h_m	height of jump on the moon, m
I	moment of inertia, N·m·sec^2
$J(q)$	Jacobian matrix
K	spring constant, N/m
L	length, m
L_F	distance through which the load moves, m
L_{SH}	shank length, m
L_{TH}	thigh length, m
L_W	distance through which the force moves, m
ΔL	change in length, m
$\mathscr{L}$	system Lagrangian
MT	muscle torque, N·m
MT_{max}	maximum muscle torque, N·m
m	mass, kg
mv	translational momentum, kg·m/sec
P_d	power to overcome drag, N·m/sec
P_i	input power, N·m/sec
P_{nm}	nonmuscular power, N·m/sec
P_{spt}	power to support body weight, N·m/sec
P_w	power to produce external work, N·m/sec
Q_i	generalized forces, N or N·m
q_i	generalized system coordinates, m or rad
r	radius, m
s	speed, m/sec
s_0	initial speed, m/sec
s_F	speed of force movement, m/sec
s_W	speed of load movement, m/sec
S_x	sex indicator, dimensionless
T	period of oscillation, sec
T	vectorial torque, N·m
t	time, sec
t_{exp}	time to exhaustion, sec
t_{rest}	resting time, sec
$\dot{V}_{O_2}$	oxygen utilization, m^3/sec
$\dot{V}_{O_2max}$	maximum oxygen uptake, m^3/sec
v	velocity, m/sec
W	weight, N
W_m	weight of person on the moon, N
X_F	horizontal foot position, m
$\dot{X}_F$	horizontal foot velocity, m
$\ddot{X}_F$	horizontal foot acceleration, m
Y	Young's modulus, N/m^2

Y_F	vertical foot position, m
$\dot{Y}_F$	vertical foot velocity, m
$\ddot{Y}_F$	vertical foot acceleration, m
ε	strain, m/m
η	muscular efficiency, dimensionless
Θ	angular difference, rad
θ	angle, rad
θ_H	hip angle, rad
θ_K	knee angle, rad
$\dot{\theta}$	time rate of change of angle, rad/sec
λ	undetermined vector
μ	friction coefficient, dimensionless
σ	stress, N/m^2
σ_{max}	maximum breaking stress, N/m^2
ϕ	angle of inclination, rad
ω	angular velocity, rad/sec

REFERENCES

Alexander, R. M. 1984. Walking and Running. *Am. Sci.* **72**: 348–354.

Alexander, R. M. 1988. Why Mammals Gallop. *Am. Zool.* **28**: 237–245.

Antonsson, E. K., and R. W. Mann. 1985. The Frequency Content of Gait. *J. Biomech.* **18**: 39–47.

Baildon, R. W. A., and A. E. Chapman. 1983. A new Approach to the Human Model. *J. Biomech.* **16**: 803–809.

Bassett, D. R., Jr., M. D. Giese, F. J. Nagle, A. Ward, D. M. Raab, and B. Balke. 1985. Aerobic Requirements of Overground Versus Treadmill Running. *Med. Sci. Sports Exerc.* **17**: 477–481.

Booyens, J., and W. R. Keatinge. 1957. The Expenditure of Energy by Men and Women Walking. *J. Physiol.* **138**: 165–171.

Davidovits, P. 1975. *Physics in Biology and Medicine.* Prentice-Hall, Englewood Cliffs, N.J., pp. 1–64.

Dean, G. A. 1965. An Analysis of the Energy Expenditure in Level and Grade Walking. *Ergonomics* **8**: 31–47.

Dul, J., and G. E. Johnson. 1985. A Kinematic Model of the Human Ankle. *J. Biomed. Eng.* **7**: 137–143.

Flashner, H., A. Beuter, and A. Arabyan. 1987. Modelling of Control and Learning in a Stepping Motion. *Biol. Cybern.* **55**: 387–396.

Freivalds, A., D. B. Chaffin, A. Garg, and K. S. Lee. 1984. A Dynamic Biomechanical Evaluation of Lifting Maximum Acceptable Loads. *J. Biomech.* **17**: 251–262.

Givoni, B., and R. F. Goldman. 1971. Predicting Metabolic Energy Cost. *J. Appl. Physiol.* **30**: 429–433.

Goldman, R. F. 1978. Computer Models in Manual Materials Handling, in *Safety in Manual Materials Handling*, C. G. Drury, ed. National Institute for Occupational Safety and Health (NIOSH), Cincinnati, pp. 110–116.

Greene, P. R. 1985. Running on Flat Turns: Experiments, Theory, and Applications. *Trans ASME* **107**: 96–103.

Haisman, M. F., and R. F. Goldman. 1974. Effect of Terrain on the Energy Cost of Walking with Back Loads and Handcart Loads. *J. Appl. Physiol.* **36**: 545–548.

Haisman, M. F., F. R. Winsmann, and R. F. Goldman. 1972. Energy Cost of Pushing Loaded Handcarts. *J. Appl. Physiol.* **33**: 181–183.

Hatze, H., and A. Venter. 1981. Practical Activation and Retention of Locomotion Constraints in Neuromusculoskeletal Control System Models. *J. Biomech.* **14**: 873–877.

Hof, A. L., B. A. Geelen, and J. Van den Berg. 1983. Calf Muscle Moment, Work, and Efficiency in Level Walking: Role of Series Elasticity. *J. Biomech.* **16**: 523–537.

Kamon, E. 1981. Aspects of Physiological Factors in Paced Physical Work, in *Machine Pacing and Occupational Stress*, G. Salvendy and M. J. Smith, ed. Taylor and Francis, London, pp. 107–115.

Kamon, E., and A. J. Goldfuss. 1978. In-Plant Evaluation of the Muscle Strength of Workers. *Am. Ind. Hyg. Assoc. J.* **39**: 801–807.

Kamon, E., D. Kiser, and J. L. Pytel. 1982. Dynamic and Static Lifting Capacity and Muscular Strength of Steelmill Workers. *Am. Ind. Hyg. Assoc. J.* **43**: 853–857.

King, A. I. 1984. A Review of Biomechanical Models. *J. Biomech. Eng.* **106**: 97–104.

Kohl, J., E. A. Koller, and M. Jäger. 1981. Relation Between Pedalling and Breathing Rhythm. *Eur. J. Appl. Physiol.* **47**: 223–237.

Martin, P. E. 1985. Mechanical and Physiological Responses to Lower Extremity Loading During Running. *Med. Sci. Sports Exerc.* **17**: 427–433.

McMahon, T. A. 1984. *Muscles, Reflexes, and Locomotion,* Princeton University Press, Princeton, N.J., pp. 194–197.

Mende, T. J., and L. Cuervo. 1976. Properties of Excitable and Contractile Tissue, in *Biological Foundations of Biomedical Engineering,* J. Kline, ed. Little, Brown, Boston, pp. 71–99.

Milsum, J. H. 1966. *Biological Control Systems Analysis.* McGraw-Hill, New York, p. 406.

Morton, R. H. 1985. Comment on "A Model for the Calculation of Mechanical Power During Distance Running." *J. Biomech.* **18**: 161–162.

Myles, W. S., and P. L. Saunders. 1979. The Physiological Cost of Carrying Light and Heavy Loads. *Eur. J. Appl. Physiol.* **42**: 125–131.

Onyshko, S., and D. A. Winter. 1980. A Mathematical Model for the Dynamics of Human Locomotion. *J. Biomech.* **13**: 361–368.

Pierrynowski, M. R., and J. B. Morrison. 1985a. Estimating the Muscle Forces Generated in the Human Lower Extremity when Walking: A Physiological Solution. *Math. Biosci.* **75**: 43–68.

Pierrynowski, M. R., and J. B. Morrison. 1985b. A Physiological Model for the Evaluation of Muscular Forces in Human Locomotion: Theoretical Aspects. *Math. Biosci.* **75**: 69–101.

Pytel, J. L., and E. Kamon. 1981. Dynamic Strength Test as an Indicator for Maximal Acceptable Lifting. *Ergonomics* **24**: 663–672.

Sargeant, A. J., E. Hoinville, and A. Young. 1981. Maximum Leg Force and Power Output During Short-Term Dynamic Exercise. *J. Appl. Physiol.* **51**: 1175–1182.

Siegler, S., R. Seliktar, and W. Hyman. 1982. Simulation of Human Gait with the Aid of a Simple Mechanical Model. *J. Biomech.* **15**: 415–425.

Soule, R. G., and R. F. Goldman. 1969. Energy Cost of Loads Carried on the Head, Hands, or Feet. *J. Appl. Physiol.* **27**: 687–690.

Tucker, V. A. 1975. The Energetic Cost of Moving About. *Am. Sci.* **63**: 413–419.

Ward-Smith, A. J. 1984. Air Resistance and Its Influence on the Biomechanics and Energetics of Sprinting at Sea Level and at Altitude. *J. Biomech.* **17**: 339–347.

Williams, K. R., and P. R. Cavanagh. 1983. A Model for the Calculation of Mechanical Power During Distance Running. *J. Biomech.* **16**: 115–128.

Winter, D. A. 1983. Biomechanics of Human Movement with Applications to the Study of Human Locomotion, in *CRC Critical Reviews in Biomedical Engineering,* J. R. Bourne, ed. CRC Press, Boca Raton Fla., vol. 9, no. 4, pp. 287–314.

Wyndham, C. H., N. B. Strydom, J. F. Morrison, C. G. Williams, G. Bredell, J. Peter, H. M. Cooke, and A. Joffe. 1963. The Influence of Gross Body Weight on Oxygen Consumption and on Physical Working Capacity of Manual Labourers. *Ergonomics* **6**: 275–286.

CHAPTER 3

Cardiovascular Responses

> The heart, consequently, is the beginning of life; the sun of the microcosm, even as the sun in his turn might be designated the heart of the world; for it is the heart by whose virtue and pulse the blood is moved, perfected, made apt to nourish, and is perceived from corruption and coagulation; it is the household divinity which, discharging its function, nourishes, cherishes, quickens the whole body, and is indeed the foundation of life, the source of all action.   —William Harvey

3.1 INTRODUCTION

The purpose of the cardiovascular system is primarily to supply oxygen and remove carbon dioxide from metabolizing tissues.[1] Perhaps this is the reason for the almost immediate cardiac response to the beginning of exercise when the metabolic needs of the muscles increase dramatically. Indeed, cardiovascular responses are so rapid that the severity of exercise stress is usually judged on the basis of an instantaneous heart rate sample.

A second important cardiovascular function during exercise is removal of excess heat (see Chapter 5). Vasodilation of surface blood vessels brings warm blood in closer contact with the cool air to facilitate heat transfer. This response does not occur at all rapidly, however. Due to the thermal mass of the body, 10–15 minutes may elapse between the start of exercise and active vasodilatory responses.

There are times when the chemical transport and heat transport functions of the blood come into direct conflict, since blood required for supply of skeletal muscle needs may be shunted to the skin for heat removal. When this happens, muscle metabolism must become at least partially anaerobic. Since there is a limit to the amount of anaerobic metabolism that can occur, this conflict can directly lead to a shortened exercise period.

It is the purpose of this chapter to detail cardiovascular mechanics and control during exercise. This book considers four elements of the cardiovascular system: the heart, the vasculature, respiratory interface, and thermal interface. Respiratory interface is treated in Chapter 4 and thermal interface in Chapter 5.

3.2 CARDIOVASCULAR MECHANICS

The cardiovascular mechanical system is composed of blood, vessels which contain the blood, and the heart to pump the blood through the vessels. In addition, the system contains substances to repair rupture.

---

[1] Because the blood permeates the entire body, it also performs a useful humoral communication function, is important in assisting transport and removal of chemical metabolites, and is useful in the body's defense against disease.

3.2.1 Blood Characteristics

Blood composition is very complex, and much beyond the scope of this book. There are, however, physical properties of the blood which are of concern to bioengineers and exercise physiologists.

Composition. A general classification separates blood into red blood cells, white blood cells, and plasma. Blood cells constitute 45% of total blood volume and plasma 55% (Ganong, 1963). Circulating blood[2] contains an average of 5.4×10^{15} red blood cells per cubic meter in men and 4.8×10^{15} per cubic meter in women (Ganong, 1963).

Oxygen-Carrying Capacity. Oxygen is transported by the blood by two different, but complementary mechanisms: as oxygen dissolved in the blood plasma and as oxygen chemically united with hemoglobin in the red blood cells (Table 3.2.1). Each human red blood cell contains approximately 29 pg (picograms) of hemoglobin. The body of a 70 kg man contains about 900 g of hemoglobin and that of a 60 kg woman, about 660 g (Ganong, 1963). Each hemoglobin molecule contains four heme units, each of which can bind with one oxygen molecule (i.e., diatomic oxygen, O_2). When fully saturated, each kilogram of hemoglobin contains $1.34 \times 10^{-3} \, m^3 \, O_2$ (1.34 mL O_2/g) (Ganong, 1963). Since average men have about 160 kilograms hemoglobin per cubic meter of blood (160 g/L blood), $0.214 \, m^3 \, O_2/m^3$ blood (214 mL O_2/L blood) is bound by their hemoglobin.

The amount of oxygen which is physically and passively dissolved in the blood plasma is usually expressed in terms of partial pressure. The partial pressure of a gas is defined as that pressure which would exist in the gas for the free gas to be in equilibrium with the gas in solution. The higher the partial pressure exerted by a gas above a solution, the more gas will dissolve in solution. For respiratory oxygen, the number of cubic meters of gas dissolved in one cubic meter of blood at 38°C at a partial pressure of one atmosphere (1 atm, $10^5 \, N/m^2$) and with gas volume corrected to conditions of standard temperature and pressure,[3] called the Bunsen coefficient, is 0.023 (Mende, 1976).

For example, if the percentage of oxygen in the alveolus is 12%, expressed as dry gas, then the percentage of oxygen, taking into account that alveolar air is saturated with water vapor, is

$$\left[\frac{(10^5 - 6266) \, N/m^2}{10^5 \, N/m^2} \right] (12\%) = 11.2\%$$

The partial pressure of oxygen[4] therefore is

$$pO_2 = (11.2/100)(10^5 \, N/m^2) = 11.2 \times 10^3 \, N/m^2 \tag{3.2.1}$$

and the amount of oxygen dissolved[5] in the pulmonary venous blood is

$$V_{O_2} = \left(\frac{11.2 \times 10^3}{10^5} \right)(0.023) = 0.00258 \, m^3 \, O_2/m^3 \text{ blood} \qquad (2.58 \text{ mL } O_2/\text{L blood}) \tag{3.2.2}$$

---

[2] The ratio of circulating blood volume, expressed as cubic centimeters, to body mass, expressed in kilograms, is about 80.

[3] Standard temperature and pressure are 0°C and 1 atm (760 mm Hg, or $10^5 \, N/m^2$). Furthermore, respiratory gases are usually expressed as dry gas and 6266 N/m² (47 mm Hg) is subtracted from total atmospheric pressure to account for water vapor in lung gases.

[4] Normal arterial pCO_2 is 5.3 kN/m² (40 mm Hg) and normal arterial pO_2 is 13.3 kN/m² (100 mm Hg).

[5] The amount of O_2 in mL per 100 mL of blood in a particular sample is usually designated by physiologists as the O_2 content of the blood. For purposes of unit consistency, we use (m³ O_2/m³ blood). To convert (m³ O_2/m³ blood) to (mL O_2/100 mL blood), multiply (m³ O_2/m³ blood) by 100.

TABLE 3.2.1 Blood Gases in Adult Humans

Variable	Blood	Sex	Whole Blood Gas Concentration, m^3/m^3 (mL/100 mL)		Blood Gas Pressure, kN/m^2 (mm Hg)	
Oxygen capacity		M	0.204	(20.4)		
		F	0.180	(18.0)		
Total oxygen	Art	M	0.203	(20.3)	12.5	(94)
		F	0.179	(17.9)	12.5	(94)
	Ven	M	0.153	(15.3)	5.33	(40)
		F	0.137	(13.7)	5.47	(41)
Free oxygen	Art	M	2.85×10^{-3}	(0.285)	12.5	(94)
		F	2.82×10^{-3}	(0.282)	12.5	(94)
	Ven	M	1.22×10^{-3}	(0.122)	5.33	(40)
		F	1.24×10^{-3}	(0.124)	5.47	(41)
Combined oxygen (HbO_2)	Art	M	0.200	(20.0)	12.5	(94)
		F	0.176	(17.6)	12.5	(94)
	Ven	M	0.152	(15.2)	5.33	(40)
		F	0.136	(13.6)	5.47	(41)
Total carbon dioxide	Art	M	0.490	(49.0)	5.47	(41)
		F	0.480	(48.0)	5.20	(39)
	Ven	M	0.531	(53.1)	6.13	(46)
		F	0.514	(51.4)	5.73	(43)
Free carbon dioxide	Art	M	0.0262	(2.62)	5.47	(41)
		F	0.0253	(2.53)	5.20	(39)
	Ven	M	0.0300	(3.00)	6.20	(46.5)
		F	0.0278	(2.78)	5.73	(43)
Total combined CO_2	Art	M	0.464	(46.4)	5.47	(41)
		F	0.455	(45.5)	5.20	(39)
	Ven	M	0.501	(50.1)	6.20	(46.5)
		F	0.486	(48.6)	5.73	(43)
Carbamino CO_2	Art	M	0.0220	(2.2)	5.47	(41)
		F	0.0190	(1.9)	5.20	(39)
	Ven	M	0.0310	(3.1)	6.20	(46.5)
		F	0.0270	(2.7)	5.73	(43)
Bicarbonate CO_2	Art	M	0.442	(44.2)	5.47	(41)
		F	0.436	(43.6)	5.20	(39)
	Ven	M	0.470	(47.0)	6.20	(46.5)
		F	0.460	(46.0)	5.73	(43)
Nitrogen	Art, ven	M	9.79×10^{-3}	(0.979)	76.3	(572)
		F	9.70×10^{-3}	(0.970)	76.5	(574)

Source: Used with permission from Spector, 1956.

In addition, hemoglobin saturation at an oxygen partial pressure of $11.2 \times 10^3 \, N/m^3$ is about 95.5%. Therefore, hemoglobin transports another $0.203 \, m^3 \, O_2/m^3$ blood. This example illustrates the extreme advantage of the presence of hemoglobin in the blood—about 100 times as much oxygen is transported as it would depending on physical solution alone. Other gases, such as nitrogen, which are not bound by carrier substances are dependent on only physical solution for movement by blood.

It is not completely known whether hemodynamic, vascular, or metabolic factors limit maximum oxygen uptake. Saltin (1985) presented evidence that the ability of the skeletal muscles to utilize oxygen (see Section 1.3) is much greater than the ability of the heart and blood to supply oxygen. At high muscle blood perfusion rates the low rate of oxygen extraction by muscle tissue is related to the low mean transit time of blood passing through the capillaries. Enlargement of muscular capillary beds which accompanies endurance training probably serves the purpose of lengthening the mean transit time, not necessarily to increase blood flow.[6] The presence of hemoglobin in the blood thus tends to narrow the gap between oxygen supply capacity and oxygen utilization capacity.

Oxygen bound to hemoglobin is in equilibrium with oxygen in plasma solution. When oxygen is removed from hemoglobin, it first passes into the plasma as dissolved oxygen before it is made available to the tissues. When oxygen is added to hemoglobin, it comes from alveolar tissue by way of solution in the plasma.

It is natural, therefore, that the oxygen-carrying capacity of hemoglobin be expressed in terms of oxygen partial pressure of the surrounding plasma. Typical oxygen dissociation curves with their characteristic sigmoid shapes are seen in Figures 3.2.1 through 3.2.3.

Blood is very well buffered to minimize sudden changes in its chemical and physical structure. The hemoglobin saturation curve does shift, however, in response to changes of P_{CO_2} (Figure 3.2.1),[7] pH (Figure 3.2.2),[8] and temperature (Figure 3.2.3). All of these are important in compensation for the oxygen demands of exercising muscle.

Figure 3.2.1 shows the direct effect of carbon dioxide on hemoglobin dissociation. For any given level of oxygen partial pressure, an increase in plasma carbon dioxide reduces the equilibrium hemoglobin saturation. Oxygen is thus removed from each hemoglobin molecule and either increases dissolved oxygen or moves to the respiring tissues. Since carbon dioxide is produced most in regions with high oxygen demand, this hemoglobin saturation shift makes extra oxygen available where it is most needed. In the muscles, this extra oxygen is stored by myoglobin (see Section 1.3.2), a molecule with function similar to hemoglobin, for use as needed by muscle cells.

When excess carbon dioxide is added to the venous blood, an important blood bicarbonate (HCO_3^-) buffering system minimizes changes to the blood and allows higher carbon dioxide–carrying capacity. This buffering occurs by means of the following reversible chemical reactions (Ganong, 1963):

$$H_2O + CO_2 \Leftrightarrow H_2CO_3 \Leftrightarrow H^+ + HCO_3^- \tag{3.2.3}$$

As carbon dioxide is added to the blood, it combines with plasma water to form a weak acid, carbonic acid. This dissociates into hydrogen ions and blood bicarbonate. At the lungs these reactions are reversed and blood bicarbonate is reduced as carbon dioxide is expelled.

Carbon dioxide production also changes acidity of the blood, as measured by pH[9], which also affects the hemoglobin saturation curve (Figure 3.2.2). The Henderson–Hasselbalch equation

---

[6] However, Saltin also adds that the capacity of the muscles to receive blood flow exceeds by a factor of 2 to 3 the capacity of the heart to supply the flow. Because of this, arterioles feeding the muscles must normally be subject to a vasoconstrictive neural control.

[7] Reduced hemoglobin is a weak acid. When combined with oxygen, hemoglobin (Hb) undergoes the chemical process

$$O_2 + HHb \Leftrightarrow HHbO_2 \Leftrightarrow HbO_2^- + H^+$$

which makes additional hydrogen ions available to drive the carbon dioxide dissociation equilibrium (Equation 3.2.3) to the left. Thus increased oxygen saturation of the hemoglobin is accompanied by increased availability of carbon dioxide. This process is called the Haldane effect (Tazawa et al., 1983).

[8] Hemoglobin has a high buffering capacity over the normal range of blood pH. Without this buffering capacity, blood pH would vary greatly as blood carbon dioxide content changed. As CO_2 is added to the blood, pH falls. With a fall in blood pH, oxygen is released from the hemoglobin molecule. This interaction between blood pH and oxygen saturation is called the Bohr effect.

[9] pH is defined as the negative logarithm of the hydrogen ion concentration. As the blood becomes more acid, hydrogen ion concentration increases and pH decreases.

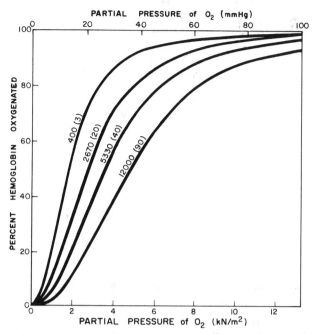

Figure 3.2.1 Effect of blood carbon dioxide on the oxygen dissociation curve of whole blood. CO_2 partial pressure for each curve is given in N/m^2 (mm Hg). An increase in CO_2 causes blood of a given oxygen saturation to increase the pO_2, thus making O_2 more readily available to dissolve in the plasma and transfer to surrounding tissues. Normal pCO_2 is taken to be 5330 N/m^2 (40 mm Hg). (Adapted and used with permission from Barcroft, 1925.)

(Woodbury, 1965) relates pH to the buffering system of Equation 3.2.3:

$$pH = 6.10 + \log\left\{\frac{c_{HCO_3^-}}{c_{H_2CO_3}}\right\} \tag{3.2.4}$$

where c_X = concentration of constituent X, mol/m^3

Normal $c_{HCO_3^-}/c_{H_2CO_3}$ ratio is 20 and normal arterial blood pH level is 7.4 (Ganong, 1963).

As long as blood oxygen levels can supply all the necessary oxygen required by exercising muscles, there is a direct correspondence between blood pH and CO_2 produced by metabolism. When metabolism becomes nonaerobic, and lactic acid is a product of incomplete metabolism (see Section 1.3.2), an increase in hydrogen ion concentration occurs, blood pH lowers, and blood pCO_2 rises. The equilibrium oxygen hemoglobin saturation curve indicates that further oxygen is then made available to the muscles.

Aberman et al. (1973) presented an equation for the oxygen hemoglobin dissociation curve which is mathematically derived and can be useful for calculation purposes:

$$S_{std} = \sum_{i=0}^{7} C_i \left(\frac{pO_{2std} - 3.6663}{pO_{2std} + 3.6663}\right) \tag{3.2.5}$$

where S_{std} = oxygen saturation for standard conditions, %
$\quad C_i$ = coefficients, %

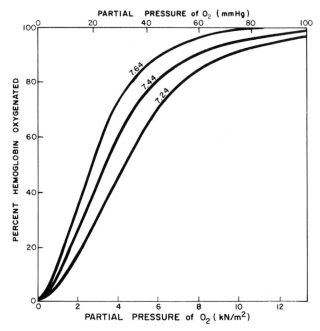

Figure 3.2.2 Effect of blood acidity level on the oxygen dissociation curve of whole blood. Blood pH is given for each curve. As blood becomes more acid, its pH falls and blood pO_2 rises for any given level of hemoglobin saturation. Thus O_2 is made more readily available to dissolve in the plasma and be transferred to surrounding tissues. Normal blood pH is usually taken to be 7.40. (Adapted and used with permission from Peters and Van Slyke, 1931.)

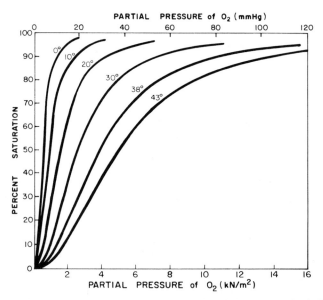

Figure 3.2.3 Effect of blood temperature on the oxygen dissociation curve of whole blood. Blood temperature is indicated on each curve. As temperature rises, blood pO_2 rises for any given saturation level. Thus O_2 is more readily available for solution in the plasma and to surrounding tissues. Normal body temperature is 37°C. (Adapted from Roughton, 1954.)

pO_{2std} = partial pressure of oxygen of the standard dissociation curve, kN/m^2
$C_0 = +51.87074$
$C_1 = +129.8325$
$C_2 = +6.828368$
$C_3 = -223.7881$
$C_4 = -27.95300$
$C_5 = +258.5009$
$C_6 = +21.84175$
$C_7 = -119.2322$

If pO_2 is measured at any conditions other than the standard temperature of 37°C, pH of 7.40, and base excess[10] of 0 Eq/m^3, a correction must be applied:

$$S_{act} = S_{std}[10^{[0.024(37-\theta)]} - 0.48\,(7.40 - pH) - 0.0013B] \qquad (3.2.6)$$

where S_{act} = actual saturation percentage
θ = temperature, °C
B = base excess, Eq/m^3 (Eq = charge equivalents)

Equation 3.2.5 fits only the standard oxygen hemoglobin dissociation curve with a pO_2 at 50% saturation of 3.546 kN/m^2 (26.6 mm Hg). It is not accurate below a pO_2 of 253 kN/m^2 (1.9 mm Hg) or above a pO_2 of 93.3 kN/m^2 (700 mm Hg) and should not be used to predict saturation when pulmonary shunts, cardiac output, or arterial-venous oxygen content differences are calculated (Aberman et al., 1973).

Hemoglobin in the red blood cells is also involved in transport of carbon dioxide (Kagawa, 1984; Mochizuki et al., 1985). Carbon dioxide reacts with amino groups, principally hemoglobin, to form carbamino compounds. Reduced hemoglobin (that which has released its oxygen and taken up more hydrogen ions) forms carbamino compounds much more readily than oxyhemoglobin (Ganong, 1963). Thus transport of carbon dioxide is facilitated in venous blood (Figure 3.2.4).

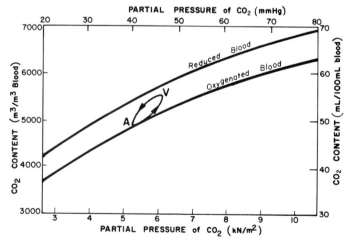

Figure 3.2.4 CO_2 titration curve of whole blood. Note that oxygenated blood contains less CO_2 than reduced blood. Blood goes through a cycle, as indicated by A (arterial blood) and V (venous blood) in the capillaries of tissues and lungs. (Adapted and used with permission from Peters and Van Slyke, 1931.)

[10]Base excess refers to the bicarbonate concentration in Equation 3.2.3 and varies directly as pCO_2.

From Table 3.2.1, we can see that male arterial blood carries a total of $0.490\,\mathrm{m^3}\ CO_2/\mathrm{m^3}$ blood. Of these, $0.026\,\mathrm{m^3}\ CO_2/\mathrm{m^3}$ blood is in free solution and $0.464\,\mathrm{m^3}\ CO_2/\mathrm{m^3}$ blood is combined in some way. Of the combined CO_2, $0.022\,\mathrm{m^3}\ CO_2/\mathrm{m^3}$ blood is transported as carbamino compounds and $0.442\,\mathrm{m^3}\ CO_2/\mathrm{m^3}$ blood is transported as bicarbonate.

Viscosity. Aside from the physicochemical characteristics of blood already described, blood must also be considered in light of its flow characteristics through the blood vessels. Since blood is a homogeneous substance from only the coarsest perspective, it cannot be expected to behave quite like truly homogeneous fluids such as water and oil.

The most important flow characteristic of blood is its viscosity, which is a measure of its resistance to motion. If two plates containing a thickness r of fluid between them are drawn apart by a force F at rate v (Figure 3.2.5), then the force F divided by the plate area A is defined as the shear stress $\tau = F/A$, and the rate of shear is defined as $\gamma = dv/dr$. Shear stress is related to the

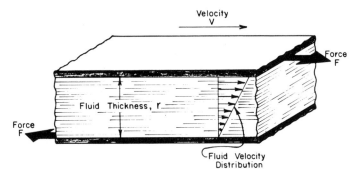

Figure 3.2.5   Conceptual apparatus for determining fluid rheological properties.

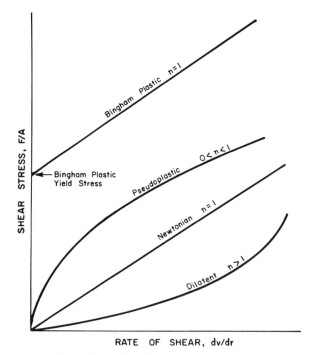

Figure 3.2.6   Fluid rheological characteristics.

force required to pump a fluid through a tube, and the rate of shear is related to the rate at which the fluid flows.

The ratio of shear stress to rate of shear is given the name viscosity:

$$\mu = \frac{\tau}{\gamma} = \frac{F/A}{dv/dr} \tag{3.2.7}$$

where μ = viscosity, kg/(m·sec)
  τ = shear stress, N/m^2
  γ = rate of shear, sec^{-1}
  v = speed of plate separation, m/sec
  r = distance between plates, m

For many fluids the viscosity is constant, and these are called Newtonian fluids. Blood plasma is a Newtonian fluid with a viscosity of 1.1–1.6 g/(m·sec) (Attinger and Michie, 1976). Fluids with nonconstant viscosities are termed non-Newtonian. Whole blood is among these.

Figure 3.2.6 is general plot of shear stress against rate of shear for various fluids (Johnson, 1980). Pseudoplastic materials generally have decreasing viscosity with increasing shear rate. These fluids are comparatively hard to start moving but easier to move once flow has been established. Dilatent fluids generally have increasing viscosity with increasing rate of shear. These fluids require more energy to keep them moving than to start them moving.[11] Bingham plastics are nearly Newtonian but require a yield stress to be overcome before they will move. Whole blood is generally considered to behave as a Bingham plastic, but mathematical properties of Bingham plastic models are inferior to those for pseudoplastics, and sometimes blood is approximated as a pseudoplastic material.

The simplest model to describe characteristics seen in Figure 3.2.6 is the power law model (Skelland, 1967):

$$\tau = K\gamma^n + C \tag{3.2.8}$$

where K = consistency coefficient, N·sec^n/m^2
  n = flow behavior index, dimensionless
  C = yield stress, N/m^2

In the case of a Newtonian fluid, $n = 1$, $C = 0$, and $K = \mu$ = viscosity. If the yield stress is ignored, then mathematical manipulation of Equation 3.2.8 becomes much easier, and thus many Bingham fluids are approximated as pseudoplastics. It has been found that measurements obtained on blood do not give constant values of n and K for more than two decades of shear rates, and thus Equation 3.2.8 has limited usefulness (Charm and Kurland, 1974).

Fluids in which particles or large molecules are dispersed are called suspensions, and suspensions often obey the Casson equation (Charm and Kurland, 1974):

$$\sqrt{\tau} = K\sqrt{\gamma} + \sqrt{C} \tag{3.2.9}$$

Whole blood appears to be in this category (Attinger and Michie, 1976; Oka, 1981).[12]

---

[11] Conceptually, pseudoplastics may be thought of as long-chain molecules suspended in a fluid bed. Upon standing they tangle and intertwine. Once moved, however, they begin to untangle and to line up parallel each other. Eventually they slide past each other with relative ease. Dilatent fluids can be thought of as densely packed hard spheres with just enough fluid between them to fill the voids. As they begin to move, there is sufficient fluid to lubricate between them. As they move faster, their dense packing becomes disrupted, and there is insufficient fluid to completely lubricate their motion. Thus they become harder to move faster. Fruit purees are pseudoplastics; quicksand is a dilatent.

[12] There are other types of non-Newtonian behavior as well. Suspensions of long-chain elastic molecules, in which the molecules add a significant elastic effect to flow of the fluid, are termed viscoelastic. Analysis of viscoelastic fluids is much beyond the scope of this book, and blood flow modeling has not usually included elasticity of particles in the blood.

Fluid time-dependent phenomena are also present. Thixotropic substances decrease viscosity with time and rheopectic substances increase viscosity as time goes on. Thixotropic behavior is closely associated with stress relaxation and creep (Attinger and Michie, 1976).

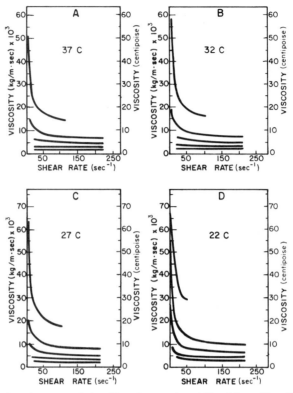

Figure 3.2.7   Viscosity–shear rate relationships of reconstituted blood from 37 to 22°C. Hematocrits of the curves in each plot are 80% (top), 60%, 40%, 20%, and 0% (bottom). The axis labeled viscosity is actually the slope of the shear stress–rate of shear diagram (Figure 3.2.6). Since viscosity appears to be higher at low rates of shear, these measurements confirm whole blood to be a pseudoplastic substance tending to Newtonian as hematocrit decreases. (Adapted and used with permission from Rand et al., 1964.)

At shear rates greater than $100 \, \text{sec}^{-1}$ normal blood behaves as a Newtonian fluid (Attinger and Michie, 1976; Haynes and Burton, 1959; Pedley et al., 1980) with a viscosity of $4–5 \, \text{g}/(\text{m} \cdot \text{sec})$ (Attinger and Michie, 1976). This value decreases by 2–3% per degree Celsius rise in temperature (Attinger and Michie, 1976). As hematocrit[13] increases, apparent viscosity increases nonlinearly (Figure 3.2.7). Because red blood cells deform so easily, blood exhibits about half the viscosity of a suspension of similarly sized and distributed hard spheres in plasma (Attinger and Michie, 1976).

Exercising individuals exhibit a so-called plasma shift due to body fluid losses mostly as sweat. Plasma volume decreases during exercise, thus concentrating suspended materials. This hemoconcentration averages less than 2% below exercise levels requiring 40% of maximum oxygen uptake (see Section 1.3); above 40% of maximum oxygen uptake hemoconcentration is

[13] Hematocrit is defined as the ratio of red blood cell volume to total blood volume, in percent. Hematocrit is usually determined by centrifugal separation. Hematocrit may vary from one vascular bed to another, where microvessels generally have lower hematocrit than their supply vessels. Fluid near the wall of blood vessels usually contains fewer red blood cells than the fluid in the center (Attinger and Michie, 1976). Hematocrit for men is usually about 0.47 and for women and children is 0.42 (Astrand and Rodahl, 1970).

directly proportional to work rate (Senay, 1979). Transient plasma volume decreases of 6–12% with the onset of exercise are corrected within 10–20 min after exercise ceases. Acclimation (see Section 5.3.5) to work in the heat is accompanied by a chronic hematocrit decrease as plasma volume increases.

3.2.2 Vascular Characteristics

Blood vessels serve the purposes of blood transport, filtering of pressure extremes, regulation of blood pressure, chemical exchange, and blood storage. They generally are classified as arteries, arterioles, capillaries, and veins, each with different storage, elastic, and resistance properties (Table 3.2.2).

Organization. The arteries are the first vessels encountered by the blood as it leaves the heart. Arteries are large-diameter vessels with very elastic walls. The large interior diameter allows a high volume of stored blood and the elastic walls store energy during heart contraction (systole) and release it between contractions (diastole). Thus the arteries play an important role in converting an intermittent blood delivery into a continuous one.

Arterioles are smaller vessels with less elastic walls containing transversely oriented smooth

TABLE 3.2.2 Characteristics of Various Types of Blood Vessels

Variable	Lumen Diameter	Wall Thickness	Approximate Total Cross-Sectional Area	Percentage of Blood Volume Contained[a]
Aorta	2.5 cm	2 mm	4.5 cm^2	2%
Artery	0.4 cm	1 mm	20 cm^2	8%
Arteriole	30 μm	20 μm	400 cm^2	1%
Capillary	6 μm	1 μm	4500 cm^2	5%
Venule	20 μm	2 μm	4000 cm^2	
Vein	0.5 cm	0.5 mm	40 cm^2	{50%}
Vena cava	3 cm	1.5 mm	18 cm^2	

Source: Used with permission from Ganong, 1963.

[a]Of the remainder, about 20% is found in the pulmonary circulation and 14% in the heart (Attinger, 1976a).

TABLE 3.2.3 Distribution of Blood to Various Organs for a Normal 70 Kg (685 N) Man at Rest

	Percentage of Total			
Variable	Weight	Blood Volume	Blood Flow	O$_2$ Consumption
Muscle	41.0	10.0	17.0	21.0
Skin	5.0	1.5	7.0	6.0
Gastrointestinal tract	4.0	23.0	27.0	22.0
Brain	2.5	0.5	13.0	8.5
Kidney	1.0	2.0	26.0	8.0
Heart	0.5	0.5	5.0	12.5
Other[a]	46.0	62.5	5.0	22.0
	100.0%	100.0%	100.0%	100.0%
Nominal total	685 N	5600 cm^3 (5.6 L)	92 cm^3/sec(5.5 L/min)	4.2 cm^3/sec (250 mL/min)

Source: Used with permission from Michie et al., 1976.

[a]Bone, fat, connective tissue, pulmonary circulation, heart chambers, larger peripheral arteries and veins.

TABLE 3.2.4 Changes in Blood Distribution to Various Organs Between Rest and Exercise

Variable	Rest	Exercise	Actual Change
Lungs	100%	100%	+ +
Gastrointestinal tract	25–30	3–5	−
Heart	4–5	4–5	+ +
Kidneys	20–25	2–3	−
Bone	3–5	0.5–1	+
Brain	15	4–6	+
Skin	5	{80–85}	+ +
Muscle	15–20		
Cardiac output	83 cm^3/sec (5 L/min)	420 cm^3/sec (25 L/min)	

Source: Used with permission from Astrand and Rodahl, 1970.

muscle fibers. Whenever these muscle fibers contract, arteriole resistance increases and blood flow decreases. Arterioles thus play an important regulating role in maintaining total blood pressure and in distributing blood flow to various organs (Tables 3.2.3 and 3.2.4).

Capillaries are very small ($5–20 \times 10^{-6}$ m diameter) vessels with very thin walls. It is through these thin walls that gas and metabolite exchange occurs.[14] Precapillary sphincter muscles control blood flow through individual capillary beds.

Venous blood return begins at the collecting venules and ends at the vena cava. As the veins become larger, greater amounts of muscle tissue are found in their walls. Larger veins also contain one-way valves, which prohibit blood from returning to smaller veins and capillaries. Muscular activity squeezes veins and moves blood toward the heart, and this blood cannot return to its former position because of the valves. Venous systems normally contain 65–70% of the total peripheral blood volume and thus act mainly as storage vessels (often termed windkessel vessels because of their considerable wall compliance) (Astrand and Rodahl, 1970).

In addition to this singular blood flow pathway are shunts, called anastomoses, between arteries or arterioles and veins. They function as return paths when the capillary structure of a particular region has been closed off during trauma or exercise.

Resistance. Basic to understanding of cardiovascular mechanics is the concept of resistance to flow in a tube. Traditionally, resistance, which is the ratio of pressure loss to flow rate, has been considered for rigid tubes of uniform cross section containing fully developed laminar flow. None of these conditions is likely to exist in actual blood vessels.

Below Reynolds numbers[15] of 1000–2000, laminar flow conditions will usually exist. Disturbances such as bifurcations, corners, and changes in cross-sectional shape or area tend to disturb laminar flow. In laminar flow, pressure loss is directly proportional to flow velocity, but

---

[14] Hydrostatic and osmotic pressure in the arteriole end of the capillaries is higher than mean interstitial pressure of surrounding tissue, and water is forced from the plasma to the extravascular fluid. On the venous end, the pressure gradient is reversed and water rejoins the plasma from the interstitial fluid. Reduced arterial pressure results in increased absorption of fluid into the blood to partially compensate for reduced pressure. Osmotic pressure of human serum was measured by Starling as 3333 N/m^2, or 25 mm Hg (Catchpole, 1966), and osmotic pressure in the interstitial space has been estimated as 667 N/m^2, or 5 mm Hg (Catchpole, 1966), thus leaving an osmotic balance of 2666 N/m^2 in favor of reabsorption of water into the blood vessel. Heart failure causes venous pressure to rise and edema results.

[15] Reynolds number is defined as

$$Re = \frac{Dv\rho}{\mu}$$

for nonlaminar or nondeveloped laminar flow, pressure loss is more closely related to the velocity squared.[16]

For fully developed laminar flow in rigid tubes,[17] the velocity profile in the tube can be described by

$$v = \frac{\Delta p \, r_o^2}{4\mu L} \left(1 - \frac{r^2}{r_o^2} \right)$$ (3.2.10)

where Δp = pressure drop, N/m²
$\quad r_o$ = outside radius of the tube, m
$\quad r$ = radial distance from the center to any point in the tube, m
$\quad \mu$ = viscosity, kg/m·sec or N·sec/m²
$\quad L$ = length of the tube, m
$\quad c$ = velocity, m/sec
Integrating this over the entire cross section gives

$$\int_0^{r_o} v(2\pi r dr) = \dot{V} = \frac{\Delta p \pi r_o^4}{8L\mu}$$ (3.2.11)

where $\dot{V}$ = volume rate of flow, m³/sec
From the definition of resistance,[18]

$$R = \frac{\Delta p}{\dot{V}} = \frac{8L\mu}{\pi r_o^4}$$ (3.2.12)

where R = tube resistance, N·sec/m⁵
This equation illustrates the extreme importance exerted by vessel radius on blood flow resistance. A decrease of only 19% in radius will halve the flow, illustrating the extremely sensitive control that can be exerted by the arterioles (Burton, 1965). This equation is indicative only, because the flow is actually pulsatile and unsteady, bends and junctions in the vessel walls do not allow sufficient distance for development of the parabolic velocity profile indicated by Equation 3.2.10 to fully develop, the vessel walls distend during systole and contract during diastole, the system is nonlinear, and blood does not possess a constant viscosity. Further

where Re = Reynolds number, dimensionless
$\quad D$ = vessel diameter, m
$\quad v$ = fluid velocity, m/sec
$\quad \rho$ = fluid density, kg/m³
$\quad \mu$ = fluid viscosity, kg/(m·sec)
For non-Newtonian fluids, like blood, where viscosity is not constant,

$$\text{Re} = \frac{\rho D^n v^{2-n}}{8^{n-1} K} \left(\frac{4n}{3n-1} \right)^n$$

where n = flow behavior index, dimensionless
$\quad K$ = consistency coefficient, N/(sec^n·m²)
for tubes of circular cross section. This latter definition is highly dependent on the model used to describe viscosity changes and the cross-sectional shape of the tube. As flow behavior index decreases, the transition to turbulent flow from laminar flow occurs at higher Reynolds numbers, up to Re = 4000–5000 for $n = 0.3$.

[16] Actually $\Delta p \propto v^{1.7}$ to $v^{2.0}$ in turbulent flow.

[17] Fully developed flow is defined in terms of the parabolic velocity profile given by Equation 3.2.10. Fully developed laminar flow in rigid tubes is often called Poiseuille flow.

[18] Resistance is usually defined as force per unit flow. Units of resistance would then be N·sec/m³. Here we are using a definition of resistance of pressure per unit flow, and thus the units are N·sec/m⁵.

analysis of the vascular system has been focused principally on the large vessels, with mean Reynolds number of 1250, peak Reynolds number of 6250, and mean blood shear rates high enough to treat blood as a Newtonian fluid (Pedley et al., 1980). Since the shear rate (dv/dr) is highest near the wall, most viscous pressure drop also occurs near the wall. Despite all this, Reynolds numbers greater than 2000 usually signify turbulent flow.

Very Small Vessels. Small vessels, such as the capillaries, are of the same diameter as red blood cells, and these cells cannot usually pass through the capillaries without some deformation. Reynolds numbers of the capillaries are about 1.0, meaning that flow is so low that Navier–Stokes equations[19] are usually applied to capillary flow. Blood flowing through capillaries cannot be considered a continuous fluid but must be treated as composed of individual cellular bodies in a surrounding fluid medium (Pittman and Ellsworth, 1986).

Apparent viscosity of blood decreases (the Fahraeus–Lindqvist effect) in tubes with diameter below about 400 μm (Pedley et al., 1980). This can be attributed to two explanations to be investigated further. First, there is a tendency of cellular components in the blood, notably red blood cells, to vacate the area next to the vessel wall. This is largely due to a static pressure difference, which is predicted by Bernoulli's equation for total energy in a moving fluid (Astrand and Rodahl, 1970; Baumeister, 1967):

$$p_2 - p_1 = \tfrac{1}{2}(v_1^2 - v_2^2) + (z_1 - z_2)\rho g \qquad (3.2.13)$$

where p_i = static pressure measured at point i, N/m^2
   v_i = fluid velocity measured at point i, m/sec
   z_i = height of point i above a reference plane, m
   ρ = density, kg/m^3
   g = acceleration due to gravity, m/sec^2

This equation states that the pressure on the side of a red blood cell will be less in the center of the vessel where the velocity is greatest than toward the side of the vessel where velocity is lower (assuming no significant difference in height). Thus cells will be pushed toward the center of the tube. However, because different local velocities cause differences in frictional drag on different sides of the red blood cell, cellular motion is a complicated maneuver. Segré and Silberberg (1962) showed that red blood cells tend to accumulate at six-tenths of the radius from the center of the vessel.

Most frictional loss in a vessel occurs near the wall where the change in velocity with radius is greatest. The "axial streaming" tendency of red blood cells removes particles from the area near the wall and replaces them with relatively low-viscosity plasma (Bauer et al., 1983). Thus friction is greatly reduced. Without this effect, the heart would be unable to maintain adequate bodily circulation.

The Navier–Stokes equations (Middleman, 1972; Talbot and Gessner, 1973) relate external

---

[19] Fundamental equations for a liquid are based on the conservation of mass, energy, and momentum. Momentum equations are identified as the Navier–Stokes equations. For a cartesian, three-dimensional steady flow of a viscous liquid, the momentum equation for the x direction is

$$\frac{\partial p}{\partial x} + \mu\left(\frac{\partial^2 v}{\partial x^2} + \frac{\partial^2 v}{\partial y^2} + \frac{\partial^2 v}{\partial z^2}\right) = \rho\left(v\frac{\partial v}{\partial x} + u\frac{\partial v}{\partial y} + w\frac{\partial v}{\partial z}\right)$$

where p = pressure, N/m^2
   x, y, z = distance along three perpendicular directions, m
   v, u, w = components of velocity in the three directions x, y, z respectively, m/sec
   μ = viscosity, N·sec/m^2
   ρ = density, kg/m^3

The left-hand side of the equation is the sum of external pressure and viscous forces, and the right-hand side is the change of momentum, or inertia (Baumeister, 1967).

forces, pressure forces, and shear forces in a moving fluid. The force balance on one-dimensional horizontal laminar flow of an incompressible fluid in a tube takes the form

$$\rho \frac{\partial v}{\partial t} = -\frac{\partial p}{\partial z} - \frac{1}{r}\frac{\partial}{\partial r}(r\,\tau_{rz}) \qquad (3.2.14)$$

where ρ = fluid density, kg/m^3
v = axial velocity, m/sec
t = time, sec
p = pressure at any point along the tube, N/m^2
z = axial dimension along the tube, m
r = radial dimension of the tube, m
τ_{rz} = shearing stress at some point in the fluid, N/m^2

For a Newtonian fluid,

$$\tau_{rz} = -\mu\frac{\partial v}{\partial r} \qquad (3.2.15)$$

and therefore Equation 3.2.14 becomes

$$\rho \frac{\partial v}{\partial t} = -\frac{\partial p}{\partial z} + \frac{\mu}{r}\frac{\partial}{\partial r}\left(r\frac{\partial v}{\partial r}\right) = -\frac{\partial p}{\partial z} + \mu\left(\frac{\partial^2 v}{\partial r^2} + \frac{1}{r}\frac{\partial v}{\partial r}\right) \cdot \qquad (3.2.16)$$

For steady-state flow, $\partial v/\partial t = 0$. For a finite tube length,

$$\frac{\Delta p}{L} = \frac{-\mu}{r}\frac{d}{dr}\left(r\frac{dv}{dr}\right) \qquad (3.2.17)$$

where Δp = pressure drop over length L of the tube, N/m^2
L = tube length over which pressure difference is measured, m

For a tube with a peripheral plasma layer and central core of whole blood, each with different viscosities, μ_p and μ_b, Equation 3.2.17 can be integrated in two parts across the tube radius with the following boundary conditions:

v is finite at $r = 0$
v at the boundary between the two layers is the same on each side of the boundary

the shear stress, $\mu(dv/dr)$, is the same for each fluid at the boundary
$v = 0$ at the wall of the tube, r_o

From these conditions, the volume flow rate $\dot{V}$ is obtained (Middleman, 1972):

$$\dot{V} = \frac{\pi r_o^4 \Delta P}{8L\mu_P}\left[1 - \left(1 - \frac{\delta}{r_o}\right)^4\left(1 - \frac{\mu_P}{\mu_b}\right)\right] \qquad (3.2.18)$$

where δ = thickness of the plasma layer, m
Since

$$\left(1 - \frac{\delta}{r_o}\right)^4 = 1 - 4\frac{\delta}{r_o} + 6\left(\frac{\delta}{r_o}\right)^2 - 4\left(\frac{\delta}{r_o}\right)^3 + \left(\frac{\delta}{r_o}\right)^4 \qquad (3.2.19)$$

and $(\delta/r_o) \ll 1$,

$$\dot{V} \simeq \frac{\pi r_o^4 \Delta P}{8L\mu_P} \left[\frac{\mu_P}{\mu_b} + 4\frac{\delta}{r_o}\left(1 - \frac{\mu_P}{\mu_b}\right) \right]$$

$$= \frac{\pi r_o^4 \Delta P}{8L\mu_b} \left[1 + 4\frac{\delta}{r_o}\left(\frac{\mu_b}{\mu_P} - 1\right) \right] \tag{3.2.20}$$

Comparing this result with Equation 3.2.11 gives an apparent viscosity of (Haynes, 1960)

$$\mu = \mu_b \left[1 + 4\frac{\delta}{r_o}\left(\frac{\mu_b}{\mu_P} - 1\right) \right]^{-4} \tag{3.2.21}$$

It is possible to use this equation with the Fahraeus–Lindqvist data to estimate the thickness of the plasma layer δ. Such estimates fall in the range of 1×10^{-6} m (Middleman, 1972). Using this value and a viscosity ratio (μ_P/μ_b) of 0.25, the apparent viscosity changes seen for very small tubes can be closely predicted.

A second explanation of the low resistance in small tubes is called the sigma effect of Dix and Scott-Blair (Attinger and Michie, 1976; Burton, 1965; Haynes, 1960).[20] According to this concept, red blood cell diameters are not insignificant compared to vessel diameter, and thus the fluid cannot be treated as a homogeneous medium (Lightfoot, 1974). This means that integration of velocity cannot be performed as in Equation 3.2.11. Rather, a summation of finite layers is more appropriate. These finite layers are cylindrical in shape with thickness equal to red blood cell diameter.

The sigma effect can be quantified by imagining the tube made of concentric hollow cylinders of thickness Δr (Dix and Scott-Blair, 1940) with the central core as a solid cylinder of either diameter $2\Delta r$ or 0 (Figure 3.2.8). Total volume flow rate is just

$$\dot{V} = \sum_{i=1}^{J} A_i v_i \tag{3.2.22}$$

where $\dot{V}$ = volume flow rate, m³/sec
  v_i = mean fluid velocity in the ith shell, m/sec
  A_i = cross-sectional area of the ith cylinder, m²
  J = total number of concentric cylinders, dimensionless

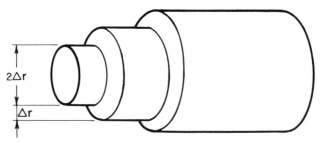

Figure 3.2.8 Concentric hollow spheres used to determine the magnitude of the sigma effect in a small tube.

[20] The sigma effect is erroneously named for the standard Greek letter denoting summation. Actually, Dix and Scott–Blair used a lowercase sigma to signify the rate of change of shear stress with rate of change of shear rate at a point (Dix and Scott–Blair, 1940). The two sigmas subsequently have been confused by other authors.

and this becomes

$$\dot{V} = \sum_{i=1}^{J} 2\pi r_i \Delta r v_i \qquad (3.2.23)$$

where Δr = thickness of ith shell = red blood cell diameter, m
     r_i = mean radius of ith shell, m
Now

$$\Delta(r_i^2 v_i) = r_i^2 \Delta v_i + 2r_i \Delta r v_i \qquad (3..2.24)$$

or

$$2r_i v_i \Delta r = -r_1^2 \frac{\Delta v_i}{\Delta r} \Delta r + \Delta(r_i^2 v_i) \qquad (3.2.25)$$

and if we assume no slip of the fluid at the wall,[21]

$$\sum_{i=1}^{J} \Delta(r_i^2 v_i) = r_i^2 v_i = 0 \qquad (3.2.26)$$

because $v = 0$ at $r_i = r_0$ and $r_i^2 v_i = 0$ when $r_u = 0$.
Therefore,

$$\dot{V} = -\pi \sum_{i=1}^{J} r_i^2 \frac{\Delta v_i}{\Delta r} \Delta r \qquad (3.2.27)$$

From Equation 3.2.17,

$$\frac{-\Delta p r}{L\mu} dr = d\left(r \frac{dv}{dr}\right) \qquad (3.2.28)$$

From which, by integrating, we obtain

$$\frac{-\Delta p r^2}{2L\mu_b} = r \frac{dv}{dr} \qquad (3.2.29)$$

or

$$\frac{-\Delta p r}{2L\mu_b} = \frac{dv}{dr} \simeq \frac{\Delta v}{\Delta r} \qquad (3.2.30)$$

Thus from Equation 3.2.26

$$\dot{V} = \frac{\pi \Delta p}{2L\mu_b} \sum_{i=1}^{j} r_i^3 \Delta r \qquad (3.2.31)$$

Since $r_i = i\Delta r$, and $J = r_o/\Delta r$,

$$\dot{V} = \frac{\pi \Delta p}{2L\mu_b} \sum_{i=1}^{J} i^3 (\Delta r)^4 \qquad (3.2.32)$$

---

[21] Isenberg (1953) treats the sigma effect as an apparent fluid slip condition at the wall with results similar to this analysis.

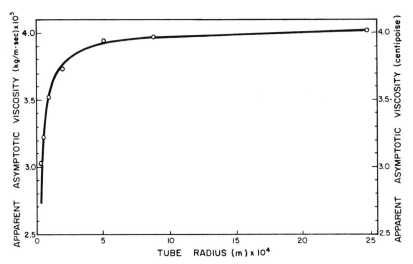

Figure 3.2.9 Fahraeus–Lindqvist data of effect of tube size on apparent viscosity. Red cell diameters of 6×10^{-6} m were used to calculate values for the curve. Data are indicated by circles. (Adapted and used with permission from Burton, 1965.)

From Hodgman (1959),

$$\sum_{i=1}^{J} i^3 = \frac{J^2(J+1)^2}{4} = \frac{\left(\dfrac{r_o}{\Delta r}\right)^2 \left(\dfrac{r_o}{\Delta r}+1\right)^2}{4} \tag{3.2.33}$$

Substituting in Equation 3.2.32 gives

$$\dot{V} = \frac{\pi \Delta p r_o^4}{8 L \mu_b} \left(1 + \frac{\Delta r}{r_o}\right)^2 \tag{3.2.34}$$

Again comparing this result to Equation 3.2.11, we obtain an apparent viscosity:[22]

$$\mu = \mu_b \left[1 + \frac{\Delta r}{r_o}\right]^{-2} \tag{3.2.35}$$

Apparent agreement between the Fahraeus–Lindqvist data and sigma effect calculations can be seen in Figure 3.2.9.

Lightfoot (1974) also mentions other reasons for the Fahraeus–Lindqvist effect. He states that because red cells are concentrated in the central, faster moving portions of the tube, their residence time is less and their mean concentration lower than in either the feed or outflowing blood. He also indicates that red cells are partially blocked from entering small tubes, thus reducing the hematocrit of the blood in small tubes. Good agreement between experimental data and prediction based on hematocrit adjustment has been found. The Fahraeus–Lindqvist effect is thus a curious example of at least three explanations which, by themselves, can each match experimental data. There is little evidence to testify to the relative importance of each of these.

---

[22] See also Schmid–Schönbein (1988) for an apparent viscosity due to blood cells in muscle microvasculature.

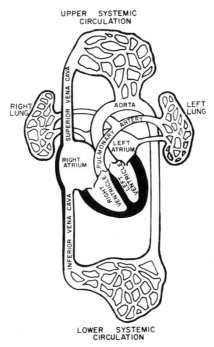

UPPER SYSTEMIC
CIRCULATION

RIGHT
LUNG

LEFT
LUNG

AORTA

SUPERIOR VENA CAVA

PULMONARY ARTERY

LEFT
ATRIUM

RIGHT
ATRIUM

RIGHT VENTRICLE

LEFT VENTRICLE

INFERIOR VENA CAVA

LOWER SYSTEMIC
CIRCULATION

Figure 3.2.10 The heart and circulation. Blood from the left ventricle is discharged through the aorta to systemic capillary beds. Blood from the head, neck, upper extremities and thorax returns to the right atrium through the superior vena cava. Blood from the lower extremities, pelvis, and abdomen returns via the inferior vena cava. The right ventricle pumps blood to the lungs through the pulmonary artery and blood returns to the left atrium through the pulmonary vein. (Adapted and used with permission from Astrand and Rodahl, 1970.)

Much more work has been done to analyze blood vessels, pulsatile flow in vessels, and systems of vessels acting together. For more information on these analyses, refer to Talbot and Gessner (1973) and Pedley et al. (1980).

3.2.3 Heart Characteristics

Central to the cardiovascular system is the motivating object, the heart. The heart is not just one pump; it is four pumps. There is one pair of pumps which service the pulmonary vascularity, and this pair is located on the right side of the heart organ. On the left side is the pair of pumps which push blood through the systemic circulation. Each of these pairs consists of a pressure pump, which develops sufficient pressure to overcome vascular resistance, called the ventricle. The atrium in each pair serves to fill its ventricle in a timely and efficient manner. Figure 3.2.10 illustrates the heart and circulation.

Each of these pumps is intermittent, being very similar to a piston pump.[23] Each contraction of the heart muscle (myocardium) is called a systole; the relaxation of myocardium is called diastole. During diastole the atria fill with venous return blood. Over two-thirds of ventricular filling at rest occurs passively during diastole. During the initial stages of systole, the atria force blood into their respective ventricles, which subsequently pump blood into the arteries during

[23] A piston pump is a positive displacement pump which delivers the same volume during each stroke. The volume delivered by the heart varies because the walls of the pump chamber are distensible.

the latter stages of systole. Blood is therefore delivered to the arteries in a pulsatile manner (Meier et al., 1980). Flaps of membrane acting as valves prohibit backflow of blood from the ventricles to atria and from the arteries to ventricles.

Starling's Law. With four pumps in a series arrangement, there must be a mechanism that allows each pump to vary the volume of blood it pumps during each contraction (called the stroke volume, or SV). Otherwise, blood outflow would be limited by the smallest stroke volume and, during periods of change, blood would pool behind the weakest pump. Fortunately, the walls of each pump are distensible and follow a length–tension relationship characteristic of other muscle tissue (see Section 5.2). That is, cardiac muscle increases its strength of contraction as it is stretched (see Figure 3.2.11), thus enabling each pump to adjust its output according to the amount of blood available to fill it. Starling's law of the heart states that the "energy of contraction is proportional to the initial length of the cardiac muscle fiber" (Ganong, 1963).

Shearing stress existing in the walls of a cylindrical pressure vessel is given by (Attinger, 1976a)

$$\tau = \frac{r_i^2 \, p_i - r_o^2 \, p_o}{r_o^2 - r_i^2} + \frac{(p_i - p_o) \, r_i^2 \, r_o^2}{(r^2 \, r_o^2 - r_i^2)} \tag{3.2.36}$$

where τ = shear stress in vessel wall, N/m^2
$\quad r_i$ = radius of inside surface, m
$\quad r_o$ = radius of outside surface, m
$\quad p_i$ = pressure of fluid inside vessel, N/m^2
$\quad p_o$ = pressure of fluid outside vessel, N/m^2
$\quad r$ = radial distance inside wall, m

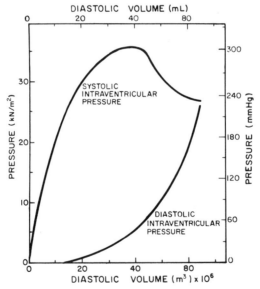

Figure 3.2.11   Length–tension relationship for dog cardiac muscle. As blood fills the ventricle during diastole, muscle fibers stretch and increase intraventricular pressure. During the subsequent systole, pressure produced in the ventricle will rise higher for cardiac muscle that has been stretched more (increased diastolic filling). With higher intraventricular pressure, more blood will be pumped in the time available. Thus the ventricle is able to adjust its output to its input. (Adapted and used with permission from Patterson et al., 1914.)

When outside pressure can be taken as zero,

$$\tau = \frac{r_o^2 p_i}{r_o^2 - r_i^2}\left(1 + \frac{r_o^2}{r^2}\right)$$ (3.2.37)

If wall thickness is small with respect to the wall radius, $\Delta r/\bar{r} < 0.1$,

$$\tau = \frac{\bar{r} p_i}{\Delta r}$$ (3.2.38)

where $\bar{r}$ = average wall radius, m

$\quad \Delta r$ = wall thickness, m

This is the so-called law of Laplace[24] relating shear stress in the wall to wall radius. Frequently it is applied to the heart and blood vessels where wall thickness is not negligible compared to average wall radius. The law of Laplace, however, does show the inverse relationship between wall tension (shear stress) and radius. It is frequently seen that cardiovascular hypertension (pressures above normal) is accompanied by cardiac hypertrophy (enlarged size) in order that the myocardium can produce the pressures required to force blood through the vasculature. The enlarged heart, caused by wall thickening, reduces the average shear stress in the wall.

Similarly, the accommodation of the heart to larger amounts of incoming blood, as represented by Starling's law, relates to the law of Laplace. A larger amount of blood in a ventricle stretches the wall more than normal and increases the wall tension. This preloads the myocardium and enables it to develop more force to more forcefully pump the blood out (see the length–tension relationship, Figure 3.2.11).[25]

Being in a closed loop, blood returning to the heart is actually pushed back to the atria by pressure developed by the ventricles. Rather than requiring a large pressure to accomplish this, a relatively small pressure is required only to overcome vascular resistance. With no changes in posture, the system acts like a syphon (Burton, 1965), without appreciable elevation difference between the inlet to the tube (aorta) and outlet from the tube (vena cava). The effect of uphill venous return is thus none at all.

With a sudden change in posture, distensibility of the veins causes pooling of blood to occur in the lowermost part of the body and venous return is momentarily reduced. During exercise, where posture changes are constantly occurring, skeletal muscle pressure on the veins pumps blood back to the heart. This is fortunate, because the heart and collapsible blood vessels could not operate effectively by attempting to create a vacuum to induce blood return. The heart is, however, an efficient organ for pressure production.

Blood Pressure. Normal resting systemic blood pressure[26] is 16.0 kN/m² (120 mm Hg) during systole and 11.0 kN/m² (80 mm Hg) during diastole in males. These values increase with age, as seen in Table 3.2.5. After the sharp rise in systolic pressure that accompanies puberty, there is a gradual increase in both systolic and diastolic pressures, probably due to a gradual decrease with age of the elesticity of arterial walls (Morehouse and Miller, 1967). In girls the sharp rise at

---

[24] The law of Laplace for an arbitrary smooth three-dimensional shape is

$$\tau = p/\Delta r (1/r_1 + 1/r_2)$$

where r_1 and r_2 are orthogonal radii of curvature. For a cylinder, $r_2 = \infty$ and $\tau = pr_1/\Delta r$. For a sphere, $r_1 = r_2$ and $\tau = pr_1/2\Delta r$.

[25] The law of Laplace has also been applied to blood vessels to show that capillaries, for instance, can withstand high internal blood pressures (see Table 3.2.6) because they are so small in diameter (see Table 3.2.2).

[26] Physiological pressures are normally measured in mm Hg. To obtain N/m² from mm Hg multiply mm Hg by 133.32.

TABLE 3.2.5   Influence of Age on Blood Pressure

Age, years	Systolic Pressure, kN/m²	(mm Hg)	Diastolic Pressure, kN/m²	(mm Hg)
0.5 male	11.9	(89)	8.0	(60)
0.5 female	12.4	(93)	8.3	(62)
4 male	13.3	(100)	8.9	(67)
4 female	13.3	(100)	8.5	(64)
10	13.7	(103)	9.3	(70)
15	15.1	(113)	10.0	(75)
20	16.0	(120)	10.7	(80)
25	16.3	(122)	10.8	(81)
30	16.4	(123)	10.9	(82)
35	16.5	(124)	11.1	(83)
40	16.8	(126)	11.2	(84)
45	17.1	(128)	11.3	(85)
50	17.3	(130)	11.5	(86)
55	17.6	(132)	11.6	(87)
60	18.0	(135)	11.9	(89)

Source: Adapted and used with permission from Morehouse and Miller, 1967.

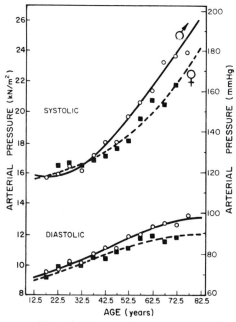

Figure 3.2.12 Arterial pressure with age in the general population. Both diastolic and systolic pressures increase, likely from a decrease in blood vessel flexibility and a decrease in vessel diameters. Open circles denote male and filled squares denote female responses. (Adapted and used with permission from Hamilton et al., 1954.)

TABLE 3.2.6   Blood Pressures Measured at Various Points in the Cardiovascular Circulation

Variable	Systolic/Diastolic, N/m^2	(mm Hg)	Mean Pressure, N/m^2	(mm Hg)
Right atrium	800/ − 400	(6/ − 3)		
Right ventricle	3,330/ − 400	(25/ − 3)		
Pulmonary artery	3,330/930	(25/7)		
Pulmonary capillaries	1,330/1,330	(10/10)		
Pulmonary veins	1,200/1,200	(9/9)		
Left atrium	1,070/0	(8/0)		
Left ventricle	16,000/0	(120/0)		
Aorta	16,000/10,70	(120/80)	13,300	(100)
Large arteries	16,700/10,30	(125/77)		
Small arteries	13,100/10,90	(98/82)	12,000	(90)
Arterioles	9,300/6,700	(70/50)	8,000	(60)
Capillaries	4,000/4,000	(30/30)	4,000	(30)
Venules	2,700/2,700	(20/20)	2,700	(20)
Veins	2,000/2,000	(15/15)	2,000	(15)
Vena cava[a]	1,300/ − 270	(10/ − 2)	1,300	(9.8)

[a] Pressures in the vena cava will fluctuate in a very pronounced manner with respiratory cycle. Flow in the vena cava will be reduced by one-third during inspiration.

puberty is less marked and is often followed by a decrease until the age of 18, after which pressure increases, as it does with males, but it is usually 1.3 kN/m^2 (10 mm Hg) higher in females (Figure 3.2.12).

Diastolic pressures given in Table 3.2.5 are pressures measured outside the heart's left ventricle.[27] Left ventricular diastolic pressures decrease to nearly zero (Scher, 1966a). Table 3.2.6 gives resting blood pressure values at many points in the cardiovascular system.

Other influences on blood pressure are emotional state (increases blood pressure), exercise [increases blood pressure from a typical systolic/diastolic value of 16/10.7 kN/m^2 (120/80 mm Hg) at rest to 23.3/14.7 kN/m^2 (175/110 mm Hg) during exercise], and body position (decreases in blood pressure accompany raising). Arm exercise causes larger blood pressure increases than leg exercise (Astrand and Rodahl, 1970). Blood pressure is generally independent of body size for nonobese individuals (Astrand and Rodahl, 1970).

Heart Rate.   Heart rate is an expression of the number of times the heart contracts in a specified unit of time. For each beat of the heart one stroke volume is pumped through the vasculature. Heart rate at rest is normally taken as 1.17 beats/sec (70 beats/min), although the normal range is 0.83–1.67 beats/sec (50–100 beats/min) (Morehouse and Miller, 1967).[28] There is a tendency for active athletes to have lower resting heart rates due to increased vagal tone, although there is not a clear correlation between resting heart rate and general physical condition in the general public. Resting heart rate usually is 0.08–0.17 beats/sec (5–10 beats/min) higher in women than in men (Morehouse and Miller, 1967).

[27] The airtight rubber cuff (sphygmomanometer) used to measure blood pressure applies sufficient pressure to the main artery of the arm to collapse the artery and stop blood flow. Sounds produced by turbulence as blood seeps through the occlusion during systole indicate that cuff pressure is just lower than systolic pressure. When all sounds disappear while cuff pressure is being released, no more turbulence is indicated, meaning that the artery is no longer partially occluded by the cuff. This cuff pressure is taken as diastolic pressure. Direct blood pressure measurements obtained from a needle inserted into the artery indicate that indirect blood pressure measurements are accurate during rest but not during exercise. For strenuous exercise, systolic pressure may be understimated by 1100–2000 N/m^2 and overestimated during the first few minutes of recovery by 2100–5100 N/m^2. Errors are even greater in the measurement of diastolic pressure (Morehouse and Miller, 1967).

[28] Elevated heart rates are normally referred to as *tachycardia*. *Bradycardia* is a heart rate lower than normal.

Heart rate increases during exercise, with heart rate accelerating immediately after, or perhaps even before, the onset of exercise. The rapidity with which heart rate returns to normal at the cessation of exercise is often used as a test of cardiovascular fitness.

In many types of work, the increase in heart rate is linear with increase in workload (Astrand and Rodahl, 1970) as related to maximal oxygen uptake (see Section 1.3). Exceptions to this relationship appear at very high work rates (Astrand and Rodahl, 1970) near the anaerobic threshold (contrasted with the aerobic threshold; see Section 1.3.5 and Ribeiro et al., 1985).

For instance, Astrand and Rodahl (1970) present data on maximum oxygen uptake for nearly 1500 males:

$$\dot{V}_{O_2max} = (4.2 - 0.03y)/60{,}000 \tag{3.2.39}$$

for 1700 females:

$$\dot{V}_{O_2max} = (2.6 - 0.01y)/60{,}000 \tag{3.2.40}$$

and for 3 exceptional male long distance runners:

$$\dot{V}_{O_2max} = (7.1 - 0.07y)/60{,}000 \tag{3.2.41}$$

where $\dot{V}_{O_2max}$ = maximum oxygen uptake, m^3/sec

y = age, yr

In each of these cases, maximum oxygen uptake corresponds to a maximum heart rate[29] for men or women given by

$$HR_{max} = (220 - y)/60 \tag{3.2.42}$$

where HR_{max} = maximum heart rate, beats/sec

Since basal oxygen consumption is only about $5 \times 10^{-7} \, m^3/sec$ (see Table 5.2.19), it is usually neglected. Therefore,

$$\frac{\dot{V}_{O_2}}{\dot{V}_{O_2max}} = \frac{HR - HR_r}{HR_{max} - HR_r} \tag{3.2.43}$$

where $\dot{V}_{O_2}$ = predicted oxygen uptake at heart rate HR, m^3/sec

HR = submaximal heart rate, beats/sec

HR_r = resting heart rate, beats/sec (HR_r = 1.17 for males and 1.33 for females)

Cardiac Output. Cardiac output (CO) is the amount of blood pumped per unit time. It is the product of stroke volume (SV) and heart rate (HR):

$$CO = (SV)(HR) \tag{3.2.44}$$

Cardiac output is approximately $92-100 \times 10^{-6} \, m^3/sec$ (92–100 mL/sec) at rest with an average stroke volume of $80 \times 10^{-6} \, m^3$ (80 mL) at a heart rate of 1.17 beats/sec (70 beats/min). Resting

---

[29] Lesage et al. (1985) conducted an experiment to determine familial relationships for maximum heart rate, maximum blood lactate, and maximum oxygen uptake during exercise. A relationship for maximum heart rate was suggested between children and mothers but not for children and fathers. A similar relationship was found for $\dot{V}_{O_2max}/kg$.

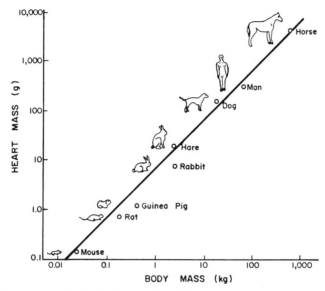

Figure 3.2.13 Heart mass related to body mass for eight species. (Used with permission from Astrand and Rodahl, 1970.)

cardiac output depends on posture: $83–100 \times 10^{-6} \, \text{m}^3/\text{sec}$ recumbent, $67–83 \times 10^{-6} \, \text{m}^3/\text{sec}$ sitting, and less for standing (Morehouse and Miller, 1967).

A dimensional analysis of cardiac output and its components, stroke volume and heart rate, is instructive in the comparison of similarly built animals of different dimensions. Astrand and Rodahl (1970), in their consideration of dimensional dependence, show that heart rate is inversely proportional to body length:

$$\text{HR} \stackrel{\triangle}{=} 1/L \tag{3.2.45}$$

where L = length dimension

and $\stackrel{\triangle}{=}$ denotes dimensional dependence. Thus a taller (and heavier) person would be expected to have a lower resting heart rate.[30]

Heart weight is directly proportional to body weight (Figure 3.2.13), and stroke volume is directly proportional to heart weight (Astrand and Rodahl, 1970). Thus

$$\text{SV} \stackrel{\triangle}{=} L^3 \tag{3.2.46}$$

Table 3.2.7 shows the increased heart volumes of trained athletes. Larger hearts are expected to have larger stroke volumes and therefore lower heart rates for any required cardiac output. This is exactly the effect seen: well-trained athletes do, indeed, have lower heart rates.

Cardiac output, being the product of stroke volume and heart rate, must therefore be proportional to body dimension squared:

$$\text{CO} \stackrel{\triangle}{=} L^2 \tag{3.2.47}$$

---

[30] The resting heart rate of a 25 g mouse is about 11.7, that of a 70 kg man is 1.17, and for a 3000 kg elephant, it is 0.42 beats/sec (Astrand and Rodahl, 1970).

TABLE 3.2.7 Effect of Training on Cardiac Parameters

Subjects	Heart Volume, $m^3 \times 10^{-6}$ (mL)		Heart Weight, N (kg)		Left Ventricular End-Systolic Blood Volume, $m^3 \times 10^{-6}$ (mL)	
Untrained	785	(785)	2.9	(0.30)	51	(51)
Trained for competition	1015	(1015)	3.4	(0.35)	101	(101)
Professional cyclist	1437	(1437)	4.9	(0.50)	177	(177)

Source: Adapted and used with permission from Ganong, 1963.

Astrand and Rodahl (1970) indicate that, if cardiac output were proportional to body mass ($\overset{\triangle}{=} L^3$), and not L^2, the blood velocity in the aorta (cross-sectional area proportional to L^2) would have to be so great in the largest mammals that the heart would be faced with an impossible task.

Cardiac output must increase during exercise to satisfy the increased oxygen needs of the body (see Section 3.2.1). If, for example, the oxygen content of mixed venous blood is 15% by volume, and that of arterial blood is 20% by volume, each $100 \, m^3$ of blood yields $5 \, m^3$ of oxygen to the tissues. With a total body oxygen consumption of $4.2 \times 10^{-6} \, m^3/sec$ (250 mL/min), $5 \times 10^{-3} \, m^3$ (5 L) of blood is required. Cardiac function during exercise is illustrated by data given in Table 3.2.8. Stroke volume increases, levels off, and then falls somewhat due to inadequate ventricular filling at high heart rates. Heart rate increases monotonically to result in increased cardiac output.

There is also a redistribution of blood flow within and between organs during exercise, from those organs relatively inactive to those with greater metabolic demands. These changes are given in Table 3.2.3.

Energetics. As fast as it beats, the heart should be expected to consume a good deal of energy. Indeed, the heart requires just under 10% of the body's resting energy expenditure (see Table 5.2.19). The transformation of chemical to mechanical energy by the heart is reflected only to a small extent by the external work done on the blood; most of it is dissipated as heat (Michie and Kline, 1976).

External work by the heart on the blood is given by a pressure energy and kinetic energy relation:

$$W = \int_{V_d}^{V_s} p \, dv + \int_{V_d}^{V_s} \tfrac{1}{2}\rho v^2 \, dV \tag{3.2.48}$$

where W = external work, N·m
$\quad$ p = ventricular pressure during ejection, N/m^2
$\quad$ V = ventricular volume, m^3
$\quad$ V_d = ventricular end-diastolic volume, m^3
$\quad$ V_s = ventricular end-systolic volume, m^3
$\quad$ ρ = density of blood, kg/m^3
$\quad$ v = blood velocity, m/sec

and

$$V_d = V_s + SV \tag{3.2.49}$$

where SV = stroke volume, m^3

TABLE 3.2.8 Changes in Cardiac Function with Exercise

Work Rate, N·m/sec (kg·m/min)	Oxygen Consumption, m³/sec × 10⁶ (mL/min)	Heart Rate, beats/sec (beats/min)	Cardiac Output, m³/sec × 10⁶ (L/min)	Stroke Volume, m³ × 10⁶ (mL)	Arteriovenous Oxygen Difference, m³/m³ blood × 10³ (mL/100 mL)
Rest	4.45 (267)	1.07 (64)	107 (6.4)	100 (100)	43 (4.3)
47.1 (288)	15.2 (910)	1.73 (104)	218 (13.1)	126 (126)	70 (7.0)
88.2 (540)	23.8 (1430)	2.03 (122)	253 (15.2)	125 (125)	94 (9.4)
147.1 (900)	35.7 (2143)	2.68 (161)	297 (17.8)	110 (110)	123 (12.3)
205.9 (1260)	50.1 (3007)	2.88 (173)	348 (20.9)	120 (120)	145 (14.5)

Source: Adapted and used with permission from Asmussen and Nielsen, 1952.

Internal work, or physiological work done by the muscle in developing tension, does not necessarily show up as external work. Isometric[31] muscle contraction, for instance, does not result in any external work but does represent a physiological oxygen cost (see Section 5.2.5). The length–tension relationship for cardiac muscle tissue (Figure 3.2.9) shows that muscle tension depends on the amount of stretching to which the muscle is subjected. In the heart, this translates into the amount of blood in the ventricular chambers before systole begins. Thus the amount of internal work of the heart depends partly on the end-diastolic volume of blood in the ventricles.

The other determinant of internal work is external work. The higher the level of external work, the higher is internal work. Muscular mechanical efficiency is defined as

$$\eta = \frac{\text{external mechanical work}}{\text{total energy used}} \qquad (3.2.50)$$

where η = mechanical efficiency, dimensionless
Mechanical efficiency of the heart is quite low, being 3–15%, and may rise to 10–15% when external work is increased (Michie and Kline, 1976). Thus when external work is doubled, internal work is also nearly doubled. With no external work performed, internal work will be minimal; with high blood pressures to overcome, or with the myocardium in a disadvantageous position on the length–tension relationship, internal work will be very high.[32]

Studies have shown that (1) stroke volume can be delivered with a minimum myocardial shortening if the contraction begins at a larger volume; (2) internal energy usage is lower for a heart at larger volume; (3) higher blood pressures can be attained by stretched muscle fibers; (4) lower amounts of energy are used for slower contraction times (lower heart rate); and (5) the greater the heart volume, the higher the muscle tension required to sustain a given intraventricular pressure (Astrand and Rodahl, 1970). All but the last factor indicates that a more efficient cardiac output would occur with higher stroke volume and lower heart rate. This has been seen to be the trend for trained athletes. For the cardiac patient, large diastolic filling is sometimes accompanied by small stroke volume and high heart rate. Heart dilatation gives improved ability of the muscle fibers to produce tension as long as they are stretched (Astrand and Rodahl, 1970). However, the high heart rate and the high muscle tension combine to use more oxygen than the capillaries of the heart can deliver during mild exercise.[33] The result is myocardial hypoxia with symptoms of angina pectoris.

It has been reported that left ventricular oxygen consumption is correlated with the product of mean ventricular ejection pressure and the duration of ejection (Michie and Kline, 1976). This is called the tension–time index.

Factors that constitute oxygen consumption (proportional to physiological work) of the heart during each beat are (1) resting oxygen consumption, (2) activation oxygen consumption, (3) contraction oxygen consumption, and (4) relaxation oxygen consumption (Michie and Kline, 1976). Resting oxygen consumption is used to maintain the muscle in its healthy, normal relaxed state. Activation oxygen consumption is that used by the muscle as the muscle is excited by a depolarization and repolarization wave (see Sections 1.3.1 and 2.2.2). Contraction oxygen consumption includes internal and external work associated with the development of muscle tension. Relaxation energy is a small (approximately 9%) amount of energy required for the muscle to return to its relaxed state (Michie and Kline, 1976).

Power output by the heart, assuming in Equation 3.2.48 a left ventricular systolic pressure of $16 \, \text{kN/m}^2$, a stroke volume of $70 \times 10^{-6} \, \text{m}^3$, a heart rate of 1.2 beats/sec, a right ventricular

---

[31] Muscle tension produced at constant length.

[32] The term *preload* is often used to describe the effect of initial fiber length, determined by intraventricular pressure and volume. *Afterload* is the term used to account for the external pressure developed by the ventricle. It is determined by intraventricular pressure and wall thickness, vascular resistance and pressure, and force–velocity relationship of the myocardium (Michie and Kline, 1976).

[33] While the cardiac muscle is contracting, capillaries in the muscle are being squeezed, allowing less blood to flow.

systolic pressure of one-sixth of the left ventricle, and a 10% increase to account for kinetic power, is about 1.8 N·m/sec (Michie and Kline, 1976). During exercise, when maximum systolic pressure may exceed 26.7 kN/m² and heart rate may be 2.5 beats/sec, kinetic power accounts for about 20% of the total cardiac power of about 8.4 N·m/sec (Michie and Kline, 1976).

It has been suggested (Hämäläinen, 1975) that blood flow and pressure can be predicted based on an optimization process. This seems to indicate that, like respiration (see Section 4.3.4), cardiodynamics are driven by a control system that tends to limit the amount of work expended during each cycle. Hämäläinen suggested a cost functional of

$$J = \int_0^{t_e} (p^2 + \alpha p \dot{V}) \, dt \tag{3.2.51}$$

where J = criterion to be minimized, N·sec/m⁴
t = time, sec
t_e = ejection time, sec
p = ejection pressure, N/m²
$\dot{V}$ = blood flow, m³/sec
α = weighting parameter, sec/m⁵

When minimized, this yields pressure curves which agree somewhat with recorded data.

3.3 CARDIOVASCULAR CONTROL

Cardiovascular control exhibits classic elements of feedback control mechanisms. There are sensors, a central controller, and actuator mechanisms. Cardiovascular control, however, has been recognized to occur on many levels (involving local control responses as well as responses imposed from central nervous system sites) and to many different organs (the capillaries, arterioles, and heart, for instance). It should be realized that cardiovascular control is composed of interrelated subunits which are integrated in such a manner as to maintain adequate chemical supply first to the brain and then to other bodily structures despite levels of demand that may vary by several orders of magnitude.

A general scheme for maintenance of blood pressure appears in Figure 3.3.1 (Scher, 1966b). Since blood pressure is

$$p = (HR)(SV)(R) \tag{3.3.1}$$

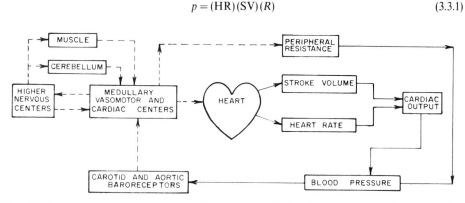

Figure 3.3.1 General scheme for regulation of blood pressure. Dashed lines indicate neural communication and solid lines indicate direct mechanical effect. Sensing occurs in the carotid and aortic baroreceptors, control in the central nervous system cardiac centers, and responses in the heart and vasculature. New evidence (Stone et al., 1985) also suggests links from the heart and working muscles which influence cardiovascular control.

TABLE 3.3.1   Cardiovascular Values at Rest and Exercise

Work Rate, N·m/sec	Mean Blood Pressure, kN/m² × 10³	Heart Rate, beats/sec	Stroke Volume, m³ × 10⁶	Cardiac Output, m³/sec × 10⁶	Peripheral Resistance, N·sec/m⁵ × 10⁻⁶
Rest	13.3	1.1	100	107	121
200	18.9	2.9	120	348	54

where p = blood pressure, N·m²

$\quad$ HR = heart rate, beats/sec

$\quad$ SV = stroke volume, m³

$\quad\quad$ R = peripheral vascular resistance, N.sec/m⁵

blood pressure can be maintained by changing heart rate, stroke volume, or peripheral vascular resistance. Table 3.3.1 includes typical values for these variables and shows that heart rate during exercise usually increases greatly and vascular resistance greatly decreases. Stroke volume does not change much. To decrease vascular resistance, most blood vessels must open wider. However, the storage vessels must close, because otherwise sufficient amounts of blood would not quickly return to the heart. This is just one illustration of the sometimes contradictory demands placed on the cardiovascular system to reestablish stable equilibrium.

3.3.1   Neural Regulation

These responses are coordinated through the central nervous system by means of cardiovascular sensors, a central controller, and various responsive organs.

Sensors. There are several different types of sensors which provide input for cardiovascular control. There is first a general class of mechanoreceptors comprised of stretch receptors and baroreceptors. Stretch receptors exist in the carotid sinus and aortic arch, baroreceptors are located in both branches of the pulmonary artery, and volume receptors are in the left and right atria. These receptors, especially in the carotid sinus and aortic arch, generally function in the maintenance of adequate arterial pressure.

$\quad$ The firing rate of these sensors reflects mean pressure as well as rates of changes in pressure. For the carotid sinus stretch receptors, the rate of impulses has been expressed (Attinger, 1976b) as

$$f = \beta_+ \frac{dp}{dt} \delta\left(\frac{dp}{dt}\right) + \beta_- \frac{dp}{dt} \delta\left(\frac{-dp}{dt}\right) + \beta_0 (p - p_{\text{th}}) \delta[p - p_{\text{th}}] \qquad (3.3.2)$$

where f = neural firing rate, impulses/sec

$\quad\quad$ p = arterial pressure, N/m²

$\quad\quad$ t = time, sec

$\quad\quad$ p_{th} = threshold arterial pressure, N/m²

$\quad$ $\delta[x] = 1, \quad x \geqslant 0$

$\quad\quad\quad = 0, \quad x < 0$

β_+, β_- = sensitivity coefficients, m²/N

$\quad$ β_0 = sensitivity coefficient, m²/(N·sec)

The magnitudes of threshold pressure and sensitivity coefficients vary with level of mean pressure. The relationship between the mean sinus pressure and average carotid sinus baroreceptor neural firing rate is sigmoid (Figure 3.3.2) with normal blood pressure in the midportion of the curve (Ganong, 1963) where the sensitivity (rate of change of firing rate to rate of change of mean arterial pressure) is greatest. Pulsating pressures result in greater firing rates.

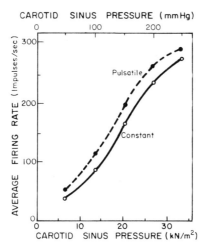

Figure 3.3.2 Average firing rate of a single carotid baroreceptor unit responding to arterial pressure. There is both an influence of pressure and rate of change of pressure on firing rate. (Adapted and used with permission from Korner, 1971.)

There are also arterial peripheral chemoreceptors in the aortic arch and carotid sinus sensitive to arterial pO_2, pCO_2, and pH (Attinger, 1976b). Although they are more important in the regulation of respiration, they do influence cardiovascular responses in extreme circumstances.

There appears to be a very small cardiovascular influence, as well, from other peripheral sensors. Lung inflation receptors represent the largest group of vagal afferent sources (Attinger, 1976b) and, since the heart is also innervated by the vagus, may play a role in the interaction seen between respiration and cardiac output. Somatic inputs through the trigeminal nerve are important in relation to the diving and nasal circulatory reflexes.[34]

Controller. The heart is capable of generation of its basic rhythm in the absence of external neural inputs and can maintain some local regulation of its output. However, the cardiovascular controller must integrate numerous pieces of afferent information into a coherent strategy for effective cardiovascular response. Much of this integration occurs in the reticular substance of the lower pons and upper medulla (Figure 3.3.3) and is called the vasomotor center. Its lateral portions are continuously sending efferent signals to partially contract the blood vessels (vasomotor tone). The medial part of the center transmits inhibitory signals to the lateral part, which results in vasodilation (Attinger, 1976b). The lateral vasomotor center also transmits impulses through sympathetic nerve fibers to the heart, which results in cardiac acceleration and increased contractility (Attinger, 1976b). The inhibitory center, on the other hand, is connected to the heart via the parasympathetic[35] fibers of the vagus nerve and tends to slow heart rate and relax the myocardium (Figure 3.3.4).

The entire cardiovascular regulatory system is not localized in one section of the central nervous system (Smith, 1966). The vasomotor center is normally influenced by peripheral baroreceptor and chemoreceptor inputs, central nervous system chemoreceptor inputs, the

[34] The diving reflex is an apparently primordial action which results in a significant lower heart rate when the face is suddenly chilled.

[35] The sympathetic nervous system is involved in reactions to stress; these include increasing heart rate, respiration rate, sweating, and secretion of adrenaline. The parasympathetic system is normally antagonistic to the sympathetic system and is used to maintain resting homeostasis: slow heart rate, maintaining gastrointestinal activity, and promoting balanced endocrine secretions. The sympathetic system acts on beta adrenergic receptors of the heart, whereas the parasympathetic system acts on gamma receptors.

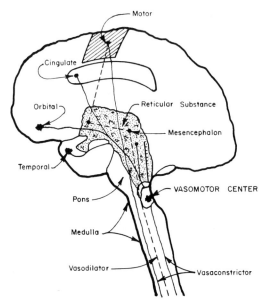

Figure 3.3.3 Areas of the brain important in cardiovascular control. The vasomotor center is located in the lower pons and upper medulla. Inputs are received in the vasomotor center from peripheral as well as other central nervous system sites. Outputs from the center connect to the heart and vasculature. (Used with permission from Guyton, 1986.)

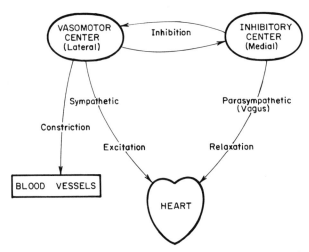

Figure 3.3.4 Basic diagram of the cardiovascular controller. The many inputs to the controller are not shown.

hypothalamus (see Section 5.3.2), the cerebral cortex, the viscera, and skin (Attinger, 1976b). Stimulation of the anterior hypothalamus, for example, results in bradycardia and a fall in blood pressure. As another example, heart rate increases during strong emotion (cortex and hypothalamic inputs). Some information is transmitted to efferent fibers at the level of the spinal cord, but these reflexes usually do not interfere with higher level control.

Every control system must have a controlled variable. In the case of cardiovascular control, as

TABLE 3.3.2 Blood Flow and Oxygen Consumption of Various Organs in a 617 N (63 kg) Adult Human with a Mean Arterial Blood Pressure of 12 kN/m² (90 mm Hg) and an Oxygen Consumption of 4.17×10^{-6} m³/sec (250 mL/min)

Region	Mass, kg	Blood Flow, m³/sec × 10⁶ (mL/min)	Arteriovenous Oxygen Difference, m³/m³ blood × 10³ (mL/L)	Oxygen Consumption, m³/sec × 10⁶ (mL/min)	Vascular Resistance,[a] N·sec/m⁵ × 10⁻⁶ (mm Hg·sec/mL)	Percentage of Total Cardiac Output	Percentage of Total Oxygen Consumption
Liver	2.6	25.0 (1500)	34 (34)	0.85 (51)	480 (3.6)	27.8	20.4
Kidneys	0.3	21.0 (1260)	14 (14)	0.30 (18)	571 (4.3)	23.3	7.2
Brain	1.4	12.5 (750)	62 (62)	0.77 (46)	960 (7.2)	13.9	18.4
Skin	3.6	7.7 (462)	25 (25)	0.20 (12)	1560 (11.7)	8.6	4.8
Skeletal muscle	31.0	14.0 (840)	60 (60)	0.83 (50)	857 (6.4)	15.6	20.0
Heart muscle	0.3	4.2 (250)	114 (114)	0.48 (29)	2880 (21.4)	4.7	11.6
Rest of body	23.8	5.6 (336)	129 (129)	0.73 (44)	2140 (16.1)	6.2	17.6
Total	63.0	90.0 (5400)	46 (46)	4.17 (250)	133 (1.0)	100.0	100.0

Source: Adapted and used with permission from Bard, 1961.

[a]Vascular resistance is mean arterial blood pressure (12 kN/m²) divided by blood flow.

in the cases of most other controlled systems discussed in this book, maintenance of a normal operating environment for the brain appears to be the controlled variable.

The cerebral vessels possess very little vasodilatory innervation, which is of little functional importance. Instead, regulatory mechanisms maintain total cerebral blood flow under widely varying conditions.[36] Total cerebral blood flow is not increased by strenuous mental activity, and it does not decrease during sleep. One reason for this may be that oxygen consumption of the human brain is very high, averaging $5.8 \times 10^{-8}\,m^3/sec$ (3.5 mL/min) per gram brain tissue, or $82 \times 10^{-8}\,m^3/sec$ (49 mL/min) for the whole brain in an adult (Ganong, 1963). This figure represents approximately 20% of the total resting oxygen consumption (Table 3.3.2). Brain tissue is extremely sensitive to anoxia, and unconsciousness occurs about 10 seconds after the blood supply is interrupted.

When blood flow to the brain is decreased, cardiovascular control mechanisms quickly attempt to return it to normal. For instance, if intracranial pressure is somehow elevated to more than $4400\,N\cdot m^2$ (33 mm Hg), cerebral blood flow is soon significantly reduced (Ganong, 1963). The resultant ischemia stimulates the vasomotor center and systemic blood pressure rises. As intracranial pressure is made to increase further, systemic blood pressure rises proportionately.

Similarly, local changes in CO_2 and O_2 partial pressures in the blood can change cerebral blood flow. A rise in pCO_2 exerts a profound vasodilator effect on the arterioles. A low pO_2 will likewise cause vasodilation. Low pCO_2 or high pO_2 results in mild vasoconstriction.[37] These effects result in a certain degree of autoregulation of blood flow to maintain the chemical milieu of the brain within tolerable limits. It therefore appears likely that the most sensitively regulated area is the brain, and that most cardiovascular regulatory responses are those associated with maintaining homeostasis of the brain.

Effector Organs. All blood vessels with the exception of capillaries and venules are innervated by sympathetic autonomic nerve fibers. The arterioles and other resistance vessels are the most densely innervated. Resistance of these vessels is regulated to control tissue blood flow and arterial pressure. The veins, which act as capacitance, or storage, vessels (Table 3.2.2), are regulated to control the amount of stored blood. Venoconstriction and arteroconstriction occur together, shifting blood to the arterial side of the circulation. In addition, vasoconstriction in the gastrointestinal area decreases blood flow to the gastrointestinal system, liver, and spleen. Other important blood reservoirs at rest are the skin and lungs. During severe exercise, constriction of the vessels in these organs, as well as decreased blood volume in the liver and splanchnic bed, may increase actively circulating blood volume perfusing the muscles by as much as 30% (Table 3.2.3). Thus vascular innervation causes two types of physical control response: (1) peripheral resistance changes to maintain blood pressure regulation and (2) blood distribution changes to maintain blood flow to tissues which require delivery of metabolites and oxygen.

Beneken and DeWit (1967) discussed with unusual clarity the role of peripheral resistance control in local and systemic regulation. Central nervous system regulation of peripheral arterial resistance occurs when arterial pressure changes and is due to baroreceptor sensing of central blood pressure. Vasoconstriction occurs when arterial pressure falls; therefore, central nervous system control can be thought of as a pressure-controlling system.

Autoregulation, the local response to inadequate tissue nutrition, allows local vascular beds to open to increase blood flow. Autoregulation mainly serves to ensure an adequate distribution of cardiac output to the various parts of the body and is so local that it has almost no direct effect on heart action and total cardiac output. Central nervous system control of arterial blood flow can be overridden by autoregulation when local tissue oxygen consumption exceeds blood oxygen delivery. Thus autoregulation can be thought of as a flow-controlling system.

[36] Cerebral blood flow in adults averages $9 \times 10^{-6}\,m^3/sec$ (0.54 L/min) per kilogram brain tissue with a normal range of 6.7–$11.2 \times 10^6\,m^3/(sec.kg)$ (0.40–0.67 L/kg min) (Ganong, 1963).

[37] The unconsciousness that results from severe hyperventilation is the result of arteriolar hypocaphic vasoconstriction, reducing the blood flow to parts of the brain.

The other major effector organ is the heart itself. Heart rate is slowed by continual firing of the vagus and speeded by sympathetic nervous discharge.[38] When sympathetic firing increases, vagus firing usually decreases. Thus the heart, which is the ultimate source of blood pressure, can be made to increase or decrease blood pressure as required.[39] As we saw in Tables 3.2.8 and 3.3.1, stroke volume does not greatly change during exercise. Increasing heart rate thus is the major means of increasing cardiac output. Coordinated control of blood pressure occurs with concomitant increases in heart rate and total peripheral resistance:

$$p = \dot{V}R \tag{3.3.3}$$

Reflexes. Among the most important of the reflex actions that occur is the systemic arterial baroreceptor reflex. If arterial pressure falls for some reason, heart rate immediately increases and peripheral vascular resistance also increases. A common example of the occurrence of this reflex is the response to standing after lying down. The head and feet are at the same level as the heart in a supine individual, and thus mean arterial blood pressure is nearly constant throughout the body at $13.3 \, kN/m^2$ (100 mm Hg). When standing, arterial blood pressure at the level of the heart is still $13 \, kN/m^2$, but the gravitational effect causes arterial blood pressure in the feet to be nearly $26 \, kN/m^2$ and at the level of the head to be $8-9 \, kN/m^2$. Blood also pools in the venous capacitance vessels of the lower extremities. If there were no compensatory mechanisms, cerebral blood flow would fall below 60% of the flow in the recumbent position, and unconsciousness would follow (Ganong, 1963).

Central arterial pressure is sensed by the baroreceptors mainly in the carotid sinus and aortic arch. Standing after lying has the effect of increasing heart rate by about 25 beats/min and increasing total peripheral resistance by about 25% (Table 3.3.3).[40] There are quite different effects on different local vascular beds, however. There are significant changes in the vascular resistance of the splanchnic and muscular beds but practically none in the skin vessels (Attinger, 1976b). The operation of the baroreflex appears to be relatively independent of central neural influences (Attinger, 1976b).

There is an inverse correspondence between carotid sinus pressure and systemic arterial pressure; that is, an increase in carotid sinus pressure causes a corresponding decrease in arterial

TABLE 3.3.3   Average Effect on the Cardiovascular System of Rising from the Supine to the Upright Position

Variable	Change
Arterial blood pressure	$0 \, kN/m^2$
Central venous pressure	$-400 \, N/m^2$
Heart rate	$+0.42$ beats/sec
Abdominal and limb flow	-25%
Cardiac output	-25%
Stroke volume	-40%
Abdominal and limb resistance	$+$ (variable)
Total peripheral resistance	$+25\%$
Small vein pressure	$+1.3 \, kN/m^2$
Pooled blood (mostly venous)	$-400 \times 10^{-6} \, m^3$

Source: Adapted and used with permission from Greg, 1961.

[38] Both parasympathetic and sympathetic systems directly affect heart rate. This rate action is called a chronotropic effect. Stimulation by the sympathetic system, moreover, increases myocardial contractility. This is called a positive inotropic effect.

[39] The vagus can affect heart rate very rapidly. Sympathetic control, however, is relatively slow (Scher, 1966b).

[40] Since vagal heart rate response is much faster than sympathetic response, initial compensation to postural change is likely to be vagal. Sympathetic effects on heart rate and blood vessel resistance occur later (Scher, 1966b).

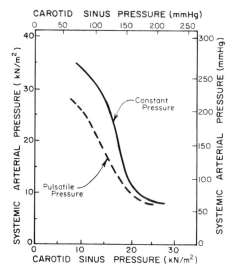

Figure 3.3.5 Relationship between mean carotid sinus pressure and mean systemic arterial pressure. The similarity between these two pressures and the neural output from the carotid sinus (Figure 3.3.2) should be noted. (Adapted and used with permission from Korner, 1971.)

pressure. There is a strong similarity between the carotid sinus firing rate curve (Figure 3.3.2) and the systemic pressure response curve (Figure 3.3.5) when the systemic pressure response curve is inverted.

Incremental gain of the system, usually defined as change in output divided by change of input, varies with pressure. It is a maximum where the slope of the systemic pressure response curve is a maximum.[41] In Figure 3.3.5, this occurs at nearly normal carotid sinus pressure of 16.7 kN/m² [data for dog (Scher, 1966b)].

Since incremental gain is not constant, it is not surprising that the arterial pressure response for a pulsatile pressure is not the same as for a constant pressure. Since incremental gain decreases away from a pressure corresponding to gain maximum, arterial pressure response is lower for a pressure pulsating between maximum gain pressure and some lower pressure.

Since pressures are sensed at two main locations (carotid sinus and aortic arch), it is of interest to know that somewhat the same systemic arterial response can be obtained from increased pressure on any one location. That is, the magnitude of the overall effect does not correspond to the algebraic sum of the individual effects (Attinger, 1976b) but instead appears to be a case of biological redundancy. The open-loop gain of the aortic arch appears to be one-quarter to one-half that of the carotid sinus receptors (Burton, 1965).

Scher (1966b) has given an analysis of the systemic arterial baroreceptor reflex. An approximation to the variable gain in Figure 3.3.5 is

$$\frac{\Delta p_\alpha}{\Delta p_s} = -\left[\frac{\Delta p_\alpha}{\Delta p_s}\Big|\text{max} + \beta_1 (p_s - p_{s\text{max}})^n \right] \qquad (3.3.4)$$

where Δp_α = change in output (arterial) pressure, N/m²
Δp_s = change in input (carotid sinus) pressure, N/m²
p_s = carotid sinus pressure, N/m²
$p_{s\text{max}}$ = carotid sinus pressure corresponding to the maximum gain, $(\Delta p_\alpha/\Delta p_s)|$max, N/m²
β_1 = coefficient, (m²/N)^n
n = an even number, dimensionless

---

[41] Scher (1966b) reports a maximal gain of 10–15 in some cats.

To account for the effects of pulsatile pressure, where a varying carotid sinus pressure decreases the resulting arterial pressure despite maintenance of a constant mean pressure, a recitification equation has been proposed. Also included in this equation is the observation that as the frequency or amplitude of these changes increases, arterial pressure falls further (Scher, 1966b).

$$\Delta \bar{p}_\alpha = -G(p_s + dp_s/dt - \beta_2)[\text{Sgn}(p_s + dp_s/dt - \beta_2)] \tag{3.3.5}$$

where $\Delta \bar{p}_\alpha$ = change in mean output pressure due to pulsating carotid sinus pressure, N/m^2

$\quad\quad t$ = time, sec

$\quad\quad \beta_2$ = constant, N/m^2

$\quad\quad G$ = amplification factor, dimensionless

$\text{Sgn}(x) = +1, \quad x > 0$

$\quad\quad\quad = -1, \quad x < 0$

Finally, to describe the pressure response to transient changes, notably square- and sine-wave inputs, Scher (1966b) presents a linear approximation. Response to an input pressure square wave is composed of a 2–4.5 sec period before any response, followed by an early overshoot and then a slow (up to 100 sec) decline to the new level.

$$\beta_3 \frac{dp_\alpha}{dt} + \beta_4 \frac{d^2 p_\alpha}{dt^2} = \frac{dp_s}{dt}[\delta(t - t_d)] \tag{3.3.6}$$

where β_3 = coefficient, dimensionless

$\quad\quad \beta_4$ = coefficient, $sec \cdot m^2/N$

$\quad\quad t_d$ = time delay

$\delta(t - t_d) = 1, \quad t > t_d$

$\quad\quad\quad = 0, \quad t_d < t$

There are other cardiovascular reflexes with neural origin. A pulmonary artery baroreceptor reflex primarily controls respiration by reducing ventilation by approximately 20% for each $130\,N/m^2$ rise in pulmonary arterial pressure; cardiovascular effects become significant when arterial pressure change exceeds $8\,kN/m^2$ (Attinger, 1976b). Cardiac mechanoreceptor reflexes are similar to, but much weaker than, the carotid sinus reflex; when strongly stimulated, epicardial and ventricular receptors produce bradycardia, hypotension, and reduced respiration (Attinger, 1976b). The arterial chemoreceptor reflex most strongly affects respiration, but it does have cardiovascular consequences; hypoxia and hypercapnia result in bradycardia, total peripheral resistance increase, arterial blood pressure increase, and catecholamine secretion increase.

Heart rate is accelerated, and consequent blood pressure is increased, by decreased baroreceptor activity, respiratory inspiration, excitement, anger, painful stimuli, anoxia, exercise, and humoral agents (Faucheux et al., 1983; Lindqvist et al., 1983). Heart rate is slowed by increased baroreceptor activity, expiration,[42] fear, grief, the diving reflex, and increased intracranial pressure (Ganong, 1963). Tranel et al. (1982) demonstrated that monetary rewards were sufficient to cause significant changes in heart rate when they were given to test subjects for desired heart rate modifications.

3.3.2 Humoral Regulation

Not all cardiovascular regulation is neural. Circulating hormones, metabolites, and regulators also have cardiovascular effects. These are effective mostly at the local level. For instance,

[42] Mehlsen et al. (1987) report that suddenly initiated (stepwise) inspiration and expiration both resulted in an increase in heart rate followed by a rapid decrease in heart rate. Heart rate was thus seen to respond to changes in lung volume. Coherent changes in heart rate and breathing are commonly referred to as respiratory sinus arrhythmia (Kenney, 1985).

chemical substances that directly act on arteriole muscle fibers to cause local vasodilation are decreased oxygen partial pressure, decreased blood and tissue pH, increased carbon dioxide pressure (especially vasodilates the skin and brain), lactic acid, and adenylic acid (Ganong, 1963).[43] Histamine released from damaged cells dilates capillaries and increases their permeability (Ganong, 1963). Bradykinin secreted by sweat glands, salivary glands, and the exocrine portion of the pancreas vasodilates these secreting tissues (Ganong, 1963).

Other substances cause vasoconstriction. Injured arteries and arterioles constrict from serotonin liberated from platelets sticking to vessel walls (Ganong, 1963). Norepinephrine has a general vasoconstrictor action. Diurnal variations of norepinephrine have been found to be associated with a mean arterial blood pressure 3700 N/m^2 (28 mm Hg) lower during the middle of the night than during the day (Richards et al., 1986). Epinephrine is also a general vasoconstrictor in all but the liver and skeletal muscle, which it vasodilates. The net effect of epinephrine is thus a decrease in total peripheral resistance (Ganong, 1963).

Norepinephrine and epinephrine both increase the force and rate of contraction of the isolated heart (Ganong, 1963). Norepinephrine increases systolic and diastolic blood pressure, which, in turn, stimulates the aortic and carotid sinus baroreceptors to produce bradycardia, leading to decreased cardiac output. Norepinephrine, epinephrine, and thyroxin all increase heart rate (Ganong, 1963). It is likely that prostaglandins will also be found to have cardiovascular regulatory roles.

3.3.3 Other Regulatory Effects

Other effects are locally important in cardiovascular regulation. We have already noted Starling's law (Section 3.2.3), which increases the contractility of myocardium in response to preload. This is important for equalization of cardiac output between the left and right hearts.

Temperature is also an important cardiovascular regulator. High environmental temperature or fever increases heart rate. A rise in temperature in muscle tissue directly causes arteriole vasodilation (Ganong, 1963).

Total blood volume is controlled indirectly through capillary pressure (see Section 3.2.2). When capillary pressure increases, fluid leaks into the cellular interstitium. When capillary pressure falls below its normal value of about 3300 N/m^2, fluid is absorbed into the circulatory system. Capillary pressure is controlled indirectly by the same artery and venous innervation that controls blood pressure.

Renal output also can be used to control total blood volume.[44] Hemorrhage usually results in a large reduction of urinary output, and fluid infusion stimulates urinary production. These adjustments are long term, however, and require a day or more to complete; capillary fluid shift requires only a few hours (Beneken and DeWit, 1967).

This mix of neural, humoral, and other local mechanisms allows cardiovascular adjustments to be very efficient. The redundancy of effects underscores the importance of the cardiovascular system.

3.3.4 Exercise

All previously presented effects are manifested during exercise (Hammond and Froelicher, 1985). Exercise increases carbon dioxide production by the muscles, which, in turn, increases venous $p\mathrm{CO_2}$, and this stimulates cardiovascular responses. Heart rate increases, stroke volume

---

[43] Adenylic acid is another term for adenosine monophosphate, or AMP, the energy-poor precursor of adenosine triphosphate, or ATP.

[44] Reeve and Kulhanek (1967) outlined an interesting, if rudimentary, model of body water content regulation. This mathematical model includes elements of urinary water excretion and drinking set in a context of a water balance for the entire body.

remains nearly the same, and cardiac output increases (Figure 3.3.6). The increase in heart rate is nearly linear with work rate (Equation 3.2.42),[45] except near maximum oxygen uptake where gains in oxygen uptake depend not only on the amount of blood delivered to the tissues (as indicated by heart rate) but also on the oxygen-carrying capacity of the blood (as indicated by pO_2). Venous pO_2 falls near maximum oxygen uptake, meaning that the muscles are increasing oxygen use without a concomitant increase in heart rate.

Blood volume is moved from the venous side of the heart to the arterial side during exercise. Stroke volume may actually fall during maximal exercise because venous return is insufficient to completely fill the atrium during each heartbeat. Venous return is enhanced by muscle pumping.

Cardiac output, composed of stroke volume and heart rate, increases to a maximum value at maximal oxygen uptake. If no differences in arterial-to-venous pO_2 occur, oxygen uptake is directly related to cardiac output.

The increase in heart rate occurring at the beginning of exercise is very rapid (Figure 3.3.7). Sometimes the increase even precedes the start of exercise, which indicates that neural control from higher nervous centers (through the sympathetic nervous system), rather than arterial pO_2 or pCO_2 changes, are at least temporarily dominant (see Jones and Johnson, 1980; Mitchell, 1985; Perski et al., 1985).

The increase of heart rate is higher for a given oxygen uptake for arm exercise compared to leg exercise. Moving the arms above the head increases heart rate more than moving the arms below the neck. Static (isometric) exercise increases heart rate disproportionately to that expected from oxygen uptake alone.

Increased muscle temperature, increased carbon dioxide concentration, decreased pH, and decreased oxygen concentration all have local vasodilatory effects. Blood flow through working muscle is thus increased. Central nervous system control of vessel caliber is added to local effects, thus shifting blood flow from regions with lower oxygen demand (especially the viscera) to regions with higher demand. Total peripheral resistance decreases. Because of this, diastolic pressures may actually decrease (although they may increase) somewhat despite higher blood flows (Comess and Fenster, 1981). Systolic pressures increase and mean blood pressure increases during exercise.

Females generally tend to exhibit higher heart rates than males at comparable percentages of maximal oxygen uptake. Trained athletes have no higher maximum heart rates than untrained individuals.[46] However, they usually develop larger hearts capable of delivering larger stroke volumes. For any rate of oxygen uptake, athletes' hearts are able to deliver the required output with lower heart rates than can untrained individuals.

The cardiac hypertrophy developed in trained individuals is difficult to distinguish from similar conditions developed by individuals with impaired cardiac function (Schaible and Scheuer, 1985). The athletic heart, however, exhibits enhanced performance,[47] whereas pathologic cardiac hypertrophy is an adjustment made by parts of the heart to overcome shortcomings of other parts of the cardiovascular system.

Chemical changes that occur improve oxygen transport to the muscles (including the myocardium). The hemoglobin dissociation curve (Figures 3.2.1 through 3.2.3) shifts with increased pCO_2, decreased pH, and increased temperature to deliver oxygen with greater ease to the working muscles. That is, for any given percentage saturation, the factors just cited tend to increase plasma pO_2 and allow more O_2 to move into the interstitial fluid and muscle cells.

Muscle oxygen consumption, by these mechanisms, can increase above resting values by 75–100 times. Even higher increases are possible for very limited amounts of time by utilizing anaerobic metabolism.

---

[45] Except for an additional increment of heart rate increase with increased deep body temperature (see Section 3.4.5).

[46] Erikssen and Rodahl (1979) showed that seasonal variations in physical fitness can exist in a population. Because of this, comparisons of results between exercise tests conducted at different times of the year may be invalid.

[47] This cardiac condition is even marked by electrocardiographic (ECG) signals that resemble those from severely ill patients.

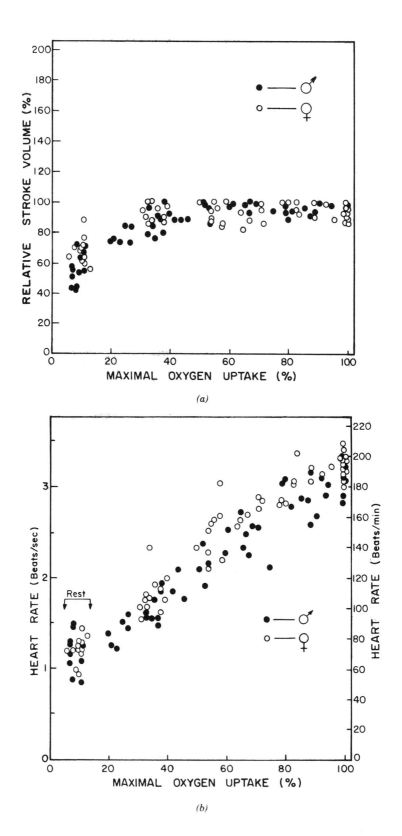

(a)

(b)

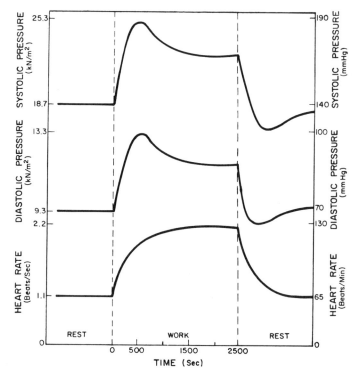

Figure 3.3.7 Somewhat idealized diagram of transient cardiovascular response to exercise. Heart rate appears to change with a single time constant, but diastolic and systolic pressures overshoot and decay toward their final values.

3.3.5 Heat and Cold Stress

Responses to heat involve cardiovascular mechanisms, most of which are described in Section 5.3.3. Vascular adjustments to heat allow more blood to reach the skin, where heat can be exchanged with the environment (Brengelmann, 1983). Cardiac adjustments include an increased heart rate when deep body temperature rises. Over a period of several days' exposure to elevated environmental temperatures, plasma volume increases to accommodate the dual demands upon the blood of heat loss and oxygen and nutrient supply to the muscles.

There are times when these dual demands cause conflict. When these adjustments cannot remove sufficient body heat, the condition of heat stroke occurs. Exactly why this occurs is open to speculation, but Hales (1986) describes the scenario in this way. The diversion of blood to the skin and the increase in cardiac output accompanying extreme heat stress greatly reduce the volume of blood in the veins supplying the heart. This reduction in central venous pressure is sensed by low-pressure baroreceptors and is responded to by a marked skin vasoconstriction. This greatly reduces the ability of the body to lose heat and a thermal overload results. Others (Brück, 1986; Kirsch et al., 1986; Senay, 1986; Wenger, 1986) have given further evidence that at times the maintenance of blood pressure takes precedence over heat loss, resulting in cutaneous vasoconstriction.

Figure 3.3.6 Stroke volume and heart rate with normalized oxygen uptake. Stroke volume quickly reaches a maximum and remains at that value. Heart rate climbs almost perfectly linearly with severity of exercise. (Adapted and used with permission from Astrand and Rodahl, 1970.)

Cardiovascular responses to cold environments are characterized by cutaneous vasoconstriction to maintain body heat. Wagner and Horvath (1985) reported that men exposed to cold air reacted with increased stroke volume and decreased heart rate. Women exposed to the same environments showed no such change [although Stevens et al. (1987) reported heart rate decreases in men but a slight increase in women, both exposed to cold stress]. Total peripheral resistance of older subjects exposed to cold environments increased more than did that of younger subjects (Wagner and Horvath, 1985). The increase in resistance was so great, in fact, that the resulting increase in mean arterial pressure could cause difficulties for hypertensive[48] or angina-prone[49] individuals exposed to the cold. They also reported a 10% increase in cardiac output to service increased oxygen demands of shivering.

3.4 CARDIOVASCULAR MECHANICAL MODELS

Cardiovascular mechanical models are intended to conceptualize the mechanics of the cardiovascular system. For physiologists, these models are more likely to be in pictorial or graphic form; for bioengineers, these models are more likely to be mathematical in nature. All models of biological systems must include the essentials of the processes described, but these models must be simplifications of reality. Because the cardiovascular system is complicated and includes much of the physical body, cardiovascular models have generally been limited to descriptions of one or two aspects of the system. We have already seen at least one model of this type in the discussion of the Fahraeus–Lindqvist effect in very small blood vessels (Section 3.2.2).

Attempts have been made to incorporate cardiodynamics into models of the vascular tree to predict parameters which can be compared to experimental observations. These attempts have included lumped-parameter mechanical models and distributed-parameter mechanical models.[50]

Use of limited models for prediction of exercise results is not very productive because of the all-inclusive nature of exercise response. We deal with some of these limited models only because it is possible that they might become elements in more comprehensive cardiovascular models. Several general cardiovascular mechanics models are described. We also briefly discuss optimization models in the heart. Finally, two models of a more unrefined, but perhaps useful nature, dealing with heart rate response to exercise challenge, are discussed.

3.4.1 Robinson's Ventricle Model

Heart mechanics, especially those of the left ventricle, have been the object of many models (Perl et al., 1986; Sorek and Sideman, 1986a, b). Robinson's model (1965; Attinger, 1976c; Talbot and Gessner, 1973) was developed to test changes of cardiac output with differences of heart muscle mechanics as given by Starling's law (see Section 3.2.3). As such, it is a lumped-parameter mechanical model of the heart and blood vessels. Robinson began at the level of the myocardium

---

[48] Hypertension is the term given to conditions marked by high blood pressure. Should blood pressure become too high, it can overcome the strength of the walls of the blood vessels and blood would burst out into surrounding tissue. The thinning, stretching, and bulging of weakened blood vessel walls is called an aneurysm, and when a ruptured aneurysm appears in the brain a stroke may result.

[49] Angina pectoris is the condition where severe chest pain due to ischemia (lack of oxygen leading to tissue necrosis) in the myocardium is caused by inadequate coronary blood circulation.

[50] Lumped-parameter models assume the entire model segment can be replaced by a very small number of elements, each usually representing one property of the segment. Any spatial dependence of these properties is neglected. Nonlinearities can be included, but waves and other spatial–temporal effects cannot be predicted. Distributed-parameter models are often similar to a large number of lumped-parameter models of subsegments and, because they can account for spatial dependence of segment properties, can reproduce wave behavior. Modeling the vascular system as one resistance, inertance, and compliance is an example of a lumped-parameter model. A distributed-parameter model would include many resistance, inertance, and compliance elements with many interconnections.

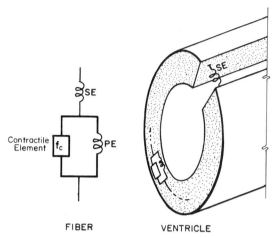

Figure 3.4.1 The three-element model of the myocardium. The output of the force source f_c depends on the length of the parallel element PE and its rate of shortening. Total muscle length equals the length of PE and the shorter length of the series element SE. The force source is assumed to be active only during systole and to be freely distensible in passive muscle. (Used with Permission from Talbot and Gessner, 1973.)

(Figure 3.4.1) by assuming each muscle fiber to be effectively given by a contractile element in parallel with an elastic element and in series with another elastic element (Mende and Cuervo, 1976; Phillips et al., 1982). The force source[51] produces a force magnitude depending on the length of the parallel elastic element and on its rate of shortening. Total muscle fiber length is the length of the parallel element (or force source) plus the length of the series element. When muscle fibers are combined into a ventricle model, force elements are all lumped together and series elastic elements are lumped together. Thus the concept of ventricular contraction consists of a force developed by the force elements forcing blood into the elastic portion with concurrent pressure buildup (Figure 3.4.2). The rate of change of volume (dV/dt) is limited by a resistance element which assumes a higher value (R_s) in systole compared to diastole (R_d). Aortic valve resistance (R_{av}) to outflow and mitral valve resistance (R_{mv}) to inflow are included. Series element compliance (C_{se}) is included in the elastic portion.

Robinson developed the following differential equation for intraventricular systolic pressure. Beginning with a pressure balance on the ventricle, intraventricular pressure equals the pressure developed by the muscle from which is subtracted pressure dissipated through viscous resistance (actually negative, since dV/dt is negative during systole) and pressure used to overcome compliance; since $V = Cp$, $C(dp/dt)$ is equivalent to dV/dt,

$$p = p_s + R_s \frac{dV}{dt} - R_s C_{se} \frac{dp}{dt} \qquad (3.4.1)$$

where C_{se} = series element compliance, m^5/N
   p = intraventricular pressure, N/m^2
   V = total ventricular volume (contractile plus elastic compartments), m^3
   R_s = internal ventricular viscous resistance during systole, N·sec/m^5
   p_s = isometrically developed muscle pressure during systole, N/m^2

[51] Force, pressure, voltage, and temperature are examples of effort variables. An ideal effort source is characterized by a constant effort no matter what the flow. Hence ideal effort sources have zero internal impedances (impedance equals change in effort divided by change in flow). Fluid flow, electrical current, and heat are examples of flow variables. Ideal flow sources are characterized by constant flow rates no matter what effort must be expended to do so. Hence ideal flow sources have infinite internal impedance.

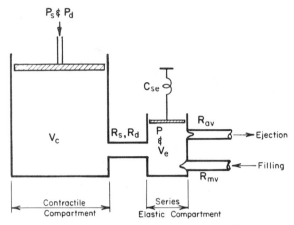

Figure 3.4.2 Principle elements of a ventricle model including internal resistance, which limits outflow velocity. Included are systolic and diastolic pressures (p_s and p_d), flow-limiting resistances during systole and diastole (R_s and R_d), aortic valve and mitral valve resistance (R_{av} and R_{mv}), and a series element compliance (C_{se}). Although this model divides the ventricle into two conceptual chambers, both together represent the entire ventricle, that is, $V = V_c + V_e$. (Used with permission from Talbot and Gessner, 1973.)

During diastole, a similar pressure balance yields an equation nearly identical to that for systole, with the exception that diastolic muscle pressure and viscous resistance replace those for systole. Robinson chose to allow the change from R_s to R_d to occur smoothly at the beginning of diastole by introducing the transition term $(R_s - R_d)e^{-t/\tau_d}$. Thus effective resistance during diastole begins as R_s and decreases rapidly to R_d.[52]

$$p = p_d + [(R_s - R_d)e^{-t/\tau_d} + R_d]\left[\frac{dV}{dt} - C_{se}\frac{dp}{dt}\right] \tag{3.4.2}$$

where R_d = internal ventricular viscous resistance during diastole, N·sec/m^5

p_d = static pressure developed by relaxed muscle, N/m^2

t = time, which begins at zero at the beginning of each diastole, sec

τ_d = time constant for myocardial relaxation, sec

Robinson solved his equations on an analog computer,[53] which switched between systole and diastole. Final values for ventricular volume V, intraventricular pressure p, and arterial pressure p_a during one stage were introduced as initial values during the next stage. After a number of cycles, an equilibrium was reached wherein no further change was noted from one cardiac cycle to the next, and this was taken to be the steady-state solution.

Robinson assumed a fixed heart rate of 2 bps, a ratio of systolic duration to diastolic duration of 2:3, and a time constant (τ_d) value of 0.05 sec. Numerical values of other constants for a 98.1 N (10 kg) dog are listed in Table 3.4.1. These values are based on experimental observations from muscle fibers, which are difficult to obtain. Therefore, these values should be considered approximate only.

The values of pressures developed by relaxed (p_d) and contracting (p_s) muscle were also developed from experimental observations on isolated myocardial fibers. Robinson approximated the elastic properties of passive heart muscle as illustrated in Figure 3.4.3. Negative pressures are required to decrease the volume below 5 cm^3 and elastic elements become stiffer at large volumes.

[52] In Robinson's original published paper, the term dV/dt is printed erroneously as dt/dV.

[53] See Appendix 3.1 for a short discussion on the means to simulate these and other model differential equations on the digital computer.

TABLE 3.4.1   Numerical Values for Robinson Model Parameters for a 98 N Dog

Parameter	Value[a]	
Heart rate	2 bps	
Systole/diastole times	2:3	
Time constant (τ_d)	0.05 sec	
Resistance of contracting muscle (R_s)	333×10^6 N·sec/m^5	(2.50 mm Hg·sec/mL)
Resistance of relaxed muscle (R_d)	12.8×10^6 N·sec/m^5	(0.096 mm Hg·sec/mL)
Total peripheral resistance (R_p)	577×10^6 N·sec/m^5	(4.33 mm Hg·sec/mL)
Resistance of aortic valve (R_{av})	4.40×10^6 N·sec/m^5	(0.033 mm Hg·sec/mL)
Resistance to filling (R_v)	2.12×10^6 N·sec/m^5	(0.0159 mm Hg·sec/mL)
Compliance of ventricle (C_{se})	19.2×10^{-9} m^5/N	(0.0256 mL/mm Hg)
Compliance of arterial system (C_p)	1.44×10^{-9} m^5/N	(0.192 mL/mm Hg)
Filling pressure (P_v)	800 N/m^2	(6 mm Hg)

[a]Compiled from Robinson, 1965.

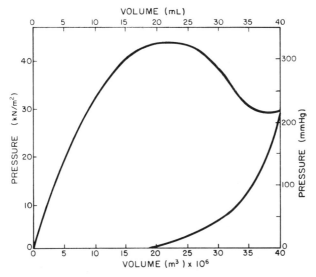

Figure 3.4.3 Isometric elastic properties of heart muscle for the 10 kg dog. Pressure–volume data for systole are given by the upper curve and data for diastole by the lower curve. The slope of a line drawn from the origin to any point on the curve gives the inverse of the static compliance. At large volumes the elastic elements in the heart become stiffer. Negative pressures are needed to reduce diastolic volume below 5 cc. (Adapted and used with permission from Robinson, 1965.)

Total available isometric pressure p_s is the sum of relaxed muscle pressure p_d and additional contractile element pressure. Robinson approximated this by the parabolic relation

$$p_s = p_d + (42.6 \times 10^3)\left[1 - \left(1 - \frac{V}{20 \times 10^{-6}}\right)^2 \right] \tag{3.4.3}$$

Atrial action was neglected in this study (Talbot and Gessner, 1973). The ventricle model received blood from a simplified mathematical model of the pulmonary veins and delivered it to a model of the systemic arterial circulation. The arterial circulation was approximated as a lumped compliance in parallel with the total peripheral resistance (Equation 3.3.3) and in series with the aortic valve resistance. Pressure balances give, for systole (Talbot and Gessner, 1973),

$$R_p C_p \frac{dp}{dt} + p + R_p R_{av} C_p \frac{d^2 V}{dt^2} + (R_p + R_{av}) \frac{dV}{dt} = 0 \tag{3.4.4}$$

where R_p = total peripheral resistance, $N \cdot sec/m^5$
$\quad C_p$ = effective arterial distensibility, m^5/N
$\quad p$ = intraventricular pressure, N/m^2
$\quad R_{av}$ = aortic valve resistance, $N \cdot sec/m^5$
$\quad V$ = ventricular volume, m^3
$\quad p_a$ = arterial pressure, N/m^2

The term $R_p R_{av} C_p$ is equivalent to an inertance as blood enters the aorta. For diastole, when no blood flows from the ventricle,

$$R_p C_p \frac{dp_a}{dt} + P_a = 0 \tag{3.4.5}$$

Numerical values for constants can be found in Table 3.4.1.

The venous inflow source is approximated by an $800 \ N/m^2$ (6 mm Hg) pressure source and a resistance representing losses in veins, atrium, and mitral valve. Inflow occurs only during diastole:

$$p = p_v - R_v \frac{dV}{dt} \tag{3.4.6}$$

where p = intraventricular pressure, N/m^2
$\quad p_v$ = filling pressure in the pulmonary venous reservoir, N/m^2
$\quad R_v$ = resistance to inflow, $N \cdot sec/m^5$
$\quad V$ = ventricular volume, m^3

Robinson found that ventricular flow was largely unaffected by changes in arterial impedance. Thus the ventricle appears to act as a flow source where flow is largely independent of peripheral load. When filling pressure was increased from $1866 \ N/m^2$ (14 mm Hg) to $3333 \ N/m^2$ (25 mm Hg), stroke volume was found to increase linearly from 12 to $14 \ cm^3$, mean arterial pressure increased from 13.3 to $15.3 \ kN/m^2$, and stroke work increased from 0.16 to $0.21 \ N \cdot m$. This is mathematical confirmation of Starling's law (see Section 3.2.3). The isolated ventricle model did not agree as well with experimental observations when peripheral resistance instead of filling pressure was increased.

3.4.2 Comprehensive Circulatory System Model

The model presented by Sandquist et al. (1982) is a comprehensive mechanical model of the entire human cardiovascular system. Three major subsystems of the heart, systemic circulation, and pulmonary circulation are included. Model equations are based on conservation of blood mass, conservation of energy of blood flow, conservation of momentum of blood flow, and equations of state describing system compliance. This model is much more comprehensive than that by Robinson, in that it includes more elaborate circulatory elements. It does not, however, treat the left ventricle in as much detail as Robinson's model, and it does not include the control aspects included in the model by Benekin and DeWit (1967) to be presented in detail in Section 3.5. This model is mentioned here, however, because of the clarity of its description, and the reader is referred to Sandquist et al. for an example of construction methods in mathematical model building.

3.4.3 Vascular System Models

Many vascular system models have been proposed (Attinger, 1976c; Linehan and Dawson, 1983; Noordergraaf, 1978; Skalak and Schmid-Schönbein, 1986; Talbot and Gessner, 1973). Most of these have been used to attempt to explain the temporal and spatial nature of pressure waves appearing in the vascular tree. Although they may include the entire systemic circulation from

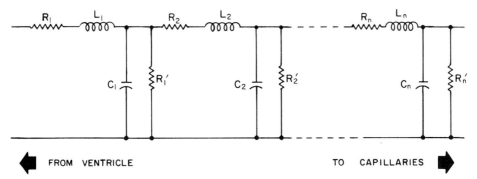

Figure 3.4.4 Transmission line analog of the arterial tree. R_i accounts for viscous resistance to fluid flow, R_i' accounts for shunt flow between arterial and venous circulation, L_i accounts for inertance of flowing blood and arterial tissue, and C_i accounts for compliance of arterial walls. These quantities, although not completely distributed along the artery analog, are nevertheless included in small enough "lumps" to act like a completely distributed parameter system.

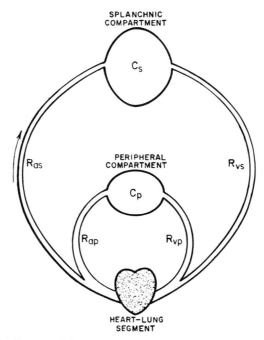

Figure 3.4.5 Schematic diagram of the two-compartment model of Green and Jackman (1984). The splanchnic compartment includes all blood flowing through the hepatic veins. The peripheral compartment comprises all other blood, including blood in the working muscles. Both compartments include elements of arterial resistance R_a, compliance C, and venous resistance R_v. Green and Jackman used their simple model to simulate the effects of exercise on cardiac output. (Adapted and used with permission from Green and Jackman, 1984.)

arteries through veins, most of these models do not elucidate mechanisms of exercise. Indeed, it is within these models that distributed parameters are most likely to be seen. Many researchers have extended the analogy between the systemic circulation and transmission lines (Figure 3.4.4). The resulting equations, although simple, are very numerous. Details are more likely to be reproduced with distributed parameters, but conceptual understanding is easier to obtain from the compact form of a few simple equations resulting from a lumped-parameter model. The reader is invited to look further into these models, but their use in exercise currently is nearly nonexistent.

Green and Jackman (1984) presented a two-compartment lumped-parameter model which depended strongly on vascular characteristics. The objective of their model was to predict changes in cardiac output occurring during exercise. The model consisted of two parallel vascular channels: the splanchnic channel, which included all blood flowing through the hepatic vein, and the peripheral channel, which included all other vascular beds (Figure 3.4.5). The exercise condition was simulated by decreasing compliances of both channels to 40% of their resting values and by adjusting each resistance such that the percentage of total cardiac output perfusing the splanchnic compartment fell from 38 to 5% while that perfusing the peripheral compartment (including skeletal muscles) increased from 62 to 95%. These combined changes increased total cardiac output from 7.3×10^{-5} to 37×10^{-5} m^3/sec (4.4 to 22 L/min), a result very similar to that found in humans. This result was achieved with active control exerted only on the vasculature and not on the heart.

3.4.4 Optimization Models

As discussed in Section 3.2.3, there is reason to suspect that cardiac events are determined by processes which optimize these events. Of the possible optimization determinants, mechanical energy expenditure is the one that has most recently received attention (Hämäläinen et al., 1982; Livnat and Yamashiro, 1981; Yamashiro et al., 1979). The oxygen cost of moving blood is very high—at least five times that for moving an equivalent amount of air (Yamashiro et al., 1979)—and the respiratory system has been shown to operate in agreement with a minimum energy expenditure criterion, so it is expected that ventricular ejection occurs in a manner which reduces ventricular energy to a minimum.

Several attempts have been made to formulate and solve this problem to yield realistic results. There is no reason to suspect that the current flurry of activity to include further refinements is over. Therefore, while the model described here reasonably accurately predicts ventricular systolic events, the promise of extensions to other cardiovascular events remains strong.[54]

Livnat and Yamashiro (1981) presented a model for prediction of left ventricular dynamics derived from a minimization of work expended during systole. Their model is seen in Figure 3.4.6. The ventricle and arterial load was assumed to consist of a time-varying ventricular compliance C_v, blood inertia I_b, valvular resistances R_{av} and R_b, total peripheral resistance R_p, and arterial compliance C_p. The equation of motion relating left ventricular pressure and aortic pressure to left ventricular outflow is

$$p - p_{ao} = (R_{av} + R_b)\frac{dV}{dt} + I_b\frac{d^2V}{dt^2}$$

(3.4.7)

where p = intraventricular pressure, N/m^2
  p_{ao} = pressure in the ascending aorta, N/m^2
  R_{av} = constant aortic valve resistance, N·sec/m^5
  R_b = nonconstant aortic valve resistance, N·sec/m^5

---

[54] Indeed, Murray (1926) discussed the size of the blood vessels in relation to the work of the flow of blood through them, their sizes seemingly determined to minimize the rates of work through them.

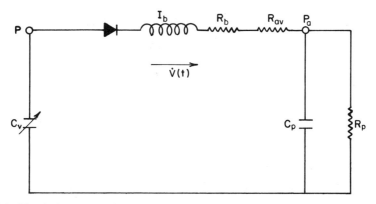

Figure 3.4.6   Electrical analog of the left ventricle and its arterial load. The ventricle is diagramed as a time-varying mechanical compliance generating a ventricular pressure p. Blood is ejected through the aortic valve, which has properties of a diode in series with a resistance, composed of a constant R_b and nonconstant R_{av} term. Total systemic circulation is diagramed as a compliance C_p in parallel with a resistance R_p. The combination of R_b and R_{av}, C_p, and R_p is commonly called the electrical analog of the modified Windkessel model. (Used with permission from Livnat and Yamashiro, 1981.)

V = ventricular volume, m³
I_b = blood inertance, N·sec²/m⁵
t = time, sec
and, from Bernoulli's equation,

$$R_b = \left(\frac{\rho}{2A^2}\right)\frac{dV}{dt} \qquad (3.4.8)$$

where ρ = blood density, kg/m³ or N·sec²/m⁴
     A = cross-sectional area of the aorta, m²
Because it is the column of blood in the aorta that must be accelerated by the ventricle, the value of blood inertance is the inertia of a column of blood having a length equal to that of the left ventricular inner radius and diameter equal to the aortic diameter.
   For the peripheral arterial circulation, a pressure balance gives

$$p_a - R_p\frac{dV}{dt} = 0 \qquad (3.4.9)$$

where R_p = total peripheral resistance, N·sec/m⁵
     V_r = volume of blood delivered to the peripheral resistance, m³

$$V_r = V - V_c \qquad (3.4.10)$$

where V_c = volume of blood delivered to peripheral compliance, m³

$$V_c = C_p p_a \qquad \text{and} \qquad \frac{dV_c}{dt} = C_p\frac{dp}{dt} \qquad (3.4.11)$$

where C_p = arterial compliance, m⁵/N

Therefore,

$$p_a - R_p \frac{dV}{dt} + C_p R_p \frac{dp_a}{dt} = 0 \qquad (3.4.12)$$

Equations 3.4.7 through 3.4.12 form a complete dynamic description of the left ventricle and systemic arterial load.

A proper variable to be optimized would be myocardial oxygen consumption rather than ventricular work. Livnat and Yamashiro (1981), however, chose to minimize external work performed by the ventricle because oxygen consumption of the myocardium is very high and a significant oxygen debt cannot be incurred. There is therefore a direct correspondence between oxygen consumption and external work. Note, however, that ventricular isovolumic contraction, basal oxygen consumption, and diastolic oxygen consumption were all ignored.

The cost functional[55] suggested by Livnat and Yamashiro (1981) is composed of a wall stress contribution to ventricular work, a term representing inotropic state contributing to the rate of oxygen consumption, external mechanical pump work, and a term penalizing the duration of contraction. In formulating the first term, Livnat and Yamashiro assumed the ventricle wall to be spherically shaped and thin. Equation 3.2.37 relates shear stress to the dimensions of a cylinder. For a sphere shear stress is

$$\tau = \frac{pr}{2\Delta r} \qquad (3.4.13)$$

where τ = shear stress, N/m^2
$\quad p$ = ventricular pressure, N/m^2
$\quad r$ = ventricular radius, m
$\quad \Delta r$ = wall thickness, m

Expressing the sphere radius in terms of the volume,

$$\tau = \left(\frac{3}{4\pi}\right)^{1/3} \frac{pV^{1/3}}{2\Delta r} \qquad (3.4.14)$$

Systolic work is proportional to the difference between wall shear stress (or tension) and the shear stress present in the wall at the end of diastole (or beginning of systole), $\tau - \tau_0$. Integrating the square of the shear stress difference over the entire surface area of the shell and then integrating the resulting term over the entire time for systole gives a term representing the stored elastic energy involved in the contraction process:

$$E_1 = \int_0^{t_s} (\tau - \tau_o)^2 4\pi r^2 dt = \alpha_1 \int_0^{t_s} (\tau - \tau_o)^2 V^{2/3} dt \qquad (3.4.15)$$

where E_1 = internal energy, N·m
$\quad \tau_o$ = end-diastolic stress, N/m^2
$\quad t_s$ = period of systole, sec
$\quad \alpha_1$ = constant, $m^3/(N \cdot sec)$

The second term in Livnat and Yamashiro's (1981) cost functional concerns the contribution of inotropic state to the rate of oxygen consumption. They used an index of contractility suggested by Bloomfield et al. (1972), which has been shown to be sensitive to both positive and negative

---

[55] The mathematical description of the costs associated with various system inputs. The cost functional is usually maximized or minimized in optimization problems. See Section 4.3.4 and Appendix 4.2.

inotropic interventions and relatively insensitive to alterations in end-diastolic volume:

$$E_2 = \alpha_2 \int_0^{t_s} \left(\frac{dp}{dt}\right)^2 dt \tag{3.4.16}$$

where E_2 = contractile energy, N·m
  α_2 = constant, m^5/(N·sec)
External work is given by

$$E_3 = \int_0^{t_s} p\left(\frac{dV}{dt}\right) dt \tag{3.4.17}$$

where E_3 = external work, N·m

Further, Livnat and Yamashiro (1981) introduced a term to demonstrate the cost of a myocardial contraction on cardiac blood flow. During systole, blood flow in the myocardium suffers a mechanical interference from the contracting muscle. Strong contraction may stop muscle blood flow entirely. Tissue oxygen partial pressure can fall to extremely low levels. The longer the duration of contraction, the lower oxygen partial pressure will become.

For a given systolic time, oxygen content of the muscle will decrease as heart rate increases. Therefore, a term is introduced to account for the reduction of oxygen availability for systolic contraction:

$$E_4 = [\alpha_3(\mathrm{HR}) + \alpha_4]t_s \tag{3.4.18}$$

where E_4 = systolic contraction penalty, N·m
  α_3 = constant, N·m/beat
  α_4 = constant, N·m/sec
  HR = heart rate, beats/sec
The entire cost functional, the expression to be minimized, is

$$J = E_1 + E_2 + E_3 + E_4 \tag{3.4.19}$$

where J = cost functional, N·m
Specified boundary conditions are

$$p(0) = p_{ao} \tag{3.4.20}$$

$$V(0) = V_o, \qquad V(t_s) = V_o - V_s \tag{3.4.21}$$

$$\frac{dV}{dt}(0) = 0, \qquad \frac{dV}{dt}(t_s) = 0 \tag{3.4.22}$$

$$p_a(0) = p_{ao} \tag{3.4.23}$$

where p_{ao} = aortic pressure at the beginning of sytole, N/m^2
  V_o = end-diastolic volume, m^3
  V_s = end-systolic volume, m^3
The solution to be found involves the time course of ventricular pressure p which will minimize the cost functional J. The term R_b injects a severe nonlinearity into Equation 3.4.7, which precludes simple methods of analysis. The Pontryagin maximum principle (see Appendix 3.2) was used to solve the preceding system of equations numerically. The reader is referred to Livnat and Yamashiro (1981) for more details of the procedure.

Model parameters and initial conditions appear in Table 3.4.2. These are based on values

TABLE 3.4.2 Model Parameters and Initial Conditions for Livnat and Yamashiro Optimization Model

Parameter	Initial Condition[a]
End-diastolic volume (V_0)	20×10^{-6} m^3 (20 mL)
Stroke volume (V_s)	12×10^{-6} m^3 (12 mL)
Heart rate	2.42 beats/sec (145 beats/min)
Cardiac output (CO)	29.0×10^{-6} m^3/sec (1740 mL/min)
Mean arterial pressure (p_a)	13.3 kN/m^2 (100 mm Hg)
Blood inertance (I)	$400 V^{1/3}$ kN·sec^2/m^5 ($0.003 V^{1/3}$ mm Hg·sec/mL)
Total peripheral resistance (R_p)	627×10^6 N·sec/m^5 (4.7 mm Hg·sec/mL)
Resistance of aortic valve (R_{av})	400×10^3 N·sec/m^5 (0.003 mm Hg·sec/mL)
Compliance of arterial system (C_p)	1.34×10^{-6} m^5/N (1.78 mL/mm Hg)
α_1	357×10^{-6} m/sec (0.0357 cm/sec)
α_2	1.78×10^{-6} sec·m^5/N (0.0178 cm^3·sec/dyn)
α_3	22.6×10^{-6} N·m/beat (226 erg·min/beat·sec)
α_4	1.393×10^{-3} N·m/sec (1.393×10^4 ergs/sec)

Source: Adapted and used with permission from Livnat and Yamashiro, 1981.
[a]Several values were given by Livnat and Yamashiro with incorrect dimensions.

appearing in the literature, especially from Robinson (1965), whose model of the left ventricle we considered in Section 3.4.1.

The results obtained by Livnat and Yamashiro (1981) are indicated in Figure 3.4.7. Ventricular systolic pressure predicted from their model is at least qualitatively similar to experimental data from Greene et al. (1973). Comparison with experimental data from other sources also showed reasonable agreement. Livnat and Yamashiro also included isovolumic contraction in their ventricle model. Thus each ventricular contraction is considered to be composed of an isovolumic period and an ejection period. Livnat and Yamashiro allowed the time for each of these to be determined by their model. Figure 3.4.8 shows a comparison between predicted and observed values of both periods in dogs as heart rate changes. Predicted and observed data both show modest decreases as heart rate increases.

Heart failure was simulated by decreasing contractile energy and increasing end-diastolic volume while maintaining cardiac output constant. Results appear in Table 3.4.3. Peak ventricular pressure decreases sharply when myocardial strength is diminished. Both isovolumic contraction and ejection times are significantly prolonged. As the heart weakens, isovolumic contraction period lengthens and the Starling mechanism (see Section 3.2.3) must be used to maintain the same level of stroke volume.

As previously discussed, the nonlinearity of this model posed difficulty for its solution. Livnat and Yamashiro (1981) were obliged to use a blood inertance value 73% higher than the experimentally observed value in order to assure stability of solution. Hämäläinen et al. (1982) also point out that the model solution is very sensitive to boundary values used and that care must be exercised in choosing proper values.

Hämäläinen and Hämäläinen (1985) further discussed this and other optimal control models of ventricular function. They showed why complete solutions to the optimality problem do not exist but could be obtained with other assumptions. Working from a set of different boundary conditions, they showed that the ejection pattern with the peak flow in the first half of ejection (e.g., that labeled experimental data in Figure 3.4.7) was optimal with respect to minimizing work external to the ventricle. The difference in ventricular work between the most efficient and least efficient patterns amounted to 4% of the optimum value.

Although this model is not yet suitable for inclusion in a global model predicting exercise performance, it is a large step in that direction. Optimization models are used to predict respiratory response to exercise (see Section 4.5.3), and the promise is that they will someday be used in prediction of cardiovascular responses to exercise. Of particular interest is the

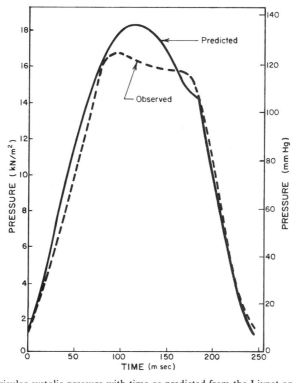

Figure 3.4.7 Ventricular systolic pressure with time as predicted from the Livnat and Yamashiro (1981) model compared to experimentally recorded data by Greene et al. (1973). Experimental data were normalized to the same systolic duration and same area under the curve as in the experimental curve. (Adapted and used with permission from Livnat and Yamashiro, 1981.)

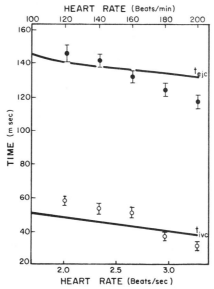

Figure 3.4.8 Predicted isovolumic contraction (lower curve) and ejection periods (upper curve) as a function of heart rate. Solid lines are model predictions and points are average measured values from Wallace et al. (1963). (Adapted and used with permission from Livnat and Yamashiro, 1981.)

TABLE 3.4.3 Results of Simulated Heart Failure

State	End-Diastolic Volume (V_0), m^3 (mL)	Contraction Energy (E_2), N·m (erg)	Maximal Rate of Ventricular Pressure Change $[(dp/dt)_{max}]$, N/(m²·sec) (mm Hg/sec)	Ventricular Elastance, kN/m⁵ (mm Hg/mL)	Isovolumic Contraction Period, sec	Ejection Time, sec
Normal	20×10^{-6} (20)	36 (3.6×10)	230×10^3 (1.722)	150×10^6 (11.6)	45×10^{-3}	138×10^{-3}
Mild dilatation	30×10^{-6} (30)	28 (2.8)	181×10^3 (1.356)	760×10^6 (5.7)	57×10^{-3}	147×10^{-3}
Severe dilatation	40×10^{-6} (40)	20 (2.0)	146×10^3 (1.093)	490×10^6 (3.7)	73×10^{-3}	154×10^{-3}

Source: Adapted and used with permission from Livnat and Yamashiro, 1981.

juxtaposition of concepts: oxygen consumption used to be thought of as a dependent variable— its magnitude was dependent upon the rate of work. This model shows that oxygen consumption can be pictured as determining, at least in part, the rate of work.

3.4.5 Heart Rate Models

Heart rate response to exercise is nearly linear. As presented in Equation 3.2.41, steady-state heart rate response can be obtained from oxygen consumption data by

$$\text{HR} = \text{HR}_r + \left(\frac{\dot{V}_{O_2}}{\dot{V}_{O_2\text{max}}}\right)(\text{HR}_{\text{max}} - \text{HR}_r) \tag{3.4.24}$$

where HR = steady-state heart rate response, beats/sec
  HR_r = resting heart rate, beats/sec
  $\dot{V}_{O_2}$ = oxygen uptake, m^3/sec
and

$$\text{HR}_{\text{max}} = (220 - y)/60 \tag{3.4.25}$$

where y = age, yr
Maximum oxygen uptake can be approximated by any of several empirical predictors such as Equation 3.3.38, 3.2.39, or 3.2.40. Oxygen uptake for any given task can be roughly calculated from other empirical equations (see Section 5.5.1) or by dividing external work rate by an assumed muscular efficiency. For leg work, muscular efficiency can be assumed to be 20% (see Section 5.2.5). Thus steady-state heart rate response to exercise can be predicted approximately.

Transient Response. Fujihara et al. (1973a, b) performed a series of experiments in which they were able to determine heart rate transient response. They were careful to begin their experiments at work rates higher than resting and terminate them before maximal efforts, thus avoiding nonlinearities at both extremes of work rates. Five healthy nonathletic laboratory personnel were studied. Impulse, step, and ramp loads were applied to the bicycle ergometer. Good agreement between experimental observations and mathematical prediction was obtained with the following step-response equation (Fujihara et al., 1973a):[56]

$$\Delta\text{HR} = k_1\delta[t - t_{d1}]\left[\frac{-\tau_1}{\tau_2 - \tau_1}(1 - e^{-t/\tau_1}) + \frac{\tau_2}{\tau_2 - \tau_1}(1 - e^{-t/\tau_2})\right] + k_2\delta[t - t_{d2}](1 - e^{-t/\tau_3}) \tag{3.4.26}$$

where ΔHR = change in heart rate, beats/sec
  k_1, k_2 = steady-state heart rate coefficients, beats/sec
  t_{d1}, t_{d2} = delay times, sec
  $\delta[t - t_d] = 0, \quad t < t_d$
    $= 1, \quad t > t_d$
  τ_1, τ_2, τ_3 = time constants, sec
Experimentally determined parameter values for step changes in work rate of 60 N·m/sec appear in Table 3.4.4. The formulation in Equation 3.4.26 is dominated by a rapid rise in heart rate

---

[56]Actually, Fujihara et al. gave their equation in the s domain (see Appendix 3.3):

$$\Delta\text{HR} = k_1 e^{-st_{d1}}[(1 + s\tau_1)(1 + s\tau_2)]^{-1} + k_2 e^{-st_{d2}}[1 + s\tau_3]^{-1}$$

which does not presuppose any specific type of forcing function such as impulse, step, or ramp. The terms e^{-st_d} are time delay terms and $(1 + s\tau)$ terms lead to exponential time responses.

TABLE 3.4.4 Subject Data and Best Fit Parameter Values[a]

Subject	Age years	Sex	Weight, N (kg)	Height, m	k_1, beats/sec (beats/min)	k_2, beats/sec (beats/min)	t_{d1}, sec	t_{d2}, sec	τ_1, sec	τ_2, sec	τ_3, sec
RA	27	M	657 (67)	1.68	0.67 (40)	−0.18 (−11.0)	1.0	14	40	2	20
YF	34	M	657 (67)	1.71	0.39 (23.5)	−0.033 (−2.0)	1.0	16	40	6	10
JH	40	M	716 (73)	1.82	0.33 (19.5)	−0.042 (−2.5)	1.0	15	18	2	8
JRH	35	F	628 (64)	1.77	0.53 (31.8)	−0.033 (−2.0)	1.0	17	25	6	8
RW	32	M	814 (83)	1.80	0.34 (20.5)	−0.017 (−1.0)	1.0	20	25	2	8
Mean					0.45 (27.1)	−0.062 (−3.7)	1.0	16.6	29.6	3.6	10.8

[a] Compiled from Fujihara et al., 1973a, b.

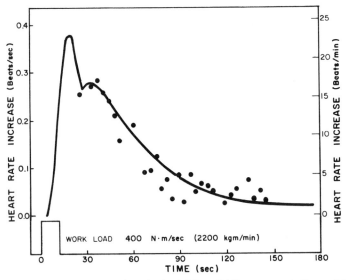

Figure 3.4.9 Heart rate response to an impulse load. The solid line represents the model prediction of Equation 3.4.26. (Adapted and used with permission from Fujihara et al., 1973b.)

determined most by τ_1 with a subsequent fall in heart rate determined by τ_3. Figure 3.4.9 shows the predicted response to an impulse load for subject Y. F.

Since Fujihara et al. (1973b) presented their parameter values for a specific work rate only, and since the steady-state change in heart rate in Equation 3.4.26 is given as $(k_1 + k_2)$, it appears reasonable to suppose that k_1 and k_2 will vary proportionately with workload. Thus

$$HR = \left\{ HR_r + \left(\frac{\dot{V}_{O_2}}{\dot{V}_{O_2 max}} \right) (HR_{max} - HR_r) \right\} \left\{ \frac{k_1}{k_1 + k_2} \delta[t - t_{d1}] \right.$$

$$\left. \cdot \left[\frac{-\tau_1}{\tau_2 - \tau_1}(1 - e^{-t/\tau_1}) + \frac{\tau_2}{\tau_2 - \tau_1}(1 - e^{-t/\tau_2}) \right] + \frac{k_2}{k_1 + k_2} \delta[t - t_{d2}](1 - e^{-t/\tau_3}) \right\} \qquad (3.4.27)$$

Heat Effects. Heart rate is influenced not only by the oxygen transport requirements of the body but also by body temperature. This reflects the additional cardiovascular burden of removing excess heat (as well as a small increase in oxygen demand to supply the increase in chemical activity which occurs with a temperature increase; see Section 3.3.5 and 5.2.5). Givoni and Goldman (1973a), obtaining experimental observations on young men in military uniforms, proposed a series of equations to predict heart rate response to work, environment, and clothing. For a more thorough discussion of the parameters involved in this model, the reader is referred to Section 5.5.

Both body temperature and heart rate respond to environmental changes by transient changes toward new final values. Of course, heart rate changes much more rapidly than body temperature. Figure 3.4.10 shows the relationship between final heart rate for four different studies. The relationship between these two demonstrates the predictability of one from the other.

The body temperature model of Section 5.5 corrects body heat load for work done on the external environment by the body.[57] No such correction is necessary for heart rate because heart rate responds to total oxygen demand, which includes that used to produce external work.

There is a limit above which the relationship between body temperature and heart rate is no longer linear. This limit occurs at a heart rate of about 2.50 beats/sec. Above this limit, body temperature can continue to increase (although the subject may expire before equilibrium is reached) while heart rate approaches a maximum of 2.83–3.17 beats/sec. Givoni and Goldman (1973a) assumed an exponential relationship between body temperature and heart rate above this limit.

Based on empirical determination, Givoni and Goldman (1973a) gave, for heat-acclimatized

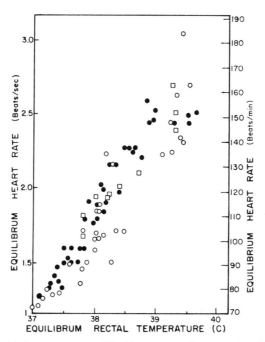

Figure 3.4.10   Relationship between measured final heart rate and computed equilibrium rectal temperature from four experimental studies. (Adapted and used with permission from Givoni and Goldman, 1973a.)

---

[57]External work is work used to move an external force, such as the weight of an object, through some distance.

men:

$$I = (6.67 \times 10^{-3})M + (6.46 \times 10^{-3}C_{cl})(\theta_a - 36) + 1.33 \exp[0.0047(E_{req} - E_{max})] \quad (3.4.28)$$

where I = heart rate index, beats/sec
  M = metabolic rate, N·m/sec (Equation 5.5.5)
  C_{cl} = thermal conductance of clothing, N·m/(m^2·sec·°C)
  θ_a = ambient temperature, °C
  E_{req} = required evaporative cooling, N·m/sec (Equation 5.5.8)
  E_{max} = maximum evaporative cooling capacity of the environment, N·m/sec (Equation 5.5.9)
and

$$HR_f = 1.08, \qquad\qquad 0 \leqslant I < 0.42 \qquad\qquad (3.4.29)$$

$$HR_f = 1.08 + 0.35\,(I - 0.42), \qquad\qquad 0.42 \leqslant I \leqslant 3.75 \qquad\qquad (3.4.30)$$

$$HR_f = 2.25 + 0.70[1 - e^{-(60I - 225)}], \qquad 3.75 \leqslant I \qquad\qquad (3.4.31)$$

where HR_f = equilibrium heart rate, beats/sec
From this system of equations, it is possible to separate the effect of exercise from the effect of body temperature on equilibrium heart rate. The first term, $(6.67 \times 10^{-3})M$, in Equation 3.4.28 represents the heart rate required to transport oxygen to support metabolism. The remaining two terms are those dealing with thermal effects on heart rate. If an incremental work rate of 5.75 N·m/sec requires an additional 0.29 m^3 oxygen per second (1 L/hr), then an extra 0.013 beats/sec is required (using Equation 3.4.30).

Givoni and Goldman (1973a) also estimated the transient responses to changes in work, environment, and clothing. At rest, heart rate is assumed to begin at 1.08 beats/sec and respond to changes with

$$HR_r = 1.08 + (HR_f - 1.08)[1 - \exp(-t/1200)] \qquad\qquad (3.4.32)$$

where HR_r = heart rate during rest, beats/sec
  t = time, beginning at a change, sec
During work, the greater the stress, or the higher the equilibrium heart rate, the longer it takes to reach the final level. Also, there is an initial elevation in heart rate when the resting subject rises and anticipates work:

$$HR_w = 1.08(HR_f - 1.08)(1 - 0.8\exp\{-[6 - 1.8(HR_f - 1.08)]t/3600\}) \qquad (3.4.33)$$

where HR_w = heart rate during work, beats/sec
  t = time, beginning when work begins, sec
After cessation of work, heart rate decreases toward the equilibrium resting level appropriate to the given climatic and clothing conditions. The rate of decrease depends on the total elevation of heart rate above its resting level and on the cooling ability of the environment:

$$HR_t = HR_w - (HR_w - HR_r)e^{-kbt/3600} \qquad\qquad (3.4.34)$$

where HR_t = heart rate during recovery, beats/sec
  HR_w = heart rate at the end of the work period, beats/sec
  k = heart rate effect on transient response, sec^{-1}
  b = colling ability on transient response, dimensionless
  t = time after beginning of recovery, sec

$$k = 2 - 6(\text{HR}_w - \text{HR}_r) \tag{3.4.35}$$

$$b = 2.0 + 12(1 - e^{0.3\text{CP}}) \tag{3.4.36}$$

where CP = cooling power of the environment, N·m/sec (see Equation 5.5.19)
For normal individuals, with 1.8 m² surface area,

$$\text{CP} = 3.11 \times 10^{-4} \, \text{im} \, C_{\text{cl}}(5866 - \phi_a p_{\text{amb}})$$
$$+ 0.027 \, C_{\text{cl}}(36 - \theta_a) - 1.57 \tag{3.4.37}$$

where im = clothing permeability index, dimensionless
  ϕ_a = ambient relative humidity, dimensionless
  p_{amb} = ambient water vapor pressure, N/m²

About a week of work in hot environments is required for nonacclimatized men to become fully acclimatized to their environment (see Sections 5.3.5 and 5.5.2). Givoni and Goldman (1973b) estimated the largest difference in heart rate between nonacclimatized and fully acclimatized subjects to be about 0.67 beat/sec. It is thus necessary to modify Equations 3.4.26 and 3.4.27 to account for acclimatization effects; no difference in resting heart rate has been noticed for acclimatization (Equation 3.4.29 remains the same).

Givoni and Goldman (1973a) assumed that equilibrium heart rate decreases exponentially with the duration of work in the heat. Also, for very restricted evaporative conditions the difference between acclimatized and nonacclimatized heart rate decreases exponentially with maximum evaporative capacity of the environment:

$$\text{HR}_{f,n} = \text{HR}_f + 0.67\{1 - \exp[-2.4(\text{HR}_f - 1.08)]\}[1 - \exp(-0.005 E_{\text{max}})]\exp(-0.3N) \tag{3.4.38}$$

where $\text{HR}_{f,n}$ = equilibrium heart rate for individuals not fully acclimatized, beats/sec
  HR_f = equilibrium heart rate for fully acclimatized individuals, beats/sec
  N = number of consecutive days spent working in hot environment, days

The number of consecutive days of work experience in the heat is to be reduced by one-half day for each day missed. Transient heart rate response to rest, work, and recovery uses $\text{HR}_{f,n}$ in place of HR_f in Equations 3.4.31 through 3.4.34.

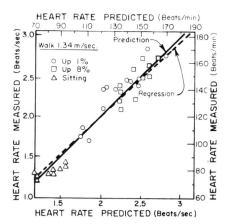 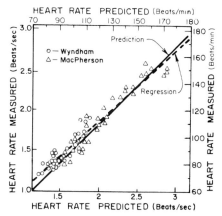

Figure 3.4.11 Correlation between predicted and observed final equilibrium heart rates. (*a*) Givoni and Goldman (1973a) studies and (*b*) studies of MacPherson (1960) on resting men and Wyndham et al. (1954) on working men. (Adapted and used with permission from Givoni and Goldman, 1973a.)

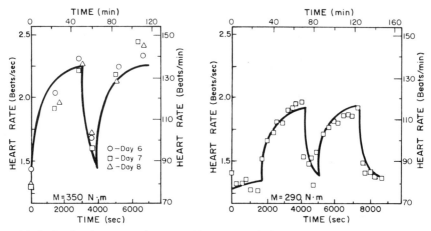

Figure 3.4.12   Predicted curves and measured heart rates during successive work–rest cycles at two different metabolic rates (M) by fully acclimatized men. (Adapted and used with permission from Givoni and Goldman, 1973a.)

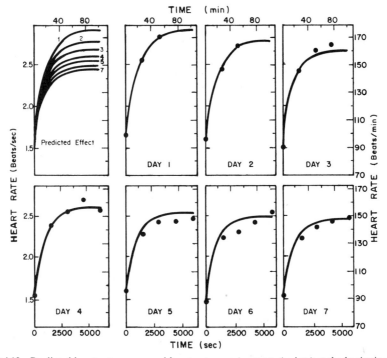

Figure 3.4.13   Predicted heart rate curves and heart rate measurements (points) at the beginning of work for successive days of work in the heat to induce acclimatization. (Adapted and used with permission from Givoni and Goldman, 1973b.)

Figure 3.4.11 shows the agreement between predicted and measured equilibrium heart rates for three different studies on fully acclimatized men from three different laboratories; Figure 3.4.12 shows measured data points superimposed on predicted curves for a complex experimental work protocol; Figure 3.4.13 shows predicted and measured heart rate for men undergoing acclimatization. Good agreement between predicted and measured results is seen for each of these conditions.

Comparison Between the Two Heart Rate Models. Transient response of heart rate was the subject for models by Fujihara et al. (1973a, b) and Givoni and Goldman (1973a, b). Both were developed from experimental data, although a greater mass of data was used by Givoni and Goldman. The difference between the two models lies in the time scale of transient response to be predicted. If the time scale is measured in seconds, that is, if very rapid heart rate events are to be predicted, the Fujihara et al. transient model should be used. If the smallest increment of time is of the order of a minute or more, the Givoni and Goldman formulation should be chosen.

3.5 CARDIOVASCULAR CONTROL MODELS

Aspects of cardiovascular control have stimulated many researchers to model development. Many of these models have concentrated on particular, limited portions of the overall system. For instance, Warner (1964) and others (Talbot and Gessner, 1973) presented models of baroreceptors and their influence on blood pressure (see Section 3.3.1). Warner (1965) modeled the effect of vagal stimulation on heart rate. Others (Talbot and Gessner, 1973) modeled local vasodilatory effects of carbon dioxide and other metabolites as well as blood volume changes due to net efflux or influx from capillary beds. A more global, but still limited approach was taken by Grodins (1959, 1963), who modeled the left and right hearts, systemic and pulmonary circulations, and resistances and compliances exhibited by the vessels. There is no doubt that this model is useful in understanding of the passive, uncontrolled cardiovascular system and its response to slow changes in pressures or flows, but it lacks the overall grand nature of a model that reproduces large-scale changes in exercise.

The model by Baneken and DeWit (1967) provides the framework for an integrated study of cardiovascular mechanics and control (Figure 3.5.1). This model includes the heart, systemic circulation, pulmonary circulation, and cardiovascular control centers. Systemic circulation is modeled as seven arterial segments including coronary blood flow, and cerebral, thoracic, abdominal, and leg arteries. The superior vena cava, returning blood to the heart from the head, and the inferior vena cava, returning blood to the heart from the lower body, are included. Each vessel includes resistance to blood flow, distensibility, resistance of the vascular wall to movement and inertance of the blood. In addition, venous valves are included (diagramed, in Figure 3.5.1, by means of a diode). Blood flow pathways are shown schematically as solid lines.

Neural pathways are shown as dashed lines. They include vasomotor effects on peripheral vascular resistance, heart rate effects, and myocardial inotropic effects (changes in contractility). Beneken and DeWit assumed vasomotor effects on peripheral resistances to be proportionately equal for all segments. It is possible, however, for the model to shift blood from one segment (e.g., viscera) to another (e.g., working muscle) through unequal proportions of resistance change (Talbot and Gessner, 1973).

3.5.1 The Heart

The Ventricles. The ventricles are modeled by Beneken and DeWit (1967) by describing the relationship among left ventricular volume, pressure, inflow, and outflow. Continuity (conserv-

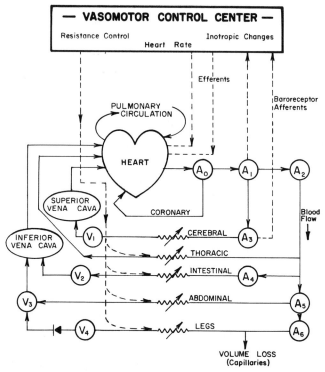

Figure 3.5.1   Beneken's model of the entire cardiovascular system, showing compartment used to simulate controlled circulation: heart, seven arterial (A_0-A_6) and six venous $(V_1-V_4$, inferior vena cava and superior vena cava) segments on the systemic side; two segments and a fairly complex pulmonary resistance on the pulmonary side. Solid lines indicate paths of blood flow. The diode indicates a valve in the venous circulation. Peripheral resistances are labelled. Neural control circuits (dashed lines) involve afferent paths from baroreceptors to vasomotor centers and efferent pathways to control peripheral resistances (arrows) and ventricular performances. Blood volume change depends on precapillary and postcapillary pressures.

ation of mass) considerations give

$$V_{LV} - V_{LV}(0) = \int_0^t (\dot{V}_{iLV} - \dot{V}_{oLV})\,dt \tag{3.5.1}$$

where V_{LV} = left ventricular volume at any time, m³
      $V_{LV}(0)$ = initial left ventricular volume, m³
      $\dot{V}_{iLV}$ = left ventricular inflow, m³/sec
      $\dot{V}_{oLV}$ = left ventricular outflow, m³/sec
      t = time, sec

Left ventricular pressure is related to pressure in the ascending aorta and ventricular outflow. This relationship is found by means of an energy balance. Work performed by the left ventricle when forcing blood into the ascending aorta is of the form pV; this work is dissipated by viscous resistance, absorbed by aortic inertance, and stored as kinetic energy:

$$\text{work} = \text{resistance energy} + \text{inertia energy} + \text{kinetic energy} \tag{3.5.2}$$

or

$$(p_{LV} - p_{ao})\Delta V_{LV} = \dot{V}_{oLV} R_L \Delta V_{LV} + I_{bL} \frac{d\dot{V}_{oLV}}{dt} \Delta V_{LV} + \frac{1}{2} m_b v_b^2 \tag{3.5.3}$$

where p_{LV} = left ventricular pressure, N/m^2
  p_{ao} = aortic pressure, N/m^2
  ΔV_{LV} = volume of blood delivered to aorta, m^3
  R_L = viscous resistance of blood, N·sec/m^5
  I_{bL} = left ventricular blood inertance, N·sec^2/m^5
  m_b = mass of blood, kg or N·sec^2/m
  v_b = blood velocity, m/sec
Dividing through by ΔV_{LV} leaves a pressure balance:

$$p_{LV} - p_{ao} = R_L \dot{V}_{oLV} + I_{bL} \frac{d\dot{V}_{oLV}}{dt} + \frac{\rho}{2} v_b^2 \tag{3.5.4}$$

where ρ = density of blood, kg/m^3
From continuity,

$$v_b = \frac{\dot{V}_{oLV}}{A_a} \tag{3.5.5}$$

where A_a = cross-sectional area of aorta, m^2
Therefore,

$$p_{LV} - p_{ao} = R_L \dot{V}_{oLB} + I_{bL} \frac{d\dot{V}_{oLV}}{dt} + \frac{\rho}{2} \frac{\dot{V}_{oLV}^2}{A_a^2}, \qquad p_{LV} > p_{ao} \tag{3.5.6}$$

If aortic pressure is less than ventricular pressure,

$$\dot{V}_{oLV} = 0, \qquad p_{LV} \leqslant p_{ao} \tag{3.5.7}$$

Blood viscous pressure drop, $R_L \dot{V}_{oLV}$, is subsequently neglected by Beneken and DeWit (1967) as being much smaller than the kinetic energy term. As previously mentioned (Section 3.4.3), blood inertance is computed as a column of blood having a length equal to the left ventricular inner radius and a diameter of the outflow vessel (I_b is given as 400 $V_{LV}^{1/3}$ kN·sec^2/m^5 in Table 3.4.4).

Similar equations for the right ventricle are

$$V_{RV} - V_{RV}(0) = \int_0^t (\dot{V}_{iRV} - \dot{V}_{oRV}) dt \tag{3.5.8}$$

$$p_{RV} - p_p = R_R \dot{V}_{oRV} + I_{bR} \frac{d\dot{V}_{oRV}}{dt} + \frac{\rho}{2A_p^2} \dot{V}_{oRV}^2, \qquad p_{RV} > p_p \tag{3.5.9}$$

where V_{RV} = right ventricular volume, m^3
  $V_{RV}(0)$ = initial right ventricular volume, m^3
  $\dot{V}_{iRV}$ = right ventricular inflow, m^3/sec
  $\dot{V}_{oRV}$ = right ventricular outflow, m^3/sec
  t = time, sec
  p_{RV} = right ventricular pressure, N/m^2

p_p = pressure in pulmonary artery, N/m^2
R_R = right ventricular resistance, $N \cdot sec/m^5$
I_{bR} = blood inertance, $N \cdot sec^2/m^5$
A_p = cross-sectional area of pulmonary artery, m^2

$$\dot{V}_{oRV} = 0, \qquad p_{RV} \leqslant p_p \qquad\qquad (3.5.10)$$

Intraventricular pressures are determined largely by muscular forces, which, in turn, depend on ventricular shape. Pressures are thus related to ventricular volumes. Beneken and Dewit (1967) assumed for the left ventricle a spherical shape with uniform wall thickness. The right ventricle is assumed to be bounded by part of the outer surface of the left ventricle together with a spherical free wall bent around part of the left ventricle (Figure 3.5.2).

Beneken and DeWit (1967) made the following assumptions in finding relations between ventricular pressure and muscular force and between ventricular volume and muscle length: (1) the muscle fibers have a uniformly directional distribution circumferential to the wall; (2) the ventricular walls retain their spherical shape throughout the cardiac cycle; (3) the wall material is isotropic and incompressible; and (4) the left ventricle determines the shape of the interventricular septum—the right ventricle does not influence left ventricular shape.

Starting from these assumptions, and continuing through an analysis of the stress–strain relationship of a thick-walled vessel (Talbot and Gessner, 1973), Beneken and DeWit give

$$p_{LV} = S_L(F_L/A_{LU}) \qquad\qquad (3.5.11)$$

where S_L = left ventricular shape factor, dimensionless
 F_L = force developed in myocardium, N
 A_{LU} = unstressed muscle cross-sectional area, m^2
and

$$p_{RV} = S_R(F_R/A_{RU}) \qquad\qquad (3.5.12)$$

where S_R = right ventricular shape factor, dimensionless
 F_R = force developed in right ventricular wall, N
 A_{RU} = unstressed muscle cross-sectional area, m^2
The value for A_{RU} and A_{LU} is taken as $10^{-6} m^2 (1 mm^2)$. Figure 3.5.3 is a graph of S_L as a function

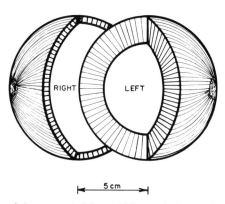

Figure 3.5.2 Cross section of the assumed right and left ventricular configuration in the end-diastolic state. The left ventricle is modeled as a thick-walled sphere and the right ventricle as a thin-walled spheroid assuming the shape of the left ventricle wall where the two join. (Used with permission from Beneken and CeWit, 1967.)

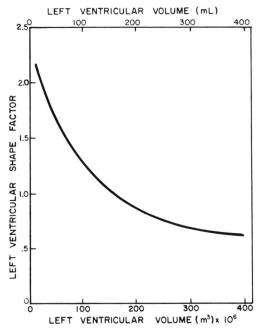

Figure 3.5.3   Relation between shape factor S_L and volume V_{LV} of the left ventricle. (Adapted and used with permission from Beneken and DeWit, 1967).

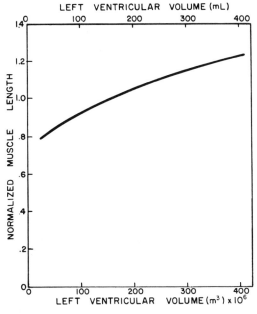

Figure 3.5.4   Relation between normalized muscle length and volume V_{LV} of the left ventricle. Actual muscle length is divided by end-diastolic muscle length. (Adapted and used with permission from Beneken and DeWit, 1967.)

of left ventricular volume. Details for calculations of S_L values can be found in Talbot and Gessner (1973).

The forces F_L and F_R are dependent on muscle length and the velocity of shortening of muscle length (see Section 5.2.5). Muscle length depends on ventricular volume. Normally, based on dimensional considerations, it would be expected that muscle length would be dependent on the cube root of the volume, but, because of the thick wall of the ventricle, there is not quite a cube root relationship. Figure 3.5.4 shows the relationship between muscle length normalized to end-diastolic length and left ventricular volume.

To determine the dependence of developed force on muscle fiber length, Beneken and DeWit (1967) used a three-element heart muscle model, composed of a series elastic element, a parallel elastic element, and a contractile element, identical to that used by Robinson (Section 3.4.1) and seen in Figure 3.4.1. Total fiber length equals the length of the series element L_s plus the length of the parallel element L_p:

$$L = L_s + L_p = L_s + L_c \tag{3.5.13}$$

where L = total length, m
L_s = series element length, m
L_p = parallel element length, m
L_c = contractile element length, m

Also,

$$F = F_p + F_c \tag{3.5.14}$$

where F = total force, N
F_p = force developed by parallel elastic element, N
F_c = force developed by contractile element, N

The relationship between total force and length of the series elastic element of cat papillary muscle appears in Figure 3.5.5. The forces developed by contractile and parallel element (see Section 3.4.1) lengths appear in Figure 3.5.6. Contractile force appearing in Figure 3.5.6 is maximum contractile force. When not activated, it is assumed that the contractile force is a small fraction of the maximum contractile force:

$$F_{\min} = \phi F_{\text{cmax}} + F_p \tag{3.5.15}$$

where $F_{\min}$ = minimum total force, N
F_{cmax} = maximum contractile force, N
ϕ = dimensionless fraction

and

$$F_{\max} = (1 + \phi)F_{\text{cmax}} + F_p \tag{3.5.16}$$

where $F_{\max}$ = maximum total force, N

A value of $\phi = 0.02$ is used by Beneken and DeWit (1967). The factor $Q = \phi$ for nonactivated muscle and $Q = (1 + \phi)$ for fully activated muscle is called the activation factor. The activation factor does not change abruptly between extremes but rises slowly and falls even more slowly. Various inotropic interventions are modeled by increasing the maximum value of Q.

To account for the effect of shortening velocity on force developed by the shortening muscle, Hill's equation is used (see Figure 5.2.12):

$$v = b(F_{\max} - F)/(F + a) \tag{3.5.17}$$

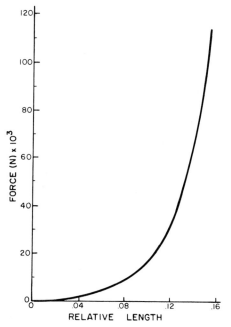

Figure 3.5.5 Length–force relation of the series elastic element of a cat papillary muscle of initial length L_U and initial cross sectional area 1 mm². L_v is the maximum length at which no force is exerted. (Used with permission from Beneken and DeWit, 1967.)

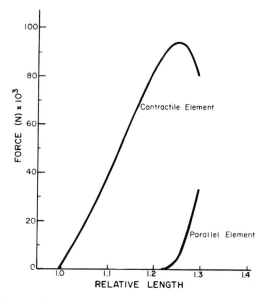

Figure 3.5.6 Length–force relations of the fully activated contractile element and of the parallel elastic element of a cat papillary muscle of initial length L_U and initial cross-sectional area 1 mm². (Used with permission from Beneken and DeWit, 1967.)

where F = muscle force, N
F_{max} = maximum muscle force, N
v = velocity of shortening, m/sec
a = constant, N
b = constant, m/sec

Velocity of shortening of the contractile element is defined as

$$v_c = \frac{dL_c}{dt} \tag{3.5.18}$$

where v_c = shortening velocity of contractile element, m/sec

Beneken and DeWit used experimental data and other analyses to modify Equation 3.5.17 to

$$v_c = \left[\frac{Qb_1L}{1 + 2.5Q} \right] \left[\frac{Q - (F_c/F_{cmax})}{Q(F_c/F_{cmax}) + a_1/F_{cmax}} \right] + U(F_c/F_{cmax}) \tag{3.5.19}$$

where Q = activation factor, dimensionless
a_1 = 18.6 N
b_1 = 4/sec
L = unstressed muscle length, m
U = muscle yielding factor, m/sec

$U = 0$ if $(Q \cdot F_{cmax}) > F_c$ and $U \cong 150$/sec times the unstressed muscle length if $(Q \cdot F_{cmax}) < F_c$. Using

$$t_{sv} = 0.16 + 0.20/HR \tag{3.5.20}$$

where t_{sv} = duration of ventricular systole, sec
HR = heart rate, beats/sec

and the previous equations and figures, Beneken and DeWit (1967) described ventricular behavior.

The Atria. Beneken and DeWit (1967) proposed a very rough approximation to atrial mechanics. Rather than include heart muscle properties and atrial shape, they included only information essential to proper model operation of the ventricles: introduction of ventricular end-diastolic volume and pressure increase of the proper amplitude, at the appropriate time in the cardiac cycle. They proposed equations to apply to the left and right atria:

$$p_{LA} = \frac{V_{LA} - V_{LA}(0)}{C_{LA}} \tag{3.5.21}$$

$$p_{RA} = \frac{V_{RA} - V_{RA}(0)}{C_{RA}} \tag{3.5.22}$$

where p_{LA} = left atrial pressure, N/m^2
p_{RA} = right atrial pressure, N/m^2
C_{LA} = time-dependent left atrial compliance, m^5/N
C_{RA} = time-dependent right atrial compliance, m^5/N
V_{LA} = left atrial volume, m^3
$V_{LA}(0)$ = left atrial end-diastolic volume, m^3
V_{RA} = right atrial volume, m^3
$V_{RA}(0)$ = right atrial end-diastolic volume, m^3

Assumed values appear in Table 3.5.1.

TABLE 3.5.1   Values Assigned to Left and Right Atrial Constants

Constant	Assigned Value[a]	
Initial right volume [$V_{RA}(0)$]	$30\,cm^3$	$(30\,mL)$
Initial left volume [$V_{LA}(0)$]	$30\,cm^3$	$(30\,mL)$
Systolic compliance of right atrium (C_{RA})	$2.7 \times 10^{-8}\,m^5/N$	$(3.8\,mL/mm\,Hg)$
Diastolic compliance of right atrium (C_{RA})	$6.2 \times 10^{-8}\,m^5/N$	$(8.3\,mL/mm\,Hg)$
Systolic compliance of left atrium (C_{LA})	$5.0 \times 10^{-8}\,m^5/N$	$(6.7\,mL/mm\,Hg)$
Diastolic compliance of left atrium (C_{LA})	$1.5 \times 10^{-7}\,m^5/N$	$(20\,mL/mm\,Hg)$

[a]Data compiled from Beneken and DeWit, 1967.

A linear approximation to the duration of atrial systole[58] was given as

$$t_{sa} = 0.10 + 0.09/HR \tag{3.5.23}$$

where t_{sa} = duration of atrial systole, sec

HR = heart rate, beats/sec

Like those for ventricles, the relations between flow and volume and between pressure and flow are

$$V_{RA} - V_{RA}(0) = \int_0^t (\dot{V}_{iRA} - \dot{V}_{oRA})\,dt \tag{3.5.24}$$

$$V_{LA} - V_{LA}(0) = \int_0^t (\dot{V}_{iLA} - \dot{V}_{oLA})\,dt \tag{3.5.25}$$

$$\dot{V}_{oRA} = (p_{RA} - p_{RV})/R_{RAV}, \qquad p_{RA} > p_{RV} \tag{3.5.26a}$$

$$\dot{V}_{oRA} = 0, \qquad p_{RA} \leqslant p_{LV} \tag{3.5.26b}$$

$$\dot{V}_{oLA} = (p_{LA} - p_{LV})/R_{LAV}, \qquad p_{LA} > p_{LV} \tag{3.5.27a}$$

$$\dot{V}_{oLA} = 0, \qquad p_{LA} \leqslant p_{LV} \tag{3.5.27b}$$

where V_{RA} = right atrial volume, m^3

$V_{RA}(0)$ = right atrial end-diastolic volume, m^3

$\dot{V}_{iRA}$ = right atrial inflow, m^3/sec

$\dot{V}_{oRA}$ = right atrial outflow, m^3/sec

V_{LA} = left atrial volume, m^3

$V_{LA}(0)$ = left atrial end-diastolic volume, m^3

$\dot{V}_{iLA}$ = left atrial inflow, m^3/sec

$\dot{V}_{oLA}$ = left atrial outflow, m^3/sec

p_{RA} = right atrial pressure, N/m^2

p_{RV} = right ventricular pressure, N/m^2

p_{LA} = left atrial pressure, N/m^2

p_{LV} = left ventricular pressure, N/m^2

R_{RAV} = resistance to flow of fully opened tricuspid valve, $N \cdot sec/m^5$

R_{LAV} = resistance of flow of fully opened mitral valve, $N \cdot sec/m^5$

---

[58]Ventricular systole starts 40 msec before the end of atrial systole.

Since the ventricles receive their blood from the atria,

$$\dot{V}_{oRA} = \dot{V}_{iRV} \tag{3.5.28}$$

$$\dot{V}_{oLA} = \dot{V}_{iLV} \tag{3.5.29}$$

Heart Rate Control. Beneken and DeWit (1967) incorporated a very simple concept of heart rate control into their model. Figure 3.5.7 is a schematic of this concept. The transfer relation between baroreceptor input (see Equation 3.3.2) and heart rate is assumed to occur through two modes. In the first mode, the baroreceptor pressure input $\mathscr{P}$ must be larger than some threshold value $\mathscr{P}_{th}$, resulting in relatively large and fast responses, predominantly of vagal origin. The transfer relation is a first-order equation with smaller time constant τ_+ for increasing pressures than for decreasing pressures τ_-. The second mode results in relatively small and slow responses caused by joint action of sympathetic and vagus nerves. The transfer relation is a second-order linear equation.

This concept of heart rate control is simplified because it is derived from observations on anesthetized animals. It does not account for the apparent action maintaining arterial mean pressure at a reference set point of $12 \, kN/m^2$ (Talbot and Gessner, 1973). This set point shifts during exercise so that mean central pressure rises higher than normal. Other neural connections (e.g., between hypothalamus and medullary vasomotor area, between motor cortex and vasomotor area, and between the respiratory control center and vasomotor area) and weightings (between sympathetic and parasympathetic afferents) are not included.

The relation between baroreceptor output and pressure input is

$$\mathscr{P} = \frac{p_{as} + p_{ad}}{2} + \phi(p_{as} - p_{ad}) - p_{th}, \qquad p > p_{th} \tag{3.5.30}$$

where $\mathscr{P}$ = baroreceptor pressure function, N/m^2
  p_{as} = systolic arterial blood pressure, N/m^2
  p_{ad} = diastolic arterial blood pressure, N/m^2
  p_{th} = threshold pressure, N/m^2
  ϕ = weighting factor, dimensionless

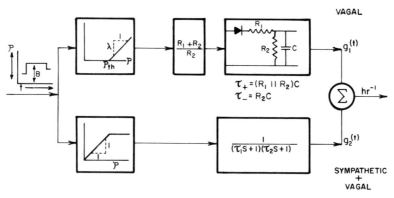

Figure 3.5.7 Two-region control of heart period incorporated in the Beneken and DeWit model. The input is from the carotid sinus baroreceptors and the output is proportional to heart rate. Two control pathways are assumed, one through the vagus (parasympathetic) nerve and the other through sympathetic and vagal action. The period of a heartbeat is the sum of the two actions caused by the two modes. (Used with permission from Beneken and DeWit, 1967.)

Systolic and diastolic pressures at the carotid sinus have been assumed to equal those at the aortic arch. Moreover, by including the pulse pressure, $(p_{as} - p_{ad})$, the differentiating effect of the baroreceptors is included.

The action of the first mode is

$$g_1 = \lambda_1(\mathscr{P} - \mathscr{P}_{th}) - \tau_3 \frac{dg_1}{dt} \tag{3.5.31}$$

where g_1 = mode 1 heart period contribution, sec
$\quad \mathscr{P}_{th}$ = threshold value of pressure function, N/m^2
$\quad \lambda_1$ = steady-state gain, m$^2 \cdot$sec/N
$\quad \tau_3$ = time constant, sec
The function g_1 is nonzero only when $\mathscr{P} > \mathscr{P}_{th}$, and there is a directional rate sensitivity, since

$$\tau_3 = \tau_+, \qquad \frac{dp}{dt} > 0 \tag{3.5.32a}$$

$$\tau_3 = \tau_-, \qquad \frac{dp}{dt} < 0 \tag{3.5.32b}$$

where τ_+, τ_- = time constants, sec, $\tau_- > \tau_+$
The action of the second mode is

$$g_2 = \lambda_2 \mathscr{P} - \tau_1 \tau_2 \frac{d^2 g_2}{dt^2} - (\tau_1 + \tau_2) \frac{dg_2}{dt} \tag{3.5.33}$$

where g_2 = mode 2 heart period contribution, sec
$\quad \tau_1$ = time constant, sec
$\quad \tau_2$ = time constant, sec
$\quad \lambda_2$ = steady-state gain, m$^2 \cdot$sec/N
Note that

$$HR = (g_1 + g_2)^{-1} \tag{3.5.34}$$

where HR = heart rate,[59] beats/sec
Table 3.5.2 gives numerical values used by Beneken and DeWit (1967).

It has been found that contractile strength of heart muscle increases as heart rate increases following an initial decline in contractility with heart rate increase (Beneken and DeWit, 1967). Furthermore, the negative inotropic effect of vagal impulses appears to be indirectly due to heart rate reduction. Therefore, as heart rate increases, there is an initial decline followed by a sustained increase in the forcefulness of blood ejection.

The activation factor Q introduced in Equations 3.5.16 and 3.5.19 is a time-varying fraction of the actual muscular force to the maximum isometric force which can be developed by the muscle. Beneken and DeWit (1967) incorporated the inotropic change in muscular contractility with

---

[59] Thus in the s domain,

$$HR(s) = \left\{ \frac{\lambda_1[\mathscr{P}(s) - \mathscr{P}_{th}]}{(1 + \tau_3 s)} + \frac{\lambda_2 \mathscr{P}(s)}{[1 + (\tau_1 + \tau_2)s + (\tau_1 \tau_2)s^2]} \right\}^{-1}$$

The similarity to the Fujihara formulation would be intriguing except that Beneken and DeWit's equation is nearly inverse to that of Fujihara (see footnote equation related to Equation 3.4.26).

TABLE 3.5.2 Numerical Values of Parameters Associated with the Relation Between Systemic Arterial Pressure and Heart Period

Parameter	Value
ϕ	1.5
p_{th}	$5.33\,\text{kN/m}^2$ (40 mm Hg)
$\mathscr{P}_{th}$	$10.7\,\text{kN/m}^2$ (80 mm Hg)
τ_+	1.5 sec
τ_-	4.5 sec
λ_1	$3.75 \times 10^{-5}\,\text{m}^2 \cdot \text{sec/N}$ (0.005 sec/mm Hg)
λ_2	$3.75 \times 10^{-5}\,\text{m}^2 \cdot \text{sec/N}$ (0.005 sec/mm Hg)
τ_1	2 sec
τ_2	1 sec

Source: Adapted and used with permission from Beneken and DeWit, 1967.

TABLE 3.5.3 Values Assigned to Activation Factor Modification Constants

Constant	Assigned Value[a]
Constant (a_1)	0.76
Coefficient (a_2)	0.2 sec
Coefficient (a_3)	0.4 sec
Time constant (τ_n)	1 sec

[a] Data compiled from Beneken and DeWit, 1967.

heart rate by forming a multipying factor H, which, when multiplied by Q, gives a new value for the activation factor Q.

$$H = a_1 + a_2(\text{HR}) - a_3(\text{HR})e^{-t/\tau_h} \tag{3.5.35}$$

where H = factor to multiply Q, dimensionless
$\quad a_1$ = constant, dimensionless
$\quad a_2$ = coefficient, sec
$\quad a_3$ = coefficient, sec
$\quad t$ = time since a change in heart rate
$\quad \text{HR}$ = heart rate, beats/sec
$\quad \tau_h$ = time constant, sec

Values of these parameters used by Beneken and DeWit (1967) are found in Table 3.5.3.

Coronary Blood Flow and Heart Performance. Adequate nutritional supply to the heart muscle is required for maintenance of contractile properties. Normally, adequate blood flow is maintained by autoregulatory mechanisms. This mechanism will fail at extremely low aortic pressure. Beneken and DeWit (1967) assumed total metabolic deficit of the heart muscle (which occurs when muscular energy requirements exceed energy delivered to the muscle by the blood) to be dependent on the decrease of aortic pressure below $8000\,\text{N/m}^2$, with the deficit accumulating with time:

$$M_c = \int (8000 - p_{ao})\,dt \tag{3.5.36}$$

where M_c = metabolic factor, N·sec/m^2
$\quad p_{ao}$ = aortic pressure, N/m^2
$\quad\quad t$ = time, sec
The activation factor Q is multiplied by M_c in the following manner:

$$Q' = Q(1 - 7.50 \times 10^{-8} M_c) \tag{3.5.37}$$

where Q' = new value of the activation factor, dimensionless
Beneken and DeWit (1967) also included a measure of cardiac damage and irreversibility, but this is not included here.

3.5.2 Systemic and Pulmonary Vessels

Mechanics. The vessels included are shown in Figure 3.5.1 and listed in Table 3.5.4. Gravitational effects are considered negligible. Pulmonary vessels are considered to be relatively short and are subdivided into arterial and venous segments only; systemic vessels will include capillaries as well. Acceleration of blood is much lower in the veins than in the arteries; consequently, venous inertial effects are neglected. Furthermore, blood volume changes in the veins are much lower than in the arteries during each cardiac cycle; therefore, venous viscous wall effects are ignored. Conceptual models of arteries and veins are seen in Figure 3.5.8.

For each segment, relations have been developed for volume, flow, and pressure. These are, for each arterial segment,

$$\Delta p_j = R_j \dot{V}_{ij} + I_j \frac{d\dot{V}_{ij}}{dt} \tag{3.5.38}$$

where Δp_j = pressure difference between entrance and outlet of segment j, N/m^2
$\quad R_j$ = resistance of segment j, N·sec/m^5
$\quad \dot{V}_{ij}$ = flow into segment j, m^3/sec
$\quad I_j$ = inertance of segment j, N·sec^2/m^5
$\quad t$ = time, sec

$$\Delta p_j = p_{ij} - p_{oj} = p_{ij} - p_i(1 + j) \tag{3.5.39}$$

where p_{ij} = entrance pressure of segment j, N/m^2
$\quad p_{oj}$ = exit pressure of segment j, N/m^2
$\quad p_i(1 + j)$ = entrance pressure to segment $(1 + j)$, N/m^2

$$V_j = V_j(0) + \int (\dot{V}_{ij} - \dot{V}_{oj})\,dt$$
$$= V_j(0) + \int [\dot{V}_{ij} - \dot{V}_i(1 + j)]\,dt \tag{3.5.40}$$

where V_j = volume of segment j, m^3
$\quad V_j(0)$ = initial volume of segment j, m^3
$\quad \dot{V}_{oj}$ = outflow from segment j, m^3/sec
$\quad \dot{V}_i(1 + j)$ = flow into segment $(1 + j)$, m^3/sec

$$p_{oj} = \frac{1}{C_j}[V_j - V_j(0)] + R'_j \dot{V}_j \tag{3.5.41}$$

TABLE 3.5.4 Numerical Values of Parameters Used in the Beneken and DeWit Cardiovascular Model

Segment	Resistance (R_b), N·sec/m^5 × 10^{-6} (mm Hg·sec/mL)	Inertance (I_b), N·sec^2/m^5 × 10^{-6} (mm Hg·sec/mL)	Compliance (C_a),[b] m^5/N × 10^9 (mL/mm Hg)	Average Transmural Pressure (p_j), N/m^2 × 10^{-3} (mm Hg)	Unextended Volume $[V_j(0)]$,[c] m^3 × 10^{6d}	Average Extended Volume $(\bar{p}_j C_j)$,[c] m^3 × 10^{6d}
Ascending aorta	—[a]	29.3 (0.22)	2.10 (0.28)	13.9 (104)	53	29
Thoracic arch	4.00 (0.03)	57.3 (0.43)	2.18 (0.29)	13.9 (104)	61	30
Thoracic aorta	120 (0.9)	507 (3.8)	2.18 (0.29)	13.9 (104)	59	30
Abdominal aorta	1,600 (12)	1,870 (14)	1.58 (0.21)	12.8 (96)	58	20
Intestinal arteries	187 (1.4)	360 (2.7)	0.45 (0.06)	12.8 (96)	17	6
Leg arteries	24,000 (180)	4,130 (31)	0.90 (0.12)	13.2 (99)	63	12
Head and arm arteries	627 (47)	1,870 (14)	2.48 (0.33)	13.2 (99)	114	33
Total systemic arterial			11.9 (1.58)		425	160
Head and arm veins	30,100 (226)		70.5 (9.4)	0.640 (4.8)	552	45
Leg veins	40,000 (300)		36.0 (4.8)	1.07 (8.0)	257	38
Abdominal veins	79,300 (595)		38.3 (5.1)	0.267 (2.0)	305	10
Intestinal veins	22,100 (166)		79.5 (10.6)	0.533 (4.0)	607	42
Inferior vena cava	2,000 (15)		62.3 (8.3)	0.667 (5.0)	488	42
Superior vena cava	8,000 (60)		62.3 (8.3)	0.667 (5.0)	488	42
Total system venous			349 (46.5)		2,697	219
Pulmonary arteries	—[a]	24.0 (0.18)	32.3 (4.3)	2.13 (16.0)	50	69
Pulmonary veins	933 (7)		63.0 (8.4)	0.853 (6.4)	460	54
Left ventricle						125
Right ventricle						125
Left atrium					30	50
Right atrium					30	50
System Total					3,692	852

Source: Adapted and used with permission from Beneken and DeWit, 1967.

[a] Resistance and inertance of these segments represent ventricular properties. Since pressure drop across opened arterial valves is flow dependent, no resistance values are given here. Refer to Equations 3.5.6, 3.5.7, 3.5.9, and 3.5.10.

[b] Viscous wall resistance is calculated as $R' = 0.04$ sec/C_a.

[c] Total segment volume is the sum of unextended and extended volumes, $V_{TOT} = V_j(0) + \bar{p}_j C_j$.

[d] Same values in mL.

144

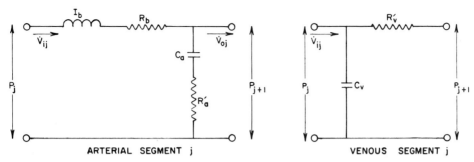

Figure 3.5.8 Schematic models of an arterial segment and a venous segment. R_b and I_b represent viscous and inertial properties of blood, C_a and R'_a represent elastic and viscous properties of an arterial segment wall, and C_v and R'_v represent the resistance to flow and compliance of a venous segment. Pressures are denoted by P and flows by $\dot{V}$. (Used with permission from Beneken and DeWit, 1967.)

where C_j = compliance of arterial segment j, m^5/N

$\qquad R'_j$ = resistance to movement of arterial wall tissue, $N \cdot sec/m^5$

Referring to Figure 3.5.8, R_b and I_b are determined by vascular dimensions, blood viscosity, and blood density. C_a, C_v, R'_a, and R'_v are related to vascular dimensions and mechanical properties of the wall. Compliance values have been determined in such a way that elastic tapering of the arterial tree is taken into account. Beneken and DeWit (1967), on the basis of published evidence, estimated the time constant $R'_a C_a$ for all systemic arterial segments to be 0.04 sec. Venous resistances have been calculated from pressure differences between adjacent venous segments. Coronary capillary resistance, although influenced by the contractile action of the heart, is assumed to be constant.

All vessel pressures are transmural; since vessels in the thoracic and abdominal cavities are subject to variations in outer pressure due to such things as respiration, these have been included for those segments that represent vessels in these cavities. Intrathoracic pressure is assumed to be constant at $-553\,N/m^2$ ($-4\,mm\,Hg$) and intra-abdominal pressure to be $+553\,N/m^2$ ($4\,mm$ Hg) with respect to atmospheric pressure. Numerical values of pertinent parameters appear in Tables 3.5.2 and 3.5.3.

Vascular Resistance Control. Beneken and DeWit (1967) included central nervous system control of vascular resistance but ignored autoregulation. For simplicity, they assumed all arteriovenous resistances change proportionately with the exception of coronary, head, and arm resistances, which are assumed to be unaffected by vasoconstrictor and vasodilator action. This proportionality would need to be changed to simulate exercise responses because blood flow distribution is different during exercise and at rest (Table 3.2.3).

Beneken and DeWit assumed a vascular resistance control function of

$$\frac{R_N}{R} = \left[1 + 0.5\left(\frac{\mathcal{P}}{\mathcal{P}_N} - 1 \right) \right] [1 - e^{-t/\tau_v}] \qquad (3.5.42)$$

where R_N = normal resistance value, $N \cdot sec/m^5$

$\qquad R$ = controlled resistance value, $N \cdot sec/m^5$

$\qquad \mathcal{P}$ = baroreceptor pressure function, N/m^2

$\qquad \mathcal{P}_N$ = normal baroreceptor pressure function, N/m^2

$\qquad t$ = time after change, sec

$\qquad \tau_v$ = vascular time constant, sec

Values of R_N can be found in Table 3.5.5. The time constant τ_v is taken as 12 sec. A change in p to one-half normal yields an eventual resistance change of four-thirds normal.

TABLE 3.5.5 Numerical Values of Arteriovenous Resistances Used in the Description of the Vascular System

Segment	Resistance of Capillary Bed,[a] $N/m^2 \times 10^6$	(mm Hg·sec/mL)
Coronary	1600	(12)
Bronchial	1600	(12)
Intestinal	307	(2.3)
Abdominal	7600	(57)
Legs	2000	(15)
Head and arms	800	(6)
Pulmonary	14.7	(0.11)

[a]Compiled from Beneken and DeWit, 1967.

Control of Capillary Pressure and Blood Volume. Capillary pressures directly influence the net flow or fluid between blood and cellular spaces. These pressures are the result of the difference between mean arteriole pressure and mean venule pressure. Both are regulated by the central nervous system as well as by local autoregulatory mechanisms.

Beneken and DeWit (1967) assumed arteriole and venule resistances to change proportionally and in a manner governed by Equation 3.5.42. Normal artery pressure is assumed to be 13,300 N/m² (100 mm Hg) and peripheral venous pressure is 800 N/m² (6 mm Hg). Then capillary pressure becomes

$$p_c = \frac{(\bar{p}_c - \bar{p}_v)p_a + (\bar{p}_a - \bar{p}_c)p_v}{(\bar{p}_a - \bar{p}_v)} \qquad (3.5.43a)$$

$$= 0.20p_a + 0.80p_v \qquad (3.5.43b)$$

where p_c = capillary pressure, N/m²
$\bar{p}_c$ = normal capillary pressure, N/m²
p_a = mean arterial pressure, N/m²

TABLE 3.5.6 Assumed Distribution of Cardiac Output Through Various Segments

Segment	Blood Flow (Fraction of Cardiac Output)			
Ascending aorta =	1.00			
Coronary arteries +		0.10		
Aortic arch =		0.90		
Head and arms arteries +			0.20	
Thoracic aorta =			0.70	
Thoracic arteries				0.10
Intestinal arteries				0.50
Abdominal arteries				0.02
Leg arteries				0.08
Leg veins				0.08
Abdominal veins			0.10	
Intestinal veins			0.50	
Inferior vena cava		0.60		
Superior vena cava		0.20		
Coronary veins		0.10		
Thoracic veins		0.10		
Atrial flow	1.00			

Source: Used with permission from Beneken and DeWit, 1967.

$\bar{p}_a$ = normal arterial pressure, N/m^2

p_v = mean venous pressure, N/m^2

$\bar{p}_v$ = normal venous pressure, N/m^2

Capillary pressure p_c becomes $3300 \, N/m^2$ (25 mm Hg) when normal values of $13,300 \, N/m^2$ and $800 \, N/m^2$ are used for arterial and venous pressures.

Net fluid flow through capillary walls occurs when capillary pressure deviates from $3300 \, N/m^2$. Beneken and DeWit used the following relationship:

$$\dot{V}_{\text{cw}} = \frac{p_c - 3300}{R_{\text{cw}}} \tag{3.5.44}$$

where $\dot{V}_{\text{cw}}$ = net flow through capillary walls, m^3/sec

R_{cw} = resistance of capillary walls to fluid flow, $N \cdot sec/m^5$

A value of 26.7×10^9 (200 mm Hg·sec/mL) is used for R_{cw}.

Blood pooling that occurs in the veins has also been taken into account (Table 3.5.6). A transient change in the pressure–volume relation of a vein vessel (Equation 3.5.41) occurs after an increase in blood volume. This can be formulated in several ways, but Beneken and DeWit chose to change the normal vessel volume $V_j(0)$ summed over all vessels:

$$V_{\text{TOT}}(t) = V_{\text{TOT}}(0) + \Delta V_{\text{TOT}}(1 - e^{-t/\tau_s}) \tag{3.5.45}$$

where $V_{\text{TOT}}(t)$ = total circulatory vessel volume as a function of time, m^3

$\qquad\qquad = \sum V_j(0)$

$V_{\text{TOT}}(0)$ = initial total circulatory vessel volume, m^3

ΔV_{TOT} = total blood volume change caused by hemorrhage or infusion, m^3

τ_s = time constant of stress relaxation in the veins, sec

Nonlinear Resistances. Highly nonlinear vascular resistances occur at the heart valves, venous valves, when veins collapse, and in the pulmonary vasculature. Heart relations were already given in Equations 3.5.6 and 3.5.7 and Equations 3.5.9 and 3.5.10. Venous valve action can be included in the model with a diode, or check-valve relation:

$$\dot{V}_j = 0, \qquad p_{oj} > p_{ij} \tag{3.5.46}$$

where $\dot{V}_j$ = flow through vein segment j, m^3/sec

p_{oj} = output pressure from vein segment j, N/m^2

p_{ij} = input pressure to vein segment j, N/m^2

Venous valve action was incorporated in the model at the junction of the leg veins and abdominal veins and at the junction of the superior vena cava and arm veins (but not head veins, which carry twice the blood flow as the total to both arms).

Vessel collapse occurs whenever vessel transmural pressure becomes negative (see Section 4.2.3 for a similar situation for respiratory exhalation). When intraluminal pressure falls, distensible walls contract. Flow velocity must increase if the same volume rate of flow is to be maintained through the reduced cross-sectional area. When velocity increases, kinetic energy increases, and potential energy of the fluid must consequently fall. When potential energy falls, fluid static pressure falls, and the vessel walls collapse still further. This has the effect, after a while, of decreasing flow velocity, and this whole scenario occurs in reverse. As a result, vessel resistance to blood flow becomes very high and outflow pressure has little effect on flow velocity.

Vessel collapse can occur when vessel transmural pressure becomes negative (with respect to the vessel interior). The inferior vena cava commonly collapses when it passes through the diaphragm and enters the thoracic cavity because intra-abdominal pressure is positive and mean right atrial pressure is zero. Beneken and DeWit (1967) included this collapse. For the model segments between the intestinal arteries and the inferior vena cava and between the abdominal veins joining the inferior vena cava,

$$R_v = \frac{p_{va} - p_{vt} - p_{ot} + p_{oa}}{\dot{V}_v}, \qquad (p_{vt} + p_{ot} - p_{oa}) > 0 \tag{3.5.47a}$$

$$\frac{p_{va}}{\dot{V}_v} = 10R_v, \qquad (p_{vt} + p_{ot} = p_{oa}) \leqslant 0 \tag{3.5.47b}$$

where p_{va} = venous transmural pressure in the abdominal cavity, N/m^2
$\quad p_{vt}$ = venous transmural pressure in the thorax, N/m^2
$\quad p_{ot}$ = outer thoracic pressure, N/m^2
$\quad p_{oa}$ = outer abdominal pressure, N/m^2
$\quad R_v$ = venous resistance, $N \cdot sec/m^5$
$\quad \dot{V}_v$ = venous flow rate, m^3/sec

Collapse is represented by a tenfold resistance increase.

Pressure–flow relations of blood vessels in the lungs are assumed to be

$$\dot{V}_p = \frac{p_{ap} - p_{vp}}{R_p}, \qquad p_{vp} > 930 \, N/m^2 \, (7 \, mm \, Hg) \tag{3.5.48a}$$

and

$$\dot{V}_p = \frac{p_{ap} - 930}{R_p}, \qquad p_{vp} < 930 \, N/m^2 \tag{3.5.48b}$$

where $\dot{V}_p$ = flow through the pulmonary vascular system, m^3/sec
$\quad p_{ap}$ – pulmonary arterial pressure, N/m^2
$\quad p_{vp}$ = pulmonary venous pressure, N/m^2
$\quad R_p$ = resistance of pulmonary vasculature, $N \cdot sec/m^5$

3.5.3 Model Performance

Beneken and DeWit (1967) tested their model to compare qualitative trends and quantitative results with experimental findings reported in the literature. These results are summarized here.

They first tested the mechanical model of the ventricles, atria, and circulation without control of heart rate, peripheral resistance, capillary pressure, and blood volume. Even without these control refinements, they found the model to maintain a homeostasis, albeit one with wide tolerances. As peripheral resistance increased by 100%, cardiac output tended to fall, but only about 20%. Individual increases in peripheral resistance, pulmonary resistance, activation factor, systemic venous compliance, and heart rate all gave caridac output changes of no more than 25% of the normal value, with a direct summation of these contributions appearing to be 61% (Table 3.5.7). However, when all changes were made simultaneously, a 110% change was seen. This illustrates the compensatory action of some of the responses to single-parameter variations.

Increasing the activation factor Q was found to result in an increase of ventricular pressure, a reduction of the time to reach peak pressure, and an increase in the rate of pressure rise.

When the aforementioned control parameters were added to the model, model reproduction of experimental circulatory response to specialized cardiovascular maneuvers and to hemorrhage was rather good. Beneken and DeWit found, for instance, that heart rate responded realistically when neural information from aortic and carotid sinus pressures was made to control effectors with equal weighting.

Although Beneken's model does appear to be able to predict rather well several cardiovascular responses, Talbot and Gessner (1973) questioned whether the model is sufficiently

TABLE 3.5.7   Individual and Combined Influence of Some Parameters on Cardiac Output in the Beneken and DeWit Model[a]

Parameter	Percent Change in Parameter	Percent Change in Cardiac Output
Peripheral resistance	60%	5%
Pulmonary resistance	50%	7%
Maximum of activation factor	200%	17%
Systemic venous compliances	50%	7%
Heart rate	200%	25%
All parameter changes simultaneously		110%

[a]Compiled from Beneken and DeWit, 1967.

complex to study exercise reactions. The model does not include peripheral resistance reaction to local concentration of oxygen, carbon dioxide, and other metabolic products. In moderate exercise, blood flow to active muscles and myocardium increases, whereas splanchnic and renal flow may decrease, as does blood flow to the skin (until an increase in body temperature causes cutaneous vasodilation; see Sections 5.3.3, 5.3.6, and 5.4.2). Cerebral blood flow remains constant unless vigorous ventilation causes a fall in carbon dioxide concentration (in which case cerebral vessels vasoconstrict; see Section 3.3.1). Central blood pressure is higher than normal in exercise, allowing higher blood flows to muscle and skin than permitted by local vasodilation alone. To account for these changes would require a more complex model including local metabolic rates and local metabolite effects.

APPENDIX 3.1
NUMERICALLY SOLVING DIFFERENTIAL EQUATIONS

Differential equations appearing in various bioengineering models can be solved on a digital computer using numerical approximations to these equations. Finite difference techniques are often used to convert differential equations into finite difference equations.

1. APPROXIMATIONS TO DERIVATIVES

A derivative such as dV/dt can be estimated at point 1 by means of the approximation

$$\frac{dV}{dt} \approx \frac{\Delta V}{\Delta t} = \frac{V_2 - V_1}{t_2 - t_1}, \qquad t_2 > t_1 \tag{A3.1.1}$$

where V_2 is the value of V corresponding to $t = t_2$. The difficulty with this approximation is that the point of interest is on the boundary of the approximation. If the point where the derivative is to be determined is point 1, then the finite difference in Equation A3.1.1 is the *forward* difference. If the point in question is point 2, then Equation A3.1.1 gives a *backward* difference. A central difference sometimes gives a better approximation:

$$\frac{\Delta V}{\Delta t} = \frac{V_2 - V_0}{t_2 - t_0}, \qquad t_2 > t_1 > t_0 \tag{A3.1.2}$$

Because information about past values of V seldom is available at the beginning of a numerical solution, the forward difference approximation must be used for the initial difference. Central differences can be used thereafter.

Second derivatives can be determined from either

$$\frac{d^2V}{dt^2} \approx \frac{\Delta\left(\dfrac{\Delta V}{\Delta t}\right)}{\Delta t} = \frac{\left[\dfrac{(V_2 - V_1)}{(t_2 - t_1)} - \dfrac{(V_1 - V_0)}{(t_1 - t_0)}\right]}{t_2 - t_0} \tag{A3.1.3}$$

or

$$\frac{d^2V}{dt^2} \approx \frac{(V_2 - V_1) - (V_1 - V_0)}{t_2 - t_0} = \frac{V_2 - 2V_1 + V_0}{t_2 - t_0} \tag{A3.1.4}$$

The second method is preferable to the first because numerically approximating a derivative tends to emphasize noise appearing in the data. If $V_2 \approx V_1$, then $(V_2 - V_1)$ will be a difference of two nearly equal numbers. The difference will be nearly zero, and round-off error, truncation error, measurement noise, and the like, will constitute a large part of the difference. Because derivative estimation emphasizes noise, taking the difference between two first-derivative estimates to form the second derivative estimate, as in Equation A3.1.3, is not recommended.

Estimation of higher order derivatives can be made using coefficients from the binomial expansion. For instance, the third derivative is given by

$$\frac{d^3V}{dt^3} \approx \frac{V_3 - 2V_2 + 2V_1 - V_0}{t_3 - t_0} \tag{A3.1.5}$$

2. INTEGRAL EQUATIONS

If derivative estimation emphasizes noise, then integration deemphasizes noise. This is because numerical integration involves summation, and errors are likely to be positive sometimes and negative at other times. In the sum, positive errors will cancel with negative errors.

Numerical integration can be performed in a number of ways. Trapezoidal integration gives

$$\int_{t_0}^{t_1} V(t)\,dt \approx \frac{(t_1 - t_0)}{2}(V_0 + V_1) \tag{A3.1.6}$$

Simpson's rule is another means of integration:

$$\int_{t_0}^{t_2} V(t)\,dt \approx \frac{(t_2 - t_0)}{3}[V_0 + 4V_1 + V_2] \tag{A3.1.7}$$

If we have a model equation of the form

$$\frac{V}{C} + R\frac{dV}{dt} + I\frac{d^2V}{dt^2} = f(t) \tag{A3.1.8}$$

then we can solve it for the highest derivative:

$$\frac{d^2V}{dt^2} = \frac{1}{I}\left[f(t) - R\frac{dV}{dt} - \frac{V}{C}\right] \tag{A3.1.9}$$

After d^2V/dt^2 is evaluated numerically, dV/dt can be formed by numerically integrating d^2V/dt^2, and V can be formed by numerically integrating dV/dt. Thus all derivatives can be found in order.

3. INITIAL VALUES

A common mistake made by students is to assume all derivatives to be initially zero. If this were the case, then lower order derivatives would never become nonzero. Returning to Equation A3.1.9, an initial estimate of d^2V/dt^2 can be made if $f(0)$, $(dV/dt)(0)$, and $V(0)$ are known or assumed. Let us assume that $f(0)$ and $f(1)$ are known. Initially we assume $V(0) = V_0 = V_1$ and $(dV/dt)(0) = dV_0/dt$. If, in addition, the parameters I, R, and C are not constant, then

$$\frac{dV_1}{dt} = \int_{t_0}^{t_1} \frac{d^2V}{dt^2} dt \approx \frac{[t_1 - t_0]}{2} \left[\frac{1}{I_1}\left(f(1) - R_1 \frac{dV_1}{dt} - \frac{V_1}{C_1} \right) + \frac{1}{I_2}\left(f(0) - R_0 \frac{dV_0}{dt} - \frac{V_0}{C_0} \right) \right]$$

(A3.1.10)

or

$$\frac{dV_1}{dt}\left[1 + \frac{R_1}{I_1}\frac{(t_1 - t_0)}{2} \right] = \frac{[t_1 - t_0]}{2} \left[\frac{1}{I_1}\left(f(1) - \frac{V_1}{C_1} \right) + \frac{1}{I_2}\left(f(0) - R_0 \frac{dV_0}{dt} - \frac{V_0}{C_0} \right) \right]$$

(A3.1.11)

If I, R, and C are constant, Equation A3.1.11 simplifies considerably. Often enough, initial values for V and dV/dt are taken to be zero, which will give a solution over time for V relative to the starting value.

After initial values of $f(t)$, dV/dt, and V are calculated, they can be substituted into the system equations to obtain all values at all times. Changes in higher order derivatives always precede changes in lower order derivatives.

4. TIME STEP

The time increment from one numerical evaluation to the next can be critical. With too large a step, inaccuracy or even instability can result. With too small a step, the entire procedure can take much longer than necessary and errors due to small differences can compound rapidly. Entire chapters in numerical technique textbooks are dedicated to this topic. In general, the more rapid the change expected in the results, the smaller the time increment must be. A useful procedure is to increase the time step by 2 and compare results from the original time increment to results from the new time step. If a difference is noted, then the increase probably cannot be made. If no appreciable difference is noted, increase the time step by another factor of 2 and repeat the procedure. No change in the results indicates that a larger time step can be used.

Instability can usually be of two kinds: results oscillate between limits and don't seem to settle down to one result, or results increase without bound. When either of these is encountered, the time increment should be decreased.

APPENDIX 3.2
PONTRYAGIN MAXIMUM PRINCIPLE

The Pontryagin maximum principle is a necessary but not sufficient condition for optimality. Beginning with the state equations for a system:

$$\frac{dx_i}{dt} = f_i(x_j), \qquad i = 1, 2, 3, \ldots, n$$
$$j = 1, 2, 3, \ldots, n \qquad \text{(A3.2.1)}$$

find the control function u which causes the functional

$$x_0 = \int_{t_0}^{t} f_0(x_j, u) \, dt \qquad \text{(A3.2.2)}$$

to take its minimum possible value.

The Pontryagin method begins with the formation of a system of linear homogeneous adjoint equations:

$$\frac{d\psi_i}{dt} = -\sum_{j=0}^{n} \frac{\partial f_j}{\partial x_i} \psi_j \qquad \text{(A3.2.3)}$$

and follows with a function H:

$$H = \sum_{j=0}^{n} \psi_j f_j(x_i, u) \qquad \text{(A3.2.4)}$$

The optimal control function u is that which causes H to take its maximum possible value for all times t. This optimal control function also causes x_0 to be minimized at all times.

A simple example shows how this scheme is applied. Consider a system described by

$$\frac{dx_1}{dt} = x_2 = f_1 \qquad \text{(A3.2.5)}$$

$$\frac{dx_2}{dt} = u = f_2 \qquad \text{(A3.2.6)}$$

with the constraint that $|u| \leqslant 1$ (Barkelew, 1975). The problem is to minimize the time for the system to reach $x_1 = x_2 = 0$ starting at any initial state $x_1(0)$, $x_2(0)$. Since the cost functional involves the time to reach zero,

$$x_0 = \int_{0}^{t} dt \qquad \text{(A3.2.7)}$$

and the minimum x_0 will give the desired condition for optimality.

Because $f_0 = 1$ does not involve x_1 or x_2, and neither do f_1 and f_2, ψ_0 is not considered. From Equation A3.2.3:

$$\frac{d\psi_1}{dt} = -\frac{\partial f_1}{\partial x_1} \psi_1 - \frac{\partial f_2}{\partial x_1} \psi_2 = -0 - 0 = 0 \qquad \text{(A3.2.8)}$$

$$\frac{d\psi_2}{dt} = -\frac{\partial f_1}{\partial x_2} \psi_1 - \frac{\partial f_2}{\partial x_2} \psi_2 = -\psi_1 - 0 = -\psi_1 \qquad \text{(A3.2.9)}$$

Integrating Equations A3.2.8 and A3.2.9 gives

$$\psi_1 = C_1 \qquad \text{(A3.2.10)}$$

$$\psi_2 = C_2 - C_1 t \tag{A3.2.11}$$

Then

$$H = C_1 x_2 + (C_2 - C_1 t)u \tag{A3.2.12}$$

The maximum value for H occurs with $u = 1$ when $(C_2 - C_1 t) > 0$ and $u = -1$ when $(C_2 - C_1 t) < 0$. Since t increases monotonically from zero, u begins with a value of $+1$ (assuming C_1 and C_2 to be positive) and changes to -1 for $t > C_1/C_2$ and then remains at -1.

The constants C_1 and C_2 can be assigned values based on initial values and ending values (ending values both zero) for x_1 and x_2. For nonlinear problems, determination of C_1 and C_2 values is not easy.

The example just given is a very simple one. For a more realistic biological model such as

$$\frac{V}{C} + R\frac{dV}{dt} + I\frac{d^2 V}{dt^2} = u \tag{A3.2.13}$$

with the objective to find u to minimize mean squared acceleration,

$$x_0 = \int_0^t \ddot{V} dt \tag{A3.2.14}$$

one proceeds to determine the first-order state equations by defining

$$x_1 = V \tag{A3.2.15}$$

$$x_2 = \dot{V} = \frac{dV}{dt} = \frac{dx_1}{dt} \tag{A3.2.16}$$

so that Equation A3.2.13 yields

$$\frac{dx_1}{dt} = x_2 \tag{A3.2.17}$$

$$\frac{dx_2}{dt} = \frac{u}{I} - \frac{x_1}{IC} - \frac{R}{I}x_2 \tag{A3.2.18}$$

From this point, finding the optimal H value proceeds in a fashion similar to the previous example, but this is very much more complicated and in all likelihood would need to be solved numerically.

The Pontryagin maximum principle attempts to find an optimal set of control values from one point in space–time. If several sets of values give local optima, the nonsufficient nature of the maximum principle does not allow the absolute optimum to be chosen from among the set of local optima.

APPENDIX 3.3
THE LAPLACE TRANSFORM

Transforms are mathematical tools that ease the solution of constant coefficient differential equations, integral equations, and convolution integrals. Laplace transforms are one type of transform used to convert ordinary differential equations into algebraic equations. This eases the work of solving these equations because algebraic operations are easily performed. The general order of solution is (1) transform the equation into its algebraic form (often called conversion into the s domain, so-called because of the Laplace transform operator symbolized by s), (2) algebraically solve the transformed equation for the dependent variable, and (3) reconvert the dependent variable into its time-equivalent function (often called conversion to the time domain). Practically speaking, the first step is usually a simple replacement of s^n for d^n/dt^n and s^{-n} for $\int_n \cdots \int (dt)^n$, and the last step can be aided by complete tables of inverse Laplace transformations (see, for example, Barnes, 1975, or Wylie, 1966).

The Laplace transform for a real function $f(t)$ which equals zero for $t < 0$ is

$$\mathcal{L}[f(t)] = \int_0^\infty e^{-st} f(t)\,dt = F(s) \tag{A3.3.1}$$

where $\mathcal{L}[f(t)] = F(s) = $ Laplace transform of $f(t)$
$\qquad\quad s = $ a complex (real + imaginary) parameter, dimensionless
and the inverse Laplace transformation is

$$\mathcal{L}^{-1}[F(s)] = \frac{1}{2\pi i} \int_{a-i\infty}^{a+i\infty} e^{st} F(s)\,ds = f(t) \tag{A3.3.2}$$

where $a = $ a real constant chosen to exclude all singularities of $F(s)$ to the left of
$\qquad\quad$ the path of integration
$\qquad i = $ the imaginary indicator
This last integral is to be completed in the complex plane and may not always exist. Fortunately, this integration need not often be carried out.

The Laplace transformation is a linear operation. This means that it obeys the rules of association and distribution:

$$\mathcal{L}[cf(t) + dg(t)] = c\mathcal{L}[f(t)] + d\mathcal{L}[g(t)]$$
$$= cF(s) + dG(s) \tag{A3.3.3}$$

$$\mathcal{L}^{-1}[cF(s) + dG(s)] = c\mathcal{L}^{-1}[F(s)] + d\mathcal{L}^{-1}[G(s)]$$
$$= cf(t) + dg(t) \tag{A3.3.4}$$

As briefly stated earlier,

$$\mathcal{L}\left[\frac{d^n f(t)}{dt^n}\right] = s^n F(s) - \sum_{m=0}^{n-1} \frac{d^m f(0^+)}{dt^m} s^{n-m-1} \tag{A3.3.5}$$

where $\dfrac{d^m f(0^+)}{dt^m} = $ the mth derivative of $f(t)$, which is evaluated at a time infinitesimally
$\qquad\qquad\qquad$ greater than zero
Often the assumption is made that the modeled system begins at rest and that all derivatives begin with a value zero. For instance, the system with a time-domain response of

$$\frac{V}{C} + R\frac{dV}{dt} + I\frac{d^2 V}{dt^2} = g(t) \tag{A3.3.6}$$

would be transformed into the equation

$$\frac{V(s)}{C} + R[sV(s) - V(0^+)] + I[s^2 V(s) - sV(0^+) - \dot{V}(0^+)] = G(s) \tag{A3.3.7}$$

If we assume the system starts completely from rest,

$$\frac{V(s)}{C} + RsV(s) + Is^2V(s) = G(s) \tag{A3.3.8}$$

Solving for the dependent variable $V(s)$,

$$V(s) = \frac{G(s)}{1/C + Rs + Is^2} \tag{A3.3.9}$$

Thus far the forcing function $G(s)$ has not been specified. If the forcing function $g(t)$ is an impulse, then $G(s) = 1$. If $g(t)$ is a unit step (the input is 0 for $t < 0$ and 1 for $t > 0$), then $G(s) = s^{-1}$. If $g(t)$ is a unit ramp $[g(t) = t]$, then $G(s) = s^{-2}$. One advantage of the Laplace transformation is that $g(t)$ need not be specified until inverse transformation is to occur, but essential information about system operation can be deduced while still in the s domain.

To obtain the inverse transformation of Equation A3.3.9, the denominator is usually factored into first-order terms:

$$V(s) = \frac{G(s)}{I(s + A)(s + B)} \tag{A3.3.10a}$$

$$A = \frac{R - (R^2 - 4IC)^{1/2}}{2I} \tag{A3.3.10b}$$

$$B = \frac{R + (R^2 - 4IC)^{1/2}}{2I} \tag{A3.3.10c}$$

and then separated into individual fractions:

$$V(s) = \frac{\alpha G(s)}{I(s + A)} + \frac{\beta G(s)}{(s + B)} = \frac{G(s)}{I(s + A)(s + B)} \tag{A3.3.11}$$

where α and β = constants to be determined
In order that Equation A3.3.11 be an equality,

$$\alpha G(s)[s + B] + \beta G(s)[I(s + A)] = G(s) \tag{A3.3.12}$$

$$(\alpha + \beta I)s + (B\alpha + \beta I A) = 1 \tag{A3.3.13}$$

Collecting like powers of s,

$$s^1: \qquad \alpha + \beta I = 0 \tag{A3.3.14a}$$

$$s^0: \qquad B\alpha + \beta I A = 1 \tag{A3.3.14b}$$

which, when solved, give

$$\alpha = (B - A)^{-1} \tag{A3.3.15a}$$

$$\beta = [I(A - B)]^{-1} \tag{A3.3.15b}$$

so that

$$V(s) = \frac{G(s)/(B - A)}{I(s + A)} + \frac{G(s)/[I(A - B)]}{(s + B)} \tag{A3.3.16}$$

If now we specify that $g(t) = 1$ and $G(s) = 1/s$,

$$V(s) = \frac{1}{(B - A)Is(s + A)} + \frac{1}{I(A - B)s(s + B)} \tag{A3.3.17}$$

which will be found from Laplace transform tables to correspond to

$$V(t) = \frac{1 - e^{-At}}{A(B - A)I} + \frac{1 - e^{-Bt}}{I(A - B)B} \tag{A3.3.18}$$

the difference of two exponential terms.

With use, Laplace transforms will be found to be easy to apply to most constant coefficient systems. Recognition that terms such as $(s + A)^{-1}$ correspond to exponentials in the time domain can come automatically. Furthermore, the frequency response of a system (i.e., the output magnitude and phase angle as input frequency is varied) can be simply obtained by replacing s by $i\omega$, where i is the imaginary operator and ω the radial frequency. This is true because the Laplace transform is a special case of the Fourier transform.

Unfortunately, many of the more realistic biological systems models are not entirely linear and may not include constant coefficients. For those models Laplace transforms can be used only for restricted conditions.

SYMBOLS

A	area, m^2
A_{LU}	unstressed left ventricular muscle cross-sectional area, m^2
A_p	cross-sectional area of pulmonary artery, m^2
A_{RU}	unstressed right ventricular muscle cross-sectional area, m^2
a	constant, N
a_1	constant, N
a_1	constant, dimensionless
a_2	coefficient, sec
a_3	coefficient, sec
B	base excess, Eq/m^3
b	constant, m/sec
b	cooling ability on transient response, dimensionless
b_1	constant, m/sec
C	yield stress, N/m^2
C_{cl}	thermal conductance of clothing, $N \cdot m/(m^2 \cdot sec \cdot °C)$
C_i	coefficient, %
C_j	compliance of segment j, m^5/N
C_{LA}	left atrial compliance, m^5/N
C_p	effective arterial distensibility, m^5/N
C_{RA}	right atrial compliance, m^5/N
C_{se}	ventricular series element compliance, m^5/N
C_v	ventricular compliance, m^5/N
CO	cardiac output, m^3/sec
CP	cooling power of the environment, $N \cdot m/sec$
c	concentration, mol/m^3
D	vessel diameter, m
E_1	internal energy, $N \cdot m$

E_2	contractile energy, N·m
E_3	external work, N·m
E_4	systolic contraction penalty, N·m
E_{max}	maximum evaporative cooling capacity of the environment, N·m/sec
E_{req}	required evaporative cooling, N·m/sec
F	force, N
F_c	force developed by muscle contractile element, N
$F_{c\,max}$	maximum contractile force, N
F_L	force developed in left ventricular myocardium, N
F_{max}	maximum force, N
F_{min}	minimum force, N
F_p	force developed by muscle parallel elastic element, N
F_R	force developed in right ventricular wall, N
f	neural firing rate, impulses/sec
G	amplification factor, dimensionless
g	acceleration due to gravity, m/sec^2
g_1	mode 1 contribution to heart period control, sec
g_2	mode 2 contribution to heart period control, sec
H	activation factor sensitivity, dimensionless
HR	submaximal heart rate, beats/sec
HR_f	final heart rate, beats/sec
$HR_{f,n}$	nonacclimated final heart rate, beats/sec
HR_{max}	maximum heart rate, beats/sec
HR_r	resting heart rate, beats/sec
HR_v	heart rate during work, beats/sec
I	heart rate index, beats/sec
I_b	blood inertance, N·sec^2/m^5
I_{bL}	left ventricular blood inertance, N·sec^2/m^5
I_{bR}	right ventricular blood inertance, N·sec^2/m^5
I_j	inertance of segment j, N·sec^2/m^5
im	permeability index, dimensionless
J	cost functional, N·m
J	ratio of red blood cell diameter to vessel radius, dimensionless
K	consistency coefficient, N·sec^n/m^2
k	heart rate effect on transient response, beats/sec
k_1	steady-state heart rate coefficient, beats/sec
L	length, m
L_c	muscle contractile element length, m
L_p	muscle parallel element length, m
L_s	muscle series element length, m
M	metabolic rate, N·m/sec
M_c	metabolic factor, N·sec/m^2
m	an even number, dimensionless
m_b	mass of blood, kg
N	number of days in heat, days
n	flow behavior index, dimensionless
$\mathscr{P}$	baroreceptor pressure function, N/m^2
$\mathscr{P}_N$	normal baroreceptor pressure function, N/m^2
$\mathscr{P}_{th}$	threshold baroreceptor function value, N/m^2
p	pressure, N/m^2
p_a	arterial pressure, N/m^2
$\bar{p}_a$	normal arterial pressure, N/m^2

p_{ad}	diastolic arterial blood pressure, N/m^2
p_{amb}	ambient water vapor pressure, N/m^2
p_{ap}	pulmonary arterial pressure, N/m^2
p_{as}	systolic arterial blood pressure, N/m^2
p_c	capillary pressure, N/m^2
$\bar{p}_c$	normal capillary pressure, N/m^2
p_d	static pressure developed by relaxed muscle, N/m^2
p_i	inside pressure, N/m^2
p_{ij}	entrance pressure of segment u, N/m^2
$p_{j(1+j)}$	entrance pressure to segment $(1 + j)$, N/m^2
p_{LA}	left atrial pressure, N/m^2
p_{LV}	left ventricular pressure, N/m^2
p_o	outside pressure, N/m^2
pO_2	partial pressure of oxygen, N/m^2
p_{0a}	outer abdominal pressure, N/m^2
p_{oj}	exit pressure of segment j, N/m^2
p_{ot}	outer thoracic pressure, N/m^2
p_p	pulmonary artery pressure, N/m^2
p_{RA}	right atrial pressure, N/m^2
p_{RV}	right ventricular pressure, N/m^2
p_s	carotid sinus pressure, N/m^2
p_s	isometric pressure during systole, N/m^2
p_{smax}	carotid sinus pressure at maximum gain, N/m^2
p_{th}	threshold pressure, N/m^2
p_v	mean venous pressure, N/m^2
p_v	filling pressure, N/m^2
p_v	normal mean venous pressure, N/m^2
p_{va}	venous transmural pressure in the abdominal cavity, N/m^2
p_{vp}	pulmonary venous pressure, N/m^2
p_{vt}	venous transmural pressure in the thorax, N/m^2
Δp	pressure drop or change in pressure, N/m^2
Δp_j	pressure difference between entrance and outlet of segment j, N/m^2
Q	activation factor, dimensionless
Q'	new value for activation factor, dimensionless
R	resistance, $N \cdot sec/m^5$
R_a	arterial resistance, $N \cdot sec/m^5$
R_{av}	aortic valve resistance, $N \cdot sec/m^5$
R_b	nonlinear aortic resistance, $N \cdot sec/m^2$
R_{cv}	resistance of capillary walls to fluid flow, $N \cdot sec/m^5$
R_d	internal ventricular resistance during diastole, $N \cdot sec/m^5$
R_j	resistance of segment j, $N \cdot sec/m^5$
R'_j	resistance to movement of wall tissue, $N \cdot sec/m^5$
R_L	viscous resistance of blood, $N \cdot sec/m^5$
R_{LAV}	mitral valve resistance, $N \cdot sec/m^5$
R_N	normal vascular resistance, $N \cdot sec/m^5$
R_p	resistance of pulmonary vasculature, $N \cdot sec/m^5$
R_p	total peripheral resistance, $N \cdot sec/m^5$
R_R	right ventricular resistance, $N \cdot sec/m^5$
R_{RAV}	tricuspid valve resistance, $N \cdot sec/m^5$
R_s	internal ventricular resistance during systole, $N \cdot sec/m^5$
R_v	resistance to inflow, $N \cdot sec/m^5$
R_v	venous resistance, $N \cdot sec/m^5$
Re	Reynolds number, dimensionless

r	distance between plates, m
r	radial distance from the center of a tube, m
r_i	inside radius of a tube, m
r_o	outside radius of a tube, m
Δr	red blood cell diameter, m
Δr	wall thickness, m
S	oxygen saturation, %
S_L	left ventricular shape factor, dimensionless
S_R	right ventricular shape factor, dimensionless
SV	stroke volume, m^3
t	time, sec
t_d	delay time, sec
t_{dv}	duration of ventricular diastole, sec
t_e	ejection time, sec
t_e	systolic period, sec
t_{sa}	duration of atrial systole, sec
t_{sv}	duration of ventricular systole, sec
U	muscle yielding factor, m/sec
V	volume, m^2
V_c	volume of blood delivered to peripheral compliance, m^3
V_d	ventricular end-diastolic volume, m^3
V_j	volume of segment j, m^3
$V_j(0)$	initial volume of segment j, m^3
V_{LA}	left atrial volume, m^3
$V_{LA}(0)$	left atrial end-diastolic volume, m^3
V_{LV}	left ventricular volume, m^3
$V_{LV}(0)$	initial left ventricular volume, m^3
V_{RA}	right atrial volume, m^3
$V_{RA}(0)$	right atrial end-diastolic volume, m^3
V_{RV}	right ventricular volume, m^3
$V_{RV}(0)$	initial right ventricular volume, m^3
V_r	volume of blood delivered to vascular resistance, m^3
V_s	ventricular end-systolic volume, m^3
$V_{TOT}(t)$	total circulatory vessel volume, m^3
$V_{TOT}(0)$	initial value of total circulatory vessel volume, m^3
ΔV_{TOT}	total blood volume change, m^3
ΔV_{LV}	volume of blood delivered by left ventricle, m^3
$\dot{V}$	volume rate of flow, m^3/sec
$\dot{V}_{cw}$	net flow through capillary walls, m^3/sec
$\dot{V}_j$	flow through segment j, m^3/sec
$\dot{V}_{ij}$	flow into segment j, m^3/sec
$\dot{V}_{iLA}$	left atrial inflow, m^3/sec
$\dot{V}_{iLV}$	left ventricular inflow, m^3/sec
$\dot{V}_{iRA}$	right atrial inflow, m^3/sec
$\dot{V}_{iRA}$	right ventricular inflow, m^3/sec
$\dot{V}_{i(1+j)}$	flow into segment $(1 + j)$, m^3/sec
$\dot{V}_{O_2}$	oxygen uptake, m^3/sec
$\dot{V}_{O_2max}$	maximum oxygen uptake, m^3/sec
$\dot{V}_{oj}$	outflow from segment j, m^3/sec
$\dot{V}_{oLA}$	left atrial outflow, m^3/sec
$\dot{V}_{oLV}$	left ventricular outflow, m^3/sec
$\dot{V}_{oRA}$	right atrial outflow, m^3/sec
$\dot{V}_{oRV}$	right ventricular outflow, m^3/sec

$\dot{V}_p$	pulmonary vessel flow rate, m^3/sec
$\dot{V}_v$	venous flow rate, m^3/sec
v	flow velocity, m/sec
v_b	blood velocity, m/sec
v_c	shortening velocity of contractile element, m/sec
W	external work, $N \cdot m$
y	age, yr
z	axial dimension along a tube, m
z	height, m
α	weighting parameter, sec/m^4
α_1	constant, $m^3/(N \cdot sec)$
α_2	constant, $m^5/(N \cdot sec)$
α_3	constant, $N \cdot m/beat$
α_4	constant, $N \cdot m/sec$
β_+	sensitivity coefficient, m^2/N
β_-	sensitivity coefficient, m^2/N
β_0	sensitivity coefficient, $m^2/(N \cdot sec)$
β_1	coefficient, $(m^2/N)^n$
β_2	constant, N/m^2
β_3	coefficient, dimensionless
β_4	coefficient, $sec \cdot m^2/N$
γ	rate of shear, sec^{-1}
δ	thickness of outer layer in two-liquid fluid flow in a tube, m
η	mechanical efficiency, dimensionless
θ	temperature, °C
θ_a	ambient temperature, °C
λ_1	steady-state gain, $m^2 \cdot sec/N$
λ_2	steady-state gain, $m^2 \cdot sec/N$
μ	viscosity, $kg/(m \cdot sec)$
μ_b	viscosity of blood, $kg/(m \cdot sec)$
μ_p	viscosity of plasma, $kg/(m \cdot sec)$
v_{O_2}	oxygen content of the blood, $m^3 O_2/m^3$ blood
ρ	density, kg/m^3
τ	shear stress, N/m^2
τ_+	time constant for increasing pressure, sec
τ_-	time constant for decreasing pressure, sec
τ_1	time constant, sec
τ_2	time constant, sec
τ_3	time constant, sec
τ_d	time constant for myocardial relaxation, sec
τ_h	time constant, sec
τ_o	end-diastolic stress, N/m^2
τ_s	time constant of venous stress relaxation, sec
τ_v	vascular time constant, sec
ϕ	dimensionless fraction
ϕ_a	ambient relative humidity, dimensionless

REFERENCES

Aberman, A., J. M. Cavanilles, J. Trotter, D. Erbeck, M. H. Weil, and H. Shubin. 1973. An Equation for the Oxygen Hemoglobin Dissociation Curve. *J. Appl. Physiol.* **35**: 570–571.

Asmusen, E., and M. Nielsen. 1952. The Cardiac Output in Rest and Work Determined by the Acetylene and Dye Injection Method. *Acta Physiol. Scand.* **27**: 217–230.

Astrand, P. O., and K. Rodahl. 1970. *Textbook of Work Physiology*. McGraw-Hill, New York, pp. 117–183.

Attinger, E. O. 1976a. The Vascular System, in *Biological Foundations of Biomedical Engineering*, J. Kline, ed. Little, Brown, Boston, pp. 163–183.

Attinger, E. O. 1976b. Cardiovascular Control, in *Biological Foundations of Biomedical Engineering*, J. Kline, ed. Little, Brown, Boston, pp. 197–216.

Attinger, E. O. 1976c. Models of the Cardiovascular System, in *Biological Foundations of Biomedical Engineering*, J. Kline, ed. Little, Brown, Boston, pp. 217–227.

Attinger, E. O., and D. D. Michie. 1976. The Structure and Rheology of Blood, in *Biological Foundations of Biomedical Engineering*, J. Kline, ed. Little, Brown, Boston, pp. 141–161.

Barcroft, J. 1925. The Respiratory Function of the Blood. Part I. Lessons from High Altitude. Cambridge University Press, Cambridge.

Bard, P. 1961. Blood Supply of Special Regions, in *Medical Physiology*, P. Bard, ed. C. V. Mosby: St. Louis.

Barkelew, C. H. 1975. Automatic Control, in *Handbook of Engineering Fundamentals*, O. W. Eshbach and M. Souders, ed. John Wiley & Sons, New York, pp. 1206–1210.

Barnes, J. L. 1975. Mathematics, in *Handbook of Engineering Fundamentals*, O. W. Eshbach and M. Souders, ed. John Wiley & Sons, New York, pp. 334–347.

Bauer, R. D., R. Busse, and E. Wetterer. 1983. Biomechanics of the Cardiovascular System, in *Biophysics*, W. Hoppe, W. Lohmann, H. Markl, and H. Ziegler, ed. Springer-Verlag, Berlin, pp. 618–630.

Baumeister, T., ed. 1967. *Marks' Standard Handbook for Mechanical Engineers*, 7th ed. McGraw-Hill, New York, pp. 355–358.

Beneken, J. E. W., and B. DeWit. 1967. A Physical Approach to Hemodynamic Aspects of the Human Cardiovascular System, in *Physical Bases of Circulatory Transport: Regulation and Exchange*, E. B. Reeve and A. C. Guyton, ed. W. B. Saunders, Philadelphia, pp. 1–45.

Berne, R. M., and M. N. Levy. 1981. *Cardiovascular Physiology*. C. V. Mosby, St. Louis.

Bloomfield, M. E., L. D. Gold, R. V. Reddy, A. I. Katz, and A. H. Boreno. 1972. Thermodynamic Characterization of the Contractile State of the Myocardium. *Circ. Res.* **30**: 520–534.

Brengelman, G. L. 1983. Circulatory Adjustments to Exercise and Heat Stress. *Ann. Rev. Physiol.* **45**: 191–212.

Brück, K. 1986. Are Non-Thermal Factors Important in the Cutaneous Vascular Response to Exercise? A Proponent's View. *Yale J. Biol. Med.* **59**: 289–297.

Burton, A. C. 1965. Hemodynamics and the Physics of the Circulation, in *Physiology and Biophysics*, T. C. Ruch and H. D. Patton, ed. W. B. Saunders, Philadelphia, pp. 523–542.

Catchpole, H. R. 1966. The Capillaries, Veins, and Lymphatics, in *Physiology and Biophysics*, T. C. Ruch and H. D. Patton, ed. W. B. Saunders, Philadelphia, pp. 617–643.

Charm, S. E., and G. S. Kurland. 1974. *Blood Flow and Microcirculation*. John Wiley & Sons, New York.

Comess, K. A., and P. E. Fenster. 1981. Clinical Implications of the Blood Pressure Response to Exercise. *Cardiology* **68**: 233–244.

Dix, F. J., and G. W. Scott-Blair. 1940. On the Flow of Suspensions Through Narrow Tubes. *J. Appl. Phys.* **11**: 574–581.

Erikssen, J., and K. Rodahl. 1979. Seasonal Variation in Work Performance and Heart Rate Response to Exercise. *Eur. J. Appl. Physiol.* **42**: 133–140.

Faucheux, B. A., C. Dupuis, A. Baulon, F. Lille, and F. Bourlière. 1983. Heart Rate Reactivity During Minor Mental Stress in Men in Their 50's and 70's. *Gerontology* **29**: 149–160.

Fujihara, Y., J. R. Hildebrandt, and J. Hildebrandt. 1973a. Cardiorespiratory Transients in Exercising Man. I. Tests of Superposition. *J. Appl. Physiol.* **35**: 58–67.

Fujihara, Y., J. Hildebrandt, and J. R. Hildebrandt. 1973b. Cardiorespiratory Transients in Exercising Man. II. Linear Models. *J. Appl. Physiol.* **35**: 68–76.

Ganong, W. F. 1963. *Review of Medical Physiology*. Lange Medical Publications, Los Altos, Calif, pp. 385–481.

Givoni, B., and R. F. Goldman. 1973b. Predicting Heart Rate Response to Work, Environment, and Clothing. *J. Appl. Physiol.* **34**: 201–204.

Givoni, B., and R. F. Goldman. 1973a. Predicting Effects of Heat Acclimatization on Heart Rate and Rectal Temperature. *J. Appl. Physiol.* **35**: 875–879.

Green, J. F., and A. P. Jackman. 1984. Peripheral Limitations to Exercise. *Med. Sci. Sports Exerc.* **16**: 299–305.

Greene, M. E., J. W. Clark, D. N. Mohr, and H. M. Bourland. 1973. A Mathematical Model of Left-Ventricular Function. *Med. Biol. Eng.* **11**: 126–134.

Greg, D. E. 1961. Regulation of Pressure and Flow in the Systemic and Pulmonary Circulation, in *The Physiological Basis of Medical Practice*, C. H. Best and N. B. Taylor, ed. Williams & Wilkins, Baltimore, pp. 274–301.

Grodins, F. S. 1959. Integrative Cardiovascular Physiology: A Mathematical Synthesis of Cardiac and Blood Vessel Hemodynamics. *Q. Rev. Biol.* **34**: 93–116.

Grodins, F. S. 1963. *Control Theory and Biological Systems.* Columbia University Press, New York.

Guyton, A. C. 1986. *Textbook of Medical Physiology.* W. B. Saunders, Philadelphia.

Hales, J. R. S. 1986. A Case Supporting the Proposal that Cardiac Filling Pressure Is the Limiting Factor in Adjusting to Heat Stress. *Yale J. Biol. Med.* **59**: 237–245.

Hämäläinen, R. P. 1975. *Optimization Concepts in Models of Physiological Systems.* Report 27, Helsinki University of Technology, Systems Theory Laboratory, Espoo, Finland.

Hämäläinen, R. P., and J. J. Hämäläinen. 1985. On the Minimum Work Criterion in Optimal Control Models of Left-Ventricular Ejection. *IEEE Trans. Biomed.* **32**: 951–956.

Hämäläinen, R. P., J. J. Hämäläinen, and U. Miekkala. 1982. Optimal Control Modelling of Ventricular Ejection—Do the Endpoint Conditions Dominate the Performance Criterion? International Federation for Information Processing Working Conference on Modelling and Data Analysis in Biotechnology and Medical Engineering, University of Ghent, Belgium.

Hamilton, M. 1954. The Aetiology of Essential Hypertension. I. The Arterial Pressure in the General Population. *Clin. Sci.* **13**: 11–14.

Hammond, H. K., and V. F. Froelicher. 1985. Normal and Abnormal Heart Rate Responses to Exercise. *Prog. Cardiovasc. Dis.* **28**: 271–296.

Haynes, R. H. 1960. Physical Basis of the Dependence of Blood Viscosity on Tube Radius. *Am. J. Physiol.* **198**: 1193–1200.

Haynes, R. H., and A. C. Burton. 1959. Role of the Non-Newtonian Behavior of Blood in Hemodynamics. *Am. J. Physiol.* **197**: 943–950.

Hodgman, C. D. 1959. *Mathematical Tables from Handbook of Chemistry and Physics.* Chemical Rubber Company, Cleveland.

Isenberg, I. 1953. A Note on the Flow of Blood in Capillary Tubes. *Bull. Math. Biophys.* **15**: 149–152.

Johnson, A. T. 1980. Biomechanics in Agriculture, in *Perspectives in Biomechanics*, H. Reul, D. N. Ghista, and G. Rau, ed. Harwood, Chur, Switzerland, pp. 399–432.

Jones, G. E., and H. J. Johnson. 1980. Heart Rate and Somatic Concomitants of Mental Imagery. *Psychophysiology* **17**: 339–347.

Kagawa, T. 1984. Programs for Solving O_2 and CO_2 Diffusions into and out of the Erythrocyte. Booklet edited by M. Mochizuki. Yamagata Medical Society, Yamagata, Japan.

Kenney, W. L. 1985. Parasympathetic Control of Resting Heart Rate: Relationship to Aerobic Power. *Med. Sci. Sports Exerc.* **17**: 451–455.

Kirsch, K. A., L. Röcker, H. B. Ameln, and K. Hrynyschyn. 1986. The Cardiac Filling Pressure Following Exercise and Thermal Stress. *Yale J. Biol. Med.* **59**: 257–265.

Korner, P. I. 1971. Integrative Neural Cardiovascular Control. *Physiol. Rev.* **51**: 312–367.

Lesage, R., J.-A. Simoneau, J. Jobin, J. Leblanc, and C. Bouchard. 1985. Familial Resemblance in Maximal Heart Rate, Blood Lactate, and Aerobic Power. *Hum. Hered.* **35**: 182–189.

Lightfoot, E. N. 1974. *Transport Phenomena and Living Systems.* John Wiley & Sons, New York, p. 31.

Lindqvist, A., E. Keskinen, K. Antila, L. Halkola, T. Peltonen, and I. Välimäki. 1983. Heart Rate Variability,

Cardiac Mechanics, and Subjectively Evaluated Stress During Simulator Flight. *Aviat. Space Environ. Med.* **54**: 685–690.

Linehan, J. H., and C. A. Dawson. 1983. A Three-Compartment Model of the Pulmonary Vasculature: Effects of Vasoconstriction. *J. Appl. Physiol.* **55**: 923–928.

Livnat, A., and S. M. Yamashiro. 1981. Optimal Control Evaluation of Left Ventricular Systolic Dynamics. *Am. J. Physiol.* **240**: R370–R383.

MacPherson, R. H. 1960. *Physiological Responses to Hot Environments*, Medical Research Council Special Report Series No. 298. Her Majesty's Stationery Office, London, England.

Mehlsen, J., K. Pagh, J. S. Nielsen, L. Sestoft, and S. L. Nielsen. 1987. Heart Rate Response to Breathing: Dependency upon Breathing Pattern. *Clin. Physiol.* **7**: 115–124.

Meier, G. D., M. C. Ziskin, W. P. Santamore, and A. A. Bove. 1980. Kinematics of the Beating Heart. *IEEE Trans. Biomed. Engr.* **BME-27**: 319–329.

Mende, T. J. 1976. Physicochemical Properties of Gases and Solutions, in *Biological Foundations of Biomedical Engineering*, J. Kline, ed. Little, Brown, Boston, pp. 17–40.

Mende, T. J., and L. Cuervo. 1976. Properties of Excitable and Contractile Tissue, in *Biological Foundations of Biomedical Engineering*, J. Kline, ed. Little, Brown, Boston, p. 97.

Michie, D. D., and J. Kline. 1976. The Heart as a Muscle and a Pump, in *Biological Foundations of Biomedical Engineering*, J. Kline, ed. Little, Brown, Boston, pp. 111–130.

Michie, D. D., J. Kline, and E. O. Attinger. 1976. Introduction to Structure and Organization [of the Cardiovascular System], in *Biological Foundations of Biomedical Engineering*, J. Kline, ed. Little, Brown, Boston, pp. 103–110.

Middleman, S. 1972. *Transport Phenomena in the Cardiovascular System.* John Wiley & Sons, New York.

Mitchell, J. H. 1985. Cardiovascular Control During Exercise: Central and Reflex Neural Mechanisms. *Am. J. Cardiol.* **55**: 34D–41D.

Mochizuki, M., T. Kagawa, K. Niizeki, and A. Shimouchi. 1985. Secondary CO_2 Diffusion Following HCO_3^- Shift Across the Red Cell Membrane, in *Oxygen Transport to Tissue*, D. Bruley, H. I. Bicher, and D. Reneau, ed. Plenum: New York, vol. 1, pp. 369–379.

Morehouse, L. E., and A. T. Miller. 1967. *Physiology of Exercise.* C. V. Mosby, Saint Louis, p. 111.

Murray, C. D. 1926. The Physiological Principle of Minimum Work. I. The Vascular System and the Cost of Blood Volume. *Proc. Natl. Acad. Sci. USA* **12**: 207–214.

Noordergraaf, A. 1978. *Circulatory System Dynamics.* Academic Press, New York.

Oka, S. 1981. *Cardiovascular Hemorheology.* Cambridge University Press, Cambridge, England.

Patterson, S. W., H. Piper, and E. H. Starling. 1914. The Regulation of the Heart Beat. *J. Physiol.* **48**: 465–513.

Pedley, T. J., T.-K. Hung, and R. Skalak. 1980. Fluid Mechanics of Cardiovascular Flow, in *Perspectives in Biomechanics*, H. Reul, D. N. Ghista, and G. Rau, ed. Harwood, Chur, Switzerland, pp. 113–226.

Perl, M., A. Horowitz, and S. Sideman. 1986. Comprehensive Model for the Simulation of Left Ventricle Mechanics. *Med. Biol. Eng. Comp.* **24**: 145–149.

Perski, A., S. P. Tzankoff, and B. T. Engel. 1985. Central Control of Cardiovascular Adjustments to Exercise. *J. Appl. Physiol.* **58**: 431–435.

Peters, J. P., and D. D. Van Slyke. 1931. *Quantitative Clinical Chemistry.* Williams & Wilkins, Baltimore.

Phillips, C. A., E. S. Grood, B. Schuster, and J. S. Petrofsky. 1982. Left Ventricular Work and Power: Circumferential, Radial and Longitudinal Components. Mathematical Derivation and Characteristic Variation with Left Ventricular Dysfunction. *J. Biomech.* **15**: 427–440.

Pittman, R. N., and M. L. Ellsworth. 1986. Estimation of Red Cell Flow in Microvessels: Consequences of the Baker-Wayland Spatial Averaging Model. *Microvasc. Res.* **32**: 371–388.

Rand, P. W., E. Lacombe, H. E. Hunt, and W. H. Austin. 1964. Viscosity of Normal Human Blood Under Normothermic and Hypothermic Conditions. *J. Appl. Physiol.* **19**: 117–122.

Reeve, E. B., and L. Kulhanek. 1967. Regulation of Body Water Content: A Preliminary Analysis, in *Physical Bases of Circulatory Transport: Regulation and Exchange*, E. B. Reeve and A. C. Guyton, ed. W. B. Saunders, Philadelphia, pp. 151–177.

Ribeiro, J. P., R. A. Fielding, V. Hughes, A. Black, M. A. Bochese, and H. G. Knuttgen. 1985. Heart Rate Break Point May Coincide with the Anaerobic and Not the Aerobic Threshold. *Int. J. Sports Med.* **6**: 220–224.

Richards, A. M., M. G. Nicholis, E. A. Espiner, H. Ikram, M. Cullens, and D. Hinton. 1986. Diurnal Patterns of Blood Pressure, Heart Rate and Vasoactive Hormones in Normal Man. *Clin. Exp.-Theory Pract.* **A8**: 153–166.

Riley, R. L. 1965. Gas Exchange and Transporation, in *Physiology and Biophysics*, T. C. Ruch and H. D. Patton, ed. W. B. Saunders, Philadelphia, pp. 761–787.

Robinson, D. A. 1965. Quantitative Analysis of the Control of Cardiac Output in the Isolated Left Ventricle. *Circ. Res.* **17**: 207–221.

Roughton, F. J. W. 1954. In *Handbook of Respiratory Physiology*, W. M. Boothby, ed. Randolph Air Force Base, Texas, Chapter 5.

Rushmer, R. F. 1966. General Characteristics of the Cardiovascular System, in *Physiology and Biophysics*, T. C. Ruch and H. D. Patton, ed. W. B. Saunders: Philadelphia, pp. 543–549.

Saltin, B. 1985. Hemodynamic Adaptations to Exercise. *Am. J. Cardiol.* **55**: 42D–47D.

Sandquist, G. M., D. B. Olsen, and W. J. Kolff. 1982. A Comprehensive Elementary Model of the Mammalian Circulatory System. *Ann. Biomed. Eng.* **10**: 1–33.

Schaible, T. F., and J. Scheuer. 1985. Cardiac Adaptations to Chronic Exercise. *Prog. Cardiovasc. Dis.* **28**: 297–324.

Scher, A. M. 1966a. Mechanical Events of the Cardiac Cycle, in *Physiology and Biophysics*, T. C. Ruch and H. D. Patton, ed. W. B. Saunders, Philadelphia, pp. 550–564.

Scher, A. M. 1966b. Control of Arterial Blood Pressure: Measurement of Pressure and Flow, in *Physiology and Biophysics*, T. C. Ruch and H. D. Patton, ed. W. B. Saunders, Philadelphia, pp. 660–683.

Schmid-Schönbein, G. W. 1988. A Theory of Blood Flow in Skeletal Muscle. *J. Biomech. Eng.* **110**: 20–26.

Segré, G., and A. Silberberg. 1962. Behavior of Macroscopic Rigid Spheres in Poiseuille Flow. *J. Fluid Mech.* **14**: 115–135, 136 157.

Senay, L. C. 1979. Effects of Exercise in the Heat on Body Fluid Distribution. *Med. Sci. Sports* **11**: 42–48.

Senay, L. C. 1986. An Inquiry into the Role of Cardiac Filling Pressure in Acclimatization to Heat. *Yale J. Biol. Med.* **59**: 247–256.

Skalak, T. C., and G. W. Schmid-Schönbein. 1986. The Microvasculature in Skeletal Muscle. IV. A Model of the Capillary Network. *Microvasc. Res.* **32**: 333–347.

Skelland, A. H. 1967. *Non-Newtonian Flow and Heat Transfer.* John Wiley & Sons, New York.

Smith, O. A. 1966. Cardiovascular Integration by the Central Nervous System, in *Physiology and Biophysics*, T. C. Ruch and H. D. Patton, ed. W. B. Saunders, Philadelphia, pp. 684–689.

Sorek, S., and S. Sideman. 1986a. A porous-Medium Approach for Modeling Heart Mechanics. I. Theory. *Math. Biosci.* **81**: 1–14.

Sorek, S., and S. Sideman. 1986b. A Porous-Medium Approach for Modeling Heart Mechanics. II. I-D Case. *Math. Biosci.* **81**: 15–32.

Spector, W. S. 1956. *Handbook of Biological Data*, WADC TR 56-273. Wright-Patterson Air Force Base, Ohio.

Stevens, G. H. J., T. E. Graham, and B. A. Wilson. 1987. Gender Differences in Cardiovascular and Metabolic Responses to Cold and Exercise. *Can. J. Physiol. Pharmacol.* **65**: 165–171.

Stone, H. L., K. J. Dormer, R. D. Foreman, R. Thies, and R. W. Blair. 1985. Neural Regulation of the Cardiovascular System During Exercise. *Fed. Proc.* **44**: 2271–2278.

Talbot, S. A., and U. Gessner. 1973. *Systems Physiology.* John Wiley & Sons, New York, pp. 345–426.

Tazawa, H., M. Mochizuki, M. Tamura, and T. Kagawa. 1983. Quantitative Analyses of the CO_2 Dissociation Curve of Oxygenated Blood and the Haldane Effect in Human Blood. *Jpn. J. Physiol.* **33**: 601–618.

Thomas, H. W. 1962. The Wall Effect in Capillary Instruments: An Improved Analysis Suitable for Application to Blood and Other Particulate Suspensions. *Biorheology* **1**: 41–56.

Tranel, D. T., A. E. Fisher, and D. C. Fowles. 1982. Magnitude of Incentive Effects on Heart Rate. *Psychophysiology* **19**: 514–519.

Wagner, J. A., and S. M. Horvath. 1985. Cardiovascular Reactions to Cold Exposures Differ with Age and Gender. *J. Appl. Physiol.* **58**: 187–192.

Wallace, A. G., J. H. Mitchell, N. S. Skinner, and S. J. Sarnoff. 1963. Duration of the Phases of Left Ventricular Systole. *Circ. Res.* **12**: 611–619.

Warner, H. R. 1964. Simulation as a Tool for Biological Research. *Simulation* **1**: 57–63.

Warner, H. R. 1965. Control of the Circulation as Studied with Analog Computer Technics, in *Handbook of Physiology, Volume 3 Section 2, Circulation*. W. F. Hamilton and P. Dow, ed. American Physiological Society, Washington, D.C., pp. 1825–1841.

Wenger, C. B. 1986. Non-Thermal Factors Are Important in the Control of Skin Blood Flow During Exercise Only Under High Physiological Strain. *Yale J. Biol. Med.* **59**: 307–319.

Woodbury, J. W. 1965. Regulation of pH, in *Physiology and Biophysics*, T. C. Ruch and H. D. Patton, ed. W. B. Saunders, Philadelphia, pp. 899–934.

Wylie, C. R. 1966. *Advanced Engineering Mathematics*. McGraw-Hill, New York, pp. 226–269.

Wyndham, C. H., N. B. Strydom, J. F. Morrison, F. D. Dutoit, and J. G. Kraan. 1954. Responses of Unacclimatized Men Under Stress of Heat and Work. *J. Appl. Physiol.* **6**: 681–686.

Yamashiro, S. M., J. A. Daubenspeck, and F. M. Bennett. 1979. Optimal Regulation of Left Ventricular Ejection Pattern. *Appl. Math. Comput.* **5**: 41–54.

CHAPTER 4

Respiratory Responses

Air which has thus served the purpose of animal respiration is no longer common air; it approaches to the nature of fixed air [air containing CO_2 and not O_2] in as much as it is capable of combining with lime-water and precipitating the lime from it, in the form of a calcareous earth; but it differs from fixed air.

—Antoine Lavoisier describing the work of Priestley

4.1 INTRODUCTION

Of all the bodily functions performed during exercise, respiration appears to be one of the most highly regulated and optimized. The amount of work performed by respiratory muscles to supply air for the exercising body can be considered to be a large part of the body's overhead. Respiratory work, which accounts for 1–2% of the total body oxygen expenditure during rest, may rise to as much as 10% or higher during exercise. This represents oxygen that is unavailable to the skeletal muscles for performing useful work. It appears reasonable, therefore, that neural mechanisms regulating respiration would aim to minimize the work of respiration. Simultaneous adjustments in airflow pattern, respiration rate, and respiratory mechanics appear to be directed toward minimizing oxygen expenditure of respiratory overhead.

Respiratory ventilation during rest is subject to a high degree of voluntary control. In exercise this does not appear to be true. Except for specialized sports such as swimming (where breathing must be synchronized to gulp air, not water) and weight lifting (where breath-holding is practiced to increase torso rigidity), respiration during exercise appears to be very highly deterministic; conscious control is difficult and usually not brought to bear. We thus find that models to predict respiratory responses usually match experimental findings very well. Even where external events such as stepping during running and pedaling during bicycling tend to synchronize breathing, many respiratory parameters can be predicted.

As in other chapters, mechanics and control are introduced before models are presented. The reader should note the similarity (and coupling; Whipp and Ward, 1982) between cardiovascular and respiratory mechanics and control. Both systems propel fluids, both have conducting passageways, and both represent support functions not directly involved in useful external work. Therefore, both are subject to some degree of optimization to reduce the burden of support during exercise.

4.2 RESPIRATORY MECHANICS

Respiratory mechanics, perhaps more than mechanics of other systems in this book, is an extremely complicated topic. The respiratory system, we all know, functions to bring air to the blood. It also functions to maintain thermal equilibrium and acid–base balance of the blood. Even while its primary function of air movement is occurring, there are gaseous fluid mechanics, physical diffusion, gas-to-liquid mass transport, muscular movement, and neural integration to consider. Although it can be argued that many of the same processes occur in the cardiovascular system, for instance, it was convenient to ignore all but those that were in consonance with the theme of this book. These mechanisms are intrinsic to respiratory functioning, however, and it is not possible to ignore them. Therefore, a slightly less integrated approach has been taken for respiratory matters compared to cardiovascular and thermal studies.

Mechanical properties of the respiratory system are best understood by first reviewing respiratory anatomy. Following that, it will be clearer how various mechanical models are formulated to account for structural considerations.

4.2.1 Respiratory Anatomy

The respiratory system consists of the lungs, conducting airways, pulmonary vasculature, respiratory muscles, and surrounding tissues and structures (Figure 4.2.1). Each of these is discussed to show the ways in which it influences respiratory responses.

Lungs. There are two lungs in the human chest; the right lung is composed of three incomplete divisions called lobes and the left lung has two.[1] The right lung accounts for 55% of total gas volume and the left lung accounts for 45%. Lung tissue is spongy because of the very small (200–300×10^{-6} m diameter in normal lungs at rest) gas-filled cavities called alveoli, which are the ultimate structures for gas exchange. There are 250 million to 350 million alveoli in the adult

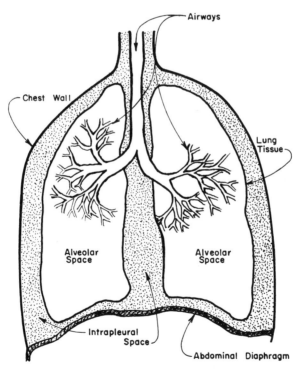

Figure 4.2.1 Schematic representation of the respiratory system.

[1]This conveniently leaves room in the chest for the heart.

TABLE 4.2.1 Classification and Approximate Dimensions of Airways of Adult Human Lung (Inflated to about 3/4 of TLC)[a]

Common Name	Numerical Order of Generation	Number of Each	Diameter, mm	Length, mm	Total Cross-Sectional Area, cm²	Description and Comment
Trachea	0	1	18	120	2.5	Main cartilaginous airway; partly in thorax.
Main bronchus	1	2	12	47.6	2.3	First branching of airway; one to each lung; in lung root; cartilage.
Lobar bronchus	2	4	8	19.0	2.1	Named for each lobe; cartilage.
Segmental bronchus	3	8	6	7.6	2.0	Named for radiographical and surgical anatomy; cartilage.
Subsegmental bronchus	4	16	4	12.7	2.4	Last generally named bronchi; may be referred to as medium-sized bronchi; cartilage.
Small bronchi	5–10	1,024[b]	1.3[b]	4.6[b]	13.4[b]	Not generally named; contain decreasing amounts of cartilage. Beyond this level airways enter the lobules as defined by a strong elastic lobular limiting membrane.
Bronchioles	11–13	8,192[b]	0.8[b]	2.7[b]	44.5[b]	Not named; contain no cartilage, mucus-secreting elements, or cilia. Tightly embedded in lung tissue.
Terminal bronchioles	14–15	32,768[b]	0.7[b]	2.0[b]	113.0[b]	Generally 2 or 3 orders so designated; morphology not significantly different from orders 11–13.
Respiratory bronchioles	16–18	262,144[b]	0.5[b]	1.2[b]	534.0[b]	Definite class; bronchiolar cuboidal epithelium present, but scattered alveoli are present giving these airways a gas exchange function. Order 16 often called first-order respiratory bronchiole; 17, second-order; 18, third-order.
Alveolar ducts	19–22	4,194,304[b]	0.4[b]	0.8[b]	5,880.0[b]	No bronchiolar epithelium; have no surface except connective tissue framework; open into alveoli.
Alveolar sacs	23	8,388,608	0.4	0.6	11,800.0	No reason to assign a special name; are really short alveolar ducts.
Aveoli	24	300,000,000	0.2			Pulmonary capillaries are in the septae that form the alveoli.

Source: Used with permission from Staub, 1963, and Weibel, 1963; adapted by Comroe, 1965.

[a]The number of airways in each generation is based on regular dichotomous branching.
[b]Numbers refer to last generation in each group.

lung, with a total alveolar surface area of 50–100 m² depending on the degree of lung inflation (Hilderbrandt and Young, 1966).

Conducting Airways. Air is transported from the atmosphere to the alveoli beginning with the oral and nasal cavities, and through the pharynx (in the throat) past the glottal opening, into the trachea, or windpipe. The larynx, or voice box, at the entrance to the trachea, is the most distal structure of the passages solely for conduction of air. The trachea is a fibromuscular tube 10–12 cm in length and 1.4–2.0 cm in diameter (Sackner, 1976a). At a location called the carina, the trachea terminates and divides into the left and right bronchi. Each bronchus has a discontinuous cartilaginous support in its wall (Astrand and Rodahl, 1970). Muscle fibers capable of controlling airway diameter are incorporated into the walls of the bronchi, as well as in those of air passages closer to the alveoli. The general tendency of airways closer to the alveoli is to be less rigid and more controllable by muscle fibers (Table 4.2.1). Smooth muscle is present throughout the respiratory bronchioles and alveolar ducts but is absent in the last alveolar duct, which terminates in one to several alveoli (Sackner, 1976a). The alveolar walls are shared by other alveoli and are composed of highly pliable and collapsible squamous epithelium cells.

The bronchi subdivide into subbronchi, which further subdivide into bronchioles, which further subdivide, and so on, until finally reaching the alveolar level. The Weibel model is commonly accepted as one geometrical arrangement of air passages (another more complicated

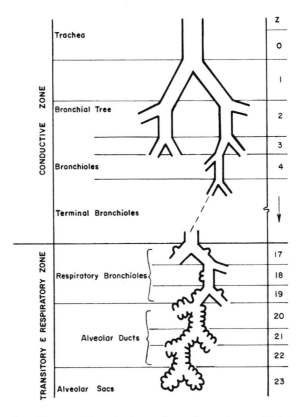

Figure 4.2.2 General architecture of conductive and transitory airways. Dichotomous branching is assumed to occur throughout, although this is not necessarily the case. (Used with permission from Weibel, 1963.)

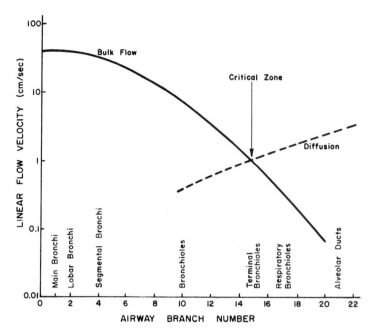

Figure 4.2.3 Linear velocity of flow in airways plotted against the airway branch number. Bulk flow is more important than diffusion in gas transport until generation 15 is reached. At that point, diffusion in the airways becomes important in gas transfer to and from the alveoli. (Used with permission from Muir, 1966.)

asymmetrical model is described in Yeates and Aspin, 1978). In this model (Figure 4.2.2), each airway is considered to branch into two subairways. In the adult human there are considered to be 23 such branchings, or generations, beginning at the trachea and ending in the alveoli.

Dichotomous branching is considered to occur only through the first 16 generations, which is called the conductive zone because these airways serve to conduct air to and from the lungs.[2] After the sixteenth generation branching proceeds irregularly dichotomously or trichotomously for three generations. A limited amount of respiratory gas exchange occurs in this transition zone. In the respiration zone, generations 20–23, most gas exchange occurs.[3]

Movement of gases in the respiratory airways occurs mainly by bulk flow (convection) throughout the region from the mouth and nose to the fifteenth generation (Figure 4.2.3). Beyond the fifteenth generation, gas diffusion is relatively more important (Pedley et al., 1977; Sackner, 1976a).[4] With the low gas velocities that occur in diffusion, dimensions of the space over which diffusion occurs (alveolar space) must be small for adequate oxygen delivery to the walls; smaller alveoli are more efficient in the transfer of gas than are larger ones.[5] Thus animals with high levels of oxygen consumption are found to have smaller diameter alveoli compared to animals with low levels of oxygen consumption (Figure 4.2.4).

[2]The airways also serve to temper air conditions by (usually) heating and humidifying the air and removing dust particles (see Chapter 5 for thermal effects). In cold weather, some of the moisture added to the air is recovered by condensation in the nostrils, thus leading to a runny nose.

[3]About 2% of the oxygen consumption at rest, and a slightly larger percentage of carbon dioxide lost, occurs in humans by diffusion through the skin (Hildebrandt and Young, 1966).

[4]Radial gaseous diffusion in the upper airways appears to be much more important in gas mixing and flow than axial gaseous diffusion (Pedley et al., 1977).

[5]When lung inflation doubles, as during exercise, the nearly spherical alveoli increase their diameters by only 1.3. Thus diffusion distances do not change greatly.

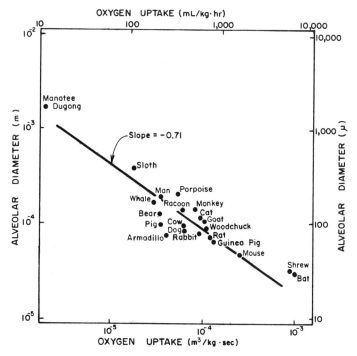

Figure 4.2.4   Alveolar diameter as a function of oxygen consumption for different animal species. (Adapted and used with permission from Tenney and Remmers, 1963.)

Alveoli. Alveoli are the structures through which gases diffuse to and from the body. One would expect, then, that alveolar walls would be extremely thin for gas exchange efficiency, and that is found to be the case. Total tissue thickness between the inside of the alveolus to pulmonary capillary blood plasma is only about 0.4×10^{-6} m (Figure 4.2.5). From the relative dimensions, it is apparent that the principal barrier to diffusion is not the alveolar membrane but the plasma and red blood cell (Hildebrandt and Young, 1966).

Molecular diffusion within the alveolar volume is responsible for mixing of the enclosed gas. Due to the small alveolar dimensions, complete mixing probably occurs in less than 10 msec (Astrand and Rodahl, 1970), fast enough that alveolar mixing time does not limit gaseous diffusion to or from the blood.

Of particular importance to proper alveolar operation is a thin surface coating of surfactant. Without this material, large alveoli would tend to enlarge and small alveoli would collapse. From the law of Laplace (see Section 3.2.3) for spherical bubbles

$$p = \frac{2\tau\Delta r}{r} \tag{4.2.1}$$

where p = gas pressure inside the bubble, N/m^2
   τ = surface tension, N/m^2
   r = bubble radius, m
   Δr = wall thickness, m

Large spherical bubbles (r large) have small internal pressures. Smaller bubbles have larger internal pressures. Connect the two bubbles together and the contents of the smaller bubble are

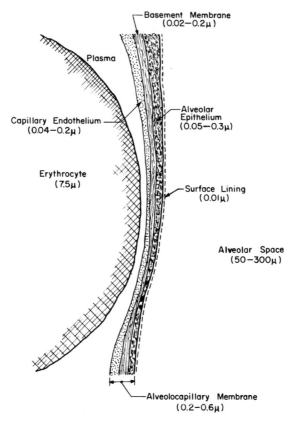

Figure 4.2.5   The fine structure of the alveolocapillary membrane. From the relative dimensions it is apparent that the principal diffusion barrier is not the membrane, but rather the plasma and red cell itself. (Used with permission from Hildebrandt and Young, 1966.)

driven into the larger one. If we generalize this instability to the lung, it is not hard to imagine the lung composed of one large, expanded alveolus and many small, collapsed alveoli. Surfactant, which acts like a detergent, changes the stress–strain relationship of the alveolar wall and stabilizes the lung (Notter and Finkelstein, 1984).[6]

Pulmonary Circulation.   The pulmonary circulation is relatively low pressure (Fung and Sobin, 1977). Because of this, pulmonary blood vessels, especially capillaries and venules, are very thin walled and flexible. Unlike systemic capillaries, pulmonary capillaries increase in diameter with any increase in blood pressure or decrease in alveolar pressure. Flow, therefore, is significantly influenced by elastic deformation.

 Pulmonary circulation is largely unaffected by neural and chemical control (Fung and Sobin, 1977). It responds promptly to hypoxia, however. And a key anatomical consideration is that pulmonary capillaries within alveolar walls are exposed to alveolar air on both sides, since alveolar walls separate adjacent alveoli.

 There is no true pulmonary analog to the systemic arterioles (Fung and Sobin, 1977). That is,

[6]Surfactant is always present on the surface of the alveoli of healthy individuals. Sighs or yawns may function by stretching closed alveoli and spreading surfactant across their surfaces so they will stay open. This contention is disputed by Provine et al. (1987). Lung surfactant is likely to be dipalmitoyl phosphatidyl choline, or DPPC (Mines, 1981).

TABLE 4.2.2 Pulmonary Capillary Transit Time

Condition	Capillary Volume $m^3 \times 10^{-4}$ (cm^3)		Cardiac Output, $m^3 \times 10^{-4}$/sec (cm^3/sec)		Transit Time, sec
Rest, sitting	1.0	(100)	1.0	(100)	1
Rest, supine	1.1	(110)	1.0	(100)	1.1
Exercise	2.0	(200)	4.0	(400)	0.5

the pressure-reduction function performed by the systemic arterioles (see Section 3.2.2) is not matched by the pulmonary arterioles. Therefore, pulmonary vessels, including capillaries and venules, exhibit blood pressures that vary approximately 30–50% from systole to diastole (Fung and Sobin, 1977).

There is also a high-pressure systemic blood delivery system to the bronchi which is completely independent of the pulmonary low-pressure ($\sim 3330 \, N/m^2$) circulation in healthy individuals (Fung and Sobin, 1977). In diseased states, however, bronchial arteries are reported to enlarge when pulmonary blood flow is reduced, and some arteriovenous shunts become prominent (Fung and Sobin, 1977).

Total pulmonary blood volume is approximately 300–500 cm^3 in normal adults (Sackner, 1976c) with about 60–100 cm^3 in the pulmonary capillaries (Astrand and Rodahl, 1970). This value is quite variable, depending on such things as posture, position, disease, and chemical composition of the blood (Sackner, 1976c).

Pulmonary arterial blood is oxygen-poor and carbon dioxide–rich. It exchanges excess carbon dioxide for oxygen in the pulmonary capillaries, which are in close contact with alveolar walls.

At rest, the transit time for blood in the pulmonary capillaries,

$$t = \frac{V_c}{\dot{V}_c}$$

(4.2.2)

where t = blood transit time, sec
$\quad V_c$ = capillary blood volume, m^3
$\quad \dot{V}_c$ = total capillary blood flow
$\qquad$ = cardiac output, m^3/sec
is somewhat less than 1 sec (Table 4.2.2).

Carbon dioxide diffusion is so rapid that carbon dioxide partial pressure in the blood is equilibrated to that in the alveolus by 100 msec after the blood enters the capillary and oxygen equilibrium is reached by 500 msec (Astrand and Rodahl, 1970).

At rest, pulmonary venous blood returns to the heart nearly 97% saturated with oxygen.[7] During exercise blood transit time in the capillaries may be only 500 msec or even less (Astrand and Rodahl, 1970), and hemoglobin saturation (see Section 3.2.1) may be limited because blood transit time is not long enough.

Respiratory Muscles. The lungs fill because of a rhythmic expansion of the chest wall. The action is indirect in that no muscle acts directly on the lung.

The diaphragm is the muscular mass accounting for 75% of the expansion of the chest cavity (Ganong, 1963). The diaphragm is attached around the bottom of the thoracic cage, arches over the liver, and moves downward like a piston when it contracts (Ganong, 1963). The external intercostal muscles are positioned between the ribs and aid inspiration by moving the ribs up and forward. This, then, increases the volume of the thorax. Other muscles (Table 4.2.3) are important in the maintenance of thoracic shape during breathing.

---

[7]This figure would be closer to 100% if pulmonary anastomoses and some nonventilated alveoli were not present.

TABLE 4.2.3 Active Respiratory Muscles

Phase	Quiet Breathing	Moderate to Severe Exercise
Inspiration	Diaphragm Internal intercostals of parasternal region Scaleni	Diaphragm External intercostals Scaleni Sternomastoids Vertebral extensors

Expiration	(Passive, except during early
	   part of expiration, when some
	   inspiratory contraction
	   persists)
		Transverse and oblique
		   abdominals
		Internal intercostals

Source: Used with permission from Hildebrandt and Young, 1965.

Quiet expiration[8] is usually considered to be entirely passive: pressure to force air from the lungs comes from elastic expansion of the lungs and chest wall. Actually, there is evidence (Hämäläinen and Viljanen, 1978a; Loring and Mead, 1982; McIlroy et al., 1963) that even quiet expiration is not entirely passive. Sometimes, too, inspiratory muscle activity continues through the early part of expiration.[9] During moderate to severe exercise, the abdominal and internal intercostal muscles are very important in forcing air from the lungs much more quickly than would otherwise occur.

Inspiration requires intimate contact between lung tissues, pleural tissues (the pleura is the membrane surrounding the lungs), and chest wall and diaphragm. This contact is maintained by reduced intrathoracic pressure (which tends toward negative values during inspiration). Any accumulation of gas in the intrapleural space in the thorax, which would ruin tissue-to-tissue contact, is absorbed into the pulmonary circulation because pulmonary venous total gas pressure is subatmospheric (Astrand and Rodahl, 1970).

The diaphragm is the respiratory muscle of most importance in developing the muscle pressure required to move air in the lungs. Its shape is largely determined because it separates the air-filled, spongy, and easily deformed lung material from the largely liquid abdominal contents. Because of the difference in height of the liquid in the abdomen across the dome shape assumed by the diaphragm, there is a significant vertical hydrostatic pressure gradient in the abdomen and a consequent difference in transdiaphragmatic pressure over the surface of the diaphragm (Whitelaw et al., 1983). Diaphragm tension should be able to be determined from its shape by the law of Laplace (Equation 4.2.1).

As the lungs fill, they become stiffer. The diaphragm must be able to produce higher pressures in order to move air into filled lungs. Normally, this would run counter to the muscular length–tension (Section 5.2.5) relationship, which indicates higher muscular tensions for longer lengths. In any case, muscular efficiencies would be expected to change during the respiratory cycle and muscle pressures exerted on the lungs would be expected to vary with position.

4.2.2 Lung Volumes and Gas Exchange

Of primary importance to lung functioning is the movement and mixing of gases within the respiratory system. Depending on the anatomical level under consideration, gas movement is determined mainly by diffusion or convection. This discussion begins with determinants of convective gaseous processes, that is, the lung volumes which change from rest to exercise.

---

[8]The terms exhalation and expiration, and the terms inhalation and inspiration, are used completely synonymously in this book. Both forms are derived from Latin roots meaning to breathe (–halare and –spirare).
[9]Producing negative work on the inspiratory muscles (see Section 5.2.5).

Lung Volumes. Without the thoracic musculature and rib cage, the barely inflated lungs would occupy a much smaller space than they occupy in situ. However, the thoracic cage holds them open. Conversely, the lungs exert an influence on the thorax, holding it smaller than should be the case without the lungs. Because the lungs and thorax are connected by tissue, the volume occupied by both together is between the extremes represented by relaxed lungs alone and thoracic cavity alone. The resting volume V_r is that volume occupied by the lungs with glottis[10] open, muscles relaxed, and with no elastic tendency to become larger or smaller.

Functional residual capacity (FRC) is often taken to be the same as the resting volume. There is a small difference between resting volume and FRC because FRC is measured while the patient breathes, whereas resting volume is measured with no breathing.[11] FRC is properly defined only at end-expiration at rest and not during exercise.

Tidal volume V_T is the amount of air exhaled[12] at each breath. Tidal volume increases as the severity of exercise increases. Dividing V_T by respiratory period (the time between identical points of successive breaths) T gives the minute volume $\dot{V}_E$, or the amount of air that would be exhaled per unit time if exhalation could be sustained. Sometimes $\dot{V}_E$ is measured as accumulated exhaled air for one minute.

Lung volumes greater than resting volume are achieved during inspiration. Maximum inspiration is represented by inspiratory reserve volume (IRV). IRV is the maximum additional volume that can be accommodated by the lung at the end of inspiration.

Lung volumes less than resting volume do not normally occur at rest but do occur during exhalation while exercising (when exhalation is active). Maximum additional expiration, as measured from lung volume at the end of expiration, is called expiratory reserve volume (ERV).

A small amount of air remains in the lung at maximum expiratory effort. This is the residual volume (RV).

Vital capacity (VC) is the sum of ERV, IRV, and V_T. Total lung capacity (TLC) equals VC plus RV. These volumes are illustrated in Figure 4.2.6.

Tidal volume ventilates both the active (alveolar) regions of the lung, composed of alveolar ventilation volume V_A, and inactive regions, called dead volume V_D, or dead space. Alveolar ventilation volume consists of air that diffuses to and from the pulmonary circulation. Respiratory dead volume is air that does not take part in gas exchange. Not all air that reaches the alveoli interacts with gases in the blood, and thus there is a portion of the total dead volume known as alveolar dead volume. The volume occupied by the respiratory system exclusive of the alveoli is normally called anatomic dead volume. The volume of gas not equilibrating with the blood is called physiological dead volume. Normally, anatomical and physiological dead volumes are nearly identical, but during certain diseases, when portions of the lung are unperfused by blood, they can differ significantly.

Dead volume is important because it represents wasted respiratory effort. During exhalation, the most oxygen-poor and carbon dioxide-rich air is the last to be expelled (so-called end-tidal air). Because of the accumulation of this air in the dead volume (Tatsis et al., 1984), this is the first air to be drawn back into the alveoli.[13] Extra respiratory effort must be expended to overcome dead volume accumulation.

Alveolar volume increases during exercise because of increased alveolar inflation and

---

[10]The glottis is the opening between the vocal cords in the larynx. The epiglottis is the small flap of cartilaginous and membranous tissue that closes off the windpipe during swallowing.

[11]At rest, exhalation is assumed to be passive, and the shape of the flow waveform is therefore exponential. It takes an infinite amount of time for all air above the resting volume to be expelled. The small amount of excess air that remains in the lungs upon initiation of inspiration, when added to resting volume, equals FRC.

[12]Some people define tidal volume as the amount of air inhaled during each breath. The two volumes are not the same because of the different temperatures of the inhaled and exhaled air, and, to a lesser extent, due to water vapor addition and different gas composition of exhaled air. Inhaled volume is somewhat easier to measure because higher resting flow rates are usually incurred.

[13]In a similar manner, when a hot-water faucet is turned on at home, the first water you get is cold water.

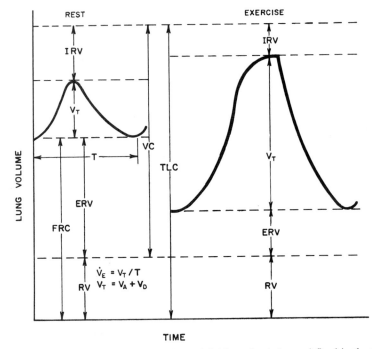

Figure 4.2.6 Representation of lung volume definitions. Symbols are defined in the text.

recruitment of additional alveolar areas. Apparent dead volume increases because of these same reasons, and because of different patterns of gas mixing in the lungs. When flow becomes turbulent, as it does in regions of the conducting air passages as flow rate increases, mixing is enhanced. Alveolar gas being mixed with freshly inhaled air is oxygen-poor and carbon dioxide–rich; thus dead volume increases. Gray et al. (1956) measured the dependence of dead volume on tidal volume for five subjects and obtained this relationship:

$$V_D = 1.8 \times 10^{-4} + 0.023V_T \qquad (4.2.3)$$

where V_D = dead volume, m^3
$\quad\;\; V_T$ = tidal volume, m^3

It can be seen, then, that the ratio of dead volume to tidal volume V_D/V_T decreases during exercise when tidal volume increases (Whipp, 1981).

Normal values[14] of all lung volumes are listed in Table 4.2.4. Subordinate volumes are indented. Lung volumes are normally given in units of liters or milliliters, but to be consistent with other chapters, cubic meters are used as primary units. Tabled volumes should be multiplied by 0.76 for healthy females because lung volumes are related to body size (see Section 5.2.6). Cerny (1987) also suggests race-related differences.

Posture affects many of these volumes through the influence of gravity. In a supine position, gravity pulls on the upper thoracic wall, depressing lung volumes. In the standing position, the effect of gravity is to expand lung volumes.

---

[14]Schorr-Lesnick et al. (1985) compared pulmonary function tests, including lung volumes, between singers, wind-instrument players, and other string or percussion instrumentalists. Contrary to popular opinion, no significant differences were found among these groups. Singers, however, generally smoked less and exercised more than the others, thus evidence of heightened awareness of health.

TABLE 4.2.4 Typical Lung Volumes for Normal, Healthy Males

Lung Volume	Normal Values	
Total lung capacity (TLC)	$6.0 \times 10^{-3}\,\text{m}^3$	$(6,000\,\text{cm}^3)$
Residual volume (RV)	$1.2 \times 10^{-3}\,\text{m}^3$	$(1,200\,\text{cm}^3)$
Vital capacity (VC)	$4.8 \times 10^{-3}\,\text{m}^3$	$(4,800\,\text{cm}^3)$
Inspiratory reserve volume (IRV)	$3.6 \times 10^{-3}\,\text{m}^3$	$(3,600\,\text{cm}^3)$
Expiratory reserve volume (ERV)	$1.2 \times 10^{-3}\,\text{m}^3$	$(1,200\,\text{cm}^3)$
Functional residual capacity (FRC)	$2.4 \times 10^{-3}\,\text{m}^3$	$(2,400\,\text{cm}^3)$
Anatomical dead volume (V_D)	$1.5 \times 10^{-4}\,\text{m}^3$	$(150\,\text{cm}^3)$
Upper airways volume	$8.0 \times 10^{-5}\,\text{m}^3$	$(80\,\text{cm}^3)$
Lower airways volume	$7.0 \times 10^{-5}\,\text{m}^3$	$(70\,\text{cm}^3)$
Physiological dead volume (V_D)	$1.8 \times 10^{-4}\,\text{m}^3$	$(180\,\text{cm}^3)$
Minute volume ($\dot{V}_e$) at rest	$1.0 \times 10^{-4}\,\text{m}^3/\text{sec}$	$(6,000\,\text{cm}^3/\text{min})$
Respiratory period (T) at rest	4 sec	
Tidal volume (V_T) at rest	$4.0 \times 10^{-4}\,\text{m}^3$	$(400\,\text{cm}^3)$
Alveolar ventilation volume (V_A) at rest	$2.5 \times 10^{-4}\,\text{m}^3$	$(250\,\text{cm}^3)$
Minute volume during heavy exercise	$1.7 \times 10^{-3}\,\text{m}^3/\text{sec}$	$(10,000\,\text{cm}^3/\text{min})$
Respiratory period during heavy exericse	1.2 sec	
Tidal volume during heavy exercise	$2.0 \times 10^{-3}\,\text{m}^3$	$(2,000\,\text{cm}^3)$
Alveolar ventilation volume during exercise	$1.8 \times 10^{-3}\,\text{m}^3$	$(1,820\,\text{cm}^3)$

Source: Adapted and used with permission from Forster et al., 1986.

A reduction in lung tissue elasticity with age increases the relative proportion of residual volume by reducing the recoil pressure driving expiration. The ratio of RV/TLC is about 20% in young individuals but doubles in individuals 50–60 years of age (Astrand and Rodahl, 1970).

Perfusion of the Lung. For gas exchange to occur properly in the lung, air must be delivered to the alveoli via the conducting airways, gas must diffuse from the alveoli to the capillaries through extremely thin walls, and the same gas must be removed to the cardiac right atrium by blood flow. The first step in this three-step process is called ventilation, and we have already been introduced to alveolar ventilation volume. When the time for alveolar ventilation to happen is taken into account, alveolar ventilation rate results. The second step is the process of diffusion.

The third step involves pulmonary blood flow, and this is called ventilatory perfusion. Obviously, an alveolus which is ventilated but not perfused cannot exchange gas. Similarly, a perfused alveolus which is not properly ventilated cannot exchange gas.[15] The most efficient gas exchange occurs when ventilation and perfusion are matched (Figure 4.2.7).

There is a wide range of ventilation-to-perfusion ratios that naturally occur in various regions of the lung (Petrini, 1986). Blood flow is greatly affected by posture because of the effects of gravity. In the upright position, there is a general reduction in the volume of blood in the thorax, allowing for larger lung volume. Gravity also influences the distribution of blood, such that the perfusion of equal lung volumes is about five times greater at the base compared to the top of the lung (Astrand and Rodahl, 1970). There is no corresponding distribution of ventilation, hence the ventilation-to-perfusion ratio is nearly five times smaller at the top of the lung (Table 4.2.5). A more uniform ventilation-to-perfusion ratio is found in the supine position and during exercise (Jones, 1984b).

Blood flow through the capillaries is not steady. Rather, blood flows in a halting manner and may even be stopped if intra-alveolar pressure exceeds intracapillary blood pressure during diastole. Mean blood flow is not affected by heart rate (Fung and Sobin, 1977), but the highly

[15]There is a much smaller blood circulation to the respiratory upper airways with the purpose of nourishing these airways. This bronchial circulation is derived from the heart left ventricle rather than the right, which supplies blood to perfuse the lung (Deffebach et al., 1987).

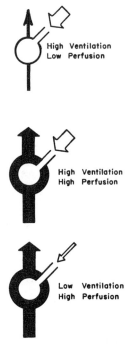

Figure 4.2.7   Schematic illustration of a lung alveolus ventilated by air and perfused by blood. Both flows are required for adequate gas exchange to occur. Only with high ventilation and high perfusion (middle condition) does the alveolus perform its intended function of adequte gas exchange.

TABLE 4.2.5   Ventilation-to-Perfusion Ratios from the Top to Bottom of the Lung of a Normal Man in the Sitting Position

Percent Lung Volume, %	Alveolar Ventilation Rate, cm³/sec	Perfusion Rate, cm³/sec	Ventilation-to-Perfusion Ratio
Top			
7	4.0	1.2	3.3
8	5.5	3.2	1.8
10	7.0	5.5	1.3
11	8.7	8.3	1.0
12	9.8	11.0	0.90
13	11.2	13.8	0.80
13	12.0	16.3	0.73
13	13.0	19.2	0.68
Bottom			
13	13.7	21.5	0.63
100	84.9	100.0	

Source: Used with permission from West, 1962.

distensible pulmonary blood vessels admit more blood when blood pressure and cardiac output increase. During exercise, higher pulmonary blood pressures allow more blood to flow through the capillaries. Even mild exercise favors more uniform perfusion of the lungs (Astrand and Rodahl, 1970). Pulmonary artery systolic pressure increases from $2670 \, \text{N/m}^2$ (20 mm Hg) at rest to $4670 \, \text{N/m}^2$ (35 mm Hg) during moderate exercise to $6670 \, \text{N/m}^2$ (50 mm Hg) at maximal work (Astrand and Rodahl, 1970).

Perfusion therefore is not steady, but average perfusion is generally all that is needed for exercise studies. Even during heavy work some parts of the lungs may be unperfused during diastole (Astrand and Rodahl, 1970). However, as long as heart rate is many times the respiration rate, average perfusion can still be close to ideal.

There are local mechanisms which tend to restore overall ventilation-to-perfusion ratios to normal when local ratios are not ideal. Inadequate alveolar ventilation results in low oxygen concentration. This, in turn, causes alveolar vasoconstriction and reduced blood flow, shunting blood to better ventilated areas (Astrand and Rodahl, 1970). Oppositely, reduced blood flow produces low concentration of alveolar carbon dioxide, and this causes local bronchiolar constriction (Astrand and Rodahl, 1970). Gas flow is thus shunted to better perfused areas. These mechanisms are far from perfect, but they seem to be adequate for matching blood flow to ventilated areas of the lung.

Gas Partial Pressures. The primary purpose of the respiratory system is gas exchange. Yet we have already seen the complexity required to perform this function. Fresh air must be brought to the alveolar gas exchange surface by an extensive piping network in order to supply oxygen to the body. On the way, the oxygen concentration is diluted in the anatomical dead volume. When it reaches the alveolus, ventilation may not be matched well enough to perfusion to accomplish the necessary gas exchange. In the gas exchange process, gas must diffuse through the alveolar space, across tissue, through plasma into the red blood cell, where it finally chemically joins to hemoglobin. A similar process occurs for carbon dioxide elimination. In this section, we deal with many of the details of gas movement.

As long as intermolecular interactions are small,[16] most gases of physiological significance can be considered to obey the ideal gas law:

$$pV = nRT \tag{4.2.4}$$

where p = pressure, N/m^2
 V = volume of gas, m^3
 n = number of moles, mol
 R = gas constant, $\text{N} \cdot \text{m/(mol} \cdot {}^\circ\text{K)}$
 T = absolute temperature, ${}^\circ\text{K}$

Errors involved in applying the ideal gas law are negligible up to atmospheric pressure ($101.3 \, \text{kN/m}^2$). Equation 4.2.4 may even be applied to vapors, although errors up to 5% may be incurred with saturated vapors (Baumeister, 1967). The ideal gas law can be applied to a mixture of gases, such as air, or to its constituents, such as oxygen and nitrogen. All individual gases in a mixture are considered to fill the total volume and have the same temperature but reduced pressures. The pressure exerted by each individual gas is called the partial pressure of the gas and is denoted by a composition subscript on the pressure symbol p (see Section 3.2.1).

Dalton's law states that the total pressure is the sum of the partial pressures of the constituents of a mixture:

$$p = \sum_{i=1}^{N} p_i \tag{4.2.5}$$

---

[16]These interactions can be considered to be significant at temperatures close to the boiling point of the gas and at pressures close to the pressure (at a particular temperature) at which the gas liquefies.

TABLE 4.2.6 Molecular Masses, Gas Constants, and Volume Fractions for Air and Constituents

Constituent	Molecular Mass, kg/mol	Gas Constant, N·m/(mol·K)	Volume Fraction In Air, m³/m³
Air	29.0	286.7	1.0000
Ammonia	17.0	489.1	0.0000
Argon	39.9	208.4	0.0093
Carbon dioxide	44.0	189.0	0.0003
Carbon monoxide	28.0	296.9	0.0000
Helium	4.0	2078.6	0.0000
Hydrogen	2.0	4157.2	0.0000
Nitrogen	28.0	296.9	0.7808
Oxygen	32.0	259.8	0.2095

Note: Universal gas constant is 8314.34 N·m/kg·mol·°K).

where p_i = partial pressure of the ith constituent, N/m^2
N = total number of constituents
Dividing the ideal gas law for a constituent by that for the mixture gives

$$\frac{p_i V}{p V} = \frac{n_i R_i T}{n R T} \qquad (4.2.6)$$

so that

$$\frac{p_i}{p} = \frac{n_i R_i}{n R} \qquad (4.2.7)$$

which states that the partial pressure of a gas may be found if the total pressure, mole fraction, and ratio of gas constants are known. For most respiratory calculations, p will be considered to be the pressure of 1 atmosphere, $101\ kN/m^2$. Avogadro's principle states that different gases at the same temperature and pressure contain equal numbers of molecules:

$$\frac{V_1}{V_2} = \frac{n R_1}{n R_2} = \frac{R_1}{R_2} \qquad (4.2.8)$$

Thus

$$\frac{p_i}{p} = \frac{V_i}{V} \qquad (4.2.9)$$

where V_i/V = volume fraction of a constituent in air, dimensionless
In Table 4.2.6 are found individual gas constants, as well as volume fractions, of constituent gases of air. From the ideal gas law[17] we can also see that

$$R = \sum_{i=1}^{N} \frac{n_i}{n} R_i \qquad (4.2.10)$$

Water vapor is added to the inhaled air. Water vapor pressure is a function of only temperature insofar as the vapor is in equilibrium with liquid water (see Table 5.2.12). At the

[17]If the volume in the ideal gas law is expressed as the volume of one molecular mass of the gas, then R is constant for all gases at 8314.34 N·m/(kg mol·K). If the volume is expressed as total volume including any mass of gas, then R will be 8314.34 divided by molecular mass of that gas.

body temperature of 37°C, water vapor pressure is 6279 N/m² (47 mm Hg). Since total pressure[18] is assumed to be 101.3 kN/m², dry gas accounts for a pressure of $101.3 - 6.3 = 95.0$ kN/m².

Since temperature, pressure, and composition of respired gas change during breathing and with position, it does not seem unusual that conventions were established to express gas properties (especially compositions and partial pressures) uniformly. There are two of these: (1) body temperature (37°C), standard pressure (101.3 kN/m²), saturated ($pH_2O = 6.28$ kN/m²), or BTPS, and (2) standard temperature (0°C), standard pressure (101.3 kN/m²), dry ($pH_2O = 0$), or STPD. Of the two, STPD is the more often used.

To calculate constituent partial pressures at STPD, total pressure is taken as barometric pressure minus vapor pressure of water in the atmosphere:

$$p_i = (V_i/V)(p - pH_2O) \qquad (4.2.11)$$

where p = total pressure, kN/m²

pH_2O = vapor pressure of water in atmosphere, kN/m²

and V_i/V as a ratio does not change in the conversion process. (The process of water addition to the air reduces partial pressures of the other constituents.

Gas volume at STPD is converted from ambient condition volume as

$$V_i = V_{amb}\left(\frac{273}{273 + \theta}\right)\left(\frac{p - pH_2O}{101.3}\right) \qquad (4.2.12)$$

where V_i = volume of gas i corrected to STPD, m³

V_{amb} = volume of gas i at ambient temperature and pressure, m³

θ = ambient temperature, °C

p = ambient total pressure, kN/m²

pH_2O = vapor pressure of water in the air, kN/m²

Oxygen consumption of the body is conventionally reported under STPD conditions. STPD conditions will be assumed in later analyses unless otherwise stated.

Partial pressures and gas volumes may be expressed in BTPS conditions. In this case, gas partial pressures are usually known from other measurements. Gas volumes are converted from ambient conditions by

$$V_i = V_{amb}\left(\frac{310}{273 + \theta}\right)\left(\frac{p - pH_2O}{p - 6.28}\right) \qquad (4.2.13)$$

TABLE 4.2.7 Gas Partial Pressures (kN/m²) Throughout the Respiratory and Circulatory Systems

Gas	Inspired Air	Alveolar Air	Expired Air	Mixed Venous Blood	Arterial Blood	Muscle Tissue
H_2O	—	6.3	6.3	6.3	6.3	6.3
CO_2	0.04	5.3	4.2	6.1	5.3	6.7
O_2	21.2	14.0	15.5	5.3	13.3	4.0
N_2[b]	80.1	75.7	75.3	76.4	76.4	76.4
Total	101.3	101.3	101.3	94.1	101.3	93.4

Source: Used with permission from Astrand and Rodahl 1970.

[a] Inspired air considered dry for convenience.

[b] Includes all other inert components.

[18] Actually, total pressure will vary slightly with position in the respiratory system and during inhalation, exhalation, or pause.

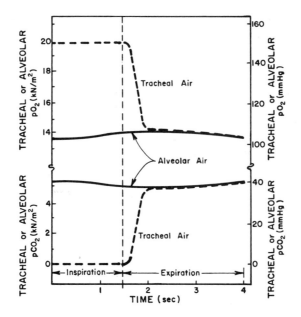

Figure 4.2.8   Variations in oxygen and carbon dioxide partial pressures in tracheal air and alveolar air during one single breath at rest. Alveolar air changes very little. (Adapted and used with permission from Astrand and Rodahl, 1970. Modified from Holmgren and Astrand, 1966.)

Minute volume $\dot{V}_E$ is conventionally measured at BTPS conditions, whereas rates of carbon dioxide production $\dot{V}_{CO_2}$ and oxygen use $\dot{V}_{O_2}$ are measured at STPD (Whipp, 1981). Ratios of $\dot{V}_E/\dot{V}_{CO_2}$ and $\dot{V}_E/\dot{V}_{O_2}$ are sometimes calculated without conversion to a consistent set of conditions. To make this conversion,

$$V_{STPD} = V_{BTPS}\left(\frac{273}{310}\right)\left(\frac{101.3 - 6.28}{101.3}\right) = 0.826 V_{BTPS} \tag{4.2.14}$$

Constituent partial pressures vary throughout the respiratory system and circulatory system. Table 4.2.7 shows some of this variation. Notice that nitrogen is considered to be inert, and in the nitrogen components are included all other inert gases.

Alveolar gas composition remains fairly constant despite large changes in composition of tracheal air (Figure 4.2.8). If this did not occur, there would be a large fluctuation in gaseous composition of blood and a serious impact on tissues sensitive to changes in blood composition (Morehouse and Miller, 1967). Partial pressures of carbon dioxide and oxygen nearly remain at 5.3 kN/m^2 (40 mm Hg) and 13.3 kN/m^2 (100 mm Hg) throughout inhalation and exhalation. These values translate into the volume fractions listed in Table 4.2.8. During exercise, the value of oxygen fraction in alveolar air decreases by nearly 2% and carbon dioxide increases by nearly 2%.

TABLE 4.2.8   Percent Composition of Dry Inspired, Expired, and Alveolar Air in Resting Men at Sea Level

Gas	Inspired Air	Alveolar Air	Expired Air
N_2	79.0	80.4	79.2
O_2	20.9	14.0	16.3
CO_2	0.04	5.6	4.5

Source: Used with permission from Riley, 1965.

Respiratory Exchange Ratio. Respiratory exchange ratio R is defined as the rate of carbon dioxide expired ($\dot{V}_{CO_2}$):

$$R = \dot{V}_{CO_2}/\dot{V}_{O_2} \tag{4.2.15}$$

In the steady state, the respiratory exchange ratio is equal to the respiratory quotient (RQ), with RQ being defined as the rate of carbon dioxide produced divided by the rate of oxygen utilized. The difference, then, between R and RQ is the difference between CO_2 exhaled and CO_2 produced. These are different during extremely heavy exercise.

RQ is measured to obtain the caloric value of oxygen consumption (see Section 5.2.5) and varies with the type of food being metabolized. For instance, carbohydrate contains multiples of carbon, hydrogen, and oxygen atoms in the ratio of 1:2:1 and is metabolized in a manner similar to glucose:

$$C_6H_{12}O_6 + 6O_2 \rightarrow 6CO_2 + 6H_2O \tag{4.2.16}$$

Six volumes of oxygen are used to produce 6 volumes of CO_2. Thus the RQ of carbohydrate is 1.00.

Fats contain less oxygen than carbohydrates and therefore require more oxygen to produce the same amount of carbon dioxide compared to carbohydrates. For instance, tripalmitin is oxidized (Ganong, 1963) by

$$2C_{51}H_{98}O_6 + 145O_2 \rightarrow 102CO_2 + 98H_2O \tag{4.2.17}$$

and, like other fats, has an RQ of 0.70.

Protein composition varies greatly, and so does protein RQ. However, an average RQ for protein is 0.82. RQ has been measured for other important substances (Table 4.2.9).

Protein is not used as a fuel by working muscles when the supply of carbohydrate and fat is adequate (Astrand and Rodahl, 1970). Nitrogen excretion in the urine, a by-product of protein metabolism, does not rise significantly following muscular work.

For subjects on normal diets exercising aerobically, 50–60% of the energy required is obtained from fats (Astrand and Rodahl, 1970). In prolonged aerobic work, fat supplies up to 70% of the energy. Fats are very concentrated energy sources[19] because they do not contain

TABLE 4.2.9 Respiration Quotients of Metabolizable Substances

Substance	Respiration Quotient
Carbohydrate	1.00
Fat	0.70
Protein	0.82 (avg)
Glycerol	0.86
β-Hydroxybutyric acid	0.89
Acetoacetic acid	1.00
Pyruvic acid	1.20
Ethyl alcohol	0.67

Source: Adapted from Ganong, 1963.

[19]Fat energy density is about 39.7 N·m/kg (9 kcal/g). Adipose tissue, which is not all fat, contains 25–29 N·m/kg (6–7 kcal/g). Carbohydrate, on the other hand, has an energy density of 17.2 N·m/kg (4 kcal/g), and stored carbohydrate (glycogen) contains about 4 N·m/kg (1 kcal/g) because of stored water of hydration (Astrand and Rodahl, 1970).

much oxygen and energy is released by oxidizing both hydrogen and carbon in fat molecules (unlike carbohydrates, which release energy, in effect, by carbon oxidation alone).

Carbohydrates are quick energy sources used predominantly at rest and at the beginning of exercise (see Section 1.3.2). Blood glucose and muscle glycogen[20] are the primary carbohydrate sources.

Resting RQ and RQ at the beginning of exercise are normally about 0.8 (Morehouse and Miller, 1967),[21] indicating that about two-thirds of the required energy is obtained from fat and one-third from carbohydrate. During strenuous exercise the RQ rises toward 1.00, indicating that more of the energy is derived from carbohydrate. Hard work for a protracted time utilizes more fat, and RQ approaches 0.7. Differing muscles and other organs probably exhibit different RQs because of different metabolism states,[22] and the overall RQ measured at the mouth is the weighted sum of these.

Total RQ depends on the individual substances metabolized:

$$RQ = \sum X_i RQ_i \qquad (4.2.18)$$

where RQ = total RQ, dimensionless
    X_i = fraction of substance i metabolized, dimensionless
    RQ_i = RQ of substance i, dimensionless
and

$$\sum X_i = 1 \qquad (4.2.19)$$

Respiratory exchange ratio R differs from respiratory quotient RQ because less information concerning fuel for metabolism can be inferred from R than from RQ. During secretion of gastric juice, for instance, the stomach has a negative respiratory exchange ratio because it uses more CO_2 from the arterial blood than it puts into the venous blood (Ganong, 1963). During anaerobic exercise, when there is not sufficient oxygen to completely metabolize the metabolic substrates, lactic acid is formed and pours into the blood from the working muscles. This excess acid drops the pH of the blood and shifts the balance of Equation 3.2.3 toward a higher amount of CO_2 available for respiratory exchange. Therefore, there is a higher amount of carbon dioxide emitted from the lungs for the same amount of oxygen used. Apparent R thus increases, many times exceeding 1.0.[23] This value is not due to the substances being oxidized: rather it is due to the manner in which they are being utilized (see Section 1.3.5).

While the respiratory exchange ratio exceeds 1.0, products of metabolism are being formed which will require oxygen to reform the original metabolites or to form carbon dioxide and water (see Section 1.3.3). This required oxygen, called the oxygen debt (Figure 1.3.2), is obtained at the cessation of exercise if the oxygen debt is large enough and widespread throughout the muscles, or it can be obtained in other parts of the body if nonaerobic metabolism is extremely localized.

At the cessation of heavy exercise, the repayment of the oxygen debt requires a large amount of oxygen to be supplied while carbon dioxide stores in the body are being rebuilt. During this time, R may drop as low as 0.50. Once the oxygen debt is repaid, the respiratory exchange ratio returns eventually to resting levels and again becomes indicative of the type of fuel being utilized.

---

[20]Glycogen is the stored form of glucose, which, unlike glucose, is not able to pass directly from the cell. Glycogen is formed from glucose by phosphorylation and polymerization in a process called glycogenesis (Ganong, 1963).

[21]Actually, this is nonprotein RQ, or RQ adjusted for metabolized protein. Since metabolized protein is usually much less than fat or carbohydrate, and the amount of protein metabolized does not greatly change during work, nonprotein RQ is often approximated by measured RQ.

[22]For example, the RQ of the brain is regularly 0.97–0.99 (Ganong, 1963).

[23]There have been efforts by many workers to correlate $R \geqslant 1.0$ with the onset of anaerobic metabolism. These correlations have not always been successful, however, due to lack of agreement on a precise definition of the onset of anaerobic metabolism.

The caloric equivalent of oxygen consumption is frequently needed for indirect calorimetry. The caloric equivalent of oxygen is often taken to be $20.18 \, N \cdot m/cm^3$ ($4.82 \, kcal/L$). However, the exact caloric equivalent depends on the fuel being burned and cannot reliably be obtained whenever an oxygen debt is being incurred or repaid.

To determine more closely the caloric equivalent of oxygen consumption, a steady-state measurement of RQ must be obtained. This RQ measurement can be converted into nonprotein RQ by determining the urinary nitrogen excretion (Ganong, 1963). Each gram of urinary nitrogen is equivalent to $6.25 \, g$ of protein. Metabolizing each gram of protein consumes $940 \, cm^3$ O_2 and produces $750 \, cm^3 \, CO_2$ (Brown and Brengelmann, 1966). These amounts of oxygen and carbon dioxide are subtracted from measured totals[24] and the results can be divided to give nonprotein RQ. Assuming, then, that carbohydrate and fat are the only other metabolized substances, it is possible to calculate the caloric equivalent of oxygen, based on RQ:

$$X_{CHO} = (RQ - 0.7)/0.3 \qquad (4.2.20)$$

where X_{CHO} = carbohydrate fraction of metabolites, dimensionless
 RQ = total, or overall respiration quotient, dimensionless

Since each $1000 \, cm^3$ of oxygen consumed corresponds to $1.23 \, g$ carbohydrate and $0.50 \, g$ fat (Ganong, 1963), and the caloric equivalent of carbohydrate has been given as $17.2 \, N \cdot m/kg$ and that of fat is $39.7 \, N \cdot m/kg$, then

$$
\begin{aligned}
U_{O_2} &= \frac{(17.2)(1.23)X_{CHO} + (1 - X_{CHO})(39.7)(0.50)}{1000} \\[2mm]
&= \frac{1.34 X_{CHO} + 19.8}{1000}
\end{aligned}
\qquad (4.2.21)
$$

where U_{O_2} = caloric equivalent of oxygen, $N \cdot m/cm^3$

Lung Diffusion. Movement of gases occurs by two basic mechanisms in the respiratory system: (1) convection transport, or bulk flow of gas, which we have seen predominates to the fifteenth airway generation, and (2) diffusion, which predominates thereafter. Diffusion of gases occurs by the well-known Fick's second equation (Geankoplis, 1978):

$$\frac{\partial c_1}{\partial t} = - D_{ij} \frac{\partial^2 c_i}{\partial x^2} \qquad (4.2.22)$$

where c_i = concentration of constituent i, mol/m^3
 t = time, sec
 D_{ij} = diffusion constant[25] of constituent i through medium j, m^2/sec
 x = linear distance, m
From Equation 4.2.4,

$$c_i = \frac{n_1}{V} = \frac{p_i}{R_i T} \qquad (4.2.23)$$

where i denotes a particular gas constituent. Therefore, the diffusion equation (4.2.22)

---

[24]Or protein RQ can be ignored for all practical purposes.
[25]Diffusion constants are also called diffusion coefficients and mass diffusivities.

becomes

$$\frac{\partial p_i}{\partial t} = -D_{ij}\frac{\partial^2 p_i}{\partial x^2} \tag{4.2.24}$$

and has the advantage that gas partial pressures, rather than concentrations, are used.

In the steady state, which is often assumed for simplicity, $\partial p_i/\partial t = 0$, and upon integrating Equation 4.2.24 we obtain

$$J_i R_i T = -D_{ij}\frac{dp_i}{dx} \tag{4.2.25}$$

where J_i = molar flux of constituent i in the x direction, mol/(m^2·sec)

Diffusion constant values, experimentally obtained by steady-state means, depend on the constituent gas i and the composition of the medium through which the gas is diffusing. Representative values of diffusion constants are given in Table 4.2.10.

Diffusion coefficients for nontabled values can be calculated (Emmert and Pigford, 1963) from

$$D_{ij} = \frac{[10.13(1/M_i + 1/M_j)^{1/2} - 24.92(1/M_i + 1/M_j)]T^{1.75}}{10^{24}pr_{ij}^2 I_D} \tag{4.2.26}$$

where D_{ij} = gas diffusivity of constituent i through medium j, m^2/sec

$\quad M_i$ = molecular weight of gas i, dimensionless

$\quad p$ = absolute pressure, N/m^2

$\quad r_{ij}$ = collision diameter, m

$\quad I_D$ = collision integral for diffusion, dimensionless

$\quad T$ = absolute temperature, °K

and

$$r_{ij} = 0.5[r_i + r_j] \tag{4.2.27}$$

TABLE 4.2.10   Diffusion Constants of Gases and Vapors in Air at 25°C and 10^3 N/m^2 Pressure

Substance	Diffusion Constant, cm^2/sec
Ammonia	0.28
Carbon dioxide	0.164
Hydrogen	0.410
Oxygen	0.206
Water	0.256
Ethyl ether	0.093
Methanol	0.159
Ethyl alcohol	0.119
Formic acid	0.159
Acetic acid	0.133
Aniline	0.073
Benzene	0.088
Toluene	0.084
Ethyl benzene	0.077
Propyl benzene	0.059

Source: Used with permission from Gebhart, 1971.

where r_i and r_j = collision diameters of the individual gases, m
Individual values of r_i for selected gases are found in Table 4.2.11.

Also needed in Equation 4.2.26 are values for I_D. These are obtained from Table 4.2.12 using individual force constant (ε_i/k) data from Table 4.2.11. ε_i is the energy of molecular interaction (N·m) and k is the Boltzmann constant (1.38×10^{-13} N·m/°K). Combined force constants are determined from

$$\frac{\varepsilon_{ij}}{k} = \left[\left(\frac{\varepsilon_i}{k} \right) \left(\frac{\varepsilon_j}{k} \right) \right]^{1/2} \tag{4.2.28}$$

Emmert and Pigford (1963) estimate the accuracy of this method of calculation of gas diffusion constants to average within 4% of the true values with a maximum deviation of 16%.

Normally, one would be mainly interested in the diffusion constants of various gases through air, and these are probably the proper values of diffusion constants to use in the upper respiratory system. In the alveoli, however, gas composition, as we have seen (Table 4.2.7), is dissimilar from ambient air. Modified diffusion constants can be calculated from Equation 4.2.26, or a somewhat simpler method proposed by Fuller et al. (1966) can be used.

The approach used by Fuller et al. (1966) begins with the Stefan–Maxwell molecular hard sphere model and additive LeBas atomic volumes. With the form of the equations thus established, they used a nonlinear least squares analysis to empirically determine coefficient values from diffusion coefficients obtained from the literature. Their equation is

$$D_{ij} = \frac{(0.0103) T^{1.75} (1/M_i + 1/M_j)^{1/2}}{p(V_i^{1/3} + V_j^{1/3})^2} \tag{4.2.29}$$

where D_{ij} = diffusion coefficient, m²/sec
T = absolute temperature, K
M_i = molecular weight, dimensionless
p = absolute pressure, N/m²
V_i = atomic diffusion volume, m³

Values of atomic diffusion volumes are found in Table 4.2.13. Errors in numerical values of

TABLE 4.2.11 Force Constants and Collision Diameters for Selected Gases

Gas	Force Constant (ε_i/k), °K	Collision Diameter (r_i), m × 10^{10}
Air	97.0	3.617
Ammonia	315.0	2.624
Argon	124.0	3.418
Carbon dioxide	190.0	3.996
Carbon monoxide	110.3	3.590
Helium	6.03	2.70
Hydrogen	33.3	2.968
Neon	35.7	2.80
Nitrogen	91.5	3.681
Nitrous oxide	220.0	3.879
Oxygen	113.2	3.433
Water	363.0	2.655

Source: Used with permission from Emmert and Pigford, 1963.

TABLE 4.2.12 Values of Collision Integral

kT/ε_{ij}	I_D	kT/ε_{ij}	I_D
0.3	1.331	3.6	0.4529
0.4	1.159	3.8	0.4471
0.5	1.033	4.0	0.4418
0.6	0.9383	4.2	0.4370
0.7	0.8644	4.4	0.4326
0.8	0.8058	4.6	0.4284
0.9	0.7585	4.8	0.4246
1.0	0.7197	5	0.4211
1.1	0.6873	6	0.4062
1.2	0.6601	7	0.3948
1.3	0.6367	8	0.3856
1.4	0.6166	9	0.3778
1.5	0.5991	10	0.3712
1.6	0.5837	20	0.3320
1.7	0.5701	30	0.3116
1.8	0.5580	40	0.2980
1.9	0.5471	50	0.2878
2.0	0.5373	60	0.2798
2.2	0.5203	70	0.2732
2.4	0.5061	80	0.2676
2.6	0.4939	90	0.2628
2.8	0.4836	100	0.2585
3.0	0.4745	200	0.2322
3.2	0.4664	300	0.2180
3.4	0.4593	400	0.2085

Source: Used with permission from Emmert and Pigford, 1963.

TABLE 4.2.13 Diffusion Volumes for Simple Molecules

Gas	Volume, $m^3 \times 10^{30}$
Air	20.1
Ammonia	14.9
Argon	16.1
Carbon dioxide	26.9
Carbon monoxide	18.9
Helium	2.88
Hydrogen	7.07
Krypton	22.8
Neon	5.59
Nitrogen	17.9
Nitrous oxide	35.9
Oxygen	16.6
Water vapor	12.7

Source: Adapted and used with permission from Fuller et al., 1966.

TABLE 4.2.14   Calculated Gas Diffusivities for Ambient Air at 298 °K (25 °C) and for Alveolar Air at 310 °K (37 °C) at 1 Atm Pressure (101.3 kNm²)

Constituent	Ambient Air		Alveolar Air	
	Mole Fraction	Diffusivity, cm²/sec	Mole Fraction	Diffusivity, cm²/sec
Water vapor	0.000	0.247	0.062	0.279
Carbon dioxide	0.000	0.154	0.052	0.178
Oxygen	0.209	0.194	0.138	0.222
Nitrogen	0.791	0.196	0.747	0.222

diffusion coefficients are expected to be slightly greater using Equation 4.2.29 compared to Equation 4.2.26.

Diffusion which occurs within a binary system of gases with equimolar counterdiffusion

$$J_{ij} = -J_{ji} \tag{4.2.30}$$

results in

$$D_{ij} = D_{ji} \tag{4.2.31}$$

Diffusion within ambient air is usually managed by considering air to be a uniform and constant medium, a binary constituent. Alveolar air is not constant or uniform, and it cannot be considered to be binary. For multicomponent diffusion, Emmert and Pigford (1963) give

$$D_i = \frac{1 - X_i}{\displaystyle\sum_{j=1}^{N} (X_j/D_{ij})} \tag{4.2.32}$$

where D_i = diffusion coefficient of constituent i in the multicomponent system, m²/sec

X_i = mole fraction of constituent i, dimensionless

Gas diffusion coefficients should be calculated for binary diffusion using Equation 4.2.29 and converted to multicomponent diffusion coefficients for alveolar air using Equation 4.2.32. Values of alveolar gas diffusivities calculated in this way appear in Table 4.2.14 and it can be seen that alveolar gas diffusivity values differ from ambient gas diffusivity values by about 15%.

During exercise, and at other times when the respiratory exchange ratio differs significantly from 1.0, the alveolar gas can no longer be considered to be a stagnant medium. There results a net movement of mass with a mean velocity $\dot{V}_m$. This case is not strictly diffusion in that a convective flow is also present.

Gas Mixing in the Airways. In any thorough consideration of gas delivery to the lungs, account must be made for the effects of combined convection (bulk movement) and diffusion (molecular movement) within the conducting airways. Although this subject can be very involved because of the complicated geometry of the air passages, it is nonetheless especially important in high-frequency ventilation.[26] There may also be an effect of non–steady-state gas mixing at the very high respiration rates achieved during heavy exercise.

---

[26]It has been found clinically that normal blood gas compositions can be maintained in patients with respiratory obstruction by assisted ventilation at high frequency (typically 5–15 cps) and low tidal volume (typically one-third of normal dead volume).

This subject has been very thoroughly presented by Pedley et al. (1977) and by Ultman (1981), and it will not be completely developed here. A few pertinent details will, however, be presented.

Flow in the conducting airways removes excess carbon dioxide during exhalation and supplies fresh oxygen during inhalation. In each case, there is a divergence between the gas composition of the flowing gas and that of the gas which is being displaced. Gas movement by convection is present for sure. Likewise, the difference in gas concentration between the displacing gas and the contacting displaced gas provides the opportunity for molecular diffusion.

Mathematical specification of axial gas transport in a conduit is given (Ultman, 1981) by

$$\dot{V}_i = F_i \dot{V} - (D_{ij} + \mathscr{D}_{ij}) A \frac{dF_i}{dx} \tag{4.2.33}$$

where $\dot{V}_i$ = volume rate of flow of constituent i, m³/sec
$\dot{V}$ = volume rate of flow of entire plug of gas, m³/sec
D_{ij} = diffusion coefficient, m²/sec
$\mathscr{D}_{ij}$ = longitudinal dispersion coefficient, m²/sec
F_i = average volume fraction of constituent i, m³/m³
A = total cross-sectional area of tube, m²
x = distance along tube, m

The ratio of material delivery by axial convection to that by radial diffusion is known as the Péclet number (Pe). The rate of supply by convective flow is given by

$$\dot{V} = vAc_i \tag{4.2.34}$$

where $\dot{V}$ = volume rate of flow, m³/sec
v = average flow velocity, m/sec
A = cross-sectional area, m²
c_i = concentration, kg/kg

Steady-state material diffusion is given by

$$\dot{V} = D_{ij} A \frac{dc_i}{dx} = D_{ij} A \frac{c_i}{l} \tag{4.2.35}$$

where (c/l) = mean concentration gradient, m⁻¹
The Péclet number is thus given by

$$Pe = lv/D_{ij} \tag{4.2.36}$$

Péclet numbers within the respiratory system vary from 10,000 at the mouth to 0.01 at the alveolar ducts.

In laminar flow through a straight tube, the profile of velocities of gas particles flowing along the tube will appear to be parabolic (see Section 4.2.3). That is, the velocity of particles in the center of the tube will be twice the average velocity and the velocity at the wall will be zero. Thus molecules of a gas in higher concentration in the displacing gas mixture will travel downstream faster in the center of the tube than at the wall. Consequently, the resulting concentration difference between tube midline and tube wall enhances radial diffusion of this constituent gas (Ben Jebria, 1984). Taylor (1953) showed that this mechanism can be described as longitudinal dispersion[27] with an equivalent virtual diffusion coefficient:

$$\mathscr{D}_{ij} = D_{ij} + \frac{(vd)^2}{192 D_{ij}} \tag{4.2.37}$$

---

[27]This mechanism of enhanced diffusion by laminar convective transport is called Taylor dispersion.

where v = mean axial velocity, m/sec

   d = tube diameter, m

The value for the number in the denominator, here shown as 192, varies with velocity profile (Ultman, 1981). For even moderate velocities and diameters, $\mathscr{D}_{ij} \gg D_{ij}$.[28] And, interestingly, the lower the molecular diffusivity D_{ij} of any gas, the higher will be the dispersion coefficient $\mathscr{D}_{ij}$.

   In turbulent flow, the velocity profile is much flatter. The equivalent dispersion coefficient is smaller (Ben Jebria, 1984):

$$\mathscr{D}_{ij} = D_{ij} + 0.73vd \qquad (4.2.38)$$

With this cursory discussion, gas mixing in the airways due to simultaneous convection and diffusion can begin to be understood.

Diffusion Capacity. As if alveolar diffusion alone were not complicated enough, there is diffusion across the alveolar membrane into the capillary plasma, diffusion through the plasma, diffusion into the red blood cell, and chemical binding of both oxygen and carbon dioxide to account for. Furthermore, nonnormal lungs[29] may not have a uniform distribution of inspired gas, thus having a nonuniform alveolar gas concentration (Sackner, 1976d). For these reasons it is often convenient to consider only the overall diffusing capacity of the lung. Certainly, it is much easier to make this measurement than the measure individual alveoli diffusion parameters.

   Lung diffusing capacity[30] is defined (Astrand and Rodahl, 1970) as

$$D_L = \frac{\text{gas flow}}{\text{mean driving pressure}} \qquad (4.2.39)$$

where D_L = lung diffusing capacity, $\text{m}^5/(\text{N} \cdot \text{sec})$

Mean driving pressure is the difference between average alveolar pressure and mean capillary partial pressure.

   Lung diffusing capacity for oxygen is of primary interest. However, mean capillary oxygen partial pressure is difficult to ascertain. It would be better to choose a gas which is held by the pulmonary capillaries at a constant partial pressure, or which disappears entirely. Carbon monoxide has 210 times the affinity for hemoglobin as does oxygen (Sackner, 1976d) and, for all purposes, is completely removed from the plasma by circulating red blood cells. Carbon monoxide, in low concentration, has thus become the standard challenge gas for determination of lung diffusing capacity:

$$D_{LCO} = \dot{V}_{CO}/p_A\text{CO} \qquad (4.2.40)$$

where D_{LCO} = lung diffusing capacity for CO, $\text{m}^5/(\text{N} \cdot \text{sec})$

   $\dot{V}_{CO}$ = CO rate of absorption in the lung, m^3/sec

   $p_A\text{CO}$ = mean alveolar partial pressure for CO, N/m^2

Steady-state lung diffusion capacity for oxygen is obtained from steady-state lung diffusion capacity for carbon monoxide by multiplying the latter by 1.23 (Astrand and Rodahl, 1970).

---

[28]For $(d/l)(\text{Pe}) > 180$, the $\mathscr{D}_{ij} < 0.05D_{ij}$, and for $(d/l)(\text{Pe}) < 20$, the $D_{ij} < 0.05\mathscr{D}_{ij}$ where l = tube length, m (Ultman, 1981).

[29]These lungs are characterized by compartments with unequal time constants (flow resistance multiplied by compliance). Regions with small time constant fill faster and empty faster. Compartments can have long time constants (usually caused by high resistance) for one phase of breathing and short time constants for the other. For example, chronic obstructive pulmonary disease (COPD) and emphysema have particularly long time constants for emptying and are called obstructive pulmonary diseases; asthma, which is a restrictive pulmonary disease, is characterized by long filling and emptying time constants.

[30]Diffusing capacity is analogous to electrical conductance. For this reason, some authors call it "transfer factor," or "transfer coefficient."

Diffusion capacity values obtained at rest are not the same as diffusion capacity values obtained during exercise. Diffusion capacity is influenced by alveolar surface area (70–90 m²), thickness of the membrane separating air from blood, and pulmonary capillary blood volume, or hemoglobin content (Astrand and Rodahl, 1970). Figure 4.2.9 shows the large increase (three times) in diffusion capacity which occurs during exercise. Most of the increase is attributable to an increase in the number of capillaries open during work (Astrand and Rodahl, 1970). For a similar reason, diffusion rates for women are lower than those for men because alveolar surface area varies with body weight (Astrand and Rodahl, 1970).

Figure 4.2.5 illustrates the diffusion pathway taken by oxygen from the alveolar space to the interior of the red blood cell. Oxygen must diffuse across the alveolar capillary membranes and into the plasma, across the red cell membrane and through the red cell interior, finally to be bound to hemoglobin. Hill et al. (1977) used the kinetics of the reactions of oxygen and carbon dioxide at various stages in this process to formulate a model of oxygen and carbon dioxide exchanges during exercise.

Carbon dioxide diffusion rates are about 20 times those for oxygen (Astrand and Rodahl, 1970). Contributing to this ratio is the fact that CO_2 molecules are larger than O_2 molecules, thus slowing diffusion, but CO_2 diffuses about 25 times more rapidly than O_2 in aqueous liquids (Astrand and Rodahl, 1970). Reaction rates of Equation 3.2.3, the equilibrium reaction between bicarbonate and carbon dioxide in the blood, are so slow, however, that all the CO_2 which must be removed from the blood would not be available to diffuse into the lungs if it were not for carbonic anhydrase, which catalyzes the reaction and allows it to proceed much more rapidly. Without carbonic anhydrase, the blood would have to remain in the capillaries for almost 4 min for the CO_2 to be given off (Astrand and Rodahl, 1970).

Diffusion capacity for carbon dioxide has been found to be an insensitive predictor of abnormal gas exchange during exercise (Sue et al., 1987). Therefore, other measures, such as arterial blood gases, must be used to determine exercise gas exchange.

Blood Gases. As the physiological interface between air and blood, the respiratory system must be studied from both aspects. We have already dealt with blood gas partial pressure in this

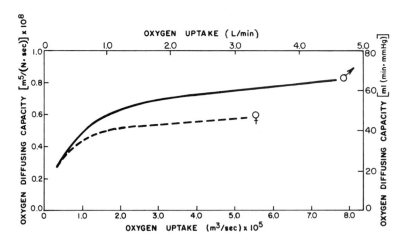

Figure 4.2.9 Variation in diffusing capacity for oxygen with increasing oxygen uptake during work on a bicycle ergometer in the sitting position for 10 trained women (bottom curve) and 10 trained men (upper curve). Increasing values on the abscissa can be considered to be increasing work rates. (Adapted and used with permission from Astrand and Rodahl, 1970.)

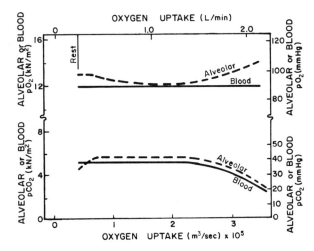

Figure 4.2.10   Alveolar and respiratory blood gas partial pressures during exercise. Carbon dioxide values track closely over the entire range of work rates used (about 0–150 N·m/sec external work), but oxygen does not.

chapter, as well as with blood gas dynamics in Chapter 3. Some details must still be introduced to complete the necessary background for study of respiratory contribution to blood gas exchange.

Carbon dioxide and oxygen are the most important gases for consideration. Other gases, such as nitrogen, do not normally play a large role in respiratory gas exchange.[31] In a general sense, blood gas levels leaving the lung remain reasonably constant: blood pO_2 is 5333 N/m² (40 mm Hg) and blood pO_2 is 13.3 kN/m² (100 mm Hg). Carbon dioxide partial pressure in mixed (pulmonary) venous blood and alveolar air is highly variable, but it begins at about 2000 N/m² at rest, decreases to about 1500 N/m² during light exercise, and increases again in severe exercise (Morehouse and Miller, 1967).

The relationships between alveolar partial pressures and respiratory blood partial pressures of oxygen and carbon dioxide are seen in Figure 4.2.10. Carbon dioxide partial pressure in the blood closely tracks carbon dioxide partial pressure in the alveolar space, and, for many practical purposes, can be considered to be the same.

There is a slight variation in arterial partial pressures of carbon dioxide and oxygen throughout the breathing cycle. Respiratory-related variations of about 900 N/m² (7 mm Hg) in pO_2 have been found in anesthetized dogs, lambs, and cats (Biscoe and Willshaw, 1981). For resting dogs, alveolar variation of pO_2, has been calculated to be 1300 N/m² (10 mm Hg) and for resting humans it has been calculated as 400 N/m² (3 mm Hg).

A variation in arterial pCO_2 has been measured indirectly[32] as 270 N/m² (2 mm Hg) in anesthetized cats (Biscoe and Willshaw, 1981). Alveolar pCO_2 changes by about 270 N/m² (2 mm Hg) in resting man, but exercise is expected to increase the excursion.

The extent of variation depends greatly on mixing occurring in the heart. The higher the number of heartbeats per breath, the less mixing occurs and the greater is the partial pressure variation. Similarly, greater end-systolic volumes attenuate the variation more than lesser volumes (Biscoe and Willshaw, 1981).

Two factors contribute to the difference between alveolar and arterial oxygen partial pressures. The first of these is shunting of venous blood around the effective alveolar volume to be

---

[31]Nitrogen exchange, as well as other so-called inert gas exchange, is important in pulmonary function measurement and abnormal respiratory or metabolic conditions.

[32]A mean variation of 0.15 pH units was recorded.

mixed consequently with arterial blood from the effective alveolar volume. Although this has a large effect on oxygen partial pressure of the resulting blood mixture, it has but a small effect on carbon dioxide partial pressure because the CO_2 dissociation curve for blood is very steep (Figure 4.2.11), indicating a small partial pressure change per unit change in concentration (also see Figure 3.2.4). The second factor contributing to oxygen partial pressure difference between alveoli and blood is the diffusion rate of oxygen across the alveolar membrane, which is much slower for oxygen than for carbon dioxide.

More importantly, oxygen saturation of mixed (pulmonary) venous blood is nearly 100% during rest and exercise up to that requiring oxygen uptake of 67×10^{-6} m^3/sec (4 L/min) (Morehouse and Miller, 1967). This comes about because pulmonary vessels closed during rest open during exercise, with the effect that the volume of blood through the lungs increases without a corresponding increase of velocity of blood through the lungs. Blood transit time through the lungs therefore remains nearly constant. The resulting improvement in distribution of ventilation to perfusion results in a decrease in oxygen partial pressure difference across the capillary and alveolar membranes. During very heavy exercise, the increased acidity and temperature of the blood (see Figures 3.2.2 and 3.2.3) reduce the ability of hemoglobin to absorb oxygen, resulting in lower blood saturation (Morehouse and Miller, 1967).

The amount of oxygen in the blood (which comes, originally, from respiration) can be obtained from (see Section 3.2.1)

$$c_{O_2} = 1340 S c_H + 0.023 \times 10^{-5} pO_2 \qquad (4.2.41)$$

where c_{O_2} = oxygen concentration of the blood, m^{3}O$_2$/m^3 blood
   S = hemoglobin saturation, fractional
   c_H = hemoglobin concentration, kg hemoglobin/m^3 blood

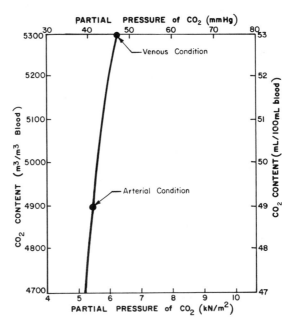

Figure 4.2.11 Physiologic CO_2 dissociation curve. The change from systemic arterial to venous concentrations of carbon dioxide is accompanied by a very small change in carbon dioxide partial pressure. (Adapted and used with permission from Riley, 1965.)

The first term on the right-hand side of Equation 4.2.41 reflects the concentration of oxygen carried by hemoglobin, and the second term represents dissolved oxygen (see Section 3.2.1). Average men have about 160 kg hemoglobin per cubic meter of blood (Ganong, 1963), and hemoglobin saturation can be calculated from Equations 3.2.5 and 3.2.6 or from a similar procedure given by West and Wagner (1977). The amount of oxygen absorbed by the pulmonary blood is

$$\dot{V}_{O_2} = (\Delta c_{O_2})(CO) \tag{4.2.42}$$

where $\dot{V}_{O_2}$ = oxygen uptake, m^3/sec
     CO = cardiac output, m^3/sec
     Δc_{O_2} = oxygen concentration difference between pulmonary arterial and pulmonary venous blood, $m^3 O_2/m^3$ blood
See Table 3.2.8 for representative values of cardiac output.

West and Wagner (1977) presented a procedure to calculate the amount of carbon dioxide taking part in respiration. They began with a procedure similar in theory to Equation 4.2.41:

$$\text{total blood } CO_2 = \text{plasma } CO_2 + \text{red blood cell } CO_2 \tag{4.2.43}$$

Based on the Henderson–Hasselbalch equation (see Equation 3.2.4) plasma CO_2 or dissolved CO_2 is calculated from

$$\text{plasma } CO_2 = \alpha_{CO_2} pCO_2(1 + 10^{(pH - pK)}) \tag{4.2.44}$$

where α_{CO_2} = solubility of CO_2 in plasma, mol/(N·m)
     pH = negative logarithm of hydrogen ion concentration, dimensionless
     pK = negative logarithm of reaction constant, dimensionless
Values of pK and α_{CO_2} may be taken as constant values of 6.10 and 0.236 (mol·m)/kN, but West and Wagner (1977) gave expressions for these as functions of temperature and pH:

$$pK = 6.086 + 0.042(7.4 - pH) + (38 - \theta)[0.0047 + 0.0014(7.4 - pH)] \tag{4.2.45}$$

where θ = temperature, °C
and

$$\alpha_{CO_2} = 0.230 + 0.0043(37 - \theta) + 0.0002(37 - \theta)^2 \tag{4.2.46}$$

Since the fractions of red blood cells and plasma in the blood are related by hematocrit, carbon dioxide concentration is

$$c_{CO_2} = 222[(Ht)(\text{red cell } CO_2) + (1 - Ht)(\text{plasma } CO_2)] \tag{4.2.47}$$

where c_{CO_2} = total CO_2 concentration in the blood, $m^3 CO_2/m^3$ blood
     Ht = hematocrit, fractional
West and Wagner (1977) calculated red blood cellular carbon dioxide as proportional to plasma carbon dioxide and oxygen saturation of hemoglobin. Thus total CO_2 concentration becomes

$$c_{CO_2} = (\text{plasma } CO_2)[222][(Ht)(B - 1) + 1] \tag{4.2.48}$$

and

$$B = B_1 + (B_2 - B_1)(1 - S) \tag{4.2.49a}$$

$$B_1 = 0.590 + 0.2913(7.4 - \text{pH}) - 0.0844(7.4 - \text{pH})^2 \qquad (4.2.49b)$$

$$B_2 = 0.644 + 0.2275(7.4 - \text{pH}) - 0.0938(7.4 - \text{pH})^2 \qquad (4.2.49c)$$

where S = fractional hemoglobin saturation, dimensionless
Fractional hematocrit is usually about 0.47 for men and about 0.42 for women and children (Astrand and Rodahl, 1970).

Similar to oxygen, the amount of carbon dioxide taking part in respiratory exchange is

$$\dot{V}_{CO_2} = (\Delta c_{CO_2})(\text{CO}) \qquad (4.2.50)$$

where $\dot{V}_{CO_2}$ = carbon dioxide evolution, m^3/sec
$\quad \Delta c_{CO_2}$ = change in carbon dioxide concentration between pulmonary
$\qquad$ arterial and pulmonary venous blood, m^3 CO_2/m^3 blood
$\quad$ CO = cardiac output, m^3/sec

Pulmonary Gas Exchange. The problem of pulmonary gas exchange is that experimental procedures limit the sites where data may be obtained. As we have seen, complex mechanisms and adjustments in the respiratory system are quite normal, but usual respiratory gas measurements can be made only at the mouth and sometimes in the systemic circulation. From these measurements must be inferred information concerning metabolic state, alveolar efficacy, pulmonary perfusion, respiratory dead volume, and a host of other interesting and clinically important processes possessed by the individual from whom the data were obtained.

Fortunately, there are mathematical means to deduce much useful pulmonary gas exchange information. The ideas in this section are relatively simple, and the algebra is not overwhelming. The problem, however, is in nomenclature; with so many subscripts and superscripts it is easy to become confused. It is hoped that the clear and straightforward presentation here will prevent that. Symbols generally follow those used by Riley (1965).

We begin with a simple steady-state mass balance, first on oxygen:

$$\text{O}_2 \text{ used} = \text{O}_2 \text{ intake} - \text{O}_2 \text{ exhausted} \qquad (4.2.51)$$

$$\dot{V}_{O_2} = \dot{V}_i F_{iO_2} - \dot{V}_e F_{eO_2} \qquad (4.2.52)$$

where $\dot{V}_{O_2}$ = oxygen uptake, m^3/sec
$\quad \dot{V}_i$ = inhaled flow rate, m^3/sec
$\quad \dot{V}_e$ = exhaled flow rate, m^3/sec
$\quad F_{iO_2}$ = fractional concentration[33] of oxygen in inhaled dry gas, m^3/m^3
$\quad F_{eO_2}$ = fractional concentration of oxygen in exhaled dry gas, m^3/m^3
And next on carbon dioxide:

$$\dot{V}_{CO_2} = \dot{V}_e F_{eCO_2} - \dot{V}_i F_{iCO_2} \qquad (4.2.53)$$

where $\dot{V}_{CO_2}$ = carbon dioxide efflux, m^3/sec
$\quad F_{eCO_2}$ = fractional concentration of carbon dioxide in exhaled dry gas, m^3/m^3
$\quad F_{iCO_2}$ = fractional concentration of carbon dioxide in inhaled dry gas, m^3/m^3
F_{iCO_2} is usually assumed to be zero for atmospheric air breathing. There are cases, especially those where masks are worn, where F_{iCO_2} cannot be assumed to be zero (Johnson, 1976). Notice, also, that all gases are assumed to be at STPD conditions (see Equation 4.2.14).

---

[33]Fractional concentration is given as volume of gas A per unit volume of mixture of gases A and B. From Equation 4.2.9 we could have given fractional concentration in terms of partial pressures.

Since there is a difference between inspired and expired volumes, a mass balance on nitrogen, which is assumed to have no net exchange across the lungs, is performed to account for volume differences:

$$\dot{V}_{N_2} = \dot{V}_i F_{iN_2} - \dot{V}_e F_{eN_2} \tag{4.2.54}$$

$$\dot{V}_i = \dot{V}_e (F_{eN_2}/F_{iN_2}) \tag{4.2.55}$$

where $\dot{V}_{N_2}$ = nitrogen uptake, m^3/sec

F_{eN_2} = fractional concentration of nitrogen in exhaled dry gas, m^3/m^3
F_{iN_2} = fractional concentration of nitrogen in inhaled dry gas, m^3/m^3

Many relationships have been developed between these variables to aid pulmonary function testing. Since measurement technique is not the object of this book, most of these relationships are ignored here. The reader is referred to Riley (1965) for further details. One useful relationship is considered, however: the determination of respiratory dead volume V_D.

During a single expiration the first air to leave the mouth is from the respiratory dead volume—the air closest to the mouth. This air has not exchanged gases with the blood and is virtually the same composition as inspired air (with the addition of water vapor, of course). Air that reaches the mouth after the dead volume air has been exhaled is considered to be from the alveolar space (see Figure 4.2.12). It is this air which is in equilibrium with the blood. Because carbon dioxide is continually evolving, the CO_2 content of alveolar air continually increases (Turney, 1983) with the rate of increase related to rate of CO_2 evolution (Newstead et al., 1980). Normally, pulmonary technicians have considered the so-called end-tidal CO_2 concentration to be representative of alveolar air. Because of the increasing CO_2 concentration, end-tidal air may not be as meaningful as previously supposed.

Considering the expired air to be composed of dead volume air and alveolar air:

$$V_e = V_{Ae} + V_{De} \tag{4.2.56}$$

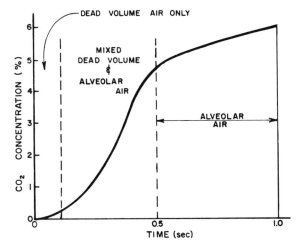

Figure 4.2.12 A typical tracing of carbon dioxide concentration with time during an exhaled breath. The first air to be removed is dead volume air and the last is alveolar air. Carbon dioxide concentration of alveolar air increasess with time because carbon dioxide from the blood is constantly being delivered to the alveoli.

where V_e = exhaled volume, m^3
  V_{Ae} = exhaled volume from alveolar space, m^3
  V_{De} = exhaled volume from dead space, m^3
total exhaled CO_2 comes from alveolar CO_2 and dead volume CO_2:

$$V_e F_{eCO_2} = V_{Ae} F_{AeCO_2} + V_{De} F_{DeCO_2} \qquad (4.2.57)$$

where F_{eCO_2} = average mixed volume fractional concentration of CO_2 from exhaled air, m^3/m^3
  F_{AeCO_2} = fractional concentration of CO_2 from alveolar space, m^3/m^3
  F_{DeCO_2} = fractional concentration of CO_2 from dead volume, m^3/m^3
Because no gas exchange occurs in the dead volume,

$$F_{DeCO_2} = F_{iCO_2} \qquad (4.2.58)$$

and F_{iCO_2} is usually assumed to be zero. Thus

$$V_{De} = \left[\frac{F_{AeCO_2} - F_{eCO_2}}{F_{AeCO_2} - F_{iCO_2}} \right] V_e \qquad (4.2.59)$$

This is called the Bohr equation. F_{AeCO_2} is usually taken to be the maximum CO_2 concentration during the exhalation, and F_{eCO_2} is the CO_2 concentration of the well-mixed total exhaled breath.

Pulmonary gas relationships will be developed for three effective pulmonary compartments (Riley, 1966): (1) effective, (2) ventilated but unperfused, and (3) perfused but unventilated. The effective compartment is considered to be the part of the lung where gas exchange occurs between alveoli and capillaries. Its volume is the alveolar volume V_A. Both second and third compartments are ineffective for gas exchange and comprise the respiratory dead volume. Compartment two corresponds to the anatomic dead volume and compartment three represents the alveolar dead volume.

Three similar compartments can be considered from the blood side of the alveolar membranes. In the respiratory circulation, however, we do not talk of blood dead volume, but rather of blood *shunting*. The effect of blood shunting is to mix unaerated mixed venous blood with aerated arterial blood.

A carbon dioxide balance of the effective volume, or alveolar volume, gives

$$\dot{V}_{CO_2} = \dot{V}_{Ae} F_{AeCO_2} - \dot{V}_{Ai} F_{AiCO_2} \qquad (4.2.60)$$

where $\dot{V}_{Ae}$ = alveolar ventilation rate during exhalation, m^3/sec
  $\dot{V}_{Ai}$ = alveolar ventilation rate during inhalation, m^3/sec
If $F_{AiCO_2} = 0$, then

$$\dot{V}_{CO_2} = \frac{\dot{V}_{Ae} p_A CO_2}{(p_B - pH_2O)} \qquad (4.2.61)$$

where $p_A CO_2$ = mean CO_2 partial pressure of effective alveolar space, N/m^2
  p_B = total barometric pressure = 101 kN/m^2
  pH_2O = partial pressure of water vapor at the temperature of the respiratory system
    = 6280 N/m^2
and, as discussed previously, alveolar and arterial CO_2 partial pressures can be considered to be the same value:

$$p_A CO_2 = p_a CO_2 \qquad (4.2.62)$$

where $p_a CO_2$ = arterial CO_2 partial pressure, N/m^2

The dead space compartments contribute no carbon dioxide to the exhaled air[34]. The dead volume compartments therefore effectively increase the volume of the exhaled breath and dilute the carbon dioxide concentration from that of the effective compartment. This condition has already been considered in the formulation of the Bohr equation (4.2.59).

A carbon dioxide balance in the blood yields

$$\dot{Q}_{\text{eff}} = \frac{\dot{V}_{CO_2}}{c_{vCO_2} \, c_{\text{effCO}_2}} \tag{4.2.63}$$

where $\dot{Q}_{\text{eff}}$ = rate of blood flow through the effective compartment, m³/sec

c_{vCO_2} = mixed venous (systemic) concentration of carbon dioxide, m³ CO_2/m³ blood

c_{effCO_2} = carbon dioxide concentration of effective blood compartment, m³ CO_2/m³ blood

The effective blood perfusion rate $\dot{Q}_{\text{eff}}$ is related to total blood flow $\dot{Q}_{\text{pulm}}$ by the addition of the shunt component of blood $\dot{Q}_s$. The concentration of carbon dioxide in the blood returning to the tissues therefore contains contributions from shunt (mixed venous pCO_2) and effective (arterial c_{CO_2}) blood flows:

$$c_{CO_2} = \frac{(\dot{Q}_{\text{pulm}} - \dot{Q}_{\text{eff}})c_{vCO_2} + \dot{Q}_{\text{eff}}c_{aCO_2}}{\dot{Q}_{\text{pulm}}} \tag{4.2.64}$$

where c_{aCO_2} = concentration of carbon dioxide in systemic arterial blood, m³ CO_2/m³ blood

Oxygen balances on alveolar and blood components give equations so similar to

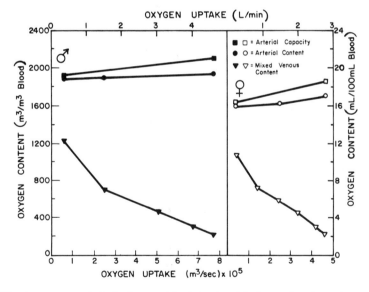

Figure 4.2.13 Oxygen content of mixed venous blood at rest and during work up to maximum on a bicycle ergometer. During maximal work the arterial saturation is about 92% compared with 97–98% at rest; the venous oxygen content is very low and simiar for women and men. (Adapted and used with permission from Astrand and Rodahl, 1970.)

[34]This is not exactly true, since carbon dioxide accumulates in the anatomic dead space during the previous exhalation and is subsequently inhaled into the remaining portions of the dead volume compartment. This small amount of carbon dioxide contributes to the carbon dioxide concentration of the following exhalation.

Equations 4.2.57–4.2.64 that they are not repeated here. An oxygen balance on the overall respiratory system gives

$$\dot{V}_{O_2} = (\dot{V}_A + V_D/T)F_{iO_2} - (\dot{V}_A + V_D/T)F_{eO_2} \tag{4.2.65}$$

where $\dot{V}_{O_2}$ = oxygen uptake, m³/sec
$\quad\dot{V}_A$ = alveolar ventilation rate, m³/sec
$\quad V_D$ = total dead volume, m
$\quad T$ = respiratory period, sec
$\quad F_{iO_2}$ = fractional concentration of oxygen in inhaled air, m³O₂/m³ air
$\quad F_{eO_2}$ = fractional concentration of oxygen in exhaled air, m³O₂/m³ air

For modeling purposes, it is usually necessary to know the return concentrations of mixed venous blood and calculate the respiratory system loading to refresh the blood (Figure 4.2.13). Partial pressure of arterial O_2 does not change greatly during exercise; arterial O_2 saturation is about 92% during exercise compared to 97–98% at rest (Astrand and Rodahl, 1970).

4.2.3 Mechanical Properties

Mechanical properties of the respiratory system play an important role in its operation. The mechanical properties normally considered are resistance, compliance, and inertance, which combine with flow rate, volume, and volume acceleration to produce pressure. The relative values of these pressures determine respiratory response to exercise in a way to be described later.

Respiratory System Models. A lumped-parameter,[35] greatly simplified analog model of the respiratory system appears in Figure 4.2.14. Three components of airways, lung tissue, and chest wall are shown.[36] Each of these components has elements of resistance (diagramed as an electrical resistor), compliance (electrical capacitor), and inertance (electrical inductor). Between components exist pressures denoted as alveolar and pleural pressures. Muscle pressure is the driving force for airflow to occur.

A pressure balance on the model of Figure 4.2.14 gives

$$(p_m - p_{atm}) + (p_{alv} - p_m) + (p_{pl} - p_{alv}) + (p_{mus} - p_{pl}) + (p_{atm} - p_{mus}) = 0 \tag{4.2.66}$$

where p_m = mouth pressure, N/m²
$\quad p_{atm}$ = atmospheric pressure, N/m²
$\quad p_{alv}$ = alveolar pressure, N/m²
$\quad p_{pl}$ = pleural pressure, N/m²
$\quad p_{mus}$ = muscle pressure, N/m²

Each pressure difference[37] can be expressed as

$$\Delta p = R\dot{V} + V/C + \ddot{V}I \tag{4.2.67}$$

---

[35]A lumped-parameter respiratory model considers similar properties collected in a small number of elements. Although these properties are really distributed throughout the respiratory system, their lumped-parameter depiction can assist understanding.

[36]Many different lumped-parameter respiratory system models have appeared in the literature. The reason for this is that different measurement methods and different model uses make other models more appropriate. Models can only approximate the true nature of the respiratory system, and the selection of an appropriate model is often based on reproduction by the model of certain kinds of data at the expense of other kinds of data. Recent respiratory modeling work has attemped to describe frequency dependencies of respiratory resistances and compliances (Dorkin et al., 1988).

[37]Except for $(p_{atm} - p_{mus})$, which is assumed to be the pressure generated by the respiratory muscles, and $(p_{alv} - p_m)$, which equals $(\dot{V}R_{aw} + \ddot{V}I_{aw})$ or V_{aw}/C_{aw}.

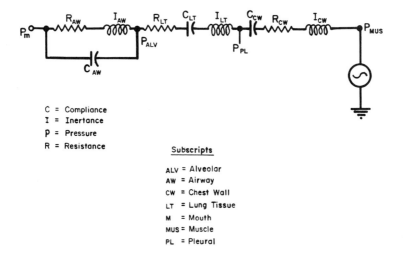

Figure 4.2.14 Lumped-parameter model of the respiratory system considered as three compartments comprising airways, lung tissue, and chest wall.

where R = resistance, $N \cdot sec/m^5$
  C = compliance, m^5/N
  I = inertance, $N \cdot sec^2/m^5$
  Δp = pressure difference, N/m^2
  V = volume, m^3
  $\dot{V}$ = flow rate, m^3/sec
  $\ddot{V}$ = volume acceleration, m^3/sec^2

Each of these terms is considered in more detail later.

The model of Figure 4.2.14 is actually too complicated for some purposes. The model seen in Figure 4.2.15 is much more useful when simple pulmonary function measurements are made or complicated mathematical expressions are used. When comparing the models in Figures 4.2.14 and 4.2.15, and noting the simplicity of the latter, one might wonder why the first model is considered at all. It is for these reasons:

1. The model of Figure 4.2.14 is more realistic than the model of Figure 4.2.15.

2. Certain respiratory disorders are localized to one of the three components in Figure 4.2.14, and specific information about that component is required.

3. Values of the elements in Figure 4.2.14 are more constant than those in Figure 4.2.15, which show strong changes with frequency of respiration.

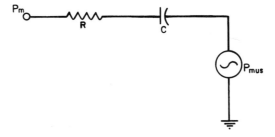

Figure 4.2.15 Simplified respiratory system model used for practical purposes at low frequencies.

TABLE 4.2.15 Mechanical Properties of Lungs and Thorax at Rest

Resistance

Total	392 kN·sec/m^5	(4.00 cm H$_2$O·sec/L)
Chest wall	196	(2.00)
Total lung	196	(2.00)
Lung tissue	39.2	(0.4)
Total airways	157	(1.6)
Upper airways	39.2	(0.4)
Lower airways	118	(1.2)

Compliance

Total	1.22×10^{-6} m^5/N	(0.12 L/cm H$_2$O)
Chest wall	2.45×10^{-6}	(0.24)
Total lung	2.45×10^{-6}	(0.24)
Airway	0.000	(0.00)
Lung tissue	2.45×10^{-6}	(0.24)

Inertance

Total	2600 N·sec^2/m^5	(0.0265 cm H$_2$O·sec^2/L)
Chest wall	1690	(0.0172)
Total lung	911	(0.0093)
Airway (gas)	137	(0.0014)
Lung tissue	774	(0.0079)
Upper airway	519	(0.0053)
Lower airway	255	(0.0026)

Table 4.2.15 gives typical values of mechanical elements appearing in the model of Figure 4.2.14. To obtain values for resistance R and compliance C appearing in Figure 4.2.15 use standard methods of combining electrical elements:

$$R = R_{aw} + R_{lt} + R_{cw} \qquad (4.2.68)$$

$$C \simeq \frac{C_{lt} C_{cw}}{C_{lt} + C_{cw}} \qquad (4.2.69)$$

This latter approximation is valid because airway compliance is nearly zero.[38]

Diurnal variation of 4–12% in lung volumes and mechanical parameters during exercise should be accounted for (Garrard and Emmons, 1986). Experimental results have shown significant diurnal variation in minute volume, respiratory exchange ratio, and carbon dioxide production rate.

Drugs, too, can significantly affect mechanical parameter values. A series of bronchoreactive drugs has been developed for use by asthmatics and others to reduce airway resistance. Even as common a drug as aspirin has been found to increase nasal resistance significantly (Jones et al., 1985), and airborne contaminants normally present in the atmosphere can have significant respiratory effects (Love, 1983).

---

[38] Airway compliance can be considered to be the compliance of the enclosed air. (Some investigators consider airway compliance to be the compliance of the tissue of the lung airways, the parenchyma.) Since $C = V/p$ and, from Equation 4.2.4, $p = nRT/R$, then $C_{aw} = V^2/nRT$. If we consider the entire lung volume to be gas entrapped within the airways, then FRC $= 2.4 \times 10^{-3}$ m^3 (Table 4.2.3), $T = 310$ °K, and $R \simeq 286.7$ N·m/kg mol °K) (Table 4.2.5). Since there are 22.4 L/kg mol at STP, there are 0.107 mol of air in the lung at FRC. Therefore, $C_{aw} \simeq 6 \times 10^{-10}$ m^5/N.

Resistance. Resistance is the energy dissipative element that appears in the respiratory system. That is, unlike compliance and inertance elements, which store energy for future use, resistance pressure losses are not recoverable.[39] Most of the energy that is developed to cause air to flow through the resistance eventually becomes heat.

Resistance in the respiratory system appears in several places: in the airways, in the lung tissue, and in the chest wall. Airway resistance occurs due to the movement of air through the conducting air passages; lung tissue and chest wall resistances appear due to viscous dissipation of energy when tissues slide past, or move relative to, one another.

These resistances are not constant (Macklem, 1980). They vary with flow rate and lung volume. One of the first attempts to quantify flow rate dependence was given by Rohrer (1915). Rohrer reasoned that pressure reduction in the airways should be due to laminar flow effects and turbulent effects (see Section 3.2.2). To account for these he postulated

$$p = K_1 \dot{V} + K_2 \dot{V}^2 \tag{4.2.70}$$

where $K_1 =$ first Rohrer coefficient, $N \cdot sec/m^5$
$\quad\quad K_2 =$ second Rohrer coefficient, $N \cdot sec^2/m^8$
$\quad\quad \dot{V} =$ flow rate, m^3/sec
From this,

$$R = P/\dot{V} = K_1 + K_2 \dot{V} \tag{4.2.71}$$

With lung volume remaining constant, resistance, as given by Equation 4.2.71, does appear to be described well in many individuals. In others, however, it appears that higher powers of $\dot{V}$ are required (Mead, 1961). This indicates that Rohrer's original concept of laminar and turbulent flows may not be entirely correct (Mead, 1961).

An alternative method of describing pressure loss was given by Ainsworth and Eveleigh (1952):

$$p = K \dot{V}^n \tag{4.2.72}$$

where $K =$ coefficient, $N \cdot sec^n/m^{(2+n)}$
$\quad\quad n =$ exponent, dimensionless
which plots as a straight line on log-log paper. Unfortunately, this description does not appear to be any more accurate than Rohrer's equation, and it has not been used as frequently.

Rohrer's equation has been applied to tissue as well as airway resistance. In applying it to tissue resistances, airflow rate is still used to obtain pressure difference despite the fact that air does not flow through the lung tissue and chest wall. Values for Rohrer's coefficients for various segments are given in Table 4.2.16. There is great variation in Rohrer's coefficients for different individuals,[40] and exhalation coefficients are generally higher than inhalation coefficients.

Standard terminology has the term respiratory resistance applied to airway plus lung tissue plus chest wall resistance. Pulmonary resistance is the term used for airway plus lung tissue resistance (respiratory resistance excluding chest wall resistance).

Most pressure–flow nonlinearities are found in the mouth and upper airways (Figure 4.2.16). Higher airflow rates occur in those segments compared to those in the lower airways, and therefore turbulence and nonlinearity are more likely to be found in the upper flow segments

---

[39]Energy stored in compliance and inertance elements is not necessarily always recovered either, if it causes the respiratory muscles to oppose the recovery. If negative work (see Section 5.2.5) is required, there may even be a greater energy expenditure because of the stored energy compared to resistive dissipation.

[40]Mead and Whittenberger (1953) give a range of 98–243 (mean 171 kN·sec/m⁵) in K_1 and a range of 12–48 (mean 28 mN sec²/m⁸) in K_2 values for seven subjects.

TABLE 4.2.16 Values of Rohrer's Coefficients[a] for Various Resistance Segments in Four Adults at Approximately 50% of Total Lung Capacity

Segment	Expiration		Inspiration	
	K_1	K_2	K_1	K_2
Total respiratory	169 (1.72)	25 (0.26)	154 (1.57)	21 (0.21)
Total pulmonary	103 (1.05)	15 (0.15)	93 (0.95)	12 (0.12)
Total airway	100 (1.02)	9.8 (0.10)	96 (0.98)	8 (0.08)

Source: Adapted and used with permission from Ferris et al., 1964.

[a]Units of K_1 are $kN \cdot sec/m^5$ ($cm\,H_2O \cdot sec/L$) and those of K_2 are $10^6\,N \cdot sec^2/m^8$ ($cm\,H_2O \cdot sec^2/L^2$).

(Table 4.2.17). Lower airway, lung tissue, and chest wall resistances are, for all practical purposes, constant (linear pressure–flow characteristic).

Steady laminar or turbulent flow profiles are established only at some distance from the inlet of a pipe. As the result of bifurcation, the previously established velocity profile is split by the wall at the branch point, and the new velocity profiles in each of the downstream segments are asymmetric for a while (Figure 4.2.17). The entrance length for laminar flow can be calculated

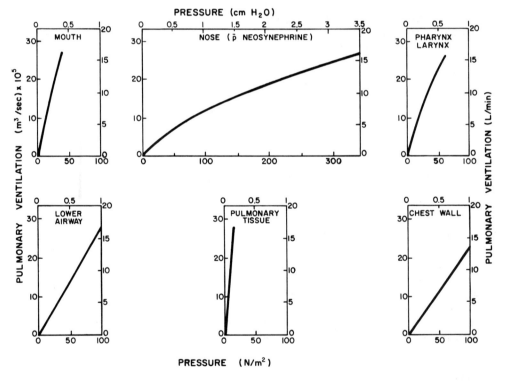

Figure 4.2.16 Flow–pressure relationships of various segments of the respiratory system. $\bar{p}$ denotes postnasal administration. Resistance of the various segments is the inverse of the slopes of the curves. Nonconstant resistances appear only in the upper airways. (Adapted and used with permission from Ferris et al., 1964.)

TABLE 4.2.17 Laminar and Turbulent Flow in Various Airway Segments of the Respiratory System

Segment	Diameter, (mm)	Linear Velocity Relative to that in Trachea	Reynolds Number at Flow Rate:		
			333	3,330	10,000
			$m^3/sec \times 10^6$		
Nasal canal	5	1.4	400	4,000[a]	12,000[a]
Pharynx	12	1.1	800	8,000[a]	24,000[a]
Glottis	8	3.4	1,600	16,000[a]	48,000[a]
Trachea	21	1.0	1,250	12,500[a]	37,500[a]
Bronchi	17	0.9	910	9,100[a]	27,300[a]
	9	1.3	700	7,000[a]	21,000[a]
	6	1.6	570	5,700[a]	17,100[a]
	4	0.8	190	1,900	5,700[a]
	2.5	0.5	74[b]	740	2,200[a]
	1	0.6	35[b]	350	1,050
Lobular bronchioles	0.4	0.1	2[b]	20[b]	60[b]

Source: Used with permission from Mead, 1961.

[a] Reynolds numbers greater than 2000 indicate turbulent flow.

[b] Denotes airway segment length longer than entrance length.

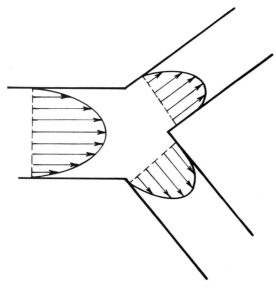

Figure 4.2.17 Resulting velocity profiles after bifurcation. Notice the asymmetry in each branch.

(Jacquez, 1979; Lightfoot, 1974; Skelland, 1967) from

$$l_e = 0.0288d\,\mathrm{Re} \tag{4.2.73}$$

where l_e = entrance length, m
$\quad d$ = tube diameter, m
$\quad \mathrm{Re}$ = Reynolds number, dimensionless

and

$$Re = \frac{dv\rho}{\mu} \tag{4.2.74}$$

where v = fluid velocity, m/sec
   ρ = fluid density, kg/m^3
   μ = fluid viscosity, kg/(m·sec)

Entrance length for turbulent flow is one-third to one-half that for laminar flow (Jacquez, 1979).

Within the entrance length, there is a great deal of turbulence and eddying, even for Reynolds numbers predicting laminar flow. Thus there is a larger amount of pressure lost than would be the case after a fully developed velocity profile is reached, and effective resistance within the entrance length is higher than would normally be expected.

For the airway segments listed in Table 4.2.17, all but the very smallest have lengths which are shorter than their calculated entrance lengths based their diameters and Reynolds numbers.[41] This would indicate that some amount of turbulence exists in most segments below Reynolds numbers of 2000.

Chang and El Masry (1982) and Isabey and Chang (1982) used a scale model of the human central airways to measure velocity profiles in the airways. They found a high degree of asymmetry in all branches, with peak velocities near the inner walls of the bifurcation. Velocity profiles were more sensitive to airway geometry, including curvature, than to flow rate. Slutsky et al. (1980) obtained measurements of friction coefficients between trachea and fourth- or fifth-generation airways on a cast model of human central airways. They found a traditional Moody diagram (Figure 4.2.18) relation between friction coefficient and Reynolds number at the trachea.

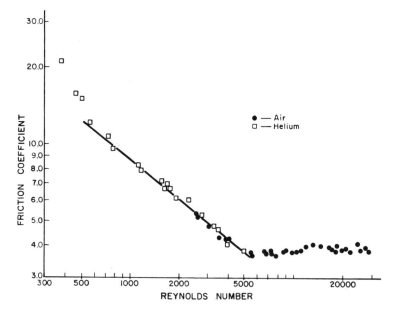

Figure 4.2.18   Moody diagram of the cast model of the human trachea. At Reynolds numbers less than 500, laminar flow exists. Fully developed turbulence exists at Reynolds numbers greater than 5000. In between is transitional flow. (Used with permission from Slutsky et al., 1980.)

---

[41]It is not until the fourteenth generation that entrance length becomes less than actual length, when total airflow is 0.001 m^3/sec (1 L/sec) (Jacquez, 1979).

TABLE 4.2.18 Percentage of Resistance Found During Mouth Breathing at 0.01 m³/sec (1 L/sec)[a]

Segment	Total Respiratory Resistance, %	Total Pulmonary Resistance, %
Mouth	12	20
Glottis-larynx	16	26
Upper airway	28	46
Lower airway	33	54
Total airway	60	98
Pulmonary tissue	1	2
Total pulmonary	61	100
Chest wall	39	
Total respiratory	100	

Source: Used with permission from Ferris et al., 1964.

[a]Values are averages for four subjects during inhalation and exhalation.

TABLE 4.2.19 Percentage of Total Respiratory Resistance Found During Quiet Nose Breathing at 4×10^{-4} m³/sec (0.4 L/sec)[a]

Segment	Resistance During Expiration, %	Resistance During Inspiration, %
Nose	47	54
Glottis and Larynx	10	4
Lower airway	24	26
Total airway	81	84
Pulmonary tissue	0	0
Total pulmonary	81	84
Chest wall	19	16
Total respiratory	100	100

Source: Used with permission from Ferris et al., 1964.

[a]Value are averages for four subjects.

Based on this, however, laminar flow was found to exist only to Reynolds numbers of 500–700, with the transition to turbulent flow occurring at Reynolds numbers higher than 700. Fully developed turbulent flow was found at Reynolds numbers greater than 10,000. This experimental evidence is important in that pressure drop in the upper airways has been shown to act as if laminar flow exists below Reynolds numbers of 700 despite the fact that entrance length of these airways is longer than the airways themselves.[42]

Airway resistance is usually measured at a flow rate of 0.001 m³/sec (1 L/sec). Table 4.2.18 gives the approximate percentage of total resistance found in each segment for mouth breathing at 0.001 m³/sec flow rate. At higher flow rates, as found during exercise, the segments with nonlinear pressure–flow characteristics would be expected to contribute a much higher proportion of the total resistance.[43] Table 4.2.19 gives similar proportions for quiet nose breathing.

---

[42]Slutsky et al. (1980) also showed that air distribution to upper lung segments is reduced compared to lower lung segments because of the more acute angles of airway branching in the upper airways. Because of this, pressure loss in the upper segment airways is greater for a given flow rate than it is for the lower segment airways. To account for experimental evidence of more even distribution of lung ventilation than would be expected from airways pressure loss, others have argued for reduced pressure loss in peripheral airways of the upper and for a higher applied pleural pressure at the upper lung than at the lower lung.

[43]Total respiratory resistance, which is about 400 N·sec/m⁵ during quiet breathing, increases to 1400 N·sec/m⁵ during rapid inspiration and to 2000–2400⁺ N·sec/m⁵ during rapid expiration (Mead, 1961).

During quiet nose breathing it has been shown that nasal resistance accounts for a large part of total airway resistance. The transition from nasal to mouth breathing during exercise seems to occur with little or no change in resistance, mouth breathing resistance at 1.67×10^{-3} m^3/sec (100 L/min) flow rate being nearly equal to nasal breathing resistance at rest. Cole et al. (1982) showed in five subjects that oral resistance was much higher when subjects were allowed to open their mouths to a natural degree than when mouthpieces required them to hold their mouths wide open. Average natural resistance decreased with increasing flow rate ($R = 2.01 \times 10^5 - 1.76 \times 10^5 \; \dot{V}$), and resistance reductions of 70–88% were found when mouthpieces were used.

Values of resistance during expiration are normally higher than those of inhalation due mainly to the effect of the surrounding tissue and pressures. During inhalation, pleural pressures are more negative than in the airways, thus pulling the conducting airways open. As they open, resistance decreases. On the other hand, exhalation is produced by positive pleural pressures, which tend to push the airways closed. Resistance increases.[44]

Different airway segments do not contribute equally to the difference in resistance during exhalation and inhalation. Because of the pressure drop as air flows through airways resistance, pressures in the upper airways are always closer to atmospheric pressure (except for positive-pressure ventilation of hospital patients and people wearing pressurized air-supplied respirator masks) than lower airways. Thus the pressure difference between airways and pleural spaces, and consequently the tendency toward airway opening during inspiration and closure during expiration, is greater in the upper airways than lower airways.

The upper airways, however, are stiffer than the lower airways, and thus can resist transmural pressure differences easier. The greatest effect of inhalation/exhalation on airway resistance is thus most likely to be felt in the middle airways, perhaps at generations 8–18. This area is usually considered to be the lower airways.

Up to now, we have dealt with measurements which were made at a thoracic gas volume V_{tg} of FRC. Airflow rate has been allowed to vary to give a pressure–flow relationship given by Equation 4.2.70. If flow rate is maintained at 10^{-3} m^3/sec (1 L/sec) and thoracic gas volume varies, airway resistance is found to be inversely proportional to lung volume for reasons similar to the preceding discussion on effect of inhalation and exhalation (see also Equation 4.4.30b). Briscoe and DuBois (1958) experimentally showed for men of different ages and body sizes[45] that

$$R_{aw} = 98{,}030/(280V - 0.204) \qquad (4.2.75)$$

where R_{aw} = airway resistance, N·sec/m^5
   V = lung volume, m^3

R_{aw} values would be expected to be divided by 0.8 for women (larger resistances than for men). Blide et al. (1964) showed that most of the effect of lung volume occurs in the lower airways.

Notice in Equation 4.2.75 that R_{aw} becomes infinite before lung volume becomes zero. This is because the lower airways close before the lung completely empties. The volume at which this occurs is termed the "closing volume" and corresponds to the residual volume in Table 4.2.3.

The combination of flow rate and lung volume effects on airway resistance requires complicated curve-fitting techniques. Consequently, very little information is available on subject averages including both effects. Johnson (1986), beginning with traditional description equations (4.2.71 and 4.2.75), matched inhalation data appearing in Bouhuys and Jonson (1967) for subject number 2 (male nonsmoker), redrawn as Figure 4.2.19:

$$p = 98{,}030 \dot{V}_i [0.744 + 426 \dot{V}_i + 6.79 \times 10^{-4}/(V - RV)] \qquad (4.2.76)$$

[44]When airway lumen diameter is larger, one would expect a larger dead volume to be present. Therefore, dead volume should be somewhat smaller during exhalation compared to inhalation.
[45]They also measured women's $R_{aw} = 98{,}030/(290V - 0.078)$ and children's $R_{aw} = 98{,}030/(140V + 0.069)$. There is a value for lung volume where men's and women's airway resistance becomes infinite (7.3×10^{-4} m^3 and 2.7×10^{-4} m^3, respectively), but there is no volume where children's airway resistance becomes infinite.

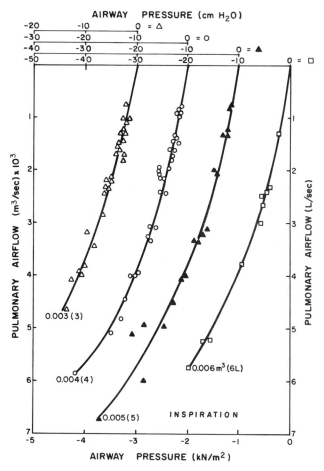

Figure 4.2.19 Inspiratory isovolume pressure–flow data in subject 2. Zero points for airway pressure on the abscissa are different for each isovolume pressure–flow curve. Lung volumes are labeled on the curves. The nonconstant slope of the lines indicates a nonlinear relationship between pressure and flow and consequent nonconstant resistance. (Adapted and used with permission from Bouhuys and Jonson, 1967.)

where p = pressure loss across airway resistance, N/m^2

$\dot{V}_i$ = inhalation flow rate (considered to be positive), m^3/sec

V = total lung volume, m^3

For subject number 5 (female smoker),

$$p = 98,030\dot{V}_i[-0.339 + 949\dot{V}_i + 1.18 \times 10^{-3}/(V - RV)] \qquad (4.2.77)$$

Description of exhalation resistance is complicated by the fact that pressures surrounding the airways tend to close them. It has been known for years that if transpulmonary pressure and expiratory flow rate are plotted along lines of equal lung volume, (1) a point is reached on each of these curves beyond which the flow cannot be increased (Figure 4.2.20), (2) sometimes flow rate is actually seen to decrease with increased pressure, and (3) the limiting flow rate decreases as lung volume decreases.[46] Since resistance is pressure divided by flow rate, resistance becomes very high once flow is limited.

[46]Peak expiratory flow rate also appears to be determined by a circadian rhythm (Cinkotai et al., 1984).

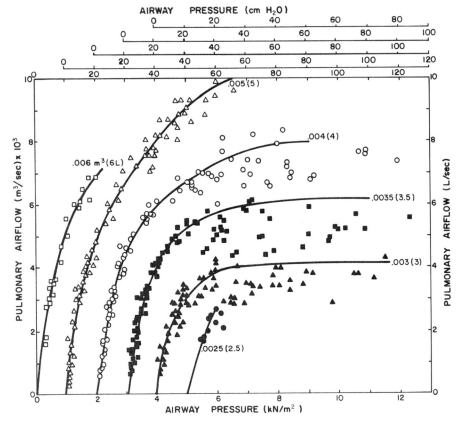

Figure 4.2.20   Expiratory isovolume pressure–flow data for the same subject as in Figure 4.2.19. Note that flow rates reach a limiting value in exhalation. When this happens, exhalation flow resistance is extremely high. (Adapted and used with permission from Bouhuys and Jonson, 1967.)

There are several explanations for this apparent increase in resistance. We have already begun the discussion with a consideration of pressures external to the tubes. To this will be added energy considerations.

An energy balance on a fluid system results in Bernoulli's equation:

$$\frac{\Delta p}{\gamma} + \Delta Z + \frac{\alpha \Delta (\dot{V}/A)^2}{2g} + h_f = 0 \qquad (4.2.78)$$

where Δp = static pressure difference between any two points in the stream, N/m^2

γ = specific weight of the fluid, N/m^3

ΔZ = height difference between two points in the stream, m

$\dot{V}$ = rate of flow, m^3/sec

A = tube cross-sectional area, m^2

$\Delta (\dot{V}/A)^2$ = difference in squared speed, m^2/sec^2

g = acceleration due to gravity, m/sec^2

h_f = frictional loss between two points in the stream, m

α = factor[47] correcting for the fact that the average velocity squared does not usually equal the average squared velocity, dimensionless

[47]Values for α depend on the profile of the velocity across the diameter of the tube and are usually taken to be 1.0 for turbulent flow and 2.0 for fully developed laminar flow. Non-Newtonian fluids (see Section 3.2.1) give other values for α.

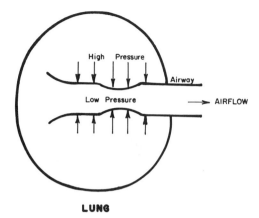

Figure 4.2.21   Collapse of airways during a forced expiration is due to external pressures exceeding internal pressures. Internal pressures diminish as flow rate increases.

For illustrative purposes, we can neglect differences in height and friction loss. The only two terms left involve pressure and flow rate. Since the sum of these two terms must be zero, any increase in one of these decreases the other. That is, if flow rate increases, as it does during a forced exhalation, static pressure must decrease. Static pressure inside a tube greater than static pressure outside a tube aids the rigidity of the tube wall in maintaining the tube opening. When static pressure decreases, tubes without totally stiff walls tend to collapse,[48] because external pressure is much greater than internal pressure (Figure 4.2.21). The same effect is seen in segments of the cardiovascular system (Section 3.5.2).

Collapse (or pinching) of the air passages increases resistance, thus increasing friction and reducing flow rate. Therefore, a dynamic balance is established, whereby flow rate remains constant. An increase in external pressure, which can occur during a particularly forceful exhalation, can actually decrease maximum flow rate because of its adverse effect on airway transmural pressure.[49] Similarly, a decrease in lung volume, which would tend to reduce tissue rigidity, would cause tube pinching, or collapse, at a lower flow rate.

Recently, these effects were quantified somewhat by the wave-speed formulation (Dawson and Elliott, 1977; Mead, 1980; Thiriet and Bonis, 1983). In this theory, the maximum velocity of airflow rate through a collapsible tube is taken to be the velocity of propagation of a pressure wave along the tube-in effect, the local sonic velocity. The speed of pressure wave propagation is

$$v_{\mathrm{Ws}} = \left\{ \left[\frac{1}{\rho} \left(\frac{dp_{\mathrm{tm}}}{dA} \right) \right] A \right\}^{1/2} \tag{4.2.79}$$

where v_{ws} = wave speed flow rate, m/sec

A = tube cross-sectional area, m^2

ρ = density of fluid, kg/m^3 (or N·sec^2/m^4)

p_{tm} = transmural pressure of the tube, N/m^2

The term (dp_{tm}/dA) is the tube characteristic, showing the rate of tube narrowing for a change in transmural pressure; it includes the stiffness of the tube wall and effect of surrounding tissue.

Rather than measuring (dp_{tm}/dA), it is easier to measure p_{tm} versus A of excised airways and take the slope of the generated curve (Martin and Proctor, 1958). In that case, however,

[48]However, Brancatisano et al. (1983) report evidence that muscular activity automatically opens the glottis during forced exhalation. The resulting lowered resistance facilitates lung emptying.

[49]Vorosmarti (1979) showed that the addition of a resistance element external to the mouth did not affect the limiting flow until its resistance exceeded the internal flow-limiting resistance.

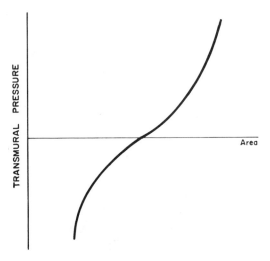

Figure 4.2.22 Tube characteristic of the airways. Actual pressures, areas, and curve shape depend on the specific airway tested.

transmural pressure or cross-sectional area must be known (Figure 4.2.22). Transmural pressure is the sum of elastic pressure (due to lung compliance) and frictional pressure drop along the tube. If these can be determined, then (dp_{tm}/dA) can be determined, A can be determined, and the wave-speed airflow rate can be known. Airflow rate through the tube cannot exceed the wave speed.

Where is flow limited? During inhalation and quiet exhalation it is not. Mead (1978, 1980) offered evidence that the only flow rates which attain a sufficiently high value to be limited occur in the neighborhood of the carina, descending perhaps to the lobar bronchi (generation 2). At very low lung volumes (around residual volume), however, the site of the flow limitation must shift[50] to the extreme lower airways, since the closing volume is taken to be an indication of the health of the lower airways.

Air is a compressible gas, but compression effects may be neglected as long as the rate of airflow does not approach the speed of sound. The Mach number indicates the importance of compression effects:

$$\text{Mc} = v/v_s \tag{4.2.80}$$

where Mc = Mach number, dimensionless
$\quad v$ = air speed, m/sec
$\quad v_s$ = sonic velocity, m/sec

Compression effects become dominant when the Mach number becomes 1.0. Since the speed of sound[51] is about 360 m/sec and mean flow speed in the trachea is about 3.9 m/sec when volume rate of flow is 10^{-3} m³/sec (1 L/sec), Mach number is 0.01, and compressibility is not important (except during breathing maneuvers such as coughs and sneezes).

Description of exhalation resistance in a manner similar to inhalation resistances of Equations 4.2.76 and 4.2.77 is difficult and somewhat arbitrary. Nevertheless, Johnson (1986) reduced airways pressure data of Bouhuys and Jonson (1967) to equation form by starting with

---

[50]This shift can be a rather abrupt one.

[51]$v_s = 14.97 \sqrt{492 + 1.8\theta}$, where θ is air temperature, °C (Baumeister, 1967).

the inhalation formulations given by Equations 4.2.76 and 4.2.77. At low flows and large lung volumes, exhalation isovolume pressure–flow (IVPF) curves are nearly coincident with mirror images of inhalation IVPF curves. Johnson therefore proposed to model exhalation IVPF curves by adding another resistive component to the inhalation IVPF formulations in Equations 4.2.76 and 4.2.77. This model is consistent with physiological evidence attributing the limiting flow rate to a local change in airway dimensions (Mead et al., 1967). It is not consistent with reports of negative effort dependence of limiting flow rate (Suzuki et al., 1982).

The general form for exhalation pressure–flow relations becomes (Johnson and Milano, 1987)

$$p_e = \hat{p}_i + K_4[(1 - \dot{V}_e/\dot{V}_L) - 1] \tag{4.2.81}$$

where p_e = exhalation pressure loss across airway resistance, N/m^2
$\hat{p}_i$ = predicted inhalation pressure loss across airway resistance at the exhalation flow rate, N/m^2
$\dot{V}_e$ = exhalation flow rate (considered to be positive), m^3/sec
$\dot{V}_L$ = limiting flow rate, m^3/sec
K_4 = constant, N/m^2
and

$$\hat{p}_i = K_1 \dot{V}_e + K_2 \dot{V}_e^2 + K_3 \dot{V}_e/(V - RV) \tag{4.2.82}$$

Specific values of the constants K_1, K_2, and K_3 are given in Equations 4.2.76 and 4.2.77.

Limiting flow rate $\dot{V}_L$ is the maximum flow rate that can be expelled from the lungs (Figure 4.2.20). Because expanded lungs hold air passages open wider than contracted lungs, limiting flow rate has been found to depend on lung volume:

$$\dot{V}_L = K_5(V - RV) \tag{4.2.83}$$

where K_5 = constant, sec^{-1}
Johnson (1986) found, for Bouhuys and Jonson (1967) subject 2,

$$p_e = \hat{p}_i + 110[(1 - \dot{V}_e/\dot{V}_L)^{-0.855} - 1] \tag{4.2.84}$$

$$\dot{V}_L = 2.63(V - 0.0013) \tag{4.2.85}$$

and for subject 5,

$$p_e = \hat{p}_i + 1235[(1 - \dot{V}_e/\dot{V}_L)^{-0.16} - 1] \tag{4.2.86}$$

$$\dot{V}_L = 2.38(V - 0.0017) \tag{4.2.87}$$

An additional body mass correction can be applied to resistance values. Since the experiments from which corrective data were obtained came from intubated animals, upper airway resistance is not included in the data. This is a severe limitation, since most resistance at the high flow rates encountered during exercise occurs in the upper airways. Notwithstanding, the relationship between pulmonary resistance (excluding upper airway resistance) and body mass is seen in Figure 4.2.23, and equations are

$$R_{aw} - R_{uaw} = (21.0 \times 10^5)m^{-0.862} \tag{4.2.88a}$$

$$R_p - R_{uaw} = (40.4 \times 10^5)m^{-0.903} \tag{4.2.88b}$$

$$R_r - R_{uaw} = (21.0 \times 10^5)m^{-0.393} \tag{4.2.88c}$$

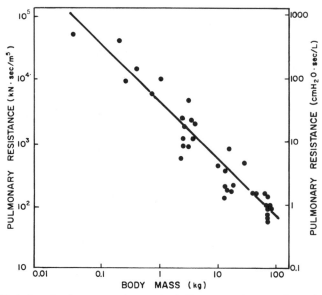

Figure 4.2.23 Variation of pulmonary resistance (excluding upper airway resistance) with body mass. (Adapted and used with permission from Spells, 1969.)

where R_{aw} = airway resistance, N·sec/m^5
  R_{uaw} = upper airway resistance, N·sec/m^5
  R_p = pulmonary resistance, N·sec/m^5
  R_r = respiratory resistance, N·sec/m^5
  m = body mass, kg

A consequence of Bernoulli's equation (4.2.78) is that when flow rate changes for any reason, an equivalent resistance must be inserted into the flow pathway. This is especially true where differential pressure measurements are made such that one side of the pressure measurement is made where there is no flow at all. Specifically, if one side of the pressure measurement is made in the atmosphere, then a resistance term must be inserted between the atmosphere and the point of pressure measurement (such as at the mouth). The value of this resistance is found from kinetic energy changes and is found to be

$$R_{equiv} = \frac{\alpha \gamma \dot{V}}{2gA^2} \tag{4.2.89}$$

where symbols are defined for Equation 4.2.78 and pressure drop caused by this resistance is

$$\Delta p = \frac{\alpha \gamma \dot{V}^2}{2gA^2} \tag{4.2.90}$$

This resistance may be significant for some systems.

Compliance. Compliance is the term that accounts for energy stored in the lungs due to elastic recoil tendencies. All muscular energy that is invested into a pure compliance vessel is returned, and this is used at rest by the respiratory system; exhalation is considered passive, requiring only stored elastic force to propel air from the lungs.

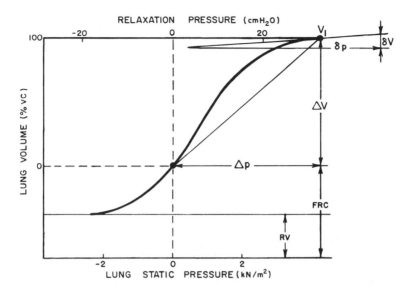

Figure 4.2.24 The volume–pressure curve for lungs plus chest wall in a living subject. Compliance is the ratio of volume to pressure and therefore is the slope of the curve. Static compliance is taken to be the slope of the line drawn from the point of zero pressure and lung volume of FRC to any other point on the curve. Dynamic compliance is the slope of the curve at any point. Static compliance at lung volume V_1 is given by $\Delta V/\Delta p$. Dynamic compliance at the same lung volume is $\delta V/\delta p$.

There are compliances in the airways, lung tissue, and chest wall. Airways compliance is often considered negligible and the other two are considered, in our mechanical models, to be effectively in series.

When both are considered together, as in Figure 4.2.15, respiratory system compliance is found by measuring mouth (or esophageal) pressure at zero flow. Figure 4.2.24 is typical volume–pressure curve for the respiratory system. Pressure measurements are referenced to relaxation pressure, at FRC. At FRC, the compliance, given as the inverse of the slope of the pressure–volume characteristic, is usually assumed to be constant (Mead, 1961). Some authors consider the compliance in the inhalation direction to be a different constant from the compliance in the exhalation direction (Yamashiro et al., 1975). As can be seen, however, the slope of the curve is not constant but depends on lung volume. At the extremes of residual volume and vital capacity, the respiratory system becomes much less compliant and large pressure changes accompany small lung volume changes.

For modeling purposes the pressure–volume curve can be described simply (Johnson, 1984) by

$$VC/V = 1.00 + \exp(b - cp) \tag{4.2.91}$$

where VC = vital capacity, m^3

V = lung volume above the residual volume (RV), m^3

b = coefficient, dimensionless

c = coefficient, m^2/N

p = mouth pressure, N/m^2

Values for the coefficient b have been found to be 1.01 (data from Jacquez, 1979) and 1.66 (data from Yamashiro et al., 1975, subject c). Values for the coefficient c were found to be 1.81×10^{-3} m^2/N and 1.03×10^{-3} m^2/N (from the same references, respectively).

Static compliance is determined during a single exhalation from maximum lung volume by simultaneously measuring lung volume and pressure. Static compliance represents a straight line connecting any desired point on the curve with one at zero pressure (Figure 4.2.24). Thus static compliance is

$$C_{stat} = \left| \frac{V_1 - V_0}{p_1 - 0} \right|$$ (4.2.92)

From Equation 4.2.91,

$$C_{stat} = \frac{V_1 - FRC}{b/c - 1/c \ln \left(\dfrac{VC}{V_1} - 1 \right)}$$ (4.2.93)

Dynamic compliance is determined during breathing by measuring lung volume and pressure whenever airflow is zero (and thus no pressure drop across resistance). This occurs at end-inspiration and end-expiration. Dynamic compliance for quiet breathing represents the slope of a line connecting a point on the curve at zero pressure with a point on the curve at end-inspiration. That is,

$$C_{dyn} = \frac{V_T}{p_1}$$ (4.2.94)

Dynamic compliance can also be considered by bioengineers to be the slope of the curve evaluated at a single point. That is,

$$C_{dyn} = dV/dp_{|p = p_1}$$ (4.2.95)

From the relationship in Equation 4.2.91,

$$C_{dyn} = \frac{VCc \exp (b - cp)}{[1 + \exp (b - cp)]^2}$$ (4.2.96)

Because the slope of the curve in Figure 4.2.24 decreases at the end points, slopes taken over wider central ranges of the curve are generally less than those over narrower ranges. Aside from other physiological conditions, this is an explanation for the general observation that $C_{dyn} < C_{stat}$ (Mead, 1961).

The actual value of compliance depends on a number of factors all relating to the stiffness of the lung and thoracic tissue. These include chest cage muscle tone, amount of blood flow through the lungs, and bronchoconstriction. Pulmonary compliance is sometimes considered to be higher during exhalation than during inhalation. Compliance in normal humans is nearly constant as breathing frequency increases but decreases with frequency in patients with chronic airway obstruction (Mead, 1961).

Lung tissue compliance and chest wall compliance are sometimes measured separately. When this is done, both compliance terms are usually based on lung volume (although chest wall compliance more properly applies to differences in chest wall posture). Lung tissue compliance is defined as

$$C_{lt} = \frac{V}{p_A - p_{pl}}$$ (4.2.97)

where C_{lt} = lung tissue compliance, m^5/N
V = lung volume, m^3
p_A = alveolar pressure, N/m^2
p_{pl} = pleural pressure, N/m^2
and chest wall compliance is

$$C_{cw} = \frac{V}{p_{pl} - p_o} \tag{4.2.98}$$

where C_{cw} = chest wall compliance, m^5/N
p_o = pressure outside the body, N/m^2
Thus, taken together in series, total compliance C is

$$C = \frac{C_{cw} C_{lt}}{C_{cw} + C_{lt}} = \frac{V}{p_A} \tag{4.2.99}$$

Like resistance terms, compliance terms vary with body mass:

$$C_{tot} = (1.50 \times 10^{-5})m \tag{4.2.100}$$

$$C_{lt} = (1.50 \times 10^{-5})m^{1.20} \tag{4.2.101}$$

$$C_{cw} = (4.79 \times 10^{-5})m^{0.898} \tag{4.2.102}$$

where m = body mass, kg
C_{tot} = total lung and chest wall compliance, m^5/N

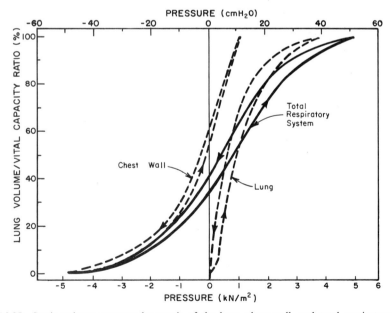

Figure 4.2.25 Static volume–pressure hysteresis of the lung, chest wall, and total respiratory system. Hysteresis is present in all measurements. (Adapted and used with permission from Agostoni and Mead, 1964.)

C_{lt} = lung tissue compliance, m^5/N

C_{cw} = chest wall compliance, m^5/N

Specific compliance, which is defined as compliance divided by FRC, appears to assume a nearly constant value of 0.00082 m^2/N (0.08/cm H$_2$O) for the whole size spectrum of mammals from bat to whale (Mines, 1981).

Figure 4.2.25 shows measurements of lung tissue, chest wall, and total respiratory compliances. Measurements consistently show hysteresis; that is, the curve traced in one direction is not the same as the curve traced in the opposite direction. Lung tissue measurements manifest much more hysteresis than chest wall measurements; this is attributable to changes in alveolar surface tension between expansion and contraction due to the surfactant coating (Section 4.2.1). Hysteresis means that all the work stored in expanding the lungs is not recovered upon contraction. This can be seen by considering work to be

$$W = pV \tag{4.2.103}$$

where W = work, N·m

p = pressure change during the process, N/m^2

V = lung volume change during the process, m^3

Work involved in expansion is the area from the left-hand axis of Figure 4.2.25 to one of the lung expansion curves (the arrow pointing up and to the right). Work involved in the subsequent contraction is the area from the left-hand axis to the contraction curve (arrow pointing down and to the left) corresponding to the expansion curve chosen before. The work involved in contraction is less than that for expansion.

Hysteresis is difficult to include in simple linear models and is therefore usually ignored. Hysteresis is a system nonlinearity which makes the present state of the lung precisely determinable only once its expansion history is known.

Inertance. Very few measurements of respiratory inertance have been made (Mead, 1961). Pressure expended on inertance in the lungs has been estimated to be about 0.5% during quiet breathing and up to 5% during heavy exercise (Mead, 1961). Most inertance is believed to exist in the gas moving through the respiratory system and very little due to lung tissues. Little information is available on chest wall inertance. Since gas, lung tissue, and chest wall inertances are considered to be in series, total inertance is the sum of these. Inertance is usually considered to be small enough to be neglected in respiratory system models. During exercise, however, where breathing waveforms have a relatively high airflow acceleration, inertia may play an important role in limiting the rate at which air can be moved.

The natural frequency of an R-I-C circuit can be given as

$$\omega_n = \sqrt{\frac{1}{IC}\left(1 - \frac{R^2}{4I/C}\right)} \tag{4.2.104}$$

where ω_n = natural frequency, rad/sec

I = inertance, N·sec^2/m^5

C = compliance, m^5/N

R = resistance, N·sec/m^5

The resistance in the circuit dissipates energy and can act to dampen any oscillations that may occur in response to a disturbance. The term $(R/2)\sqrt{C/I}$, called the damping ratio, is usually given the symbol ζ. If the damping ratio is less than 1, the circuit is said to be underdamped, and oscillations can occur. With values of R, I, and C that appear in Table 4.2.15, the damping ratio of the respiratory system is about 4.3, making this system extremely overdamped: oscillations do not spontaneously occur and the gas and tissue of the respiratory system closely follow the respiratory muscles. If the respiratory system were not overdamped, a very disconcerting and uncontrollable flow of air in and out of the mouth would occur when the system was jarred in the slightest way.

The respiratory system is recognized to have a natural frequency, however, but this is recognized only when the inertance and compliance terms disappear from measurements and only resistance remains.

Reactance of a compliance is given by

$$X_c = \frac{1}{j\omega C} \tag{4.2.105}$$

where X_c = reactance of compliance, $N\cdot sec/m^5$
ω = frequency, rad/sec
j = imaginary operator, denoting a phase angle between pressure and flow
Reactance of an inertance is given by

$$X_I = j\omega I \tag{4.2.106}$$

where X_I = reactance of inertance, $N\cdot sec/m^5$
When $X_I = X_L$,

$$\frac{1}{j\omega_n C} = j\omega_n I \tag{4.2.107}$$

and

$$\omega_n = 1/\sqrt{IC} \tag{4.2.108}$$

The frequency ω_n, called the undamped natural frequency, represents the frequency at which oscillations would occur if no damping were present. Natural frequencies of the respiratory systems of normal individuals are in the range 38–50 rad/sec (6–8 cycles/sec). Using a mean value of 45 rad/sec and a pulmonary compliance of $1.22 \times 10^{-6}\,m^5/N$ gives a calculated pulmonary inertance of $405\,N\cdot sec^2/m^5$.

Time Constant. When inertance is ignored, the inverse of the product of resistance times compliance, which has the units of seconds, is called the time constant of the lung:

$$\tau = 1/RC \tag{4.2.109}$$

where τ = time constant, sec
R = resistance, $N\cdot m^5/sec$
C = compliance, m^5/N
Lung time constant determines the time required for filling and emptying the lungs. This is especially seen during passive exhalation, which has an exponential airflow waveshape (Figure 4.3.35a). The time constant of the exhalation is $1/RC$ and has a value of about 0.66 sec (Mead, 1960).

Since dynamic compliance values have been found to be independent of breathing frequency from 0 to 1.5 breaths/sec, Mead (1961) argues that this implies that the time constants for various lung segments must be the same. Dynamic compliance would be independent of frequency only if the volume change in each of the pathways to various parts of the lung remained in fixed proportion to the total volume change of the lungs at all frequencies. If not, the nonlinear pressure–volume characteristic would cause a change in measured compliance. The only way this could be expected to occur is if each lung portion filled at the same rate, thus implying equal time constants. In abnormal patients—those with bronchoconstriction, asthma, and chronic emphysema, where time constants of filling are known to differ in different parts of the lung—dynamic compliance measurements vary with breathing rate. In central regions of the lung, which are expected to have less flow resistance than peripheral regions, the condition of equal time constants requires that central compliance is greater than in peripheral regions (Mead, 1961).

Respiratory Work. The work of the respiratory muscles is composed of two components: the work of breathing and the work of maintaining posture. Although not a great amount of work has been done concerning the latter, it has been stated that a considerable amount of respiratory muscular work is involved in the maintenance of thoracic shape (Grodins and Yamashiro, 1978). For instance, as the diaphragm pulls air into the lungs, the intercostal muscles move the ribs up and out to further increase chest volume. The coordination of this effort requires both positive and negative work (see Section 5.2.5).

The work of breathing can be expressed as

$$W = p_{pl} V = \int p_{pl} \dot{V} dt \qquad (4.2.110)$$

where W = work, N·m

p_{pl} = intrapleural pressure, N/m^2

V = lung volume, m^3

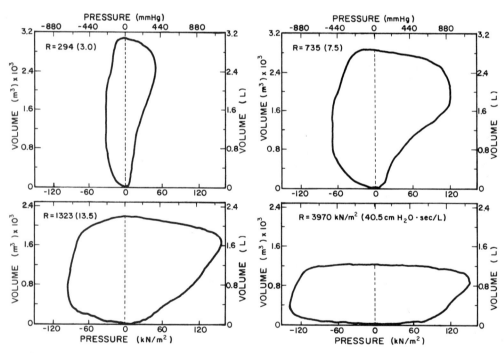

Figure 4.2.26 Pressure–volume loops for maximum breathing effort with four levels of airway resistance. As resistance increases the area enclosed by the loops, and thus the respiratory work, increases. Muscular inefficiencies increase the required respiratory work even more. When resistance is so high that required pressures cannot be generated by the respiratory muscles, respiratory work again decreases. (Adapted and used with permission from Bartlett, 1973.)

$\dot{V}$ = airflow rate, m^3/sec

t = time, sec

This amount of work can be seen as the enclosed area of the loop in Figure 4.2.26.

Since the efficiency of the respiratory muscles (see Section 5.2.5) has been estimated at 7–11% (mean 8.5%) in normal individuals and at 1–3% (mean 1.8%) for emphysemic individuals (Cherniack, 1959), the amount of oxygen consumption that the body spends on respiration can be considerable (Tables 4.2.20 and 4.2.21) during exercise.

The pressure–volume curves of Figure 4.2.26 directly indicate respiratory work for four different breathing resistances. In each of these figures appears a loop. If there were no resistance in the respiratory system, the loops would be very narrow, almost a diagonal line from the upper left-hand corner to the lower right-hand corner of the loop. These narrow loops would correspond to the compliance curves of Figure 4.2.25. With resistance, however, more work must be expended to inhale and less energy is recovered during exhalation. Because the resistive component of pressure requires that negative inspiratory pressures become more negative and positive expiratory pressures become more positive, the loops widen. From Equation 4.2.107 we see that the area enclosed by the loops represents work done by the respiratory system on the air and tissues being moved. It does not represent total physiological work, however, because muscular efficiency is not included.

At low resistance (294 kN·sec/m^5 or 3.00 cm H$_2$O·sec/L) the area under the curve of Figure 4.2.26 is relatively small. For higher resistance of 735 and 1323 kN·sec/m^5 (7.50 and 1.350 cm H$_2$O·sec/L) the volume of air remains nearly the same, but exerted pressures are increased. Mechanical work therefore increases. With a still higher resistance of 3970 kN·sec/m^5 (40.5 cm H$_2$O·sec/L), the respiratory muscular pressure becomes limited and work decreases. All curves are maximum exertion at 0.67 breath/sec, and therefore respiratory volume decreases for the largest resistance (to maintain the same volume, a longer time would have been required, an

TABLE 4.2.20 Oxygen Cost of Breathing as Related to Total Oxygen Cost of Exercise

Total Oxygen Cost of Exercise, cm^3/sec (L/min)	Oxygen Cost of Ventilation, cm^3/sec (mL/min)	Cost of Breathing Compared of Total, %
5.0 (0.30)[a]	0.10 (6)[a]	2.0[a]
19.5 (1.17)	0.40 (24)	2.1
26.7 (1.60)	0.60 (36)	2.25
39.7 (2.38)	0.97 (58)	2.1
89.5 (5.37)	7.17 (430)	8.0

Source: Adapted and used with permission from Bartlett, 1973.

[a] Oxygen cost at rest.

TABLE 4.2.21 Respiratory Dynamics

Flow rates		
Maximum expiratory flow rate	6700 cm^3/sec	(402 L/min)
Maximum inspiratory flow rate	5000 cm^3/sec	(300 L/min)
Maximum minute ventilation	2000 cm^3/sec	(120 L/min)
Pressures		
Maximum inspiratory pressure	4400 N/m^2	(45 cm H$_2$O)
Maximum expiratory pressure	6900 N/m^2	(70 cm H$_2$O)
Maximum respiratory power	80 N·m/sec	(820 cm H$_2$O·L/sec)

effect which is seen during spontaneous breathing). It can be seen that there is a maximum work output which occurs at the intermediate resistance values.

The oxygen cost of breathing through these resistances was found to be relatively constant across the range of breathing resistances (Bartlett, 1973). Since the caloric equivalent of oxygen remains nearly constant at about $0.0202 \, N \cdot m/cm^3$, respiratory efficiency is highest where the mechanical work is highest.

4.3   CONTROL OF RESPIRATION

Regulation of respiration means different things to different people. To some, it means the way in which the periodic breathing pattern is generated and controlled; to others, respiratory regulation means the control of ventilation, and the reciprocating nature of airflow could just as well be considered to be continuous flow; to yet others, respiratory regulation deals with optimization and the means with which various respiratory parameters are determined.

In a sense, this multiplicity of views has hindered development of comprehensive respiratory models. In surveying the recent literature, it can be said (although it is difficult to substantiate) that more information is known about the respiratory system than about any of the other systems dealt with in this book. Yet less is known about how pieces of this information relate to each other. The difficulty to be encountered, then, is one of integration and synthesis.

The nature of respiratory control causes this to be a very complex topic. Unlike cardiovascular control, the basic act of breathing is not initiated within the respiratory muscles; therefore, external inputs cannot be considered to be modifying influences only. Unlike the thermoregulatory system, the details of the process of respiration are considered to be important, and the amount of pertinent information therefore cannot be reduced to a relatively few coarse measurements. Thus on the one hand much is known about regulation of respiration, but on the other hand not enough is known to serve as the basis for comprehensive models.

In this chapter, as well as the chapters on other physiological systems, we deal with sensors, controller, and effector organs. However, as will be seen, the respiratory system sometimes acts as

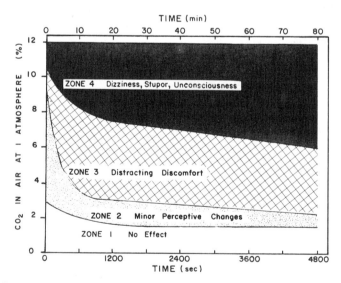

Figure 4.3.1 Symptoms common to most subjects exposed for various times to carbon dioxide–air mixtures at 1 atm pressure. Acute changes are more profound than chronic changes. (Adapted and used with permission from Billings, 1963.)

if there are sensors which have not yet been found to exist, control is not localized to one particular region, and the effector organs are many.

It has been seen in Chapter 3 that cardiovascular control appears to be directed toward maintenance of adequate flow first to the brain and then to other parts of the body. Likewise, it will be seen in Chapter 5 that thermoregulation appears to regulate first the temperature of brain structures and then the remainder of the body. In a similar fashion, respiratory control appears to be coordinated such that an adequate chemical milieu is provided to the brain and other structures are subordinate to that goal. Because chemical supply to the brain comes through the blood, cardiovascular and respiratory control are often entwined, with complementary or interactive responses occurring in both systems.

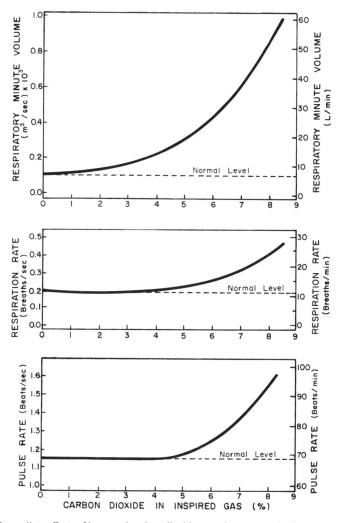

Figure 4.3.2   Immediate effects of increased carbon dioxide on pulse rate, respiration rate, and respiratory minute volume for subjects at rest. Percent carbon dioxide is converted to partial pressure by multiplying by total atmospheric pressure: $101 \, kN/m^2$ or 760 mm Hg. (Adapted and used with permission from Billings, 1973.)

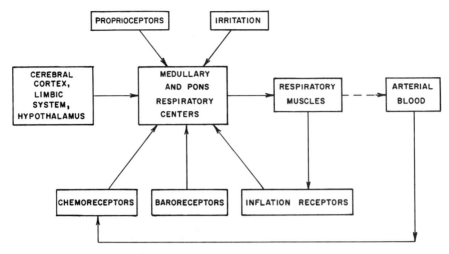

Figure 4.3.3   General scheme of respiratory control.

If a single controlled variable had to be identified for the respiratory controller, it would have to be pH of the fluid bathing areas of the lower brain. This relates directly to the carbon dioxide partial pressure of the blood. A very small excess of carbon dioxide in inhaled air produces severe psychophysiological reactions (Figure 4.3.1), and respiratory responses to inhaled carbon dioxide are profound (Figure 4.3.2). Surprisingly, lack of oxygen does not evoke strong responses at all, leading one to believe that in the environment where respiratory control evolved, oxygen was almost always in plentiful supply and carbon dioxide was not; the threat to survival came from carbon dioxide excess and not from oxygen lack. The controlling process is considered in detail in the remainder of this section.

Dejours (1963) notes that "when a subject starts easy dynamic exercise, ventilation increases immediately; then, during the next 20–30 seconds following the onset of exercise, ventilation remains constant. After this lag, it increases progressively and eventually, if the exercise is not too intense, reaches a steady state." He termed the initial, fast ventilatory increase as the neural component, and the second, slower increase as the humoral, or chemical, component. There is wide agreement today that both neural and humoral components contribute to respiratory control; there is no such agreement about the relative speed of each (Whipp, 1981), and it may be that both neural and humoral components act both fast and slowly.

Figure 4.3.3 shows the general scheme for respiratory control. The system is highly complex, with each block of the diagram corresponding to several major sites. The location and function of each of these are discussed in succeeding sections.

4.3.1   Respiratory Receptors

As seen in Figure 4.3.3, there is a host of receptor types which have been identified as having importance to respiration. Since respiration is a complex function, with ventilatory control superimposed on the basic respiratory rhythm, each group of sensors is required to properly regulate the respiratory system. We deal with these receptors in two groups: sensors functioning in chemical control and sensors relaying mechanical information.

Chemoreceptors. It is generally believed that chemoreceptors important to respiratory control exist peripherally in the aortic arch and carotid bodies and centrally in the ventral medulla

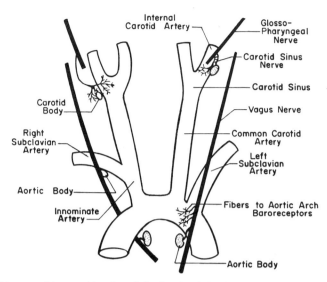

Figure 4.3.4 Diagram of the carotid and aortic bodies. Aortic bodies are located in the chest near the heart and carotid bodies are located in the neck. (Used with permission from Ganong, 1963.)

oblongata of the brain (Bledsoe and Hornbein, 1981). These receptors appear to be sensitive to partial pressures of CO_2 and O_2 and to pH.

Some peripheral chemoreceptors have been localized to the carotid bodies (Hornbein, 1966; McDonald, 1981), tiny and very vascular nodules located in the neck near the ascending common carotid arteries (Figure 4.3.4). On an equal mass basis, blood flow in the carotid body is about 40 times greater than through the brain and 5 times greater than through the kidney (Ganong, 1963),[52] and thus these bodies are very sensitive to sudden changes in blood composition. Information from glomus cells within the carotid bodies is transmitted to the brain through the glossopharyngeal nerve (Hornbein, 1966).

Carotid bodies appear to be sensitive to changes in arterial pO_2,[53] pCO_2, and pH. Figure 4.3.5 and 4.3.6 show neural responses[54] of the carotid sinus nerve of the cat for varying arterial oxygen and carbon dioxide partial pressures. Carotid bodies are much more sensitive to changes in pO_2 than to changes in pCO_2.

It is not entirely clear that the carotid body response to pCO_2 is independent of pH response or that both responses are manifestations of the same effect (Biscoe and Willshaw, 1981). Hornbein (1966) asserts that steady-state responses to CO_2 are entirely due to pH (Figures 4.3.7–4.3.9). Increased pCO_2 evokes a prompter response than a change in acidity, probably because CO_2 diffuses more readily into the chemoreceptor cells to produce a more rapid fall in pH. Combined hypoxia (below normal pO_2) and hypercapnia (above normal pCO_2) produce an interaction which is greater (Figure 4.3.7) than the added effects of both taken singly (Hornbein, 1966).

[52]Each carotid body has a mass of 2 mg and receives a blood flow of 0.33 cm^3/g of tissue per second; the brain averages 0.009 cm^3/g·sec blood flow (Ganong, 1963).

[53]The blood flow through the carotid body is so great that oxygen demands are met by dissolved oxygen only. The carotid bodies do not seem to be sensitive to oxygen bound to hemoglobin except as it affects pO_2. Thus hemoglobin abnormalities produce no exceptional response (Ganong, 1963).

[54]These neural responses are averages taken over a relatively long time. There is actually a good deal of irregularity in single unit discharges, which seems to follow a Poisson probability distribution. The probability of the occurrence of an action potential is never zero, meaning that there is no threshold level of chemical input below which the fiber cannot respond (Biscoe and Willshaw, 1981).

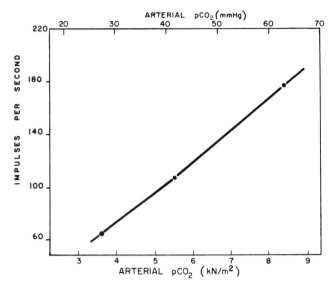

Figure 4.3.5 Changes in neural output from the carotid sinus nerve of the cat when arterial carbon dioxide partial pressure is changed. The relation between carbon dioxide partial pressure and nervous discharge is linear. Normal changes in carbon dioxide are very small and normal values are about $5.2\,kN/m^2$ (40 mm Hg) in man. (Adapted and used with permission from Lambertsen, 1961. Modified from Bartels and Witzleb, 1956.)

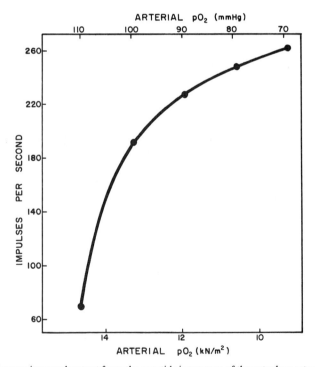

Figure 4.3.6 Changes in neural output from the carotid sinus nerve of the cat when arterial oxygen partial pressure is changed. The relationship is decidedly nonlinear, with maximum sensitivity at high oxygen partial pressures. Normal values are $13.3\,kN/m^2$ (100 mm Hg) in man. (Adapted and used with permission from Lambertsen, 1961. Modified from Witzleb et al. 1955.)

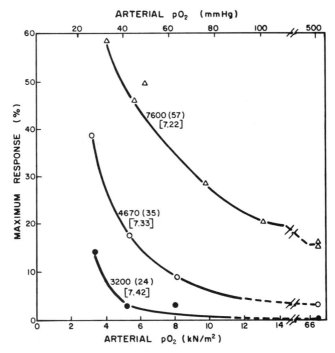

Figure 4.3.7   Average neural discharge from the carotid body of the cat in response to changes of arterial oxygen partial pressure. Each curve was elicited with a carbon dioxide partial pressure given in N/m^2 (mm Hg) and [pH] units. Carbon dioxide was varied by altering ventilation. The presence of these different curves indicates interaction between oxygen and carbon dioxide sensitivity. (Adapted and used with permission from Hornbein and Roos, 1963.)

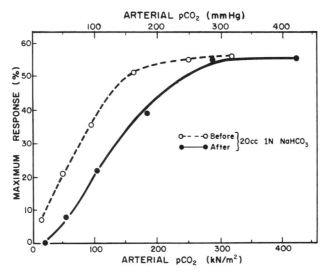

Figure 4.3.8   Average neural discharge from the cat's carotid body responding to step increases in inspired carbon dioxide. The nearly linear portion of the curve compares to that in Figure 4.3.5. Addition of sodium bicarbonate to change blood pH alters the carbon dioxide response. (Adapted and used with permission from Hornbein and Roos, 1963.)

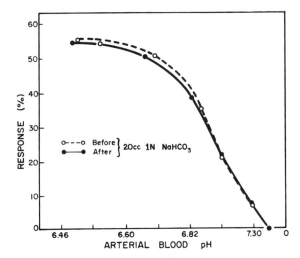

Figure 4.3.9 Average neural discharge from the cat's carotid body responding to step increases in inspired carbon dioxide. Sodium bicarbonate was added to change blood pH. When neural discharge is plotted against blood pH, sodium bicarbonate does not have the effect seen in Figure 4.3.8. (Used with permission from Hornbein and Roos, 1963.)

Carotid chemoreceptors have very rapid response. They can follow tidal changes in arterial blood gas tensions (Biscoe and Willshaw, 1981) which occur during each breath (see Section 4.2.2). Whether or not there is an output frequency component related to the rate of change of pCO_2 and pH is still open to question (Biscoe and Willshaw, 1981), although many other somatic receptors do exhibit transient components (see Sections 3.3.1 and 5.3.1) and it would be somewhat surprising if the carotid bodies were not similar.

There are neural and chemical means to alter the output of the carotid body. Catecholamines injected into the arterial supply of the carotid body of cats cause transient depression of chemoreceptor output (Biscoe and Willshaw, 1981); carotid sinus nerve excitation can cause depression of chemoreceptor activity; and excitation of the sympathetic nerve supply to the carotid body causes an increase in chemoreceptor output (Biscoe and Willshaw, 1981).[55]

The other major peripheral chemosensitive area is in the region of the aortic arch. Because of their anatomical location, the aortic bodies have not been studied in as much detail as the carotid bodies. They are assumed to respond similarly to carotid bodies.

Other peripheral receptors play a minor role in respiratory regulation. Among these are chemoreceptors in the coronary and pulmonary vessels (Ganong, 1963). There is also a great deal of interaction between cardiovascular sensors and responses and pulmonary sensors and responses.

There is located within 0.5 mm of the ventral surface of the medulla oblongata (at the junction of spinal cord and brain) a central chemoreceptive site (Bledsoe and Hornbein, 1981; Ganong, 1963; Hornbein, 1966). This site does not appear to be sensitive to anoxia and may have limited sensitivity to carbon dioxide. By far its greatest, and perhaps its only practical sensitivity is to pH, or hydrogen ion concentration in the brain extracellular fluid (Bledsoe and Hornbein, 1981).

An indirectness occurs here, however. There are epithelial layers between the blood and cerebrospinal fluid which are poorly permeable to most polar solutes (ions), and which have specialized transport systems to facilitate carriage of glucose, lactate, and amino acids (Bledsoe and Hornbein, 1981). These are called the "blood–brain barrier" and appear to serve as

---

[55]This could be at least part of the link among psychological state, exercise, and respiration.

protection for the brain against harmful substances or changes which occur in the blood. Hydrogen ions do not easily cross the blood–brain barrier.

Carbon dioxide, probably in hydrated form, can easily move across this barrier, and, by means of the buffer equation (3.2.3),

$$H_2O + CO_2 \Leftrightarrow H_2CO_3 \Leftrightarrow H^+ + HCO_3^- \tag{3.2.3}$$

change the hydrogen ion concentration of cerebrospinal fluid. Furthermore, there appears to be some active buffering of bicarbonate (HCO_3^-) levels by brain cells to minimize HCO_3^- concentration differences in the brain extracellular fluid (Bledsoe and Hornbein, 1981).[56]

These mechanisms seem to indicate that the composition of the fluid bathing the brain cells is controlled to a high degree but can lead to some interesting, and somewhat paradoxical, results. For instance, pH shifts in the cerebrospinal fluid must always be slower than $p\mathrm{CO}_2$ and pH shifts in the blood. Such shifts will likely be much smaller in cerebrospinal fluid than in blood. Also, metabolic acidosis, occurring naturally during exercise above the anaerobic threshold, stimulates ventilation (presumably from peripheral chemoreceptor excitation), thereby lowering

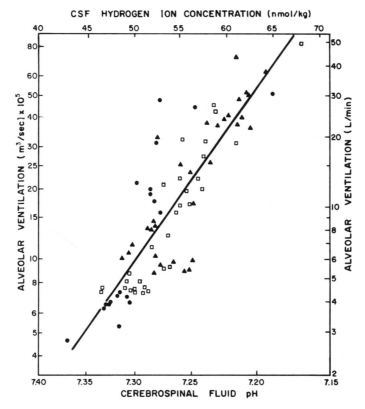

Figure 4.3.10 Alveolar ventilation in awake goats as a function of cerebrospinal fluid hydrogen ion concentration. Arterial bicarbonate levels seem to have little effect on the basic linear relationship. (Adapted and used with permission from Fencl et al., 1966.)

[56]The distinction between brain extracellular fluid and cerebrospinal fluid is that the former is more local than the latter, and concentrations which cannot be maintained in the bulk fluid can be maintained locally.

arterial pCO_2. When pCO_2 is lowered, Equation 3.2.3 indicates that H^+ concentration will be lowered. Thus the blood will be observed to be acidic and the cerebrospinal fluid alkaline (Hornbein, 1966).

Measurements of alveolar ventilation were made on conscious goats while cerebrospinal fluid composition was monitored during various metabolic states (Jacquez, 1979). The results appear in Figure 4.3.10 and the relation between these variables can be described as

$$\log \dot{V}_A = 48.1 - 7.14 \, pH \qquad (4.3.1)$$

where $\dot{V}_A$ = alveolar ventilation rate, m^3/sec
   pH = acidity, pH units (dimensionless)
Notice the amount of scatter in the data and the very small change in pH which produces a large change in alveolar ventilation.[57]

Mechanoreceptors. Mechanoreceptors produce inputs which are responsible for nonchemial respiratory regulation. Such things as the basic rhythmic respiratory oscillation, initial respiratory stimulation at the onset of exercise, removal of irritants in the respiratory pathway, and control of airway caliber are influenced by these receptors.

Active and passive movement of the limbs stimulates respiration (Celli, 1988; Ganong, 1963; Jammes et al., 1984.[58] Proprioceptor afferent pathways from muscles, tendons, and joints to the brain normally function to inform the brain of the positions and conditions of bodily members (Duron, 1981). These proprioceptors appear to exert an influence on the increase of ventilation during exercise.

A host of different mechanoreceptors are located throughout the respiratory tract (Widdicombe, 1981, 1982). Nasal receptors are important in sneezing, apnea,[59] bronchodilation/bronchoconstriction, secretion of mucus, and the diving reflex (see footnote 79, Section 3.3.1). Laryngeal receptors appear to be important in coughing, apnea, swallowing, bronchoconstriction, airway mucus secretion, and laryngeal constriction. Tracheobronchial receptors are important in coughing, pulmonary hypertension, bronchoconstriction, laryngeal constriction, and production of mucus. Information about each of these receptor types is abundant but incomplete. There is no clear distinction between these receptors and those serving other functions, such as smell. The overall function of these receptors appears to be respiratory system support, including protection from irritants, but does not appear to be involved with control of respiratory rhythm or ventilation (Widdicombe, 1981).

There is a class of mechanoreceptors which seems to be somewhat important in the generation of the respiratory rhythmic pattern. Some are present in the tracheobronchial tree and some within the respiratory muscles (Duron, 1981; Widdicombe, 1981; Young, 1966). Some of these receptors increase their output discharge frequencies with increasing lung and chest inflation; others increase their outputs when the lung or chest is underinflated. Slowly adapting receptors fire with relatively slight degrees of lung distension, whereas rapidly adapting receptors respond only to rapid and forcible lung distension. The outputs of both types eventually decrease to zero with no further change in lung distension. The sensitivity of these receptors is enhanced by a decrease in lung compliance (Widdicombe, 1981). These receptors are joined to the brain via the vagus nerve.

---

[57]The reader should be cautioned that whereas the form of Equation 4.3.1 may be correct for other species, the actual predicted values are not to be construed as applicable to humans. pH values for human cerebrospinal fluid is normally 7.4, with a range of 7.35–7.70 (Spector, 1956). These values do not appear on the abscissa of Figure 4.3.10.

[58]Presumably, this mechanism could be used in conjunction with cardiopulmonary resuscitation to stimulate breathing. It has been used to help revive animals overdosed with anesthesia.

[59]*Apnea* is the term used for lack of breathing; *hypernea* means the deeper and more rapid breathing during exercise; *eupnea* is easy, normal respiration at rest; *dyspnea* is stressful breathing; *tachypnea* is rapid breathing; and *bradypnea* is abnormally slow respiration.

Baroreceptors (actually stretch receptors) in the carotid sinuses, aortic arch, and heart atria and ventricles influence the respiratory system as well as the cardiovascular system (see Section 3.3.1). This influence, increasing vascular pressure leading to inhibition of respiration, is very slight, however (Ganong, 1963).

Other Inputs. There are excitatory and inhibitory afferent[60] nerve fibers from the neocortex to the respiratory controller, since breathing can become voluntarily controlled (although respiration is more difficult to control voluntarily during exercise). Pain and emotional stimuli affect respiration, presumably through a pathway from the hypothalamic area in the brain (see Section 5.3.2).

4.3.2 Respiratory Controller

The respiratory controller must integrate many inputs from many outputs. That is, respiratory control is very complex because it must first form the basic pattern of respiration and then regulate it to respond appropriately to varying mechanical and chemical conditions.

Respiratory Rhythm. Generation of the basic respiratory rhythm has been generally accepted to occur in the brainstem in the region of the pons and medulla (Mines, 1981; Young, 1966). Most published works mention three centers: (1) the respiratory center (composed of both inspiratory and expiratory centers), located bilaterally in the medulla, which generates the basic respiratory oscillation; (2) the apneustic center,[61] located caudally in the pons, which supports an inspiratory drive; and (3) the pneumotaxic center, located in the pons, which inhibits the respiratory center and supports expiration (Ganong, 1963; Mines, 1981). There is a good deal of uncertainty concerning the locations and functions of these centers (Mitchell and Berger, 1981), and much has been written concerning and interrelating experimental evidence.

Even the site of the generation of the basic respiratory rhythm is no longer clear. There is new evidence that periodic nervous discharges can occur as low in the central nervous system as the spinal cord, and how many of the three aforementioned centers are required to maintain breathing is not well defined (Mitchell and Berger, 1981). It is possible that this oscillatory discharge could come from pacemaker cells, similar to those in the heart, or from nonlinearly acting, mutually inhibiting neural arrangements similar to electronic circuits.

Also unclear is the site and mechanism of controller implications of P_{CO_2} effects, either directly on the central chemosensitive area or indirectly through the carotid bodies. Although it is known that the glossopharyngeal nerve (the 9th cranial nerve) joins the brain in the area of the medulla, pathways have not been established to ascertain exactly how afferent impulses affect the respiratory drive.

With such a control system, diffused and detailed yet not conceptually assembled, we must be somewhat more schematic rather than specific in our description. Refer, then, to Figure 4.3.11 for a functional schematic of the respiratory system controller.

In this schematic, based on evidence and concepts presented by Mitchell and Berger (1981), all known influences are not included. And, as previously mentioned, not enough is known about some of the interconnections to be completely sure of all the details shown. However, the essential actions are these: a central pattern generator, probably located in the upper spinal cord, produces a series of repeating clusters of neural discharge, which is the basic respiratory rhythm. By itself, the central pattern generator would produce a gasping type of irregular breathing (severe apneusis). The central nervous pattern is modified by two groups of respiratory neurons located in the medulla (together they are equivalent to the medullary respiratory center). The dorsal group mainly controls the inspiratory muscles, whereas the ventral respiratory group

---

[60]*Afferent* refers to input, *efferent* to output.

[61]*Apneusis* is an abnormal form of respiration consisting of prolonged inspirations alternating with short expirations.

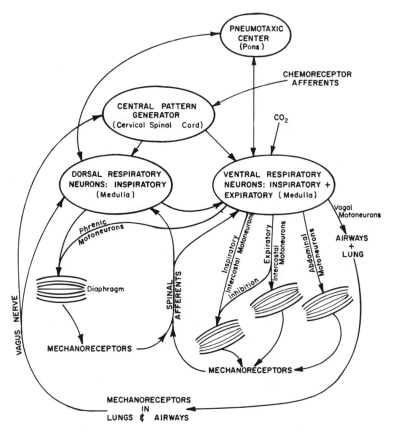

Figure 4.3.11 Functional schematic of the more outstanding elements of the respiratory controller.

regulates both inspiratory and expiratory muscles. Both neural groups are influenced by the pneumotaxic center in the pons. The pneumotaxic center primarily inhibits output from the inspiratory center and acts to shape inspiration into a smooth, coordinated action. Output from the dorsal inspiratory center, through phrenic motoneurons, controls diaphragmatic movement. Output from the ventral group controls the intercostal and abdominal muscles, and, through vagal motoneurons, airway muscle tone and lung actions. Feedback from mechanoreceptor inputs is provided from the muscles by means of spinal nerve afferent fibers and from the lungs and airways by means of vagal afferent fibers. Carbon dioxide (or brain extracellular fluid pH) has a close and almost direct effect on the respiratory center, and chemoreceptor glossopharyngeal nerve afferents affect the generated pattern.

Airflow Waveshape. Breathing waveform, durations of inspiration and expiration, and end-expiratory volume (ERV; see Section 4.2.2) are all controlled as primary variables by the respiratory controller. Air flows into the lungs whenever

$$p_{\text{mus}(i)} - p_{\text{mus}(e)} - p_{\text{el}} > 0 \tag{4.3.2}$$

where $p_{\text{mus}(i)}$ = lung pressure developed by inspiratory muscles, N/m^2
  $p_{\text{mus}(e)}$ = lung pressure developed by expiratory muscles, N/m^2
    p_{el} = pressure of elastic recoil of the respiratory system, N/m^2

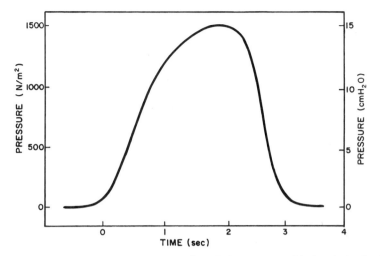

Figure 4.3.12   Typical shape of respiratory muscle occlusion pressure with time during inspiration.

At FRC, $p_{el} = 0$; during quiet breathing, inspiratory and expiratory muscles will not be simultaneously contracting, and therefore $p_{mus(e)} = 0$; inspiration will thus occur whenever $p_{mus(i)} > 0$. The shape with time of $p_{mus(i)}$ can be approximately obtained by measuring pressure in the respiratory system during occlusion (i.e., when no air is flowing).[62] This shape during quiet breathing is characterized by a finite rate of rise, a rounded peak, and rapid fall (Figure 4.3.12). The shape appears to be relatively constant from cycle to cycle in one individual in any particular state but varies considerably between individuals and between different conditions for one individual (Younes and Remmers, 1981). This shape is largely due to diaphragmatic activity in response to phrenic nervous discharge: the greater the rate of discharge, the greater the muscular force. The relation between inspiratory muscular pressure $p_{mus(i)}$ and neural output is not linear or constant, however, and will depend on other factors to be discussed in Section 4.3.3.

Hypercapnia increases the rate of rise of $p_{mus(i)}$ with time without changing its shape (Younes and Remmers, 1981). If there is a plateau in $p_{mus(i)}$, it also rises. Body temperature changes affect the rate of rise without changing the level of the plateau. Hypoxia and limb movements, both active and passive, increase the rate of rise, but anesthetics and narcotics depress the rate of rise (Younes and Remmers, 1981). Vagal volume feedback has been reported to have little effect on inspiratory output prior to inspiratory termination (Younes and Remmers, 1981).

Awake humans under steady-state conditions display substantial interbreath variation in tidal volume, which is due mainly to inspiratory duration variability. Mean inspiratory flow rates are also scattered, presumably from interbreath variation in the rate of rise of neural output.[63]

Younes and Remmers (1981) present equations relating the volume–time profiles of the lungs to neural output. Inspiratory flow rate can be computed from

$$\dot{V}_i = \frac{\eta N_i - v(V - V_r) - (V - V_r)/C - p_{mus(e)}}{\phi R} \tag{4.3.3}$$

---

[62]With no airflow, mouth pressure is assumed to equal alveolar pressure.

[63]It is interesting to speculate about a connection between the irregular carotid body afferent discharge and the irregular phrenic nerve efferent discharge. If the second is a direct result of the first, it could be a "dithering," or slight variation, about the mean control point, resulting in faster response and relying on sufficient inertia by the body CO_2 stores to absorb small CO_2 variations.

where $\dot{V}_i$ = inspiratory flow rate, m^3/sec

$\quad N_i$ = neural output, neural pulses

$\quad (V - V_r)$ = lung volume above resting volume, m^3

$\quad p_{mus(e)}$ = pressure generated by expiratory muscles, N/m^2

$\quad C$ = respiratory compliance, m^5/N

$\quad R$ = respiratory resistance, $N \cdot sec/m^5$

$\quad \eta$ = conversion of neural output to muscle isometric pressure at FRC, N/m^2/neural pulses

$\quad v$ = muscle force–length and geometric effects, N/m^5

$\quad \phi$ = muscle force–velocity effect, $N \cdot sec/m^5$

If $v(V - V_r) > \eta N_i$, then the muscle cannot generate an inspiratory pressure because of its mechanical disadvantage. In this case, which occurs in the early part of inspiration when lung volume is above the resting volume V_r, flow is still in the exhalation direction, and

$$\dot{V}_e = \frac{V - V_r}{RC} \tag{4.3.4a}$$

where $\dot{V}_e$ = expiratory flow rate, m^3/sec

If $[v(V - V_r) + (V - V_r)/C + p_{mus(e)}] > \eta N_i$, flow is also in the exhalation direction. This situation is encountered when $V > V_r$ and ηN_i has not become sufficiently strong to overcome elastic recoil:

$$\dot{V}_e = \frac{\eta N_i - v(V - V_r) - (V - V_r)/C}{R} \tag{4.3.4b}$$

If $(V - V_r)/C < 0$, then inspiratory flow is both passive and active. Flow is calculated in two steps, with passive flow calculated from

$$\dot{V}_{i\,passive} = \frac{-[(V - V_r)/C + p_{mus(e)}]}{R} \tag{4.3.4c}$$

and active flow from

$$\dot{V}_{i\,active} = \frac{\eta N_i - v(V - V_r) - \phi \dot{V}_{i\,passive}}{\phi + R} \tag{4.2.4d}$$

and

$$\dot{V}_i = \dot{V}_{i\,passive} \qquad \text{if } \dot{V}_{i\,active} < 0 \tag{4.3.4e}$$

$$\dot{V}_i = \dot{V}_{i\,passive} + \dot{V}_{i\,active} \qquad \text{if } \dot{V}_{i\,active} > 0 \tag{4.3.4f}$$

Volume is obtained by integrating flow rate.

Coefficient values were obtained from the literature: ηN_i was chosen to give a peak isometric pressure of $1470 \, N/m^2$ ($15.0 \, cm \, H_2O$) with a neural input of 15.0 arbitrary units ($\eta = 98.03 \, N/m^2$/arbitrary unit). Compliance C was taken to be $1.3 \times 10^{-6} \, m^5/N$ ($0.13 \, L/cm \, H_2O$) and two values of resistance R used were $196 \, kN \cdot sec/m^5$ ($2.0 \, cm \, H_2O \cdot sec/L$) and $588 \, kN \cdot sec/m^5$. The muscle length–tension effects represent the difference between passive elastance[64] and effective elastance obtained in normal human subjects during electrophrenic stimulation. The

---

[64]Elastance is the inverse of compliance.

value for v thus becomes 5.4×10^5 N/m^5 (5.4 cm H$_2$O/L). Although taken to be a constant, the actual value of v probably varies with level of inspiratory activity (Younes and Remmers, 1981). The value for muscle force–velocity effect ϕ is taken from human subject data at a lung volume close to FRC. Its value is 573 kN·sec/m^5 (5.85 cm H$_2$O·sec/L), and, again, it would probably be more correct not assumed constant.

Younes and Remmers (1981) report that inspiration, as determined by flow rate, is different from inspiration from a neural standpoint. Inspiratory flow rate is delayed from the onset of neural output if beginning lung volume is above resting lung volume: expiration continues until the neural output overcomes opposite elastic tendencies. If beginning lung volume is below resting lung volume, then inspiratory flow may precede neural output. The amount of delay or anticipation depends on the rate of rise of the neural output as well as resistance and compliance of the respiratory system.

The end of inspiratory flow is always delayed beyond the peak of neural output. The extent of delay depends on rate of decline of neural output and respiratory resistance and compliance (Younes and Remmers, 1981). Changes in the shape with time of the neural output can overcome large increases in respiratory resistance and compliance.

Inspiratory duration appears to be determined by the respiratory controller. Although the exact mechanism of inhalation time control is unknown, it appears that inhalation can be ended abruptly in a manner similar to a switch (Younes and Remmers, 1981). This switch appears to have a variable threshold to such input factors as lung volume, chest wall motion, blood gases, muscular exercise, body temperature, sleep, disease, and drugs. Figure 4.3.13 shows that the

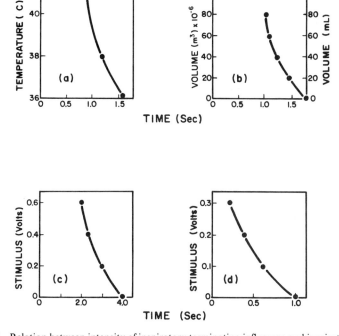

Figure 4.3.13 Relation between intensity of inspiratory terminating influences and inspiratory duration in the cat. As each stimulus (clockwise from upper right: lung volume, electrical stimulus to the rostral pons, electrical stimulus to the intercostal nerves, and body temperature) increases in magnitude, inspiratory time shortens. Conversely, as inspiratory time accumulates, a lower stimulus is necessary to halt inspiration. No lung volume feedback was present for voltage and temperature stimuli. (Adapted and used with permission from Younes and Remmers, 1981.)

threshold to terminate inspiration decreases with inspiratory time. For instance, the longer inspiration progresses, the smaller the lung volume must be in order to conclude inspiration. Sustained lung volume changes have little or no effect (Younes and Remmers, 1981).

Similarly, electrical stimuli to intercostal nerves will shorten inspiration with a time-varying threshold. It would be expected that this effect would be analogous to the effect produced by intercostal muscle mechanoreceptors operating naturally within a feedback loop. It has been reported that airway occlusion, chest wall distortion, and vibration all cause shortening of inspiration (Younes and Remmers, 1981).

Stimulation of the rostral pons area (in the region of the pneumotaxic center) of the brain can decrease inspiratory duration, as can body temperature. Hypercapnia decreases inspiratory duration, and at least part of this may be due to increased participation of chest wall reflexes as the result of more vigorous inspiration. Many of the preceding factors seem to interact to reduce inspiration discontinuance threshold below the level that would exist if several factors were not present (Younes and Remmers, 1981).

This effect of body temperature on inspiratory time is clearly of importance to an animal that pants when overheated, like a cat. Although humans are not known to rely on this same heat loss mechanism, an effect such as this would give rise to a respiratory–thermal exercise limitation interaction as discussed in Section 1.5.

Control of expiratory time is somewhat different from that of inspiratory time. Unlike inspiration, which is always actively initiated by muscular action, exhalation is considered to be passive at rest and active during exercise. Control of expiration appears to differ, therefore, in the dependence of expiratory duration on the previous inspiratory time, and in the active control of expiratory flow by respiratory resistance regulation (Martin et al., 1982; Younes and Remmers, 1981).

The transition from exhalation to inhalation also exhibits switching behavior with variable threshold (Figure 4.3.14).[65] The switch characteristic can be determined by stimulus of the rostral pons area (nucleus parabrachialis medialis) and by chemical stimulation of the carotid bodies. Subthreshold stimuli cause a translocation of the stimulus–time characteristic toward the left (Younes and Remmers, 1981). Because of this, repetitive subthreshold stimuli can have a cumulative effect and change the overall shape of the stimulus–time switching characteristic. Hence static lung volume changes (as stimuli) do affect the exhalation switching characteristic (Figure 4.3.15), unlike the inhalation switch where static lung volume did not affect inhalation time (Younes and Remmers, 1981).

Exhalation time is essentially linked to the preceding inhalation time (Grunstein et al., 1973; Younes and Remmers, 1981). Evidence shows a central neural linkage between these two times, which probably acts through the central expiratory excitation threshold illustrated in Figure 4.3.14.

Since expiratory time and lung volume are interrelated, it should not be surprising to note that expiratory reserve volume (ERV; see Section 4.2.2) also appears to be under respiratory control. An increase in exhalation time would be expected to increase ERV because of the curve in Figure 4.3.15. Changes in ERV are minimized by active resistance changes, to be discussed later, but decreases in ERV have been reported in humans with hypercapnia (Younes and Remmers, 1981).

Evidence from cats indicates that an important expiratory flow rate–regulating mechanism, called expiratory braking, is due to contraction of the inspiratory musculature during exhalation and due to active regulation of upper airway resistance (Younes and Remmers, 1981). The role of each of these in humans is not clear, but it is likely that expiratory braking does occur,[66] probably by inspiratory muscular action. Vagal discharge to upper airway muscles causes changes in glottal opening. Rapid changes in resistance, as through opening and closing of a tracheostomy

---

[65]Although this evidence was obtained from resting animals, there is no reason to believe it is not true during exercise.
[66]For instance, there appears to be an optimal resistance to exhalation in humans, and switching from nose breathing at rest to mouth breathing during exercise occurs when nasal resistance exceeds mouth resistance.

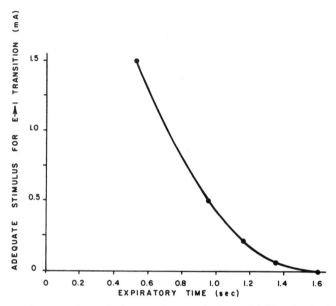

Figure 4.3.14 Stimulus strength required to terminate expiration and initiate inspiration as related to expiratory time. The stimulus was current applied to the rostral pons area of the brain. As current increases, expiratory time shortens. (Used with permission from Younes and Remmers, 1981.)

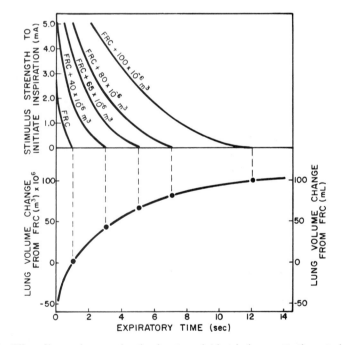

Figure 4.3.15 Effect of lung volume on the stimulus strength (electrical current to the rostral pons) required to terminate expiration and initiate inspiration. As lung volume increases, so does expiratory time (lower plot). A series of splayed curves of the type found in Figure 4.3.14 (upper plot) will result in exhalation time varying with lung volume. Thus stimulus strength must also be influenced by lung volume. For higher volumes a larger amount of current is required to terminate exhalation at any specific time. (Adapted and used with permission from Younes and Remmers, 1981.)

tube, result in rapid and continuous changes in generated muscle pressure. Expiratory flow rate thus appears to have a regulated level. Hypercapnia seems to decrease expiratory braking.

Control Signals. Most models to be considered later use as the controlled variable a level of some chemical component such as arterial or venous pCO_2. Yamamoto (1960) has suggested, however, that the magnitude of oscillations of pCO_2 throughout the respiratory cycle may be involved in respiratory control. We have seen that there are discernible oscillations in blood gas levels during respiration (Section 4.2.2) and that peripheral chemoreceptor outputs follow these oscillations (Section 4.3.1). We have also noted that cardiovascular control is influenced by pulse pressure (Section 3.3.1). It would therefore not be surprising if respiratory-produced blood gas fluctuations had a role in respiratory regulation. Because this fluctuation would dampen more severely by mixing as distance from the pulmonary circulation increases, it is suggested that it is detected by peripheral chemoreceptors (Jacquez, 1979).

Some authors have suggested that, instead of the excursion of the oscillation, the meaningful input is the derivative, or rate of change, of arterial pCO_2.

4.3.3 Effector Organs

Many actions are associated with respiration, and there are interfaces between things internal to the body and external, between cardiovascular and respiratory systems, and between various and often contradictory functions such as swallowing, smelling, and breathing. It is no wonder, then, that respiratory regulation is so complex and deals with so many effector organs.

Respiratory Muscles. The most obvious effector organs are the respiratory muscles, consisting of the diaphragm and external intercostals for inspiration and the abdominals and internal intercostals for expiration. These muscles are responsible for causing the rhythmic mechanical movement of air. Respiratory function of these muscles is superimposed on their functioning to maintain correct posture of the thoracic cage.

Respiratory muscles, like all other skeletal muscles, react by contraction to a neural input discharge. In general, the force of contraction varies with degree of neural input (both firing rate and number of fibers firing). However, the degree of reaction varies with geometrical configuration of the muscles. There is a length–tension relationship, whereby force generated by the contracting muscle is directly related to its length: the longer the respiratory muscle, the greater the force that can be produced (see Section 5.2.5). Thus the smaller the thoracic volume, the more vigorous is the inspiratory drive. There is also a force–velocity relationship, whereby contractile force is maximum when the velocity of shortening of the muscle is zero (see Section 5.2.5). At any given lung volume the generated inspiratory pressure is greatest for the lowest inspiratory flow rate. It is clear, then, that inspiratory and expiratory muscle pressures are not simple translations of neural output.

Inspiratory muscles, which actively pull against the force of expiration, and expiratory muscles, which pull against inspiration, help to stabilize respiratory control and can be important in expiratory braking. It frequently happens during respiration that muscles are pulled by other muscles against their developed forces. When a muscle length is increasing while it is actively developing a force tending to shorten itself, the muscle is said to be developing negative work (see Section 5.2.5). All of the energy expended by a muscle undergoing negative work becomes heat.

Airway Muscles. Airway muscles must be coordinated in their actions with the major respiratory muscles in order to perform the actions of swallowing, sneezing, coughing, and smelling. The muscles of the pharynx are used to prevent the passage of food and gastric materials into the lungs (Comroe, 1965). When specific chemical irritants pass below the larynx, there is a pulmonary chemoreflex consisting of apnea, bradycardia, and hypotension often followed by a cough (Comroe, 1965). Bronchoconstriction also occurs in response to chemical irritants such as sulfur dioxide (SO_2), ammonia (NH_3), high levels of carbon dioxide (CO_2), inert dusts, and smokes. The degree of response adapts rapidly to repeated stimuli and becomes weaker with age (Comroe, 1965). Smoking a cigarette induces an immediate twofold to threefold increase in airway resistance which lasts from 10 to 30 minutes (Comroe, 1965).

Local Effectors. Many other local effector organs are used to deal with specific respiratory problems and operate within the overall context of respiratory control and coordination. We have already mentioned the reflex control of ventilation and perfusion in local areas of the lung (see Section 4.2.2). There is also a local control of mucus secretion and movement of cilia to remove dust particles from the lower reaches of the lung and move them toward the throat, where they can be swallowed.[67]

4.3.4 Exercise

Although a great deal of research has been performed investigating the nature of ventilatory responses to exercise, at this time there is no final explanation for experimental observations. This is not due to a lack of ingenious or elegant experiments; enough of these appear to have been performed to possibly elucidate respiratory controller details [see especially the results of Kao (1963) and Casaburi et al. (1977)]. Rather, the difficulty appears to lie in the complex nature of respiratory control and the multitude of possible inputs and outputs. Because of these, details of respiratory responses are difficult to reproduce, and there appear to be significant influences of the degree of sophistication of the subjects, prior work history, ages of the subjects, and individual variation (Briscoe and DuBois, 1958; Whipp, 1981). Responses to be described in this section are, therefore, to be considered to be responses of normal, healthy, young adult males, with cautious application to any one particular individual. Application of these ideas to young females can probably be made without much reservation—fine details may vary—and application to older adults must take into account changes of mechanical properties and responsiveness that occur with age (Berger et al., 1977).

A schematic representation of the ventilatory response with time during exercise appears in

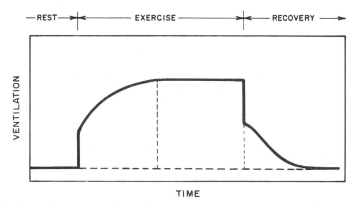

Figure 4.3.16 Schematic representation of the ventilatory response to exercise. The immediate rise is probably due to muscular stimulation, and the plateau value will depend on the level of exercise. When exercise stops, the immediate fall probably indicates that the muscles have ceased moving. Residual carbon dioxide production keeps ventilation above resting levels at least until the oxygen debt is repaid.

[67]To be sure that the upper airway cilia are not overwhelmed by the larger amounts of mucus received from the lower airways, upper airway cilia beat (move repetitively) at a higher frequency than lower airway cilia (Iravani and Melville, 1976).

Figure 4.3.16. Immediately after the onset of exercise there is a sudden rise of minute volume, followed by a slower rise to some steady-state value. When exercise ceases, there is an abrupt fall in minute volume, followed by a recovery period.

Initial Rise. The immediate rise is thought by most researchers to be neurogenic (Tobin et al., 1986), possibly arising from the exercising muscles themselves (Adams et al., 1984) and possibly involving the rapid transient increase in blood flow (Weiler–Ravell et al., 1983). There are several reasons for this view: first, the response occurs too abruptly to allow for the carriage of metabolites from exercising muscles to known chemoreceptor sites; and, second, passive stimulation of the muscles will also induce hyperpnea. There is typically no change seen in end-tidal CO_2 (and, by inference, no change in arterial pCO_2 or pH) or respiratory exchange ratio (R) at the onset of exercise. Yet there is a sudden and significant rise in ventilation, the magnitude of which has been found to sometimes, but not always, depend on the severity of exercise (Miyamoto et al., 1981; Whipp, 1981). Passive limb movement (limbs moved by other than the muscles of the person himself) will also result in this immediate ventilatory response (Jacquez, 1979).

There has been no convincing confirmation of the muscular sensors or neural pathways that induce this immediate rise. Also, for work increments imposed on prior work, no additional abrupt change is observed; that is, the sudden hyperpnea occurs only upon the transition from rest to exercise despite the fact that, when it occurs, its magnitude appears to vary with exercise level. Also, this immediate hyperpnea can be abolished by prior hyperventilation (Whipp, 1981). Nevertheless, it is generally conceded that muscular movement induces an immediate exercise hyperpnea that remains constant for 15–20 seconds after the onset of exercise.[68] Sudden cessation of exercise is accompanied by a similar abrupt fall in ventilation.

Transient Increase. Following the first phase of exercise response, there is an exponential increase in ventilation toward a new, higher level, which occurs with a time constant of 65–75 sec (Whipp, 1981). There is a very similar time constant for carbon dioxide production, as measured at the mouth. The time constant for oxygen uptake, however, is only about 45 sec (Whipp, 1981). Thus there appears to be a much higher correlation between $\dot{V}_{CO_2}$ and $\dot{V}_E$ than between $\dot{V}_{O_2}$ and $\dot{V}_E$. This implies the importance of carbon dioxide in respiratory control.

Whipp (1981) notes, however, that $\dot{V}_{CO_2}$, as measured at the mouth, differs considerably from $\dot{V}_{CO_2}$ as produced by the muscles. There is a large capacity for CO_2 storage in the muscles and blood.[69] Thus the high correlation between $\dot{V}_E$ and $\dot{V}_{CO_2}$ involves CO_2 delivery to the lungs and not CO_2 production by exercising muscles. Carotid body function is essential for this close association to take place.

Figure 4.3.17 shows measured responses to sinusoidally varying exercise level in a healthy subject. Minute volume, oxygen uptake, carbon dioxide production, and end-tidal CO_2 partial pressure (and pCO_2) all show sinusoidal variations. Minute volume is highest when arterial pCO_2 is the highest, but the ratio between $\dot{V}_E$ and $\dot{V}_{CO_2}$ does not remain constant and can be seen to decrease when $\dot{V}_E$ increases. The reason for this is that V_E is not zero when V_{CO_2} is zero; thus the effect of the initial constant value for $\dot{V}_E$ is made smaller as $\dot{V}_E$ increases.

Whipp (1981) unequivocally states that the transient increase in ventilation appears to have a first-order linear response. That is, the increase in minute volume obeys the characteristic differential equation

$$\tau \frac{d\dot{V}_E}{d(t - t_d)} + \dot{V}_E = 0 \qquad (4.3.5)$$

[68]See Saunders (1980) for an alternative explanation of the immediate ventilatory rise based on the time rate of change of CO_2 at the carotid bodies. An increase in heart rate at the beginning of exercise changes this rate of rise almost immediately.
[69]There is very little oxygen storage capacity compared to oxygen needs.

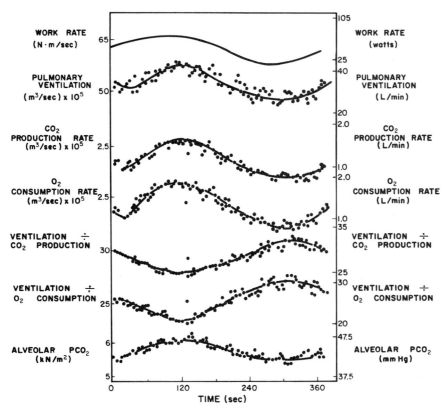

Figure 4.3.17 Average responses to sinusoidal exercise in a healthy subject. Phase lags are evident. Those responses with no phase lag are assumed to be directly related to the exercise stimulus. (Adapted and used with permission from Whipp, 1981.)

where τ = time constant of the response, sec
$\quad t_d$ = delay time, sec
The value for τ, as mentioned before, is about 65–75 sec. The solution to Equation 4.3.5 will be found from both complementary and particular solutions. For instance, if, at the beginning of time, a step change in work rate is incurred, the solution to Equation 4.3.5[70] is

$$\dot{V}_E = (\dot{V}_{E_\infty} - \dot{V}_{E_0})(1 - e^{-(t - t_d)/\tau}) \qquad (4.3.6)$$

where $\dot{V}_{E_\infty}$ = steady-state minute volume after the step change, m³/sec
$\quad \dot{V}_{E_0}$ = steady-state minute volume before the step change, m³/sec
Jacquez (1979) cites evidence that the transient response to increasing concentrations of CO_2 in the inspired breath does not appear to come from a linear system (Figure 4.3.18). As the magnitude of the steady-state response increases, so does the time constant (Table 4.3.1).

Steady State. If the work rate performed is not too high (less than the anaerobic threshold), a steady state is finally reached wherein minute volume does not change appreciably. Relationships between respiratory ventilation and percentage of inhaled CO_2, percentage of

---

[70]Whipp et al. (1982) state that this equation can also be used for $\dot{V}_{O_2}$ and $\dot{V}_{CO_2}$. Powers et al. (1985) give evidence that caffeine slows the response.

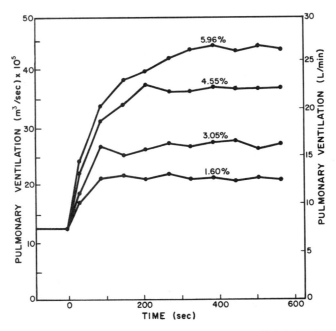

Figure 4.3.18 The response of one individual to different percentages of inhaled carbon dioxide. As the steady-state response increases, so does the apparent time constant. (Adapted and used with permission from Padget, 1927.)

TABLE 4.3.1 Approximate Time Constant Values Taken from the Curves of Figure 4.3.18

Percent CO_2	Final $\dot{V}_E$, m³/sec (L/min)	Time Constant, sec
5.96	4.38×10^{-4} (26.3)	78
4.55	3.70×10^{-4} (22.2)	74
3.05	2.76×10^{-4} (16.6)	58
1.60	2.14×10^{-4} (12.8)	50
	Initial $\dot{V}_E = 1.25 \times 10^{-4}$ (7.50 L/min)	

inhaled O_2, and blood pH are seen in Figure 4.3.19. Since normal percentages of carbon dioxide in the exhaled breath are 4.2–4.5% (Tables 4.2.7 and 4.2.8), the large increase in minute volume with carbon dioxide increase occurs at percentages very close to normal values. On the other hand, the range of percentage of oxygen in the exhaled and inhaled air is 15–21%, but minute volume does not begin to respond to oxygen lack until the 6–8% level. Therefore, carbon dioxide appears to be a much more potent stimulus for respiratory adjustments than is oxygen.

One reason for this may be the dramatically adverse psychophysiological effects of increased atmospheric carbon dioxide content (Figure 4.3.2). As little as 2–4% can cause measurable changes in perception, and 20–30% CO_2 in the inhaled gas can cause coma (Jacquez, 1979). Oxygen concentration of inhaled air would have to be reduced to 10% or less for any noticeable effect, and normally the only feeling that is described is one of euphoria.

Opinion on the driving input for ventilatory response has been divided for a number of years. Jacquez (1979) summarized experimental data which relate minute volume to alveolar partial

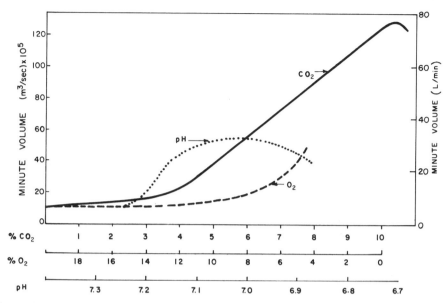

Figure 4.3.19 The responses of healthy men to increasing inhaled carbon dioxide levels, decreasing blood pH levels, and decreasing oxygen levels. The response to carbon dioxide is linear over a wide range beyond the threshold value of 3.5%. Above 10% CO_2 the respiratory system can no longer compensate by increased ventilation. Responses to pH and O_2 are, in general, smaller and nonlinear. (Adapted and used with permission from Comroe, 1965.)

pressure of carbon dioxide (arterial pCO_2 is strongly related). Whipp (1981) maintains, however, that the true driving input is carbon dioxide evolution at the lungs, not arterial pCO_2. We will return to Whipp's formulation after a while. Both authors agree that there is a linear relationship between $\dot{V}_E$ and either arterial pCO_2 or $\dot{V}_{CO_2}$ for the normal control range above some threshold value and below an upper extreme. To be clearer about this, we note that *slope* of the response graph relating $\dot{V}_E$ to some measure of carbon dioxide production is linear, but the value of the ratio between $\dot{V}_E$ and the carbon dioxide measure diminishes because of the initial value for $\dot{V}_E$.

Figures 4.3.20 and 4.3.21 show this linear relationship between alveolar partial pressure of CO_2 and minute volume. Above a threshold value called the "dog-leg," or "hockey-stick," portion, ventilation is seen to be a linear function of arterial pCO_2.[71] The family of curves results from different values of arterial pO_2. Since the slopes of these curves change, the interaction between carbon dioxide and oxygen appears to be multiplicative. Within a small amount of error, all curves above the dog-leg intersect the abscissa at a common point. Jacquez (1979) presents the form for carbon dioxide control of ventilation above the dog-leg as

$$\dot{V}_E = \kappa(p_A CO_2 - \beta)\left(1 + \frac{\alpha}{p_A O_2 - \gamma}\right) \qquad (4.3.7)$$

where $\dot{V}_E$ = minute volume, m^3/sec

$p_A CO_2$ = alveolar partial pressure of carbon dioxide, N/m^2

$p_A O_2$ = alveolar partial pressure of oxygen, N/m^2

$\alpha,\beta,\gamma,\kappa$ = constants which vary between individuals, α,β,γ, N/m^2; κ, $m^5/(N \cdot sec)$

---

[71] Cunningham (1974) reports that in the hypoxia of exercise the $\dot{V}_E$ vs. pCO_2 curves are displaced greatly to the left and upward, may no longer be linear, may have slopes less than those of the curves at rest, and show no sign of a dog-leg.

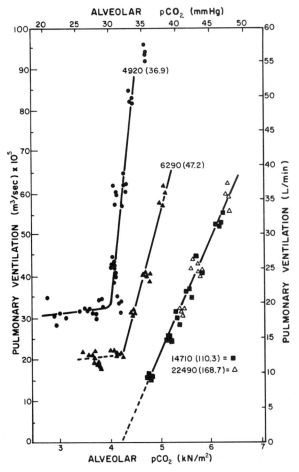

Figure 4.3.20 Ventilatory responses to alveolar levels of carbon dioxide for four levels of alveolar oxygen. In this plot is shown the abrupt change in sensitivity that occurs at some threshold value called the dog-leg. (Adapted and used with permission from Nielsen and Smith, 1952.)

Changes in blood pH also affect minute ventilation, and, because of the relation between pCO_2 and pH (Equation 3.2.3), pH effects are difficult to separate from CO_2 effects. Somewhat slower transient response of ventilation to pH compared to pCO_2 indicates that pH effects are not identical to pCO_2 effects (Jacquez, 1979). This is not surprising in view of the chemoreceptor mechanisms discussed earlier (Section 4.3.1).

If a steady-state response is reached, Cunningham et al. (1961) showed that the ventilatory response to pCO_2 in ammonium chloride acidosis is shifted toward increased alveolar pCO_2 with no significant change in slope. In metabolic acidosis,[72] they concluded, there is only a minor change in the parameters α, κ, γ in Equation 4.3.7 but the parameter β changes significantly. Data

---

[72]Metabolic acidosis occurs whenever blood pH is lowered by natural metabolic or pathogenic means. Inhaling air enriched in CO_2 produces metabolic acidosis; blood bicarbonate movement to replace chloride lost in vomiting produces metabolic acidosis; metabolizing large quantities of protein containing sulfur (metabolized into sulfuric acid) produces metabolic acidosis; excessive ketone production during lipolysis and fatty acid liberation in diabetes can produce metabolic acidosis; incomplete oxidation of glycogen into lactic acid causes metabolic acidosis.

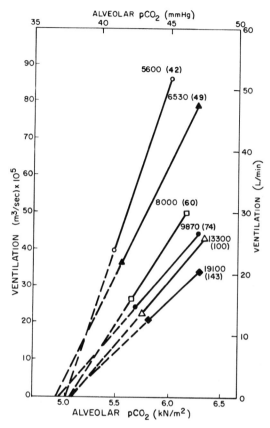

Figure 4.3.21 Ventilatory responses to alveolar levels of carbon dioxide for six levels of alveolar oxygen partial pressures in N/m² (mm Hg). All curves intersect roughly at the same point. Note also the highly nonlinear interaction between CO_2 and O_2. (Adapted and used with permission from Comroe, 1965.)

by Cunningham et al. (1961) show

$$\beta = \beta_0 + \beta_1 c_{HCO_3^-} \tag{4.3.8}$$

where β = parameter in Equation 4.3.5, N/m²

β_0 = intercept of β sensitivity, N/m²

β_1 = sensitivity of β to bicarbonate concentration changes, N·m/kg

$c_{HCO_3^-}$ = bicarbonate concentration,[73] kg/m³

Average values for β_0 and β_1 for five subjects are 2400 N/m² and 1.75 N·m/kg, respectively. The term $(p_A CO_2 - \beta)$ in Equation 4.3.7 now becomes $(p_A CO_2 - \beta_0 - \beta_1 c_{HCO_3^-})$; in this sense the effects of CO_2 and pH are additive (Jacquez, 1979).

One main difficulty with Equation 4.3.7 is that it does not predict the ventilatory response to exercise (Jacquez, 1979). In fact, the response to increased carbon dioxide in the blood caused as a result of metabolism is an almost imperceptible change in arterial pCO_2 but a large increase in

---

[73]Plasma and urine concentrations are frequently expressed in terms of milligrams percent (mg of the species/100 mL solution) or milliequivalents per liter (millimoles of the species times electrical charge/volume of solution in liters). The value for β_1 was originally expressed as 0.8 mm Hg·L/meq.

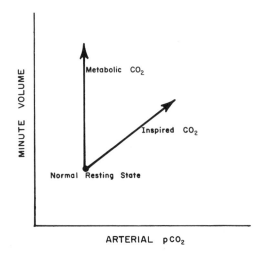

Figure 4.3.22   The ventilatory response to carbon dioxide depends on its source. Inhaled CO_2 causes an increase in ventilation with a concomitant increases in arterial partial pressure of CO_2. Metabolic CO_2 produced within the working muscles results in an isocapnic increase of ventilation. The difference between these two sources of CO_2 may be due to the remoteness of the CO_2 respiratory sensor.

ventilation. The response to inhaled carbon dioxide is a much larger change in arterial pCO_2 and a smaller increase in ventilation (Figure 4.3.22). Swanson (1979) gives a possible controller equation for ventilation as

$$\dot{V}_e = K_1 p_a CO_2 + K_2 \dot{V}_{CO_2} + K_3 \tag{4.3.9}$$

where $\dot{V}_{CO_2}$ = the rate of carbon dioxide production, m^3/sec
  $p_a CO_2$ = arterial partial pressure of carbon dioxide, N/m^2
K_1, K_2, K_3 = coefficients, $m^5/(N \cdot sec)$, unitless, and m^3/sec, respectively
The first term related to arterial pCO_2 is a feedback term, which indicates to the system that ideal levels have not been maintained and that ventilation must be increased proportionately to the error which appears in $p_a CO_2$. The second term is a feedforward term which indicates to the system that a ventilatory adjustment must be made to anticipate future changes in $p_a CO_2$ (see also Section 2.4.2 for further discussion of feedback and feedforward control applied to stepping motion). The K_2 coefficient must be very much larger than K_1 if the situation illustrated in Figure 4.3.22 is to hold true. During exercise, there are both an increased level of metabolic CO_2 and an increased level of inhaled CO_2 due to respiratory dead volume.

Below the dog-leg, carbon dioxide sensitivity is drastically reduced. The reason for this is not now known, but several hypotheses have been offered (Jacquez, 1979). One possibility involves the estimate that 80% of the CO_2 response results from central receptors and the remaining 20% from peripheral receptors. It may be that below the dog-leg, central receptors are not contributing to CO_2 response. Another possibility is that the low arterial pCO_2 below the dog-leg causes constriction of the cerebral blood vessels so that local cerebral pCO_2 depends on local CO_2 production and not on arterial pCO_2.

Similarly, the interaction between hypercapnia and hypoxia illustrated in Figure 4.3.20 has been postulated to arise in peripheral chemoreceptors (Cunningham, 1974). Outputs from these receptors then sum with outputs from central receptors in the final determination of minute volume. Lloyd's (Cunningham, 1974) formulation of this activity takes the form

$$\dot{V}_{E_a} = \frac{\lambda_0 + \lambda_H \log(H_a^+/H_{a0}^+)}{(p_A O_2 - \gamma)} \qquad (4.3.10a)$$

where $\dot{V}_{E_a}$ = minute volume contribution due to arterial chemoreceptors, m^3/sec
λ_0 = hypoxia threshold, $m^5 \cdot sec/N$
λ_H = hypoxia sensitivity, $m^5 \cdot sec/N$
γ = constant, N/m^2 (see Equation 4.3.7)
H_a^+ = arterial hydrogen ion concentration, kg/m^3
H_{a0}^+ = arterial threshold hydrogen ion concentration, kg/m^3
If $H_a^+ < H_{a0}^+$, then

$$\dot{V}_{E_a} = \frac{\lambda_0}{(p_A O_2 - \gamma)} \qquad (4.3.10b)$$

The use of hydrogen ion concentration rather than carbon dioxide partial pressure merely indicates the normally close relationship between them. This use treats these receptors as the same whether or not they respond separately to arterial pCO_2 or H^+. Response to central (brain) receptors is given by

$$\dot{V}_{E_c} = \mu_0 + \mu_v \log(H_c^+/H_{c0}^+) \qquad (4.3.11a)$$

where $\dot{V}_{E_c}$ = intracranial receptor contribution to minute volume, m^3/sec
μ_0 = central receptor response independent of H^+, m^3/sec
μ_v = central receptor sensitivity to H^+, m^3/sec
H^+ = central hydrogen ion concentration, kg/m^3
H_{c0}^+ = central threshold hydrogen ion concentration, kg/m^3
If $H^+ < H_{c0}^+$, then

$$\dot{V}_{E_c} = \mu_0 \qquad (4.3.11b)$$

Total minute ventilation is the sum of $\dot{V}_{E_a}$ and $\dot{V}_{E_c}$:

$$\dot{V}_E = \dot{V}_{E_a} + \dot{V}_{E_c} \qquad (4.3.12)$$

Whipp (1981) argues strongly for considering minute ventilation to be related to carbon dioxide production[74] rather than to arterial pCO_2. Any change in arterial pCO_2 "is a consequence of the ventilatory change, not the cause of it." Mean arterial pCO_2 and H^+ during moderate exercise are typically unchanged from control values; therefore, there must be a different control mechanism in this instance compared to CO_2 inhalation studies where arterial pCO_2 and H^+ increase (Whipp, 1981).

Most investigators have indicated that arterial pCO_2 does not change during exercise from its normal value of $5.33 \, kN/m^2$ (40 mm Hg; Comroe, 1965). Berger et al. (1977), however, report on a study that shows small but measurable increases in pCO_2 accompanied by increased oxygen

---

[74]Whipp (1981) reviews evidence that the type of metabolized food is important in determining ventilation. When fats are metabolized, with a respiratory exchange ratio of 0.7, about 7 molecules of CO_2 are produced for every 10 molecules of O_2 utilized. When carbohydrates are used, $R = 1.0$, and 10 molecules of CO_2 are produced for each 10 molecules of O_2 utilized. The CO_2 output is considerably higher for a given metabolic load when carbohydrates are the predominant fuel source. It has been demonstrated that minute volume is proportionately higher for larger proportions of carbohydrate metabolized.

uptake. Martin et al. (1978) and Filley et al. (1978) suggest an increased sensitivity to pCO_2 during exercise. Mahler (1979) presents the view that muscular exercise and other neural influences shift the intercept of the CO_2 response curve without shifting the slope. Therefore, the basic control of ventilation during exercise is through these shifts in CO_2 sensitivity.

Response to severe oxygen lack is difficult to elicit from humans without changes in ventilation, which, in turn, decrease arterial partial pressure of carbon dioxide. When care is taken to assure constant arterial pCO_2, curves similar to those in Figure 4.3.23 result. For constant alveolar pCO_2, the ventilatory response is nonlinear and shows the multiplicative interaction discussed earlier. When plotted against arterial hemoglobin saturation percentage, minute ventilation response curves become linear (Figure 4.3.24).

Oxygen sensitivity is wholly a result of peripheral chemoreceptors. From the instant a subject is given a breath of pure oxygen, a decrease in ventilation is seen after a short delay of about 5 sec (3.45–10.5 sec for different individuals, longer delays for older subjects; Jacquez, 1979). This is equivalent to 0.83–3.89 respiratory cycles and is the appropriate amount of time for the circulating blood to reach the peripheral chemoreceptors. Maximum response occurs after 10–20 sec.

Hypoxic sensitivity is somewhat more variable than hypercapnic sensitivity in normal subjects (Berger et al., 1974). The change in respiratory minute volume can be expressed as (Cunningham, 1974)

$$\dot{V}_E = \dot{V}_{E_0} + \frac{\alpha}{p_a O_2 - \gamma} \tag{4.3.13}$$

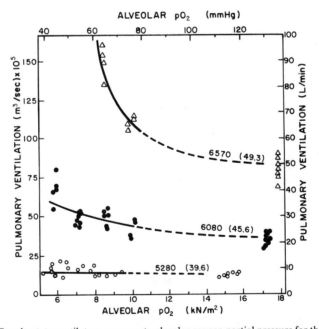

Figure 4.3.23 Steady-state ventilatory response to alveolar oxygen partial pressure for three fixed levels of alveolar carbon dioxide partial pressure given in N/m^2 (mm Hg). The oxygen ventilatory response is nonlinear and interrelated to carbon dioxide response. (Adapted and used with permission from Lloyd and Cunningham, 1963.)

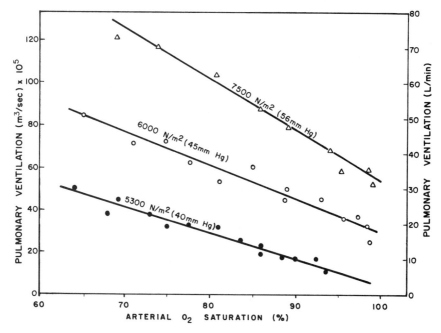

Figure 4.3.24   Steady-state ventilatory response to arterial oxygen saturation of hemoglobin. For each of the three different levels of alveolar carbon dioxide partial pressure, the oxygen ventilation response is linear. (Adapted and used with permission from Rebuck and Woodley, 1975.)

where $\dot{V}_{E_0}$ = minute volume in response to a very high p_aO_2, m^3/sec

$\quad p_aO_2$ = arterial partial pressure of oxygen, N/m^2

$\quad \alpha$ = constant, $N \cdot m/sec$

$\quad \gamma$ = threshold value, N/m^2 (see Equation 4.3.7)

The value for γ is approximately 4.27 kN/m^2 (or 32 mm Hg; Cunningham, 1974) and the value for α has been found to range from 0.153 to 0.911 $N \cdot m/sec$ (69–410 mm Hg·L/min) with an average value of 0.400 $N \cdot m/sec$ (Berger et al., 1974). Martin et al. (1978) found an almost tenfold increase in the value of α between rest and exercise.

Although minute volume is not a linear function of oxygen partial pressure, it is often considered to be linearly related to oxygen uptake below the anaerobic threshold (Figure 4.3.24). Arterial pCO_2 is not maintained at set levels during these exercise tests.

Other inputs have been found to influence the steady-state level of ventilation. Ammonia has been found to produce hyperventilation, and significant amounts of ammonia are found in the blood during exercise and some pathological states (Jacquez, 1979). Body temperature, which increases during exercise, is known to affect ventilation mainly through an increase in sensitivity to alveolar pCO_2 (Jacquez, 1979; Whipp, 1981). This increased sensitivity appears as an increase in parameter κ in Equation 4.3.7.

Emotion and stress can induce hyperpnea. Increased catecholamine concentrations, which often accompany high levels of emotion, have been shown to increase ventilation by increasing hypoxic sensitivity. In Equation 4.3.7, the effect is seen mainly in a change in parameter α (Whipp, 1981).

Sleep, high blood pressure, anesthetics, and some drugs decrease ventilation levels (Jacquez, 1979; Whipp, 1981). Other drugs, such as aspirin, increase CO_2 sensitivity and thus increase ventilation (Jacquez, 1979).

Acclimatization can modify ventilatory responses to CO_2, O_2, and pH. Figure 4.3.25 presents

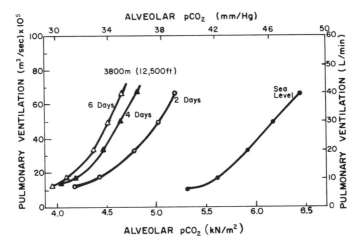

Figure 4.3.25 Average ventilatory response of three subjects to inhalation of carbon dioxide as they acclimatize to 3800 m altitude. As with many bodily functions, response to change is greatest immediately after the imposition of the change, and the response slows with time. (Adapted and used with permission from Severinghaus et al., 1963).

carbon dioxide sensitivity curves as they change over the course of eight days at 3800 m altitude (hypoxic conditions). It is also known that patients with chronic obstructive pulmonary disease (COPD) usually exhibit abnormally low carbon dioxide sensitivities (Anthonisen and Cherniack, 1981), but there is a question whether existing low CO_2 sensitivity predisposes humans to suffer from COPD (Forster and Dempsey, 1981). Age appears to decrease CO_2 sensitivity (Altose et al., 1977) and the practice of yoga breathing exercise has also been found to reduce CO_2 sensitivity (Stănescu et al., 1981).

Cessation of Exercise. When exercise ceases, there is often an immediate fall in minute ventilation (Figure 4.3.16), although this may be masked by a long, gradual decline. Ventilation rates remain elevated because carbon dioxide and lactate are not removed immediately from the blood (see Section 1.3.3). For subjects recovering from maximal exercise (90–100% $\dot{V}_{O_2max}$), breathing is typically more rapid and shallow than for lower exercise rates. Younes and Burks (1985) attribute this to pulmonary interstitial edema (fluid in the lung tissue) occurring only at very severe exercise rates, but Martin et al. (1979) assert that the rise in rectal temperature associated with exercise reduces tidal volume compared to its value without heating.

Anaerobic Ventilation. During very heavy exercise there is an additional respiratory drive caused by increased blood lactate (see Section 1.3.5).[75] Incomplete oxidation of glucose results in lactic acid, which then produces increased arterial pCO_2 through the buffering reaction:

$$H^+ + La^- + Na^+ + HCO_3^- \Leftrightarrow Na^+ + La^- + H_2CO_3 \Leftrightarrow Na^+ + La^- + CO_2 + H_2O$$

$$(4.3.14)$$

where La^- = lactate anion = $CH_3 \cdot CHOH \cdot COO^-$

Bicarbonate levels are reduced and carbon dioxide production is increased beyond that

---

[75]Cunningham (1974) reports negligible steady-state changes in blood lactate at work intensities below 60–75% of aerobic capacity (60–75% of $\dot{V}_{O_2max}$), but lactate concentration increases more than tenfold in severe exercise. In mild exercise, blood lactate concentrations increase transiently and reach a significant peak 5–10 min after the start.

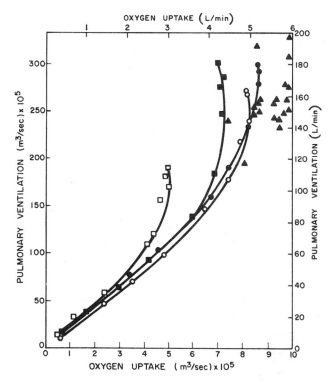

Figure 4.3.26   Pulmonary ventilation for various levels of oxygen consumption during rest and exercise. There is a linear portion until the aerobic threshold is reached. Four individual curves show the scatter to be expected between individuals. (Adapted and used with permission from Astrand and Rodahl, 1970.)

predicted by the respiratory quotient (see Section 3.2.2).[76] During this phase, the respiratory exchange ratio will exceed the respiratory quotient.

There is a narrow range of work rates over which nearly complete ventilatory compensation can be made for the increased levels of CO_2 produced (Figure 4.3.26). The relationship between oxygen uptake and work rate will still appear to be linear, but the relationship between minute volume and oxygen uptake will become nonlinear in this region. If a steady state can be reached, end-tidal pCO_2 decreases, but the blood pH level appears to be regulated at its previous normal value. At even higher work rates (see Section 1.3.5), ventilation increases ever more rapidly, arterial pCO_2 falls even more, and blood pH declines (Whipp, 1981). This condition cannot be maintained.

Kinetics of this process are very poorly understood. Aside from the practical problems of pushing test subjects to their limits to obtain meaningful data, many aspects of the problem cannot be easily measured. With a reduction in arterial pCO_2, one would expect, on the basis of information in Figure 4.3.20, that a decrease in ventilation would result. Instead, minute volume appears to be related to the rate of CO_2 evolution. In addition, the blood–brain barrier is much more permeable to CO_2 relative to H^+ and HCO_3^-. Therefore, while the peripheral chemoreceptors are reacting to increased blood H^+ (metabolic acidosis) and carbon dioxide production, the cerebrospinal fluid (and thus fluid surrounding the central chemoreceptors) becomes alkaline. These conditions are sure to produce conflicting regulatory tendencies.

[76]Approximately $4 \times 10^{-7} \, m^3$ (400 mL) of CO_2 is produced as a result of a decrease of 61 g/m^3 (1 meq/L) of HCO_3^- in the extracellular fluid (Whipp, 1981).

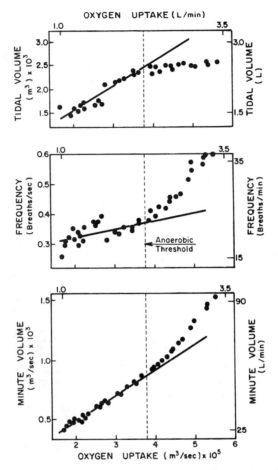

Figure 4.3.27 Respiratory measures with progressive work rate. Minute volume increases linearly with work rate up to the anaerobic threshold, when it begins increasing disproportionately. Tidal volume can be seen to reach a limit after the anaerobic threshold, but respiration rate increases greatly. (Adapted and used with permission from Martin and Weil, 1979.)

If work rate increases at a rate too high for equilibrium to be established, blood pH no longer appears to be regulated but instead falls (Whipp, 1981). Respiration is much less efficient, and the respiratory muscles begin to require much more oxygen to perform the work of breathing than they require below the anaerobic threshold. It has been reported that at a ventilation rate of $0.0023 \, m^3/sec$ (140 L/min) a small increase in ventilation requires an increment of oxygen utilization greater than that which can be provided by the increase in ventilation (Abbrecht, 1973). Figure 4.3.27 illustrates another interesting facet: below the anaerobic threshold, increased minute volume comes as a result mainly of tidal volume increase; above the anaerobic threshold, tidal volume remains nearly constant, and the increase of minute volume is supplied by an increase in respiration rate.

Ventilatory Loading. It has been stated, and commonly assumed, that exercise performance is not limited by respiration in healthy subjects (Astrand and Rodahl, 1970). The same cannot be said for humans suffering the effects of respiratory disease, or those who are wearing respiratory apparatus for protection or testing. The addition of various mechanical devices, such as masks or J-valves, can have severe consequences on respiratory responses and exercise performance.

Various types of ventilatory loads can be applied. The first is resistive: adding elements to the respiratory pathways which increase resistance in ways similar to airways, lung tissue, and chest wall resistance. Breathing through contaminant filters, tubes of small diameter, perforated disks, or screens, breathing during bronchoconstriction, and breathing gases of high density or viscosity (Cherniack and Altose, 1981)—all increase resistance loading.

Elastic loading changes pressure–volume relationships of breathing. Examples of this are breathing from rigid containers, during chest strapping, or with a pneumothorax or atelectasis.[77] For both of these, higher pressures are required of the respiratory muscles in order to inhale or expel any given volume.

Pressure loading involves the application of gas which opposes inspiration or expiration. This can be accomplished by breathing from pressurized cylinders of gas and is frequently found in positive pressurized, air- (or oxygen-) supplied masks.

Threshold loads prevent flow at the beginning of inspiration or expiration until a threshold pressure is exceeded (Cherniack and Altose, 1981). Examples of this type of loading occur when breathing through a tube inserted to a fixed depth underwater, or when wearing a pressure-demand respirator mask.

Many of these ventilated loads can be externally applied. Usually, some amount of dead volume is applied simultaneously.

When ventilatory loading is applied to a human, several compensatory mechanisms can operate. The first of these are the various mechanical properties of the chest wall and muscles themselves. The muscles can intrinsically increase their forces as their resting lengths are increased (see Section 5.2.5). Because the diaphragm is dome shaped, increasing resting volume shortens inspiratory muscle resting length and decreases the inspiratory force that can be produced. Increasing resting volume has exactly the opposite effect on the expiratory muscles — expiratory forces are increased. The elastic nature of the chest wall and lung tissue also aids expiration and hinders inspiration as the resting volume is increased. Some respiratory response to ventilatory loading would thus be expected to be a change in resting volume of the lungs. Posture affects the size and shape of the respiratory muscles, and thus affects load compensation.

Ventilatory loading that reduces the velocity of shortening of the muscles can increase the forces produced by those muscles, which serves to maintain tidal volume.[78] Respiration rate falls and minute volume also falls.

Another compensatory mechanism deals with the neural input to the muscles of the chest, abdomen, and respiratory airways. These inputs arise from chemoreceptors, mechanoreceptors (mainly stretch receptors in the lung and chest), and from higher centers in the brain. With these diverse inputs, the response to ventilatory loading becomes very complex.

For example, hypoxia or hypercapnia leads to an increased output from chemoreceptors. This tends to shorten exhalation time, which induces an increased resting volume. Laryngeal resistance decreases, however, and postinspiratory braking of the diaphragm diminishes, tending to preserve the normal level of resting volume (Cherniack and Altose, 1981).

Without pulmonary mechanoreceptor input, stimulation of the chemoreceptors increases tidal volume without change in inspiratory time. With pulmonary mechanoreceptor input, tidal volume changes are inversely proportional to changes in the inspiratory time (Cherniack and Altose, 1980). In general, elastic loads decrease tidal volume and increase the respiration rate, due mostly to an increase in neuronal discharge to the inspiratory muscles. During exercise, elastic

---

[77]A pneumothorax occurs whenever air is introduced between the lung and pleura, or between the pleura and thoracic wall. Since tissue-to-tissue contact is no longer present, the affected lung may partially or fully collapse. Atelectasis refers to an airless state of the interior of a part or all of the lung. Air is often replaced by fluid.

[78]As exercise progresses, higher respiratory flow rates increase airways resistance. Lind (1984) states that a higher respiratory muscle pressure is automatically applied to overcome this increased resistance.

loads decrease the vital capacity and decrease the maximum tidal volume (see Figure 4.3.26) which is reached. Respiration rate increases above that of the unloaded condition. Elastic loads can be perceived by humans, although not as readily as resistive loads. Changes on the order of 10–25% are readily detected (Cherniack and Altose, 1981).

Resistive loads generally increase inhalation time and/or exhalation time and decrease flow rate. Inspiratory loading increases inhalation time, decreases respiration rate, and lowers minute volume. The duration of the succeeding exhalation is influenced by the prior inhalation, longer inspiratory times leading to long expiratory times (Cherniack and Altose, 1981). Expiratory resistance loading increases the exhalation time and reduces expiratory flow rate without influencing the next inspiration. Resistance loading during exercise does not decrease the maximum tidal volume reached during exercise (see Figure 4.3.26) but does limit the respiration rate.

The ability to detect increases in resistance depends on the prior level of airway resistance. Burki et al. (1978) and Gottfried et al. (1978) concluded that the minimum detectable external resistance is always a constant proportion (25–30%) of the resistance already present.[79] Since the level of resistance present in the airways of those with respiratory disease, and in the old (Campbell and Lefrak, 1978), is higher than in young, healthy adults, the inability to detect small changes in added resistance may be a valid reason why ventilatory compensation for resistance loads is less complete in these individuals (Cherniack and Altose, 1981; Rubin et al., 1982).

The detection of resistive loads has been found to be impaired by elastic loading (Shahid et al., 1981; Zechman et al., 1981), the minimum detectable difference of resistive loads being a fixed proportion of both resistive and elastic loading. Detection of elastic loads does not appear to depend at all on resistive loads present.

Ventilatory responses to hypoxia and hypercapnia are reduced during resistive loading. The more severe the resistive load, the greater is the fall in minute volume (Cherniack and Altose, 1981). Increasing the percentage of CO_2 in the inhaled air increases inspiratory time, whereas increased CO_2 in the exhaled air has no effect on inspiratory time and results in an increase in exhalation time only after a time delay.

Occlusion pressure increases during resistive loading in healthy, normal subjects. It does not increase in chronic obstructive lung disease patients (Cherniack and Altose, 1981). There is a limit, however, to the maximum pressures that can be developed even in healthy subjects (see Table 4.2.21).

Respiratory responses to ventilatory challenges depend on previous experience and personality traits. Inexperienced subjects increase their abdominal muscle force during positive pressure breathing to minimize the change in resting volume and maintain the diaphragm in an optimal mechanical position. Experienced subjects allow their resting volumes to enlarge and maintain adequate minute volumes despite the mechanical disadvantage of the diaphragm by increases in the neural drive to inspiration (Cherniack and Altose, 1981).

Psychometrically identified neurotic individuals tend to breathe more rapidly and shallowly than normal individuals. Neurotics tend to increase minute volume in response to expiratory threshold loading more than do normals (Cherniack and Altose, 1981). Anxiety has been shown to shorten inspiratory and expiratory times as tidal volume increases (Bechbache et al., 1979). Circulating catecholamine levels normally affect respiration and may influence the response to loading. Performance of difficult arithmetic tasks has been shown to cause increases in respiratory resistance (Kotses et al., 1987).

Dyspnea and Second Wind. Dyspnea is difficult, labored, uncomfortable breathing (Astrand and Rodahl, 1970). Dyspnea can occur during exercise, at rest in humans with respiratory diseases, or in normals with ventilatory loading. Elements of chest tightness, awareness of

---

[79]Katz-Salamon (1984) found that the just-noticeable difference in lung volume was also 25–29% of lung volume present before the change.

excessive ventilation, excessive frequency of breathing, and difficult breathing are all present (Campbell and Guz, 1981).

No one knows for sure what causes the sensation of dyspnea (Wasserman and Casaburi, 1988). It appears not to be pain, it is not directly related to work or effort by the respiratory muscles, nor does respiratory muscle fatigue appear to be a direct cause (Campbell and Guz, 1981).

Respiratory sensation appears to depend on mouth pressure, inspiratory time, and respiration rate (Jones, 1984):

$$\psi = K p_m^{1.4} t_i^{0.52} f^{0.26} \tag{4.3.15}$$

where ψ = sense of respiratory effort, dimensionless
  p_m = mouth pressure, N/m^2
  t_i = inspiratory time, sec
  f = respiration rate, breaths/sec
  K = coefficient, m$^{2.8}$/(N$^{1.4}$·sec$^{0.26}$)

Involved in determination of the coefficient K are respiratory muscle strength and resting lung volume. Sensation is increased with volume and decreased with strength. Experience seems to modify the amount of respiratory sensation, and age seems to be accompanied by a change of sensation based on volume to that based on respiratory muscle force (Tack et al., 1983).

O'Connell and Campbell (1976) studied three groups of subjects (patients with airways obstruction who complained of dyspnea at rest, a control group of patients with airways obstruction but no symptoms of dyspnea, and a group of normal subjects). They determined that normal subjects experiencing dyspnea could be separated from normal subjects experiencing no dyspnea by forming the ratio of respiratory muscle pressure required to produce the highest inspiratory flow during breathing p to maximum developed muscle pressure p_{max}. When the ratio p/p_{max} was greater than 0.1, the sensation of dyspnea was felt in all but two cases (Figure 4.3.28). Likewise, there was a separation between patients with and without dyspnea at p/p_{max} ratios of about 0.14. However, there was considerable overlap of the ratios for normal subjects with dyspnea and the ratios of patients without dyspnea.

This relationship between muscle pressure and dyspnea is consistent with the concept of the feeling of mechanical appropriateness of the respiratory muscles. This hypothesis suggests that mechanoreceptors in the lung and chest wall send information to the central nervous system about the length–tension relationship of the muscles. If too much force must be developed in the muscles for any particular lung volume, a conscious feeling of labored breathing results. Higher pressures must be developed when breathing through higher resistances, into lower compliances, or when breathing at higher than normal lung volumes.

Where this information originates, how it is transmitted, and where it is felt are open to speculation. The information pathway probably involves the vagus nerve (Campbell and Guz, 1981).[80] The actual sensation can be modified by expectations about the load and by anxiety states (Campbell and Guz, 1981).[81]

Second wind is the feeling of respiratory relief that is experienced after exercise has progressed for a short time. Although not everything is known about second wind, it appears to be the result of time lags in the accommodation to exercise conditions. Although there is an immediate increase in minute volume when exercise begins, the rise to steady-state levels does not occur

---

[80]Mohler (1982) attempted to quantify dyspnea by voice pitch analysis. He found that the fundamental frequency of speaking during exercise was related to a feeling of dyspnea. The mechanism of this linkage may involve vagal signals to the larynx.

[81]See Section 2.4.2 for a model of stepping with similar concepts. In that model, steps are normally performed with feedforward programming. Special steps require feedback and more conscious awareness. Breathing could act in a similar way.

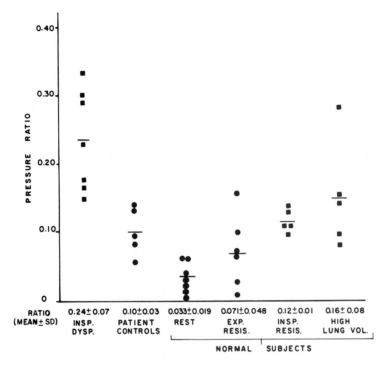

Figure 4.3.28   Ratio of the pressure required to produce the highest inspiratory flow during quiet breathing to the muscle strength in those with (squares) and without (circles) inspiratory dyspnea. INSP. DYSP. indicates patients complaining of inspiratory dyspnea at rest. PATIENT CONTROLS are obstructive patients matched as well as possible without dyspnea complaints. NORMAL SUBJECTS were tested at rest, with additional expiratory resistance, with additional inspiratory resistance, and with high resting lung volume (to decrease muscle strength). Bars indicate average values for the group. In patients and normal subjects at rest, there is no overlap in the ratios of those with and without inspiratory dyspnea. With two exceptions, all the ratios of the normal subjects in whom inspiratory dyspnea was induced were higher than those without dyspnea. (Adapted and used with permission from O'Connell and Campbell, 1976.)

instantaneously (Figure 4.3.16). The relief of this initial hypoventilation may contribute to second wind Astrand and Rodahl, 1970).

The redistribution of blood from the gut and kidneys to the working muscles (Table 3.2.4) may also take some time to develop. It thus appears that the respiratory muscles are forced to work anaerobically at the beginning of heavy exercise (Astrand and Rodahl, 1970).

Second wind appears to be strongly related to the temperature of the working muscles (Morehouse and Miller, 1967). When they have attained their higher temperatures, muscle metabolism appears to return to a more normal state, efficiency increases, and muscular demand on the respiratory system diminishes somewhat. This is reflected by a decrease in respiratory rate and minute volume and a small decrease in oxygen consumption. Second wind can be delayed by cool environmental temperatures (Morehouse and Miller, 1967).

Optimization of Breathing.   Respiratory work, which accounts for only 1–2% of the total body oxygen consumption at rest, may rise to as much as 10% or higher during exercise (see Table 4.2.20). For moderately exercising patients with chronic obstructive pulmonary disease, the portion of the body's total oxygen consumption used by the respiratory muscles to support the act of breathing rises to 35–40% (Levison and Cherniack, 1968). Since this is work that does

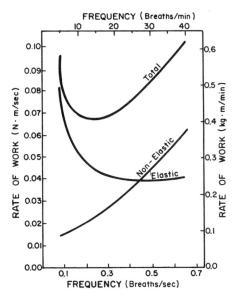

Figure 4.3.29 Breathing work rate with different respiration rates. Both elastic (compliance) and nonelastic (resistance) components comprise total respiratory work rate. Because these components have opposite trends, total respiratory work rate exhibits a minimum value at one specific frequency. This leads to the optimization of respiration at the frequency corresponding to the minimum. (Adapted and used with permission from Otis et al., 1950.)

not aid primarily the completion of the muscular task being performed during exercise, it appears reasonable that the neural mechanisms regulating respiration would aim toward minimizing the work of respiration. Many of the physical adjustments in breathing, as measured during exercise, appear to be the same adjustments that would be made to minimize the power expenditure of breathing, or some very similar quantity.[82] Adjustments in breathing airflow pattern, frequency, relative durations of inhalation and exhalation, expiratory reserve volume, and perhaps airways resistance, dead volume, and compliance appear to be the result of some integrated neural optimization.

Whereas respiratory ventilation during rest is sometimes subject to a high degree of voluntary control, this is usually much less true during exercise. One of the most noticeable changes that occurs happens to respiration rate, which becomes much higher during exercise: a resting respiration rate of 0.25 breath/sec (15 breaths/min) will normally progress to 0.7 breath/sec (42 breaths/min) during maximal sustained exertion.

There appears to be good reason for his change in respiration rate. Otis et al. (1950) were among the first to speculate on the basis of the adjustment in respiration rate. To that speculation they added a simple quantitative analysis based on a criterion of minimization of average inspiratory power.

Most optimization models are based on the fact that as flow rate increases, dissipation of power across respiratory resistance increases. However, elastic power, represented by the amount of power needed to stretch the lungs and chest wall, increases as depth of breathing increases. To minimize resistive power and still maintain the required minute volume, long, slow breaths with low flow rates are implied. To minimize elastic power, rapid, shallow breaths with relatively high flow rates are required. Since these requirements oppose each other, a minimum should be found between the two extremes. This is illustrated in Figure 4.3.29. The frequency

[82]Kennard and Martin (1984), however, failed to observe any oxygen uptake differences from subjects exercising while breathing at different frequencies.

corresponding to minimum respiratory work is nearly equal to the spontaneous frequency of breathing at rest. Christie (1953) showed that the frequency corresponding to minimum respiratory power increases during exercise, despite the fact that the actual magnitude of the respiratory power minimum is much higher than nonminimum values during rest.

Otis et al. (1950) based their modeling on several assumptions:

1. The pattern of breathing is sinusoidal.
2. Breathing occurs at a rate required to minimize the average inspiratory power.
3. Alveolar ventilation rate does not vary with respiratory period.
4. Inertia of tissues and air is neglected.
5. Expiration is passive or at least does not enter into the determination of respiratory period.

They formulated the expression for inspiratory work as

$$W_i = \int_0^{V_T} p_i \, dV \tag{4.3.16}$$

where W_i = inspiratory work, N·m
$\quad V_T$ = tidal volume, m³
$\quad p_i$ = pressure developed by the inspiratory muscles, N/m²
$\quad V$ = lung volume, m³

$$p_i = V/C_i + R_i \dot{V}_i \tag{4.3.17}$$

where C_i = inspiratory compliance, m⁵/N
$\quad R_i$ = inspiratory resistance, N·sec/m⁵
$\quad \dot{V}_i$ = inspiratory flow rate, m³/sec

and

$$\dot{V}_i = \dot{V} \sin \frac{2\pi t}{T} \tag{4.3.18}$$

where $\dot{V}$ = peak inspiratory flow rate, m³/sec
$\quad t$ = time, sec
$\quad T$ = respiratory period, sec

Because of the constraint that the accumulated inspiratory airflow must equal the tidal volume,

$$V_T = \int_0^{T/2} \dot{V} \sin \frac{2\pi t}{T} \, dt \tag{4.3.19}$$

then

$$\dot{V} = \pi V_T / T \tag{4.3.20}$$

From equations 4.3.15 and 4.3.16,

$$W_i = \int_0^{V_T} \frac{V}{C_i} \, dV + \int_0^{T/2} p_{ir} \dot{V}_i \, dt \tag{4.3.21}$$

where p_{ir} = inspiratory pressure contribution of resistance, N/m²
$\quad = R_i \dot{V}_i$

and

$$W_i = \frac{V_T^2}{2C_i} + \frac{\pi^2 V_T^2}{4T} R_i \qquad (4.3.22)$$

Average inspiratory power is

$$\bar{W}_i = W_i/T = \frac{V_T^2}{2C_i T} + \frac{\pi^2 V_T^2}{4T^2} R_i \qquad (4.3.23)$$

where $\bar{W}_i$ = average inspiratory power, N·m/sec
Since alveolar ventilation rate, not tidal volume, is considered to be constant, and

$$\dot{V}_A = (V_T - V_D)/T \qquad (4.3.24)$$

where $\dot{V}_A$ = alveolar ventilation rate, m^3/sec
V_D = dead volume, m^3

then

$$\bar{W}_i = \frac{1}{2C_i T}(\dot{V}_A T + V_D)^2 + \frac{\pi^2 R_i}{4}(\dot{V}_A + V_D/T)^2 \qquad (4.3.25)$$

The first term on the right-hand side represents elastic power and increases as T increases. The second term represents viscous power and decreases as T increases. Figure 4.3.29 demonstrates these effects and shows that $\bar{W}_i$ becomes a minimum at approximately $T = 4$ sec.

Solving for T at the minimum[83] requires differentiation of $\bar{W}_i$ with respect to T, and setting the result to zero. We obtain an equation involving T:

$$T^2 - \frac{V_D}{\dot{V}_A} T - \pi^2 R_i C_i (V_D/\dot{V}_A) = 0 \qquad (4.3.26)?$$

T can be obtained by solution of the quadratic equation (Mead, 1960) as

$$T = \frac{1 + \sqrt{1 + 4\pi^2 R_i C_i (\dot{V}_A/V_D)}}{2(\dot{V}_A/V_D)} \qquad (4.3.27)$$

---

[83]Most authors solve their equations in terms of respiratory rate f, which is equal to $1/T$. However, solution for the respiratory period T has advantages in graphical determination of true minima. In graphing respiratory power or force against frequency, a broad minimum is usually obtained. From the chain rule,

$$\frac{\partial \dot{W}_i}{\partial T} = \frac{\partial \bar{W}_i}{\partial f} \frac{\partial f}{\partial T} \quad \text{and} \quad \frac{\partial f}{\partial T} = -1/T^2$$

Since T is often given in minutes, and $T \ll 1$ min,

$$|-1/T^2| \gg 1 \quad \text{and} \quad \frac{\partial \bar{W}_i}{\partial T} \gg \frac{\partial \bar{W}_i}{\partial f}$$

Therefore, the slope of average respiratory power graphed against T is greater than the slope or power against f, and the minimum point should be graphically better defined.

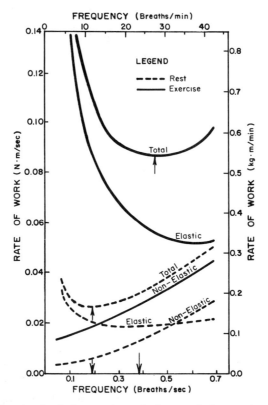

Figure 4.3.30 An explanation for the increase in respiration rate during exercise. Although total rate of respiratory work is higher during exercise than at rest, the minimum point moves to a higher frequency. (Adapted and used with permission from Christie, 1953.)

No optimal value for T can be found if total cycle work rather than inspiratory work is used as the optimization parameter. This is because elastic work stored during inspiration is completely used during expiration. If expiration is not passive, stored elastic work reduces the amount of exhalation work expended, with a net result of no elastic work term appearing in total cycle work expression. Without elastic work, there can be no optimal respiratory period.

Recognizing the shortcomings of assuming a sinusoidal waveform, Otis et al. (1950) indicated that if the actual airflow velocity pattern were known, actual respiratory power could be calculated. One procedure they suggested is to calculate pressures corresponding to points on the velocity curve and then obtain work by graphical or numerical solution of Equation 4.3.16. A similar procedure was used by Christie (1953) to produce curves demonstrating that the observed respiratory frequency increase during exercise is due to a shift in the minimum average inspiratory work (Figure 4.3.30).

Mead (1960) proposed that, instead of minimizing inspiratory work rate, respiratory period is controlled by a criterion of minimum average respiratory muscle force. In an elaborate and thorough paper, he derived an expression for respiratory frequency based on the force criterion, and he proceeded to demonstrate that most observations were more consistent with his hypothesis than with the minimum power hypothesis. Mead assumed;

1. The pattern of breathing is sinusoidal.
2. Breathing occurs at a rate required to minimize the average respiratory muscle force.

3. Alveolar ventilation rate does not vary with respiratory period.

4. Inertia of tissues and air is neglected.

5. Average force is proportional to the peak-to-peak amplitude of force for the cycle.

6. Nonconsistent resistance and compliance terms are neglected.

Average amplitude of muscle pressure was expressed by Mead as

$$\bar{p}_{\text{mus}} = \bar{V}|Z_m| \tag{4.3.28}$$

where $\bar{p}_{\text{mus}}$ = average muscle pressure, N/m^2
$\quad\quad |Z_m|$ = amplitude of the mechanical impedance, $N \cdot sec/m^5$
$\quad\quad\quad = [R^2 + (T/2\pi C)^2]^{1/2}$
$\quad\quad \bar{V}$ = average inspiratory flow rate, m^3/sec
$\quad\quad\quad = 2\pi V_T/T$

Therefore,

$$\bar{p}_{\text{mus}} = \frac{V_T}{C}\sqrt{(2RC/T)^2 + 1} \tag{4.3.29}$$

When tidal volume is substituted by its equivalent alveolar ventilation rate and dead space, Equation 4.3.29, and the resulting expression for $\bar{p}_{\text{mus}}$, is differentiated to find the extremum. Average respiratory period which minimizes pressure amplitude and hence average muscle force is

$$T = (2\pi RC)^{2/3} (\dot{V}_A/V_D)^{-1/3} \tag{4.3.30}$$

Figure 4.3.31 shows frequency plotted from Equation 4.3.29 as minimum force amplitude,

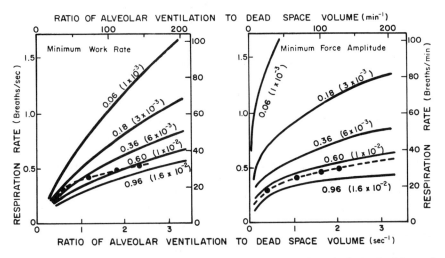

Figure 4.3.31 Data on actual respiratory rates match curves computed on the basis of minimum force amplitude (*right*) better than curves computed on the basis of minimum work rate (*left*). These curves were computed for various respiratory time constants in seconds (minutes). Data points are connected by the dashed line. (Adapted and used with permission from Mead, 1960.)

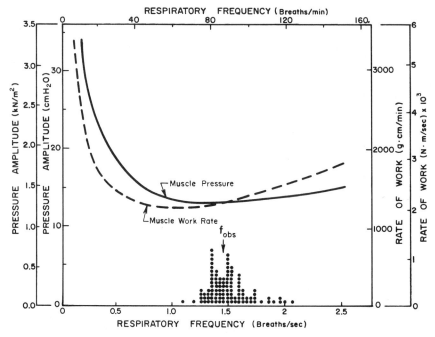

Figure 4.3.32 Comparison of optimization lines for respiratory work rate and respiratory muscle pressure with actually observed respiratory rate. Observed frequencies fall closer to the minimum of the curve for pressure than for power, leading Mead to the conclusion that respiratory force, not power, is minimized. (Adapted and used with permission from Mead, 1960.)

and frequency plotted from Equation 4.3.27 as minimum work rate. Plotted as data points are values of respiratory frequency observed on resting and lightly exercising (up to 102 N·m/sec) humans. As Mead (1960) points out, data values appear to be more consistent with the force amplitude criterion than the minimum work criterion. Mead also reports that respiratory time constant measurements on seven resting humans averaged 0.642 sec, which is extremely close to the time constant isopleth[84] of 0.66 sec upon which the data points fell in the force amplitude graph.

As mentioned earlier, the optimum frequency is not sharply defined. Figure 4.3.32 shows how broad the minimum is in each case. Because the minimum is so broad, frequency deviations from the optimum can occur without severe penalty of increased respiratory power or force amplitude. It is not surprising, then, that considerable breath-to-breath variability is observed in respiratory period in humans and animals.

Although Mead (1960) has presented considerable evidence that force amplitude, rather than respiratory power, controls respiratory period, present modeling is based on the latter criterion. The work by Ruttimann and Yamamoto (1972) showed that force amplitude as a criterion could not successfully predict airflow waveshape. Yamashiro and Grodins (1971, 1973) demonstrated considerable differences between waveshape and period at rest and exercise (Figures 4.3.33 and 4.3.34). Despite the fact that no direct evidence has been entered disclaiming Mead's hypothesis (modeling results excluded), perhaps these points can account for such large differences between

---

[84]The line on which lie corresponding values of the dependent and independent variables, here used as the line of unvarying time constant, *RC*.

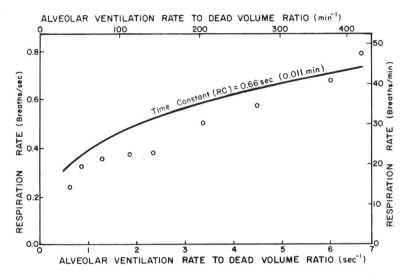

Figure 4.3.33 Comparison of theoretically predicted respiratory frequency for minimum force determination (line) with data from Silverman et al. (1951). (Adapted and used with permission from Yamashiro and Grodins, 1973.)

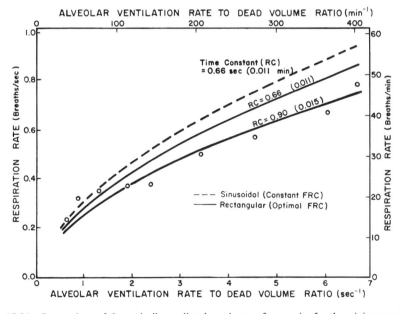

Figure 4.3.34 Comparison of theoretically predicted respiratory frequencies for the minimum work rate criterion (lines) with data from Silverman et al. (1951). Other assumptions about respiratory airflow waveshape and lung volumes are included. (Adapted and used with permission from Yamashiro and Grodins, 1973.)

force amplitude and minimum power predictions:

1. It is possible that force amplitude is minimized during rest and respiratory power is minimized during exercise.
2. Respiratory power predictions may be more sensitive to the assumption of sinusoidal waveform.
3. Mead's derivation contains a hidden constraint of constant midinspiratory position (Ruttimann and Yamamoto, 1972), which does not occur in reality.

More recently, in a series of papers Hämäläinen and co-workers (Hämäläinen 1973, 1975; Hämäläinen and Sipilä, 1980; Hämäläinen and Viljanen, 1978a,b,c) outlined a conceptual model of the optimal control of the respiratory system and provided a criterion for optimization which includes elements of minimum force and minimum power.

Hämäläinen's criterion for optimization, called the cost functional or performance functional, in the inhalation direction is

$$J_i = \int_0^{t_i} [\ddot{V}_i^2(t) + \alpha_i p_i(t) \dot{V}_i(t)] \, dt \tag{4.3.31}$$

where J_i = inspiratory cost functional, m^6/sec^3
   t_i = inhalation time, sec
   $\ddot{V}_i(t)$ = volume acceleration of the lung, m^3/sec^2
     = rate of change of lung airflow
   $p_i(t)$ = inspiratory pressure developed by the respiratory muscles, N/m^2
   $\dot{V}_i(t)$ = airflow rate, m^3/sec
   t = time, sec
   α_i = weighting parameter, $m^5/(N \cdot sec^3)$
and in the exhalation direction is

$$J_e = \int_{t_i}^{t_i + t_e} [\ddot{V}_e^2(t) + \alpha_e p_e^2(t)] \, dt \tag{4.3.32}$$

where J_e = expiratory cost functional, m^6/sec^3
   t_e = exhalation time, sec
   $\ddot{V}_e(t)$ = rate of change of airflow during exhalation, m^3/sec^2
   $p_e(t)$ = expiratory pressure developed by the respiratory muscles, N/m^2
   α_e = expiratory weighting parameter, $m^{10}/(N^2 \cdot sec^4)$

These cost functionals were developed based on some physiological considerations and with the goal of producing realistic respiratory waveforms.

The inspiratory criterion may be interpreted as the weighted sum of the average square of volume acceleration and the mechanical work produced by the inspiratory muscles. We have already discussed optimization based on muscular work, but it should be noted that muscular work may not be the ideal indicator of muscular load. In Sections 5.2.5 and 3.2.3, we see that muscular efficiency varies with the velocity of shortening and with the length of the muscle. Thus external work, as calculated from $p(t) V(t)$, as in Section 4.2.3, is not always a good indicator of the physiological load that the respiratory muscles represent. As we saw in Table 4.2.20, the oxygen cost of respiratory muscular work increases drastically during exercise. Oxygen consumption and external mechanical work are related through muscular efficiency, which varies. There is no clear indication whether the physiological optimization process operates to minimize mechanical work or oxygen consumption. The distinction between these two is not too important at this stage of our knowledge but may become important later as models are reconciled to physiological reality.

The average squared volume acceleration in J_i penalizes rapid changes in airflow rate. Inclusion of this term is based on:

1. The likely reduction in respiratory muscular efficiency with high accelerations [although Hämäläinen and Viljanen (1978a) indicate that no direct experimental verification of this effect in respiratory muscles has been reported].
2. The possibility of overstraining and tissue rupture at high accelerations.
3. The possibility of instability and poor control if rapid accelerations were tolerated.

In a later work, Hämäläinen and Sipilä (1980) modified the inspiratory cost functional yet further by including a term that accounted for the loss of efficiency with muscular load:

$$J'_i = \int_0^{t_i} \{ \ddot{V}_i^2(t) + [(1 + \beta_i p_i(t)) \{ \alpha_i p_i(t) \dot{V}_i(t) \}] \} \, dt \tag{4.3.33}$$

where β_i = a constant coefficient, m^2/N

The loss of efficiency has been assumed to be linear with muscular load, as represented by muscular pressure $p_i(t)$.

The expiratory cost functional is not the same as the inspiratory cost functional. Hämäläinen indicates that this is because the inspiratory muscles perform negative work by opposing expiration at the beginning of expiration. Thus muscular oxygen consumption is not represented well by the external mechanical work. Because the oxygen cost of negative work is different from the oxygen cost of positive work, these two types of work cannot be directly summed, even if absolute values are taken. Hämäläinen thus replaced the mechanical work term with the mean squared driving pressure as an index of the total cost of breathing.

The parameters α_i, α_e, and β_i are considered to be individual constants, the values of which differ from person to person. There is no direct means of measuring their values except to compare measured respiratory waveshapes with those predicted by modeling, and to adjust their values in the model until differences become minimal.

The force and power criteria of optimization are merged in these cost functionals. The first term in J_i can be seen to minimize something akin to mean squared force, and the second term to minimize respiratory work. The unity of this approach is appealing, as are the results of this approach, which show the transitions that occur in respiratory waveform from rest to exercise.

Breathing waveshapes are typified by those seen in Figure 4.3.35. Part A shows a typical resting breathing waveshape. Inhalation is sinusoidal and exhalation, being largely passive, is exponential. Part B shows a typical waveshape for moderate exercise. Both inhalation and exhalation are now active, and both appear to be nearly trapezoidal with rounded corners. The trapezoidal waveshape was shown to result from a minimization of respiratory power if airways resistance is taken to be inversely related to lung volume (Ruttimann and Yamamoto, 1972) or a result of minimizing J'_i with constant respiratory resistance (Hämäläinen and Sipilä, 1980). The rounded corners are probably a result of penalizing rapid accelerations, as included in both J_i and J'_i.

Typical respiratory waveforms for heavy exercise are seen in part C. Inhalation waveforms are still nearly trapezoidal, indicating that the same optimization process active in moderate exercise still governs heavy exercise. Exhalation, however, has reverted to exponential waveshapes. This is because exhalation flow rate is limited (Figure 4.2.19), and the value of the limiting flow rate decreases as lung volume decreases. The exhalation waveshape is no longer completely determined by neural control but is determined mainly by respiratory mechanical events. For any given tidal volume, exhalation time cannot decrease any further, and whether or not exhalation is still optimized has not been determined.

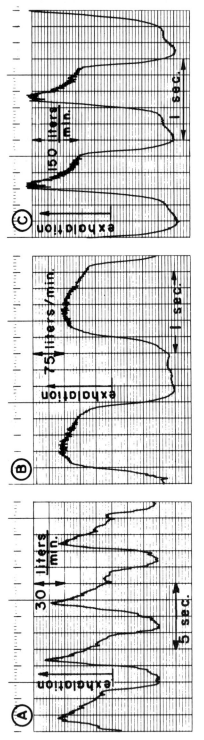

Figure 4.3.35 Typical progression of breathing waveshapes as exercise intensifies. Part *A* is a typical flow pattern at rest, with sinusoidal inhalation and exponential (passive) exhalation. During moderate exercise (*B*), inhalation and exhalation waveforms become trapezoidal in shape. Severe exercise (*C*) is accompanied by expiratory flow limitation resulting again in an expiratory exponential waveshape.

The dimples appearing in inhalation waveforms in parts B and C of Figure 4.3.35 are also seen quite often. The exact meaning of this topographical feature is not known, but, under some conditions of minimizing J_i', a dimple does appear in midinspiration.

Hämäläinen and Viljanen (1978b) presented a hierarchical context for respiratory optimization models to fit within (Figure 4.3.36). They assumed no details of the ventilatory demand process, but, once the demand for a certain alveolar ventilation rate is made known, the system is considered to provide this rate of alveolar ventilation within the framework of an optimal solution. First, the system is assumed to directly set respiration rate and inhalation time–exhalation time ratio (Johnson and Masaitis, 1976; Yamashiro et al., 1975). At this time, as well, the system may set respiratory dead volume. Widdicombe and Nadel (1963) were the first to propose that, since dead volume is proportional to airways volume but resistance is inversely related to airways volume, an optimal balance could be achieved. Other possibly optimized parameters include expiratory reserve volume (similar to preload on the heart: inspiration is made easier at the expense of expiration) and perhaps respiratory compliance (as respiratory muscle tone increases, compliance decreases). It may be that there are several control levels within this set of parameters, and that some of this set are conceptually determined before others. For instance, respiratory period must be settled before inhalation time can be determined.

Once these parameters are fixed, the lower level criteria (such as the J_i and J_e previously discussed) determine breathing waveshape. Considered to be constants at this lower level are the optimized parameters of the upper level. This can be seen, for example, in Equation 4.3.31, where inhalation time is assumed to be fixed.

Optimization models are considered further in Section 4.5. But for now, we summarize this discussion by noting that it appears to be true that respiratory responses to exercise are optimized; this is a reasonable presumption, but evidence for the optimization assertion rests

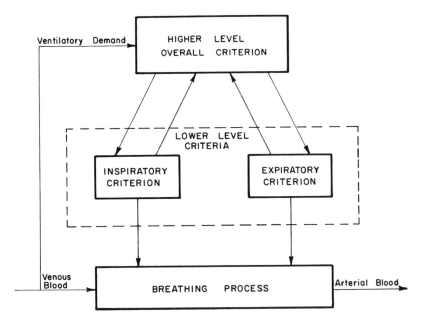

Figure 4.3.36 A schematic diagram of the hierarchical model of respiratory control. Ventilatory demand can be determined by chemoreceptors. Such basic quantities as respiration rate are optimized to reduce ventilatory muscle oxygen demand. Once respiration rate is determined, such variables as inhalation time/exhalation time ratio and breathing waveshape are optimized as well. (Used with permission from Hämäläinen and Viljanen, 1978b.)

with correspondence between modeling results and experimental measurements. At present, a total picture of the optimal controller is not available (Bates, 1986), nor is it clear that the correspondence between model results and experimental results is the consequence of an active optimization process or some preprogrammed genetic code.

Summary of Control Theories. There are certainly enough theories of respiratory control to explain exercise hyperpnea (Whipp, 1981). None, however, can account for all details of respiratory response. At the same time, none of the surviving theories has been conclusively proven to be false.

If there are weaknesses in these theories, two seem to be paramount. First, those control schemes proposed by bioengineers, and which appear to be reasonably successful in their modeling results, cannot be easily translated into physiological mechanisms with known sites, actions, and interconnections which can subsequently be tested by physiological experiment. Second, proposed control schemes do not appear to account for the tremendous amount of redundancy built into respiratory control: there may not be one important input as much as one hundred; there may be many different ways in which any given output state may be determined. Therefore, it is not surprising that each of these control theories only partly explains respiratory response to exercise, since each theory proposes the preeminence of a limited number of mechanisms.

Physiologists have for years debated the relative importance of neural and humoral mechanisms of control. The humoral component is presumed to be related to one or more of the following: $\dot{V}_{CO_2}$, pCO_2, pH, $\dot{V}_{O_2}$, metabolites, and oxygen saturation blood hemoglobin. Most physiologists assume that the humoral component of respiratory regulation is too slowly developed to be responsible for the rapid increase in ventilation at the onset of exercise, but they also assume that the humoral component is the major contributor to the steady-state respiratory response (Whipp, 1982). This assumption is still the subject of controversy because some scientists claim that humoral causes also control rapid responses at the onset of exercise.

Neural control mechanisms are thought to arise in muscle spindles, joint proprioceptors, muscle thermoreceptors, the cerebral cortex, and elsewhere. Because these inputs are thought to be connected directly and indirectly by means of the nervous system to the respiratory control areas of the brain, they are considered to result in rapid ventilatory responses. They are usually not considered to be the major contributor to steady-state respiratory response. Again, there is some controversy over that assumption, and we have already seen in this section that neurogenic mechanisms can underlie at least part of the steady-state response.

More specific theories have been advanced to explain steady-state and slow responses of respiration. The first of these involves some amount of steady-state error in the mean arterial level of pCO_2 or H^+. The steady-state ventilatory response would then be proportional to this error.

$$\dot{V}_E = k(pCO_2 - p_nCO_2) \tag{4.3.34}$$

where $\dot{V}_E$ = minute volume, m^3/sec

$\quad k$ = coefficient of proportionality, m^5/(sec·N)

p_nCO_2 = "normal," or set-point, value of arterial partial pressure of carbon dioxide, N/m^2
As simple as this theory is, however, it does not seem to reflect the true situation in normal subjects, where changes (which, if any, are small) in mean arterial pCO_2 or pH are viewed as a consequence, rather than the cause, of ventilatory adjustments (Whipp, 1981).

A variation of this theory asserts that a steady-state error in pH can exist at chemoreceptor sites without a measurable change in arterial pH. This is because carbonic anhydrase is found in the interior of the erythrocyte but not in the plasma. Due to differences in the time it takes to establish equilibrium between CO_2, H_2CO_3, and HCO_3^- (see Equation 3.2.3) in plasma and red blood cells, blood perfusing the carotid bodies could be more acid than whole blood (Whipp,

1981). Whereas this effect has been demonstrated theoretically and in the laboratory, it has yet to be proved important in real life.

It has been mentioned previously that Whipp (1981) and others (Miyamoto et al., 1983) observed that ventilation follows CO_2 delivery to the lungs. That is, the cardiac output (or rate of blood flow to the lungs) times blood concentration of carbon dioxide must be matched by an appropriate alveolar ventilation rate or a change in blood pCO_2 is bound to occur. This change would then act as a powerful stimulant to the respiratory controller to correct the pCO_2 error. While this particular idea of respiratory control begs the question of control mechanisms, it is a simple statement of respiratory reaction. From a simple mass balance,

$$CO_2 \text{ delivered to the lung} = CO_2 \text{ removed by the blood} + CO_2 \text{ removed by air} \quad (4.3.35)$$

$$\dot{Q}_{\text{pulm}} c_{vCO_2} = \dot{Q}_{\text{pulm}} c_{aCO_2} + \dot{V}_A F_{eCO_2}|_{\text{alv}} \quad (4.3.36)$$

where $\dot{Q}_{\text{pulm}}$ = pulmonary perfusion, or cardiac output, m^3/sec
c_{CO_2} = carbon dioxide concentration, m^3/m^3
$\dot{V}_A$ = alveolar ventilation rate, m^3/sec
$F_{eCO_2}|_{\text{alv}}$ = fraction of CO_2 in alveolar air, m^3/m^3
a, v = subscripts denoting arterial and venous values

From Table 4.2.2, resting cardiac output is $10^{-4}\, m^3/\text{sec}$, and from Table 4.2.8, alveolar mass fraction of carbon dioxide is $0.056\, m^3/m^3$. From Table 3.2.1, resting values of carbon dioxide concentration in arterial and venous blood for males are 0.490 and $0.531\, m^3\, CO_2/m^3$ blood, respectively. Therefore,

$$\dot{V}_A = \frac{Q_{\text{pulm}}(c_{vCO_2} - c_{aCO_2})}{F_{eCO_2}|_{\text{alv}}} \quad (4.3.37)$$

$$= 7.32 \times 10^{-5}\, m^3/\text{sec}$$

By adding the dead volume ventilation rate

$$\dot{V}_D = V_D/T \quad (4.3.38)$$

where $\dot{V}_D$ = rate of dead volume ventilation, m^3/sec
V_D = dead volume, m^3
T = respiratory period, sec
we obtain

$$\dot{V}_E = \dot{V}_A + \dot{V}_D \quad (4.3.39)$$

where $\dot{V}_E$ = minute volume, m^3/sec
From Table 4.2.4, $V_D = 180 \times 10^{-6}\, m^3$, and $T = 4\, \text{sec}$. Calculated $\dot{V}_E$ then becomes $118 \times 10^{-3}\, cm^3/\text{sec}$, which compares favorably to the tabled (approximate) value of 100×10^{-3} cm^3/sec. The conclusion of this calculation is that alveolar ventilation rate appears to be calculable from cardiac output and pulmonary arterial–venous carbon dioxide concentration difference.

The last theory of respiratory regulation which is to be summarized here is based not on steady-state carbon dioxide values but on the oscillations that occur in the blood during the normal respiratory cycle. This theory of control was proposed by Yamamoto (1960). It is the contention of this theory that average values of pCO_2 and pH can remain constant, but because exercising conditions produce more CO_2 and lower pH compared to rest, the depth of

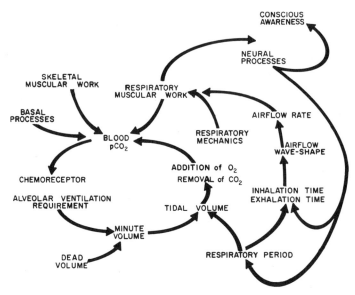

Figure 4.3.37   Control loops for respiration. The chemical loop assures adequate ventilation to remove excess CO_2 and the neural loop ensures that ventilation is maintained at least cost. If, for some reason such as a limitation on exhalation flow rate, least cost cannot be preserved, ventilation is forced to increase. Such a situation can lead to instability in respiratory control for respiratory-impaired subjects. (Adapted from Johnson, 1980.)

oscillations increases. These oscillations are felt at the level of the carotid bodies, and it has been shown that carotid chemoreceptors are rate sensitive (Whipp, 1981). Indeed, there has been demonstrated a periodicity in carotid chemoreceptor discharge which matches the oscillations in the blood (Whipp, 1981).

There seems to be other supporting evidence for this mechanism of control. Decreasing blood oscillations of pCO_2 and pH by means of a mixing chamber has been found to decrease minute volume in cats (Whipp, 1981). Results of this experiment are not so easy to interpret, however, because other conditions, besides oscillations, also changed. The fact that subjects without carotid bodies respond to exercise with steady-state values of minute volume which are not significantly different from those of control subjects casts doubt on the importance of oscillations, at least in the steady state (Whipp, 1981).

A schematic diagram of respiratory control (Johnson, 1980) seen in Figure 4.3.37 illustrates the two main control loops for respiration. The two control criteria seem to be to (1) maintain CO_2 levels (2) at least cost. When these two control criteria cannot be maintained, the situation certainly calls for alarm. Normally, no degree of exercise is sufficient to cause this lack of control. But maximal exercise being performed in a respiratory protective mask can be one instance when control is lost.

To give some idea of the problems that might be encountered, imagine this scenario: the subject works on a bicycle ergometer at a constant rate of 250 N·m/sec while wearing a mask. The mask has enough resistance and dead volume to roughly double the resistance and dead volume he must breathe through without the mask. As his muscles work, they produce CO_2, which, in turn, requires a higher minute ventilation.[85] His respiratory system answers the need by breathing faster and somewhat deeper, as dictated by the minimization of respiratory power. The

[85]Martin et al. (1984) showed that respiratory muscles are required to anaerobically metabolize energy to sustain high exercise levels. This would cause an even greater ventilatory stimulus due to lowered blood pH.

mask makes his respiratory muscles work harder than usual. The slow trend toward faster breathing is suddenly interrupted by a limitation on the rate at which he can exhale. The respiratory response is no longer optimized, and his respiratory muscles become less efficient, producing more CO_2 for a given minute ventilation increment than they did before. This requires faster breathing, which produces more CO_2, which requires faster breathing, and so on. The system is now effectively out of control.

The result, as we have seen in the laboratory, is an end point which is characterized by:

1. Panic—a strong feeling of breathlessness is developed.
2. Persistence—the feeling continues for several minutes after the cessation of exercise.
3. Pointedness—there is a clear indication that the mask is a major contributor to the feeling of breathlessness. (Remove the mask and the feeling goes away.)

Interestingly, we have not been able to duplicate this end point in any subject who once experienced it. This could mean that there are unconscious physiological clues which the subject learns to seriously heed to avoid ever having to face that situation again.

This scenario is a practical illustration of respiratory control and its limitations.

4.4   RESPIRATORY MECHANICAL MODELS

Respiratory mechanical models are many and varied. For the sake of presentation, these models are classified as (1) models of respiratory mechanics, including airflow models and mechanical parameter models, (2) gas transport models, and (3) other types of models, including models of pulmonary vasculature (Heijmans et al., 1986; Linehan and Dawson, 1983), muscle mechanics (Macklem et al., 1983), and lung deformation (Ligas, 1984; Vawter, 1980). The third classification of models is not included here, because these models are too specific for our discussion. Nevertheless, they may appear to be of extreme interest to some respiratory mechanical modelers.

4.4.1   Respiratory Mechanics Models

Again, some discrimination between models must be performed to distinguish between the many respiratory mechanical models which have been proposed. Some models have as their sole purpose the improved measurement of respiratory mechanical parameters (Clément et al., 1981; de Wilde et al., 1981; Johnson et al., 1984; Lorino et al., 1982; Nada and Linkens, 1977; Peslin et al., 1975). That is, measurements are forced to conform to general model schemes in order to extract best estimates of resistance, compliance, and other respiratory mechanical parameters. These models are not reviewed here because their general predictive ability is limited. Some other models have special purposes, such as improved design and use of hospital ventilators (Barbini, 1982), estimation of lung diffusing capacity (Prisk and McKinnon, 1987), and deposition of aerosol particles (Kim et al., 1983). These models are not reviewed here. Of the models not included, the one by Hardy et al. (1982) is worthy of note because of its inclusiveness, but its emphasis is circulatory, and it is not as illustrative as those included here.

The two types of models reviewed here are examples of general predictive respiratory mechanical models and several more specific flow-determining models.

Jackson–Milhorn Computer Model. This model is a comprehensive model of respiratory mechanics which responds realistically. Jackson and Milhorn (1973) modeled the lungs as two compartments within the pleural space and chest wall (Figure 4.4.1). Figure 4.4.1 shows the various pressures that act on model elements.

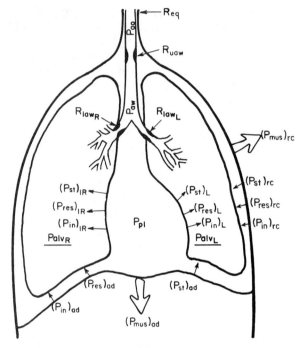

Figure 4.4.1   Schematic diagram of the respiratory system showing the pressures acting on the lungs, rib cage, and abdomen–diaphragm. Resistance and pressure symbols are defined in the text. (Used with permission from Jackson and Milhorn, 1973.)

As with many of these models, Jackson and Milhorn began with a basic pressure balance:

$$p_{app} = p_{st} + p_{res} + p_{in} \qquad (4.4.1)$$

where p_{app} = pressure applied to any element of the respiratory system, N/m^2
$\quad p_{st}$ = static recoil pressure due to compliance, N/m^2
$\quad p_{res}$ = pressure loss due to resistance, N/m^2
$\quad p_{in}$ = pressure loss due to inertance, N/m^2

As in Figure 4.4.1, they portrayed the respiratory system with two lung compartments, representing right and left lungs, and two thoracic components, representing rib cage and abdomen–diaphragm.

Pressure balances on each of these components yields, for the lungs,

$$p_{alvR} - p_{pl} = (p_{st})_{lR} + (p_{res})_{lR} + (p_{in})_{lR} \qquad (4.4.2a)$$

$$p_{alvL} - p_{pl} = (p_{st})_{lL} + (p_{res})_{lL} + (p_{in})_{lL} \qquad (4.4.2b)$$

where p_{alv} = alveolar pressure, N/m^2
$\quad p_{pl}$ = pleural pressure, N/m^2

and the subscript l denotes lungs, subscripts L and R specify left or right. Then for the rib cage

$$p_{pl} + (p_{mus})_{rc} - p_{bs} = (p_{st})_{rc} + (p_{res})_{rc} + (p_{in})_{rc} \qquad (4.4.3)$$

where p_{mus} = respiratory muscle pressure, N/m^2
$\quad p_{bs}$ = body surface pressure, N/m^2

and the subscript rc denotes rib cage. Then for the abdomen–diaphragm

$$p_{pl} + (p_{mus})_{ad} - p_{bs} = (p_{st})_{ad} + (p_{res})_{ad} + (p_{in})_{ad} \qquad (4.4.4)$$

where the subscript ad denotes abdomen–diaphragm.

Static recoil pressure due to compliance can be calculated from

$$p_{st} = (V - V_r)/C \qquad (4.4.5)$$

where V = lung volume, m^3

V_r = resting, or stable, volume, m^3

C = compliance, m^5/N

Instead, it appears that Jackson and Milhorn numerically evaluated recoil pressure from pressure–volume characteristics, as given later.

Resistive pressure is calculated from

$$p_{res} = \dot{V} R \qquad (4.4.6)$$

where $\dot{V}$ = flow rate, m^3/sec

R = resistance, N·sec/m^5

and inertial pressure is calculated from

$$p_{in} = \ddot{V} I \qquad (4.4.7)$$

where $\ddot{V}$ = volume acceleration, m^3/sec^2

I = inertance, N·sec^2/m^5

Jackson and Milhorn included nonlinear and time-dependent compliance characteristics within their model. The three static recoil pressures, $(p_{st})_l$, $(p_{st})_{rc}$, and $(p_{st})_{ad}$, are estimated in different ways. Rib cage and abdomen–diaphragm pressure–volume characteristics (the slope is compliance) were assumed to be those in Figure 4.4.2. Their model determined static recoil pressures once lung volume was known.

Static recoil pressure of the lungs was developed from lung tissue and lung surfactant (see Sections 4.2.1 and 4.2.3):

$$(p_{st})_l = (p_{st})_{sur} + (p_{st})_{lt} \qquad (4.4.8)$$

where $(p_{st})_{sur}$ = surfactant static recoil pressure, N/m^2

$(p_{st})_{lt}$ = lung tissue recoil pressure, N/m^2

Jackson and Milhorn (1973) based their lung surfactant model on the results of Archie (1968), who developed an equation defining elastic recoil pressure as a result of surface tension forces of a thin surfactant film at the air–liquid interface. The equation assumes that a film of constant thickness lines the alveolar surfaces and that surface tension of this film is inversely proportional to the concentration of two different macromolecules diffusing to and from this film from an underlining bulk phase having constant concentration. The equations they used are

$$(p_{st})_{sur} = MV \left(1.0 - \sum_{i=1}^{z} \left\{ L_i \left[1.0 - \frac{1.0}{H_i(t) + G_i(t)} \right] \right\} \right) \qquad (4.4.9)$$

and

$$H_i(t) = (V_{A\infty}^2 / V^2)(c_{i0}/c_{i\infty})e^{-t/\tau_i} \qquad (4.4.10)$$

and

$$G_i(t) = [e^{-t/\tau_i}/V^2] \int_0^t (V^2/\tau_i)e^{t/\tau_i} dt \qquad (4.4.11)$$

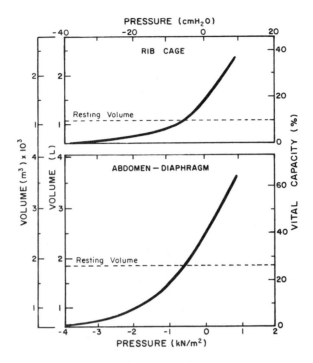

Figure 4.4.2 Static pressure–volume relationships for the rib cage and the abdomen–diaphragm. (Adapted and used with permission from Jackson and Milhorn, 1973.)

where M = proportionality constant, N/m^5

V = lung volume, m^3

$(c_{i0}/c_{i\infty})$ = ratio of initial concentration to the equilibrium concentration of the ith constituent, dimensionless

L_i = dimensionless constant

τ_i = diffusion time constant of the ith constituent, sec

t = time, sec

$V_{A\infty}$ = alveolar volume where thermodynamic equilibrium occurs, m^3

Values for these parameters are listed in Table 4.4.1. These equations predict hysteresis, the gradual decline in compliance with constant tidal volume, and the return to greater compliance following a deep breath or sigh.

The tissue component of lung compliance pressure was obtained empirically by matching model results to published experimental results. Tissue recoil pressure was obtained by subtraction of calculated surfactant pressure from experimental stop-flow results. The result appears in Figure 4.4.3, where the curve represents the tissue pressure–volume characteristic for each lung.

Tissue resistance values used by Jackson and Milhorn are similar to those presented in Table 4.2.15. They used a minimum value for lung tissue resistance, which became very small compared to airway resistance. They did not mention the value used.

Because they intended to simulate high breathing rates, Jackson and Milhorn included inertial pressures. In partitioning total respiratory inertance, they assumed that pulmonary inertance and chest wall inertance appear in series, but that rib cage and abdomen–diaphragm inertance (together comprising chest wall inertance) act in parallel with each other. Pulmonary inertance is composed mainly of inertance of the gases in the airways and a somewhat smaller amount of lung tissue inertance. Inertance values are given in Table 4.4.1.

TABLE 4.4.1   Parameter Values for the Jackson–Milhorn Respiratory Mechanical Model[a]

Parameter	Value	Units	
$(c_{i0}/c_{i\infty})$	1.0	Dimensionless	
L_1	0.7	Dimensionless	
L_2	0.7	Dimensionless	
τ_1	600	sec	(10 min)
τ_2	0.6	sec	(0.01 min)
M	294	kN/m^5	(3.0 cm H_2O/L)
$V_{A\infty}$	0.003	m^3	(3.0 L)
R_{rc}	196	$kN \cdot sec/m^5$	(2.0 cm $H_2O \cdot sec$/L)
R_{ad} (abdomen diaphragm)	196	$kN \cdot sec/m^5$	(2.0 cm $H_2O \cdot sec$/L)
R_{lt} (lung tissue)	(unspecified minimum value)		
I_{ad}	8.60	$kN \cdot sec^2/m^5$	(0.08 cm $H_2O \cdot sec^2$/L)
I_{rc}	2.10	$kN \cdot sec^2/m^5$	(0.02 cm $H_2O \cdot sec^2$/L)
I_g (gas)	774	$N \cdot sec^2/m^5$	(0.0079 cm $H_2O \cdot sec^2$/L)
I_{lt}	137	$N \cdot sec^2/m^5$	(0.0014 cm $H_2O \cdot sec^2$/L)
I_{uaw}	519	$N \cdot sec^2/m^5$	(0.0053 cm $H_2O \cdot sec^2$/L)
I_{law}	255	$N \cdot sec^2/m^5$	(0.0026 cm $H_2O \cdot sec^2$/L)
I_m (mouthpiece 20 cm long by 1.5 cm dia)	911	$N \cdot sec^2/m^5$	(0.0093 cm $H_2O \cdot sec^2$/L)
K_{1e}	37	$kN \cdot sec/m^5$	(0.38 cm $H_2O \cdot sec$/L)
K_{2e}	77	$MN \cdot sec^2/m^8$	(0.79 cm $H_2O \cdot sec^2/L^2$)
K_{1i}	30	$kN \cdot sec/m^5$	(0.31 cm $H_2O \cdot sec$/L)
K_{2i}	34	$MN \cdot sec^2/m^8$	(0.35 cm $H_2O \cdot sec^2/L^2$)
G_2	222	Dimensionless	
G_1	1265	cm^3	(1.265 L)
V_{uaw}	70	cm^3	(70 mL)
G_3	0.50	$(N \cdot sec/m^2)^{1/2}$	(0.05 (cm $H_2O \cdot sec)^{1/2}$)
C_{p1}	51×10^{-9}	m^5/N	(0.005 L/cm H_2O)

[a] Compiled from Jackson and Milhorn, 1973.

Air movement in each of the conducting airways was assumed to occur as a unit of mass. This air was assumed to be incompressible (compliance therefore is zero). A pressure difference between two successive compartments causes movement of the air column connecting them. Jackson and Milhorn assumed four distinct airway compartment types: alveolar space, lower airways, upper airways, and mouthpiece. There are two (left and right) alveolar and lower airways compartments in parallel. These compartments are schematically diagramed in Figure 4.4.4.

Considering first the mouthpiece and associated equipment gives

$$p_{bs} - p_{ao} = R_m(dV_1/dt) + I_m(d^2V_1/dt^2) \tag{4.4.12}$$

where p_{bs} = body surface pressure, N/m^2

p_{ao} = airway opening pressure, N/m^2

R_m = mouthpiece resistance, $N \cdot sec/m^5$

I_m = mouthpiece inertance, $N \cdot sec^2/m^5$

V_1 = volume of air moving from mouthpiece to atmosphere (across point 1), m^3

To determine p_{ao}, the upper airway compartment must be considered. During inspiration there is a mass of air entering the upper airway compartment equal to the air density ρ times V_1. Likewise, the mass of air leaving the compartment is ρV_2. The rate of change of mass is thus

$$dm_{uaw}/dt = \rho_1 \dot{V}_1 - \rho_2 \dot{V}_2 \tag{4.4.13}$$

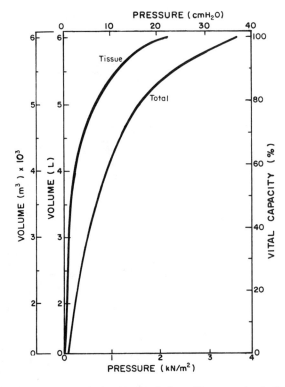

Figure 4.4.3 Static pressure–volume relationships for the lung. Shown are the elastic recoil pressure due to elastic tissue and the total static elastic recoil pressure of the lung. (Adapted and used with permission from Jackson and Milhorn, 1973.)

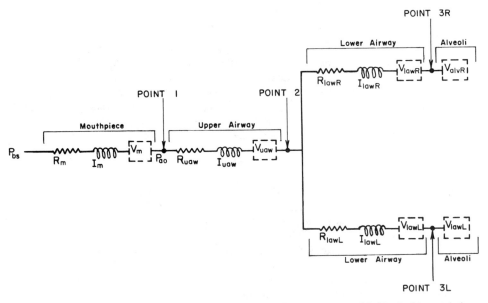

Figure 4.4.4 Schematic representation of the Jackson and Milhorn airway model. (Used with permission from Jackson and Milhorn, 1973.)

where m_{uaw} = mass in upper airway compartment, kg

ρ = air density, kg/m^3

$\dot{V}_2$ = rate of change of volume moving from upper airway to mouthpiece (across point 2), m^3

and

$$dm_{uaw} = (\rho_1 \dot{V}_1 - \rho_2 \dot{V}_2)dt \qquad (4.4.14)$$

$$\Delta m_{uaw} = \rho_1 V_1 - \rho_2 V_2 \qquad (4.4.15)$$

where Δm_{uaw} = change of mass in the upper airway compartment in an arbitrary time interval Δt, kg

The change of density within the upper airway compartment is

$$\Delta \rho_{uaw} = \Delta m_{uaw}/V_{uaw} = (\rho_1 V_1 - \rho_2 V_2)/V_{uaw} \qquad (4.4.16)$$

where V_{uaw} = upper airway volume, m^3

The bulk modulus B is defined (Anderson, 1967) as

$$B = \rho \, dp/d\rho \qquad (4.4.17)$$

where B = bulk modulus, N/m^2

This becomes

$$dp_{ao} = B(d\rho/\rho) = (B/\rho_{uaw})(\rho_1 V_1 - \rho_2 V_2)/V_{uaw} \qquad (4.4.18)$$

where $dp_{ao} \cong \Delta p_{ao}$ – the change in airway opening pressure between any two instances of time, N/m^2

Substituting Equation 4.4.18 into Equation 4.4.12 yields

$$I_m(d^2 V_1/dt^2) + R_m(dV_1/dt) + (B\rho_{bs} V_1/\rho_{uaw} V_{uaw}) - (BV_2/V_{uaw}) - p_{bs} = 0 \qquad (4.4.19)$$

Since airway density changes by no more than 1% with a pressure change of 980 N/m^2 (10 cm H$_2$O), Equation 4.4.19 can be simplified by assuming all densities to have the same value. Thus for the mouthpiece

$$I_m(d^2 V_1/dt^2) + R_m(dV_1/dt) + (B/V_{uaw})V_1 - (B/V_{uaw})V_2 - p_{bs} = 0 \qquad (4.4.20)$$

A similar equation for the upper airway is

$$I_{uaw}(d^2 V_2/dt^2) + R_{uaw}(dV_2/dt) + [(B/V_{law} + B/V_{uaw})] V_2$$
$$- (B/V_{law})V_{aL} - (B/V_{law})V_{aR} - (B/V_{uaw})V_1 = 0 \qquad (4.4.21)$$

where I_{uaw} = upper airway inertance, N·sec^2/m^5

R_{uaw} = upper airway resistance, N·sec/m^5

V_{law} = lower airway volume, m^3

V_{aL} = volume of air moving between left lung lower airways compartment and upper airways, m^3

V_{aR} = volume of air moving between right lung lower airways compartment and upper airways, m^3

For the lower airways (left lung)

$$I_{lawL}(d^2V_{aL}/dt^2) + R_{lawL}(dV_{aL}/dt) + [(B/V_{AL}) + (B/V_{law})]V_{aL}$$
$$- (B/V_{law})V_2 + (B/V_{law})V_{aR} - (B/V_{AL})\Delta V_{AL} = 0 \qquad (4.4.22)$$

where I_{lawL} = lower airway inertance of left compartment, $N \cdot sec^2/m^5$
R_{lawL} = lower airway resistance of left compartment, $N \cdot sec/m^5$
V_{AL} = alveolar volume of left lung, m^3
ΔV_{AL} = change in alveolar volume, m^5

A similar equation for the right lung lower airways is

$$I_{lawR}(d^2V_{aR}/dt^2) + R_{lawR}(dV_{aR}/dt) + [(B/V_{AR}) + (B/V_{law})]V_{aR}$$
$$- (B/V_{law})V_2 + (B/V_{law})V_{aL} - (B/V_{AR})\Delta V_{AR} = 0 \qquad (4.4.23)$$

Solution of these closely coupled equations must begin with a known change in alveolar volume and then volume changes may be successively calculated between each of the other compartments.

Pressure changes within each compartment are calculated from

$$\Delta p_{ao} = (B/V_{uaw})(V_1 - V_2) \qquad (4.4.24)$$

$$\Delta p_{aw} = (B/V_{law})(V_2 - V_{aR} - V_{aL}) \qquad (4.4.25)$$

$$\Delta p_{alvR} = (B/V_{alvR})(V_{aR} - \Delta V_{alvR}) \qquad (4.4.26)$$

$$\Delta p_{alvL} = (B/V_{alvL})(V_{aL} - \Delta V_{alvL}) \qquad (4.4.27)$$

Values for constants in Equations 4.4.12–4.4.27 appear in Table 4.4.1. From the ideal gas law, the value for bulk modulus of a gas is equal to the static pressure of the gas for isothermal compression. For adiabatic compression, the bulk modulus for air is 1.4 times the static pressure.[86]

To describe airway resistance, Jackson and Milhorn considered upper and lower airway resistances separately. Upper airway resistance was described using the Rohrer model with different values for inhalation and exhalation coefficients:

$$R_{uawi} = K_{1i} + K_{2i}\dot{V}_i \qquad (4.4.28a)$$

$$R_{uawe} = K_{1e} + K_{2e}\dot{V}_e \qquad (4.4.28b)$$

where i denotes inspiration and e denotes expiration. Lower airway resistances (left and right) are described by

$$R_{lawR} = 2/(G_2 V_{AR} - G_1) \qquad (4.4.29a)$$

$$R_{lawL} = 2/(G_2 V_{AL} - G_1) \qquad (4.4.29b)$$

where G_2 and G_1 are constants.

The use of these equations to describe lower airways resistances thus includes the effect of lung volume on the sizes of the very distensible small airways. Since these airways are thought to close when lung volume reaches residual volume, the ratio G_1/G_2 must represent residual volume in each lung because at $V_A = G_1/G_2$, R_{law} tends to ∞.

---

[86]The value 1.4 is the ratio of specific heat at constant pressure to specific heat at constant volume. This value holds approximately for all diatomic gases (Hawkins, 1967).

Upper airways volume was assumed to be a constant $70 \, cm^3$. Lower airways volume, on the other hand, was assumed to vary significantly. Jackson and Milhorn derived their relationship between lower airways volume and lower airways resistance in the following manner.

The volume of a tube with circular cross section is

$$V_{law} \propto r^2 l \qquad (4.4.30a)$$

where r = tube radius

l = tube length

If airflow in these airways obeys Poiseuilles' law (see Section 3.2.2), then resistance is proportional to length and inversely proportional to the radius to the fourth power:

$$R_{law} \propto l/r^4 \qquad (4.4.30b)$$

Thus

$$V_{law} \propto (l^3/R_{law})^{1/2} \qquad (4.4.30c)$$

Jackson and Milhorn cite some evidence that the length of the lower airways in excised lungs is a function of the cube root of the lung volume.[87] Thus

$$V_{law} = G_3 [V_A/R_{law}]^{1/2} \qquad (4.4.30d)$$

where G_3 = constant coefficient, $(N \cdot sec)^{1/2}/m$

V_A = alveolar volume of left and right lungs, m^3

The next compartment to be considered is the pleural cavity. Changes in respiratory system volume can be generated only by movement of rib cage and/or abdomen–diaphragm. This volume change must be accompanied by a change in either or both lung and pleural cavity. Therefore, changes in volume of abdomen–diaphragm and/or rib cage are reflected by a change in volume of pleural cavity and/or lungs:

$$\Delta V_{ad} + \Delta V_{rc} = \Delta V_{pl} + \Delta V_A \qquad (4.4.31)$$

The pleural space is depicted as very stiff (has low compliance of $53 \times 10^{-9} \, m^5/N$):

$$\Delta p_{pl} = - \Delta V_{pl}/C_{pl} \qquad (4.4.32)$$

where C_{pl} = pleural compliance, m^5/N

The negative sign preceding the change in pleural volume indicates that a smaller volume is accompanied by an increase in pressure.

Two driving pressures were used by Jackson and Milhorn. These driving pressures take the form of time-varying muscle pressures applied to the model. The first condition describes normal resting breathing [oxygen consumption $5 \times 10^{-6} \, m^3/sec$ (300 mL/min)]:

$$p_{mus} = 671t + 574t^2 - 474t^3, \qquad 0 \leqslant t \leqslant 1.25 \text{ sec} \qquad (4.4.33a)$$

$$p_{mus} = 1760 - 980t + 130t^2, \qquad 1.25 \leqslant t \leqslant 3.5 \text{ sec} \qquad (4.4.33b)$$

$$p_{mus} = 0, \qquad 3.5 < t \qquad (4.4.33c)$$

where p_{mus} = muscle pressure, N/m^2

---

[87] One would expect tube length to vary with the cube root of lung volume on purely dimensional grounds. Tube length has a dimension of length, L. Lung volume, which comprises many of these tubes and their alveolar extensions, has a dimension of L^3. Thus tube length would be expected to vary as volume to the one-third power. The same general philosophy is used in calculation of binary mixture diffusivities (Equation 4.2.29).

During exercise [oxygen consumption 56.88×10^{-6} m^3/sec (3413 mL/min)]

$$p_{\text{mus}} = 784 + 2210 \sin(5.03t - 0.179) \tag{4.4.34}$$

Jackson and Milhorn assumed parallel rib cage and abdomen–diaphragm contributions to muscle pressure, so that

$$p_{\text{mus}} = (p_{\text{mus}})_{\text{ad}} = (p_{\text{mus}})_{\text{rc}} \tag{4.4.35}$$

where $(p_{\text{mus}})_{\text{ad}}$ = abdomen–diaphragm contribution to muscle pressure, N/m^2
    $(p_{\text{mus}})_{\text{rc}}$ = rib cage contribution to muscle pressure, N/m^2

The structure of their model requires implicit, or iterative, methods of solution at several points. Unfortunately, details of this process were not given in their original paper (see Appendix 3.1 for solution methods). Jackson and Milhorn programmed their model on a digital computer and simulated respiratory system response to spontaneous breathing at rest and during exercise. They also simulated two very rapid disturbances produced by (1) the interrupter technique for estimating dynamic alveolar pressure and (2) the stop-flow technique for determining the quasistatic pressure–volume relationships of the lung. Two pathological conditions which were simulated were (1) decreased concentration of surfactant and (2) unilateral partial airway obstruction. Results from these simulations are described only partially here.

Figure 4.4.5 shows experimental and model results of alveolar volume, airflow, and muscle pressure for spontaneous breathing at rest. The calculated experimentally derived driving pressure produced a tidal volume of 480×10^{-6} m^3 and maximum volume occurring at 1.55 sec. Experimental peak airflow rates were 450×10^{-6} m^3/sec (expiration) and 500×10^{-6} m^3/sec (inspiration); model peak airflow rates were 350×10^{-6} m^3/sec (expiration) and 550×10^{-6} m^3/sec (inspiration). Other results simulating rest were reasonably good as well.

Exercise simulation did not yield as close agreement between model and experiment. In Figure 4.4.6 are shown some of these comparisons between experimental and model results for muscle pressure, airflow, and lung volume. The authors attribute the disagreement mainly to the driving pressure used, since it was derived with airway resistance assumptions different from those used in their model.

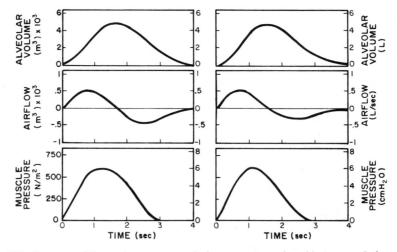

Figure 4.4.5   Response of the respiratory system during spontaneous breathing at rest. Leftmost curves were determined experimentally. Righmost curves were obtained from the computer model. (Adapted and used with permission from Jackson and Milhorn, 1973.)

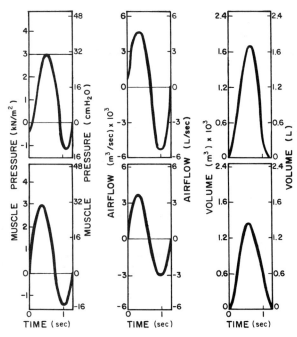

Figure 4.4.6 Response of the respiratory system during spontaneous breathing while exercising. Upper curves were determined experimentally. Lower curves were obtained from the computer model. (Adapted and used with permission from Jackson and Milhorn, 1973.)

One notable result involves calculated airway resistance values. During rest, upper airway resistance and lower airway resistance are of nearly equal magnitude. During exercise, however, most of the airway resistance occurs in the upper airways. Indeed, resistance pressure drops during rest and exercise were very great compared to inertance pressure drops, and the inclusion of inertances probably was not necessary to satisfactory model results for all but the rapid airway interruption maneuver.

Expiratory Flow Model. The notion of expiratory flow limitation has already been introduced in Section 4.2.3. Lambert et al. (1982) produced a model which has been adjusted to yield good agreement with experimental results.

Lambert et al. began by assuming the ideal lung geometry given by Weibel (Section 4.2.1), where the conducting airways form a symmetric bifurcating tree. Airway mechanics were assumed to change more or less smoothly from one generation to the next, with lower airways being more compliant than upper airways. The trachea was assumed to have the same mechanical properties as the bronchi. Within this system, flow was considered to be steady and incompressible. All pressures were referenced to pleural pressure, and peribronchial pressure was assumed equal to pleural pressure. Alveolar gas pressure was assumed to be uniform and equal to static recoil pressure at each lung volume:

$$p = p_{st} - p_{kin} - p_{fric} \qquad (4.4.36)$$

where p = net lateral airway pressure, N/m^2
  p_{st} = static pressure (no flow), N/m^2
  p_{kin} = kinetic pressure component, N/m^2
  p_{fric} = friction pressure loss, N/m^2

This can be expanded to give

$$p = p_{st} - \tfrac{1}{2}\rho(\dot{V}/A)^2 - \int_0^x f\,dx \qquad (4.4.37)$$

where ρ = gas density, kg/m^3
$\quad \dot{V}$ = volume rate of flow, m^3/sec
$\quad A$ = total cross-sectional area of all airways in the nth generation, m^2
$\quad f$ = friction pressure loss per unit distance, N/m^3
$\quad dx$ = distance along airway axis, m

The pressure gradient along the airway axis is obtained by differentiating Equation 4.4.37 with respect to x:

$$\frac{dp}{dx} = 0 + (\rho \dot{V}^2/A^3)\frac{dA}{dx} - f \qquad (4.4.38)$$

Here, the volume rate of flow cannot vary with x unless flow is unsteady, but total generational cross-sectional area is assumed to vary from generation to generation (see Table 4.2.1).

$$\frac{dp}{dx}\left[1 - (\rho \dot{V}^2/A^3)\frac{dA}{dp} \right] = -f \qquad (4.4.39)$$

and

$$\frac{dp}{dx} = -f\left/\left[1 - (\rho \dot{V}^2/A^3)\frac{dA}{dp} \right]\right. \qquad (4.4.40)$$

From Equation 4.2.79,

$$\dot{V}_{ws}^2 = v_{ws}^2 A^2 = \left(\frac{1}{\rho}\frac{dp}{dA}\right)A^3 \qquad (4.2.79)$$

which combines with Equation 4.4.40 to give

$$dp/dx = -f/(1 - \dot{V}^2/\dot{V}_{ws}^2) \qquad (4.4.41)$$

As the flow speed $\dot{V}$ approaches wave speed $\dot{V}_{ws}$, the pressure gradient along the direction of the conducting airways becomes very large. Apparent resistance of the airways thus becomes very large as well.

Since the geometry of the bronchial tree is so complicated, it is difficult to obtain an accurate expression for the distribution of viscous pressure loss f. An empirical formula used by Lambert et al. is

$$f = \frac{8\pi\mu\dot{V}}{A^2}(3.4 + 2.1 \times 10^{-3}\,\mathrm{Re}) \qquad (4.4.42)$$

where μ = fluid (air) viscosity, kg/(m·sec)
$\quad \mathrm{Re}$ = local Reynolds number, dimensionless

$$\mathrm{Re} = 2\rho\dot{V}/\mu\sqrt{\pi A} \qquad (4.4.43)$$

where ρ = density, kg/m^3

As Lambert et al. explain, the coefficient $8\pi\mu\dot{V}/A^2$ is the pressure loss per unit length in Poiseuille flow (see Equations 3.2.12 and 4.4.30b). At low Reynolds numbers, laminar viscous pressure losses in the branching network are 3.4 times larger than for flow in a long, smooth-walled, straight rigid pipe. At high Reynolds numbers, the second term in parentheses in Equation 4.4.42 predominates. This term, which describes fully turbulent dissipative losses, gives a pressure loss quadratic in $\dot{V}$. Both terms are equivalent at a local Reynolds number of 1600. Both terms together give a pressure loss in the airways similar to the Rohrer equation (4.2.61) in that pressure loss is determined by a term linear in $\dot{V}$ and another quadratic in $\dot{V}$.[88]

Pressure is computed in steps, beginning at the periphery (alveolus) and working toward central airways (bronchi and trachea). Equation 4.4.41 is integrated over the length of the nth generational airway to obtain a pressure drop along that airway. The friction pressure loss is calculated using the empirical relationship in Equation 4.4.42. At the junction between generations, transitional flow is assumed to take place over such a short distance that frictional dissipation $f\,dx$ is considered negligible. Equation 4.4.37 can thus be evaluated at the two points represented by the end (distance $= L$) of the $(n+1)$th generation and the beginning (distance $= 0$) of the nth generation. The pressure difference at the junction is thus

$$p_{n+1}(L) - p_n(0) = \tfrac{1}{2}\rho\,\dot{V}^2[1/A_n^2(0) - 1/A_{n+1}^2(L)] \tag{4.4.44a}$$

where $p_n(0)$ = pressure at beginning of nth generation airway, N/m^2
  $p_{n+1}(L)$ = pressure at end of $(n+1)$th generation airway, N/m^2
  $A_n(0)$ = cross-sectional airway area at beginning of nth generation, m^2
  $A_{n+1}(L)$ = cross-sectional airway area at end of $(n+1)$th generation, m^2

Equation 4.4.44a is assumed true if the area at the convergence of the airways decreases, that is, if $A_n(0) \leqslant A_{n+1}(L)$. If, on the other hand, intergenerational airways area increases, no pressure difference is assumed:

$$p_{n+1}(L) - p_n(0) = 0, \qquad A_n(0) \geqslant A_{n+1}(L) \tag{4.4.44b}$$

As seen in Tables 4.2.1 and 4.4.2, total cross-sectional area of all airways in any generation increases from the nth generation to the $(n+1)$th generation. Therefore, Equation 4.4.44a would be expected to be used at every junction. However, due to certain combinations of airway distensibility and pressure drops, the condition $A_n(0) \geqslant A_{n+1}(L)$ may hold, and Equation 4.4.44b would be required. Since the choice between these two equations demands knowledge of airway area, Lambert et al. developed a model of airway dimensions.

Airways are described as characterized by a maximum area modified by transmural pressure. The assumed shape of this relation, as illustrated in Figure 4.2.21, is similar to the pressure–volume characteristics for the entire lung, seen in Figure 4.2.23. This relationship is described by two rectangular hyperbolas matched in value and slope at zero pressure. These curves are normalized by dividing airway by maximum airway area:

$$\alpha = A/A_m \tag{4.4.45}$$

where α = normalizing model parameter, dimensionless
  A_m = maximum total cross-sectional generational airway area, m^2

---

[88]In an airway cast model, Slutsky et al. (1980) found the Moody friction factor for central human airways to decrease linearly with tracheal Reynolds number until the Reynolds number became 500. Above a Reynolds number of 5000, there was no further change in friction factor. In between was an extended transition zone where the friction factor decreased at a rate proportional to the square root of the Reynolds number. Because branching angles of the airways in the upper lobes were greater than those of the lower lobes, resistances to the upper lobes were greater and flow was less than to the lower lobes.

TABLE 4.4.2 Model Parameters of Bronchial Mechanical Properties

Z^a	α_0	α'_0	n_1	n_2	A_m, cm^2	L,^{b} cm
0	0.882	0.000011	0.50	10.00	2.37	12.00
1	0.882	0.000011	0.50	10.00	2.37	4.76
2	0.686	0.000051	0.60	10.00	2.80	1.90
3	0.546	0.000080	0.60	10.00	3.50	0.76
4	0.450	0.000100	0.70	10.00	4.50	1.27
5	0.370	0.000125	0.80	10.00	5.30	1.07
6	0.310	0.000142	0.90	10.00	6.50	0.90
7	0.255	0.000159	1.00	10.00	8.00	0.76
8	0.213	0.000174	1.00	10.00	10.20	0.64
9	0.184	0.000184	1.00	10.00	12.70	0.54
10	0.153	0.000194	1.00	10.00	15.94	0.47
11	0.125	0.000206	1.00	9.00	20.70	0.39
12	0.100	0.000218	1.00	8.00	28.80	0.33
13	0.075	0.000226	1.00	8.00	44.50	0.27
14	0.057	0.000233	1.00	8.00	69.40	0.23
15	0.045	0.000239	1.00	7.00	113.00	0.20
16	0.039	0.000243	1.00	7.00	180.00	0.17

Source: Used with permission from Lambert et al., 1982.

$^a Z$ = airway generation
$^b L$ = length of airway.

These two hyperbolas are given by

$$\alpha = \alpha_0(1 - p/p_1)^{-n_1}, \qquad p \leqslant 0 \qquad (4.4.46a)$$

and

$$\alpha = 1 - (1 - \alpha_0)(1 - p/p_2)^{-n_2}, \qquad p \geqslant 0 \qquad (4.4.6b)$$

where α_0 = value of α at $p = 0$, dimensionless
p_1, p_2 = vertical asymptotes for the two hyperbolas, N/m^2
n_1, n_2 = hyperbola parameters, dimensionless
They are chosen to match in value at $p = 0$. They are also chosen so that their slopes match at the intersection point (Figure 4.4.7). This produces equations for the vertical asymptotes p_1 and p_2:

$$p_1 = \alpha_0 n_1/\alpha'_0 \qquad (4.4.47a)$$

$$p_2 = -n_2(1 - \alpha_0)/\alpha'_0 \qquad (4.4.47b)$$

where $\alpha'_0 = d\alpha/dp$ at $p = 0$, m^2/N

Values of α_0, α'_0, n_1, n_2, A_m, and airway length L used in the model are given in Table 4.4.2. Values were chosen to match, as closely as possible, experimental data from Weibel (1963) and Hyatt et al. (1980). Estimates for α_0 for central airways (low generational numbers) were easily obtained from these experimental data and appear to have an approximately logarithmic decrease with generation number. For peripheral airways, however, no experimental data were available to guide the choice of α_0. The logarithmic decrease was thus extrapolated, although the slope was increased somewhat for the smaller airways. Lambert et al. argued that if the airways behaved isotropically with the lung, airway dimensions would vary with the cube root of lung volume. However, for the smaller airways, the finite wall thickness becomes important, and airway luminal diameter would decrease much more than the cube root of lung volume. The value for α_0, which refers to lumen area, would be very low. Estimates of α'_0 were chosen to bring the airway area–pressure curves to near maximal area at reasonable pressures. The complete set

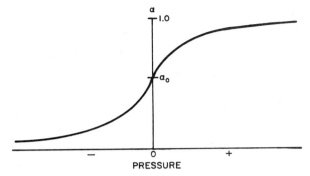

Figure 4.4.7 Matched rectangular hyperbolas used to describe airway pressure–area behavior. Fractional airway area α is plotted against transmural pressure. Separate equations are utilized for positive and negative values of pressure, and two hyperbolas are matched in value and slope at α_0, the value at zero pressure. (Used with permission from Lambert et al., 1982.)

of model A/A_m versus p curves, as outlined in Figure 4.4.7, appears in Figure 4.4.8. The curve for the trachea (generation 0) was assumed to be identical to that for the bronchi (generation 1).

The calculation procedure used by Lambert followed this general course: for each static recoil pressure, a relatively small value of $\dot{V}$ was chosen, and Equations 4.4.44a or b and 4.4.46a and b were solved at the entrance of generation 16. Equation 4.4.41 was integrated along the airway, using an airway area from the curves in Figure 4.4.8 for each local value of p at each point. This procedure was repeated for each generation to the end of the trachea. The value of $\dot{V}$ was then

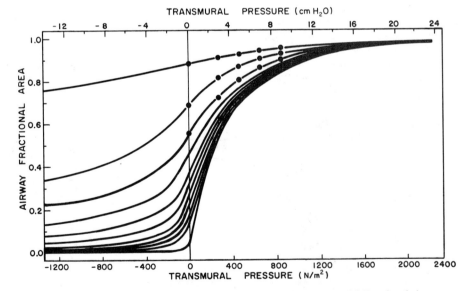

Figure 4.4.8 Airway mechanical properties utilized in the expiratory flow model. Fractional airway cross-sectional area α is plotted against transmural pressure for each airway generation from trachea (top curve), second through tenth, and sixteenth generation (bottom curve). (Adapted and used with permission from Lambert et al., 1982.)

increased, and the procedure was repeated. This continued until one of these three conditions was met:

1. Local velocity came within 99.9% of wave speed at some point in the bronchial tree.
2. There was no simultaneous solution to Equations 4.4.44a or b and 4.4.46a and b, indicating that wave speed would be exceeded at the junction.
3. The pressure became less than -9803 N/m^2 ($-100 \text{ cm H}_2\text{O}$).

When one of these occurred, a smaller increment of flow was tried until a flow increment of $10^{-8} \text{ m}^3/\text{sec}$ (0.01 L/sec) exceeded maximal flow, where the calculation was halted. Therefore, all maximal flows are within $10^{-8} \text{ m}^3/\text{sec}$ of wave speed or else a pressure decrease of -9803 N/m^2 was produced. The location where one of these conditions occurs is the flow-limiting site.

Figure 4.4.9 presents some results from the Lambert study. The upper portion shows the isovolume pressure–flow relationships which Lambert et al. calculated. Notice the similarity between these curves and those of Figure 4.2.19. In Figure 4.4.10 airway resistance is plotted from the slopes of the curves in Figure 4.4.9 at a flow rate of $5 \times 10^{-8} \text{ m}^3/\text{sec}$ for corresponding lung volumes. Figure 4.4.11 presents model predictions of the flow-limiting site as a function of static recoil pressure. At high recoil pressures (and high lung volumes), expiratory airflow is limited in the central airways of main bronchi or trachea. At low recoil pressures (and low lung volumes), expiratory flow is limited more and more peripherally. Although the movement of flow-limiting segments has been confirmed experimentally (Smaldone and Smith, 1985), this type of predictive ability best illustrates the use of models in biological systems.

Ventilation Distribution Model with Nonlinear Components. A considerably different sort of mechanical model was presented by Shykoff et al. (1982). This model, although relatively simple in overall construction, differed from many other respiratory models by incorporating nonlinearities into its respiratory components.

The intention of the model was to determine what differences in gas distribution within the lung can be expected from variations of pleural pressure in different parts of the lung. Unequal lung filling had previously been blamed mainly on unequal time constants in different portions of the lung. New experimental evidence had suggested, however, that pleural pressures were distributed unevenly between upper and lower chest, that these differences were affected by the patterns of muscle use during spontaneous breathing, and that these pressure differences might, indeed, produce variations in lung filling.

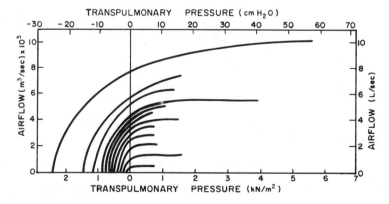

Figure 4.4.9   Model predictions of isovolume pressure–flow (IVPF) relationships. (Adapted and used with permission from Lambert et al., 1982).

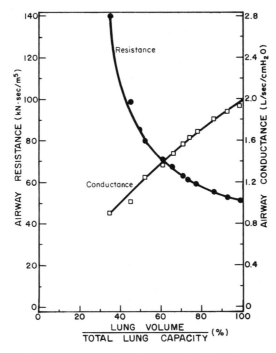

Figure 4.4.10 Airway conductance computed from the slope of individual IVPF curves in Figure 4.4.9 at a flow rate of 5×10^{-4} m^3/sec (0.5 L/sec). Lung volume was obtained from the model pressure–volume curve. (Adapted and used with permission from Lambert et al., 1982.)

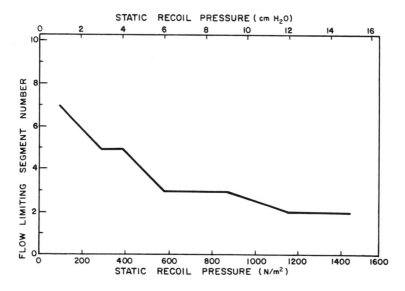

Figure 4.4.11 Location of flow-limiting segments in the lung as determined from the model. As lung volume (and static pressure) increases, the flow-limiting segment nears the mouth. (Adapted and used with permission from Lambert et al., 1982.)

To test the hypothesis of a connection between pleural pressure differences and lung filling, Shykoff et al. proposed a two-compartment lung model. The upper and lower compartments were treated in a parallel arrangement, and each was considered to be represented by a resistance and compliance in series. Each was exposed to a different variable pleural pressure. A common resistance connected the two compartments (Figure 4.4.12).

Model equations for the common pathway are

$$p_m - p_b = R_c \dot{V} \tag{4.4.48}$$

where p_m = pressure at the entrance to the common airway, N/m²
  p_b = pressure at exit from common airway, N/m²
  R_c = common airway resistance, N·sec/m⁵
  $\dot{V}$ = volume flow rate, m³/sec
and

$$\dot{V}_i = \dot{V}_1 + \dot{V}_2 \tag{4.4.49}$$

where $\dot{V}_i$ = flow rate to compartment i, m²/sec ($i = 1$ or 2)
For each compartment,

$$p_b - p_i = R_i \dot{V}_i \tag{4.4.50}$$

$$dV_i = C_i d(p_i - p_{\text{pl}i}) \tag{4.4.51}$$

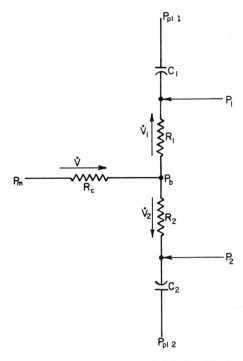

Figure 4.4.12 Shykoff et al. (1982) two-compartment model of the lung. Resistances and compliances are considered to be nonlinear. Symbols are defined in the text.

where p_i = pressure in compartment i, N/m^2
R_i = resistance in compartment i, N·sec/m^5
V_i = volume in compartment i, m^3
p_{pli} = pleural pressure on compartment i, N/m^2
C_i = compliance in compartment i, m^5/N
Equations used for compliance were

$$C_i = \frac{(V_{max}^* - V^*)^2 (V_{min}^* - V^*)^2}{\lambda_1 (V_{min}^* - V^*)^2 + \lambda_2 (V_{max}^* - V^*)^2} \frac{VC}{100} \qquad (4.4.52)$$

$$V^* = 100(V - RV)/VC$$

where V_{max}^*, V_{min}^* = constants, dimensionless
λ_1, λ_2 = constants, N/m^2
VC = vital capacity, m^3
RV = residual volume, m^3
Resistance was given by

$$R = \frac{k_1 + k_2 \dot{V}}{k_3 + k_4 V} \qquad (4.4.53)$$

where R = resistance, N·sec/m^5
k_1 = constant, N·sec/m^5
k_2 = constant, N·sec^2/m^8
k_3 = constant, dimensionless
k_4 = constant, m^{-3}
Values for these constants are found in Table 4.4.3.

TABLE 4.4.3 Constants of the Compliance and Resistance Relationships Used by Shykoff et al.

Constant	Value	
Compliance (lobes 1 and 2)		
λ_1	147.05 kN/m^2	(1500 cm H$_2$O)
λ_2	4901 N/m^2	(50.0 cm H$_2$O)
V_{max}^*	135	(135% VC)
V_{max}^*	−2.0	(−2.0% VC)
Resistance (common)		
k_1	29.4 kN·sec/m^2	(0.3 cm H$_2$O·sec/L)
k_2	39.2 × 10^6 N·sec^2/m^8	(0.4 cm H$_2$O·sec^2/L^2)
k_3	1.0	(1.0)
k_4	0.0 m^{-3}	(0.0 L^{-1})
Resistance (lobes 1 and 2)		
k_1	29.4 kN·sec/m^2	(0.3 cm H$_2$O·sec/L)
k_2	39.2 × 10^6 N·sec^2/m^8	(0.4 cm H$_2$O·sec^2/L^2)
k_3	0.17	(0.17)
k_4	300 m^{-3}	(0.3 L^{-1})

Source: Adapted and used with permission from Shykoff et al., 1982.

Airflow into these compartments was driven by sinusoidal, square, or triangular waveforms superimposed on a static pressure difference. The amplitudes of the pressures were independently varied on the two compartments; a range of static pressures and frequencies was used; and a phase lag between compartments was introduced for sinusoidal and square-wave pleural pressure variations.

The authors found that at low pleural pressure amplitudes and frequencies (up to 490 N/m^2 at 0.25 breath/sec), there was essentially no difference between results using constant compliance and resistance values and those using nonlinear values. At higher frequencies the differences become greater at lower amplitudes, and at higher amplitudes the differences become greater at lower frequencies. Compliance nonlinearities are more important at low flow rates, but resistance nonlinearities are increasingly more important at higher flow rates.

The ratio of volumes in compartments 1 and 2 does not change appreciably for sinusoidal, square, or triangular pleural pressure waveforms. Thus Shykoff et al. conclude that the waveform of the pleural pressure swing has no effect on the distribution of tidal volumes, unless very high initial flow rates are generated.

Oscillatory intralung airflow which does not involve the source is called pendelluft. Pendelluft occurs in the lungs when one compartment, lobe, or portion fills faster than another and eventually delivers part of its volume to another compartment, lobe, or portion. Pendelluft was demonstrated in the model of Shykoff et al. and is illustrated in Figure 4.4.13 for the case of a sinusoidal pleural pressure variation and no phase angle between compartments. As seen in

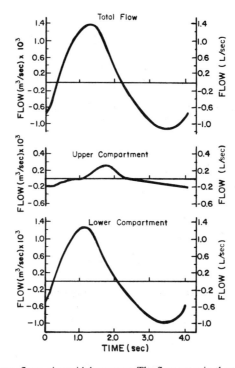

Figure 4.4.13 Instantaneous flows, sinusoidal pressure. The flow rates in the total lung model, the upper compartment, and the lower compartment are shown as a function of time. The pressure amplitude on the upper compartment is 98 N/m^2 (1.0 cm H$_2$O) and that on the lower is 735 N/m^2 (7.5 cm H$_2$O). The static pleural pressure difference is 392 N/m^2 (4 cm H$_2$O), and the pleural pressure variations on the compartments are in phase. (Adapted and used with permission from Shykoff et al., 1982.)

Figure 4.4.13, the lower compartment fills first, followed by emptying into the upper compartment.

Although this model is a very simple one in structure as well as results, it has yielded important information. The effects of nonlinearities are perhaps best highlighted by a model as limited in scope as this one is.

Theory of Resistive Load Detection. The last of the respiratory mechanical models to be included here is interesting because of the way it illustrates how modeling can be used to suggest mechanisms of action. In this case, the model suggests, in a more rigorous manner than previously attempted, how addition of resistance to the respiratory system can be detected.

The model by Mahutte et al. (1983) begins with the general concept of length–tension inappropriateness discussed previously (see Section 4.3.4). This concept involves the detection of a mismatch between the demanded motor act and the achieved result. What Mahutte et al. did was to show how this detection could occur. Note, however, that even the most rational model results may differ from reality by huge amounts.

Mahutte et al. began by assuming muscle pressure as a function of time to be a single sinusoidal pulse:

$$p_{mus} = p_{max} \sin(2\pi f t), \qquad 0 < t < \frac{1}{2f} \qquad (4.4.54)$$

$$= 0, \qquad t < 0 \text{ and } t > \frac{1}{2f}$$

where p_{mus} = muscle pressure, N/m^2
$\quad p_{max}$ = maximum muscle pressure amplitude, N/m^2
$\quad f$ = respiratory frequency, breaths/sec
$\quad t$ = time, sec

A simple mechanical description of the respiratory system was assumed:

$$R \, dV/dt + V/C = p_{mus} \qquad (4.4.55)$$

where R = resistance, $N \cdot sec/m^2$
$\quad C$ = compliance, m^5/N
$\quad V$ = lung volume, m^3

The resulting airflow is thus

$$\dot{V} = dV/dt = (p_{max}/R) \sin\theta \, [\cos(2\pi f t - \theta)$$
$$- (\cos\theta) \exp(-2\pi f t/\tan\theta)] \qquad (4.4.56)$$

where θ = phase angle between applied pressure and resting flow, rad

$$\theta = \tan^{-1}(2\pi f R C) \qquad (4.4.57)$$

Adding a small resistance, ΔR, would change the phase angle to θ_R:

$$\theta_R = \tan^{-1}[2\pi f C(R + \Delta R)] \qquad (4.4.58)$$

Mahutte et al. assumed that resistive load detection occurs if a critical change occurs in phase angle. That is, if $(\theta_R - \theta) \geqslant \theta_{crit}$,

$$\tan^{-1}[2\pi f(R + \Delta R)C] - \tan^{-1}[2\pi f R C] \geqslant \theta_{crit} \qquad (4.4.59)$$

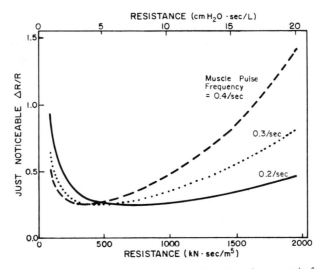

Figure 4.4.14 Effects of increasing resistance on the just-noticeable resistance ratio for three values of muscle pulse frequency. The shape of each of these curves is the same as the characteristic of the Weber–Fechner law. (Adapted and used with permission from Mahutte et al., 1983.)

Solving for $\Delta R/R$ yields

$$\frac{\Delta R}{R} = \frac{1}{2\pi f RC} \tan\left[\theta_{\text{crit}} + \tan^{-1}(2\pi f RC)\right] - 1 \tag{4.4.60a}$$

$$= \cot\theta \tan\left[\theta_{\text{crit}} + \theta\right] - 1 \tag{4.4.60b}$$

The just-noticeable added resistance must satisfy the preceding equation.

Mahutte et al. added another insight to their model. This phase angle can be detected by a time difference, and since we know the brain contains a sense of time, probably resulting from a neural oscillator and a counter mechanism,[89] the just-noticeable additional resistance could possibly be detected by a time delay schema. Use of the following reasonable values of respiratory parameters:

$R = 294 \text{ kN} \cdot \text{sec/m}^5 (3 \text{ cm H}_2\text{O} \cdot \text{sec/L})$
$C = 980 \text{ kN/m}^5 (10 \text{ cm H}_2\text{O/L})$
$f = 0.27 \text{ breath/sec} (16 \text{ breaths/min})$
$\Delta R/R = 0.3$

give $\theta_{\text{crit}} = 0.11 \text{ rad} (6.5°)$, or a critical delay time of $0.08–0.1$ sec. The authors discuss this result as highly reasonable in view of experimental observations on neural circuit times.

This model also predicts (Figure 4.4.14) a nonconstant ratio of just-noticeable added resistance to previously existing resistance ($\Delta R/R$). This is an interesting result, one which has been observed with biological threshold phenomena (Weber–Fechner law) other than resistance detection,[90] but which has yet to be confirmed with added respiratory resistance. Model results

[89]Or, more likely, it result from the potentiation of a neural outburst by summation of many subthreshold transmembrane potentials.
[90]For instance, the sensitivity to sound level has a characteristic similar to the shape in Figure 4.4.14.

also predict an effect of respiratory compliance on $\Delta R/R$, which, again, has yet to be experimentally confirmed.

4.4.2 Gas Concentration Models

The objective of these models is to reproduce the distribution of various gas species within the respiratory gas-conduction passages, and to demonstrate the dependence of this distribution on the respiratory mechanical properties considered in previous models. Visser and Luijendijk (1982) presented a drawing of an old Chinese model (Figure 4.4.15) which incorporates nine bronchial segments and six lobes. They indicated that at that time divisibility by 3 was more important than reality for the number of elements of a model. More modern models have certainly reproduced reality much better than the old Chinese model and, because of this, have come to be depended upon for predictions that cannot be easily measured.

Concentration Dynamics Model. The one model to be considered in detail involves pulmonary mechanics and gas concentration dynamics in a nonlinear model (Lutchen et al., 1982). The objective of this model is to show how mechanical parameters of the lung produce pendelluft, the distribution of dead volume gas to other lung compartments, the distribution of compartmental resting and tidal volumes, and differences in compartmental gas concentrations.

This model begins with a multicompartmental analysis of the lung, as seen in Figure 4.4.16. The three distinct compartments are the conducting airway and dead volume (1) and two parallel alveolar compartments (2 and 3). Each alveolar compartment is assumed to possess perfect gas mixing and to vary in volume. The dead space compartment does not possess gas mixing during flow—that is, gas flow through the dead volume occurs as a slug of gas displaces the previously resident gas—and is of constant volume. There is a mixing point at the common junction of all three compartments where gas from the dead volume mixes with gas in the alveolar compartments. Effects of gas compression are neglected and only inert, insoluble tracer gases which take no part in alveolar-capillary transport are considered. Only small tidal volumes

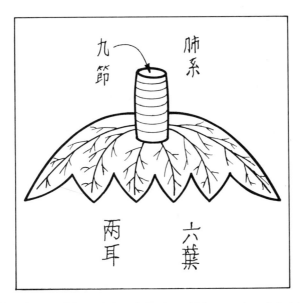

Figure 4.4.15 Chinese lung model, consisting of nine bronchial segments and six lobes. (Redrawn from Visser and Luijendijk, 1982.)

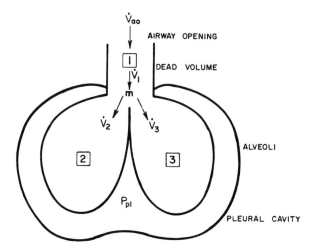

Figure 4.4.16 Lutchen et al. (1982) model structure with conducting airway (1) and alveolar compartments (2 and 3). V_1 equals the dead space volume. (Used with permission from Lutchen et al., 1982. © 1982 IEEE.)

(compared to end-expiratory volume) and low breathing rates (less than 1 breath/sec) are considered.

Because dead volume is assumed to be constant, lung volume changes occur only by means of changes in the alveolar compartments, or

$$\dot{V}_L = \dot{V}_2 + \dot{V}_3 \qquad (4.4.61)$$

where $\dot{V}_L$ = total lung flow rate, m³/sec
$\dot{V}_i$ = flow rate into compartment i, m³/sec
A pressure balance on the model yields

$$p_{tp} = (p_{ao} - p_m) + (p_m - p_{pl}) \qquad (4.4.62)$$

where p_{tp} = transpulmonary pressure, N/m²
p_{ao} = pressure at the airway opening, N/m²
p_{pl} = pleural pressure, N/m²
To describe each pressure difference appearing on the right-hand side of Equation 4.4.62, relatively simple yet nonlinear impedances were used. Considering the upper airways to be rigid (no compliance) and breathing rates to be low (negligible inertance) gives

$$(p_{ao} - p_m) = R_{uav} \dot{V}_L \qquad (4.4.63)$$

where R_{uaw} = constant upper airway resistance, N·sec/m⁵
Pressure drop across each alveolar compartment was assumed to depend on resistance and compliance. Resistance of the peripheral airways within these alveolar compartments is assumed to be inversely related to compartment volume (see Section 4.2.3):

$$R_{law} = r_i/V_i \qquad (4.4.64)$$

where R_{law} = lower airway resistance for compartment i, N·sec/m⁵
r_i = specific resistance of compartment i, N·sec/m²
V_i = volume of each compartment, m³

An exponential equation form was used to describe the elastic behavior of the lung parenchyma:

$$C_i = V_i/[h_i \exp(V_i/\varepsilon_i)] \tag{4.4.65}$$

where C_i = compartment compliance, m^5/N
h_i = pressure coefficient, N/m^2
ε_i = volume coefficient, m^3
Transpulmonary pressure becomes

$$p_{tp} = R_{uaw}\dot{V}_L + r_i\dot{V}_i/V_i + h_i \exp(V_i/\varepsilon_i) \tag{4.4.66}$$

Transpulmonary pressure will be used as the input forcing function causing flow into or out from compartments. This flow becomes

$$\dot{V}_2 = \left(\frac{V_2}{V_2 R_{uaw} + r_2}\right)[-R_{uaw}\dot{V}_3 - h_2 \exp(V_2/\varepsilon_2) + p_{tp}] \tag{4.4.67a}$$

$$\dot{V}_3 = \left(\frac{V_3}{V_3 R_{uaw} + r_3}\right)[-R_{uaw}\dot{V}_2 - h_3 \exp(V_3/\varepsilon_3) + p_{tp}] \tag{4.4.67b}$$

Two forms for the forcing function were used. The one giving values closest to most reported results consists of a periodic exponential rise and exponential fall:

$$p_{tp} = p_0 + p\left\{1 - \exp[-(t - t_e(k))]/\tau_r\right\}, \qquad t_e(k) \leqslant t \leqslant t_i(k) \tag{4.4.68a}$$

$$p_{tp} = p_0 + P\exp\{-[t - t_i(k)]/\tau_f\}, \qquad t_i(k) \leqslant t \leqslant t_e(k+1) \tag{4.4.68b}$$

where p_0 = pressure constant, N/m^2
P = pressure factor, N/m^2
$t_e(k)$ = starting time for expiration k, sec
$t_i(k)$ = starting time for inspiration k, sec
τ_r = time constant of pressure rise, sec
τ_f = time constant of pressure fall, sec
Using values listed in Table 4.4.4, the inspiratory time was 2.67 sec, expiratory time was 1.33 sec, and respiration rate was 0.25 breath/sec.

The transpulmonary pressure was also simulated using a sinusoid:

$$p_{tp} = p_0 + P_s[1 - \cos(2\pi f t)] \tag{4.4.69}$$

where P_s = sinusoidal pressure factor, N/m^2
f = breathing frequency, breaths/sec
Gas transport equations were developed for the inert tracer gas. Axial diffusion is neglected and plug transport occurs in the dead volume. Therefore, the volume of gas entering at the airway opening does not reach the mixing point (at the junction of compartments 1, 2, and 3) until after a time delay. For the first breath of the tracer gas,

$$c_{im} = \begin{cases} c_0, & \Delta V_L < V_D \\ c_{in}, & \Delta V_L > V_D \end{cases} \tag{4.4.70}$$

TABLE 4.4.4   Parameter Values Used in the Gas Dynamical Model[a]

Parameter	Value	
R_{uaw}	$133 \, kN \cdot sec/m^5$	$(1.36 \, cm \, H_2O \cdot sec/L)$
r_2 (normal)	$159 \, N \cdot sec/m^2$	$(1.62 \, cm \, H_2O \cdot sec)$
r_3 (normal)	$159 \, N \cdot sec/m^2$	$(1.62 \, cm \, H_2O \cdot sec)$
r_2 (obstructed)	$159 \, N \cdot sec/m^2$	$(1.62 \, cm \, H_2O \cdot sec)$
r_3 (obstructed)	$2.45 \, kN \cdot sec/m^2$	$(25.00 \, cm \, H_2O \cdot sec)$
h_2 (normal)	$54.1 \, N/m^2$	$(0.552 \, cm \, H_2O)$
h_3 (normal)	$54.1 \, N/m^2$	$(0.552 \, cm \, H_2O)$
h_2 (obstructed)	$54.1 \, N/m^2$	$(0.552 \, cm \, H_2O)$
h_3 (obstructed)	$235 \, N/m^2$	$(2.400 \, cm \, H_2O)$
ε_2 (normal)	$680 \times 10^{-6} \, m^3$	$(0.68 \, L)$
ε_3 (normal)	$680 \times 10^{-6} \, m^3$	$(0.68 \, L)$
ε_2 (obstructed)	$680 \times 10^{-6} \, m^3$	$(0.68 \, L)$
ε_3 (obstructed)	$2050 \times 10^{-6} \, m^3$	$(2.05 \, L)$
τ_r	$0.11 \, sec$	
τ_f	$0.22 \, sec$	
P	$392 \, N/m^2$	$(4 \, cm \, H_2O)$
p_0	$490 \, N/m^2$	$(5 \, cm \, H_2O)$
P_s	$196 \, N/m^2$	$(2 \, cm \, H_2O)$
f	$0.25/sec$	
$[t_e(k) - t_i(k)]$	$2.67 \, sec$	
$[t_i(k) - t_e(k)]$	$1.33 \, sec$	
Initial V_L	$3150 \times 10^{-6} \, m^3$	$(3.15 \, L)$
V_D	$150 \times 10^{-6} \, m^3$	$(0.15 \, L)$
Initial V_i	$1500 \times 10^{-6} \, m^3$	$(1.5 \, L)$

[a]Compiled from Lutchen et al., 1982.

where c_{im} = gas concentration entering the mixing point from the dead volume compartment, M^3/m^3

c_0 = initial concentration throughout the lung, m^3/m^3

c_{in} = input concentration, m^3/m^3

ΔV_L = change in lung volume from the beginning of an inspiration, m^3

V_D = dead volume, m^3

Equation 4.4.70 thus states that the concentration of gas at the mixing point does not change from the initial lung concentration unless a sufficient change in lung volume clears old gases from the dead volume.

Similarly, during expiration, the first gas delivered to the airway opening has the input concentration of the tracer gas. If the input gas had reached the mixing point during the previous inspiration, then exhaled gas at the airway opening would have the concentration

$$c_{ao} = \begin{cases} c_{in}, & \Delta V_L < V_D \\ c_m, & \Delta V_L > V_D \end{cases} \qquad (4.4.71)$$

where c_{ao} = gas concentration at the airway opening, m^3/m^3

c_m = concentration at mixing point, m^3/m^3

The time required before airway opening gas concentration changes from c_{in} to c_m is t_d, where

$$t_d = V_D/\dot{V}_L \qquad (4.4.72)$$

Flow rate $\dot{V}_L$ is not constant throughout the breath cycle.

Ventilation of both alveolar compartments may not be in synchrony or in the same direction, thus leading to pendelluft. There are six possible directions of flow among the conducting airway and alveolar compartments. A mass balance at the mixing point gives

$$- \dot{V}_1[c_m u(-\dot{V}_1) + c_1 u(\dot{V}_1)] + \dot{V}_2[c_m u(\dot{V}_2) + c_2 u(-\dot{V}_2)]$$
$$+ \dot{V}_3[c_m u(\dot{V}_3) + c_3 u(-\dot{V}_3)] = 0 \qquad (4.4.73)$$

where c_i = mixed concentration in compartment i, m^3/m^3

$$u(\dot{V}_i) = \begin{cases} 1, & \dot{V}_i > 0 \\ 0, & \dot{V}_i < 0 \end{cases} \qquad (4.4.74)$$

where $u(\dot{V}_i)$ = unit step function, dimensionless

A mass balance on each alveolar compartment with negligible alveolar-capillary transport gives

$$\frac{d}{dt}(c_i V_i) = \dot{V}_i[c_m u(\dot{V}_i) + c_i u(-\dot{V}_i)] \qquad (4.4.75)$$

For some reason not explained by the authors, alveolar compartment i volume was assumed to be invariant with time. Therefore, during inspiration they obtained

$$\frac{dc_i}{dt} = \frac{\dot{V}_i}{V_i}(c_m - c_i), \qquad \dot{V} > 0 \qquad (4.4.76)$$

and during expiration,

$$\frac{dc_i}{dt} = 0, \qquad \dot{V}_i < 0 \qquad (4.4.77)$$

Lutchen et al. (1982) used their model to investigate the effects of mechanical parameters on concentration differences between the two compartments and to determine the effects of pendelluft on concentration differences. They considered the standard nitrogen washout maneuver for normal mechanical property values (equal time constants) and values corresponding to obstructive pulmonary conditions. The nitrogen washout procedure consists of suddenly breathing pure oxygen and recording the decline in nitrogen concentration accompanying each succeeding exhalation. By determining the total amount of nitrogen exhaled, the functional residual capacity of the lung can be calculated.

In Figure 4.4.17 is seen flow, volume, and concentration during multibreath nitrogen washout for the uniform (normal) lung model. The double exponential pressure forcing function was used to achieve these results. The decrease of nitrogen concentration with time can be seen.

A nonuniform, obstructive lung was simulated by increasing R_3, h_3, and ε_3. This caused the mechanical time constant RC of compartment 3 to be much larger than that of compartment 2. A considerable amount of pendelluft occurs, and the nitrogen concentration in compartment 2 is always less than the concentration in compartment 3. Because compartment 3 is slower to empty than compartment 2, there is a distinct rise in nitrogen concentration during each exhalation (Figure 4.4.18).

An interesting result shown by the Lutchen et al. model is that there is a natural compensation for the concentration effects which accompany compartments with unequal time constants. The unobstructed compartment with the smaller time constant fills faster, but the first air to enter the compartment is dead volume air. Dead volume air is largely made of air from the slower emptying compartment with the higher nitrogen concentration. Thus a large portion of the air

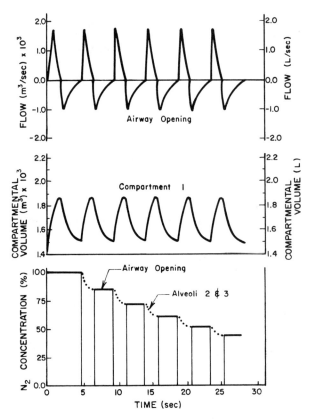

Figure 4.4.17 Flow, volume, and concentration dynamics during multibreath nitrogen washout for the uniform (normal) model. Normalized nitrogen concentrations are shown for the airway opening and for alveolar compartments 1 and 2. The alveolar compartment outputs are identical. On inspiration, alveolar concentration is shown as the dotted line and is distinct from airway opening concentration, shown as a solid line. (Adapted and used with permission from Lutchen et al., 1982. © 1982 IEEE.)

filling the faster compartment does not dilute the air in that compartment as much as it would have if the dead volume air had been evenly distributed. On the other hand, the slower filling compartment fills mostly with fresh air, which has filled the dead volume compartment after the stale air largely filled the faster compartment. Thus air in the slower compartment is diluted more than it would be otherwise. Pendelluft flow between compartments further reduces concentration differences between them.

There are other cases studied by the authors, and further clinical significance which they discuss. The significance of this model, however, is that respiratory dysfunction can be easily modeled and respiratory parameters normally inaccessible can be closely watched. Because some model assumptions preclude application of these results to exercise, a model to investigate similar parameters during exercise would require further complexity.

4.5 RESPIRATORY CONTROL MODELS

Models of respiratory control are abundant. Many models have been proposed which proceed from a premise of material balances. These models seek to define respiratory control in terms of the maintenance of blood property homeostasis. They may involve removal of excess carbon dioxide, return of blood acidity to normal levels, or resupply of hemoglobin oxygen saturation.

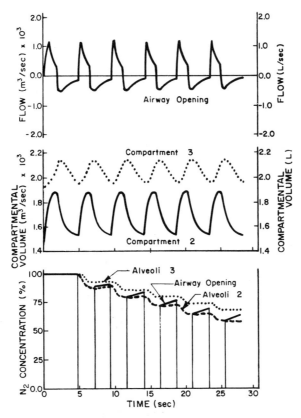

Figure 4.4.18 Flow, volume, and concentration dynamics during multibreath washout for the nonuniform (obstructive) model. Normalized N_2 concentrations are shown for the airway opening and for alveolar compartments 1 and 2. The obstructive model demonstrates clearly different behavior from the normal model. (Adapted and used with permission from Lutchen et al., 1982. © 1982 IEEE.)

They propose mechanisms by which experimental results are recreated. In general, the output of these models is respiratory ventilation. They are seldom concerned with respiratory details more minute than ventilation.

Contrarily, there is a large set of models which begin with a ventilation requirement and are concerned with the prediction of such variables as respiration rate, ratio of inhalation time to exhalation time, and breathing waveshape. This class of models proceeds along the line of parameter optimization.

In both control model types, there are strong appearances of elements of the respiratory mechanical models reviewed earlier (Section 4.4). For the most part, respiratory mechanical properties are included in a very rudimentary fashion, usually including constant resistances and compliances and one lung compartment. This is necessary because most model mathematics become extremely complicated once more realistic mechanical properties are included.

In this section, several of the more important models are reviewed. Degrees of similarity appear, but differences have been the cause for discussion in the field.

4.5.1 System Models

There are several models that encompass the entire respiratory system, including the controlled system and respiratory controller. The two major models presented here have been used as the basis for further model refinements.

Grodins Model. Of the models included in this book, the Grodins model (Grodins et al., 1967) is probably the most complex. Yet it will be clear that many simplifications were included in the model, and correction of these is the aim of later work (e.g., Saunders et al., 1980). The model has existed in several forms, each a variant or improvement of those coming before. The version reviewed here was published in 1967 and has been the object of much subsequent work. This version was still subject to variation when it was published, and its authors left no doubt that there were still significant imperfections in the model. Grodins (1981) indicated that whereas some modern models satisfactorily reproduce respiration and gas inhalation at rest, no model has yet to satisfactorily reproduce exercise effects.

The model of Grodins et al. (1967) was split into two components: (1) a controlled system, called the plant or process, and (2) a controller. Of the two, the controlled system was far more fully described.

The controlled system comprised three major compartments: the lung, brain, and tissue, connected by circulating blood (Figure 4.5.1). Blood gas pressures in arterial blood leaving the lung were assumed to equal alveolar pressures in the expired air. Total oxygen content of arterial blood is the sum of physically dissolved and oxyhemoglobin components (see Section 3.2.1). Similarly, the total carbon dioxide content of the blood consists of dissolved CO_2 and that chemically incorporated into blood bicarbonate, carboxyhemoglobin, and other blood proteins. Nitrogen is present exclusively in dissolved form. Gas partial pressures in each compartment were assumed constant and equal to those in exiting venous blood.

Following a transport delay, which depends on vascular volume and blood flow rate, arterial blood arrives from the lungs at brain or tissue compartments. Oxygen is removed from the blood and carbon dioxide added according to metabolic rate. Addition of carbon dioxide can change blood bicarbonate concentration, which, in turn, can influence pH.

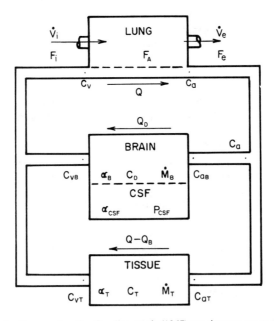

Figure 4.5.1 Schematic diagram for the Grodins et al. (1967) respiratory control model. The lung is assumed to have one-way airflow. Two other compartments are the brain (with CSF subcompartment) and body tissue. All compartments are linked through the cardiovascular system. (Used with permission from Grodins et al., 1967.)

The brain compartment is separated from a cerebrospinal fluid (CSF) section by a semipermeable membrane passing respiratory gases only. These diffuse across the membrane at rates proportional to their pressure gradients. Unlike the brain blood section, the CSF section contains no protein capable of buffering carbonic acid. The CSF section bicarbonate content is assumed to remain constant at all CO_2 pressures above $1333 \, N/m^2$ (10 mm Hg).

Venous blood leaving the brain and blood leaving the tissue combine, after appropriate time delays, to form mixed venous blood. After another delay, this blood enters the lung to complete the circle of gas transport.

The lungs were regarded as a box of constant volume, uniform content, and zero dead space. This box was ventilated by a continuous unidirectional stream of gas. There was no cyclic respiratory movement or change in gas composition.

Total cardiac output and local brain flow vary as functions of arterial CO_2 and oxygen partial pressures. Since circulatory delays are functions of blood flow, delay times were treated as dependent variables.

The controller was not described in terms of its physical details of receptors, locations, neural pathways, and muscles, but instead was described as consisting of a chemical concentration input transferred into a ventilation output. Controller equations were not given in much detail, probably because correct equations were not exactly known.

System equations begin with material balance equations for carbon dioxide, oxygen, and nitrogen for each of the three compartments of lung, brain, and tissue. For the lung,

$$V_A \dot{F}_{ACO_2} = \dot{V}_i F_{iCO_2} - \dot{V}_e F_{ACO_2} + \frac{\kappa_s}{(p_{atm} - pH_2O)} \dot{Q}(c_{vCO_2} - c_{aCO_2}) \tag{4.5.1}$$

$$V_A \dot{F}_{AO_2} = \dot{V}_i F_{iO_2} - \dot{V}_e F_{AO_2} + \frac{\kappa_s}{(p_{atm} - pH_2O)} \dot{Q}(c_{vO_2} - c_{vO_2}) \tag{4.5.2}$$

$$V_A \dot{F}_{AN_2} = \dot{V}_i F_{iN_2} - \dot{V}_e F_{AN_2} + \frac{\kappa_s}{(p_{atm} - pH_2O)} \dot{Q}(c_{vN_2} - c_{aN_2}) \tag{4.5.3}$$

where F_{Ax} = fractional concentration of constituent x in alveolar air, m^3/m^3

F_{ix} = fractional concentration of constituent x in inspired air, m^3/m^3

$\dot{F}_{Ax}$ = rate of change of fractional concentration of constituent x in alveolar air, $m^3/(m^3 \cdot sec)$

V_A = alveolar volume, m^3

$\dot{V}_i$ = inspired flow rate, m^3/sec

$\dot{V}_e$ = expired flow rate, m^3/sec

$\dot{Q}$ = blood flow rate, m^3/sec

c_{vx} = venous blood concentration of constituent x, m^3/m^3

c_{ax} = arterial blood concentration of constituent x, m^3/m^3

κ_s = conversion factor from STPD to BTPS conditions (see Equation 4.2.14)

= $115.03 \, kN/m^2$

p_{atm} = atmospheric pressure, N/m^2

pH_2O = partial pressure of water vapor at body temperature

= $6.28 \, kN/m^2$

For the brain compartment, mass balances give

$$V_B \dot{c}_{BCO_2} = \dot{M}_{BCO_2} + \dot{Q}_B(c_{aBCO_2} - c_{vBCO_2}) - D_{CO_2}(p_B CO_2 - p_{CSF} CO_2) \tag{4.5.4}$$

$$V_B \dot{c}_{BO_2} = -\dot{M}_{BO_2} + \dot{Q}_B(c_{aBO_2} - c_{vBO_2}) - D_{O_2}(p_B O_2 - p_{CSF} O_2) \tag{4.5.5}$$

$$V_B \dot{c}_{BN_2} = \dot{Q}_B(c_{aBN_2} - c_{vBN_2}) - D_{N_2}(p_B N_2 - p_{CSF} N_2) \tag{4.5.6}$$

where V_B = volume of the brain compartment, m^3

$\dot{c}_{Bx}$ = rate of change of concentration of constituent x in the brain, $m^3/(m^3 \cdot sec)$

$\dot{M}_{Bx}$ = rate of use or evolution of constituent x, m^3/sec (STPD)

$\dot{Q}_B$ = blood flow rate through the brain, m^3/sec

c_{aBx} = brain arterial concentration of constituent x, m^3/m^3

c_{vBx} = brain venous concentration of constituent x, m^3/m^3

D_x = diffusion coefficient for constituent x across the blood–brain barrier $m^5/(N \cdot sec)$

$p_B x$ = partial pressure of constituent x in brain, N/m^2

$p_{CSF} x$ = partial pressure of constituent x in cerebrospinal fluid, N/m^2

For the tissue compartment, mass balances give

$$V_T \dot{c}_{TCO} = \dot{M}_{TCO_2} + \dot{Q}_T (c_{aTCO_2} - c_{vTCO_2}) \tag{4.5.7}$$

$$V_T \dot{c}_{TO_2} = -\dot{M}_{TO_2} + \dot{Q}_T (c_{aTO_2} - c_{vTO_2}) \tag{4.5.8}$$

$$V_T \dot{c}_{TN_2} = \dot{Q}_T (c_{aTN_2} - c_{vTN_2}) \tag{4.5.9}$$

where V_T = tissue volume, m^3

$\dot{c}_{Tx}$ = rate of change of concentration of constituent x in tissue, $m^3/(m^3 \cdot sec)$

$\dot{M}_{Tx}$ = rate of use or evolution of constituent x in tissue, m^3/sec (STPD)

$\dot{Q}_T$ = blood flow through the tissue, m^3/sec

$\quad = \dot{Q} - \dot{Q}_B$

c_{ax} = concentration of constituent x in arterial blood, m^3/m^3

c_{vx} = concentration of constituent x in venous blood, m^3/m^3

For the cerebrospinal fluid, mass balances give

$$\dot{p}_{CSF}CO_2 = \left(\frac{D_{CO_2}}{V_{CSF}\, \alpha_{CSFCO_2}}\right)(p_B CO_2 - p_{CSF}CO_2) \tag{4.5.10}$$

$$\dot{p}_{CSF}O_2 = \left(\frac{D_{O_2}}{V_{CSF}\, \alpha_{CSFO_2}}\right)(p_B O_2 - p_{CSF}O_2) \tag{4.5.11}$$

$$\dot{p}_{CSF}N_2 = \frac{D_{N_2}}{V_{CSF}\, \alpha_{CSFN_2}} p_B N_2 - p_{CSF}N_2 \tag{4.5.12}$$

where $\dot{p}_{CSF} x$ = rate of change of partial pressure of constituent x in the cerebrospinal fluid, $N/(m^2 \cdot sec)$

V_{CSF} = volume of cerebrospinal fluid, m^3

α_{CSFx} = solubility coefficient of constituent x in the cerebrospinal fluid, m^2/N[91]

Since there are only three gaseous constituents,

$$F_{ACO_2} + F_{AO_2} + F_{AN_2} = 1 \tag{4.5.13}$$

The same is true for inspired and expired gas. Also, because lung volume is assumed constant,

$$\dot{F}_{ACO_2} + \dot{F}_{AO_2} + \dot{F}_{AN_2} = 0 \tag{4.5.14}$$

Solving for expired air volume gives

$$V_E = V_I + \left[\frac{\kappa_s}{P_{atm} - pH_2O}\right]\dot{Q}(c_{vCO_2} - c_{aCO_2}) + (c_{vO_2} - c_{aO_2}) + (c_{vN_2} - c_{aN_2}) \tag{4.5.15}$$

---

[91] All solubility coefficients are m^3 gas (STPD)/[(m^3 blood) (N/m^2 atmospheric pressure)].

Equilibrium between alveolar and arterial concentrations of the three gaseous constituents are described next. Carbon dioxide is present in blood bicarbonate (and carbonic acid), carbamino hemoglobin, and physical solution. In addition, there is an interaction between carbon dioxide-carrying capacity of the hemoglobin and oxygen saturation, called the Haldane effect. The carbon dioxide balance between systemic arteries and alveoli gives

$$c_{aCO_2} = B_b + 0.375\,(K_{O_2} - c_{aHbo_2}) - (0.16 + 2.3\,K_{O_2})\log\frac{c_{aCO_2} - \alpha_{CO_2}(p_{atm} - pH_2O)F_{ACO_2}}{0.01(p_{atm} - pH_2O)F_{ACO_2}}$$

$$- 0.14 + \alpha_{CO_2}(p_{atm} - pH_2O)F_{ACO_2} \tag{4.5.16}$$

where B_b = blood bicarbonate content, $m^3\ CO_2/m^3$ blood, CO_2 at STPD, blood at $37°C$

K_{O_2} = total blood oxygen capacity, $m^3\ O_2/m^3$ blood

c_{aHbo_2} = systemic arterial (pulmonary venous) concentration of oxyhemoglobin, m^3/m^3

α_{CO_2} = solubility coefficient for CO_2 in blood, m^2/N

The oxygen balance between systemic artery and alveolus is

$$c_{aO_2} = \alpha_{O_2}(p_{atm} - pH_2O)F_{AO_2} + c_{aHbo_2} \tag{4.5.17}$$

where oxyhemoglobin concentration is

$$c_{aHbo_2} = K_{O_2}\{1 - \exp[-S(p_{atm} - pH_2O)F_{Ao_2}]\}^2 \tag{4.5.18}$$

where S = oxygen saturation of hemoglobin, m^2/N

$$S = 0.0033694(pH_a) + 0.00075743(pH_a)^2 + 0.000050116(pH_a)^3 + 0.00341 \tag{4.5.19}$$

where pH_a = acidity level of blood leaving the lung, dimensionless

$$pH_a = 9 - \log c_{aH^+} \tag{4.5.20}$$

where c_{aH^+} = arterial concentration of hydrogen ions, $\mu mol/m^3$

To determine arterial blood hydrogen ion concentration,

$$c_{aH^+} = K_{H^+}\left[\frac{\alpha_{CO_2}(p_{atm} - pH_2O)F_{ACO_2}}{c_{aCO_2} - \alpha_{CO_2}(p_{atm} - pH_2O)F_{ACO_2}}\right] \tag{4.5.21}$$

where K_{H^+} = dissociation constant for carbonic acid, $\mu mol/m^3$

An alveolar–arterial nitrogen balance gives

$$c_{aN_2} = \alpha_{N_2}(p_{atm} - pH_2O)F_{AN_2} \tag{4.5.22}$$

The foregoing arterial equations were fitted empirically to standard data on human blood.

Venous blood–brain equilibria for the three gases follow. For carbon dioxide,

$$c_{BCO_2} = B_B - 0.62\left(\log\frac{c_{BCO_2} - \alpha_{BCO_2}p_BCO_2}{1.33\,p_BCO_2} - 0.14\right) + \alpha_{BCO_2}p_BCO_2 \tag{4.5.23}$$

where c_{BCO_2} = brain concentration of carbon dioxide, m^3/m^3

B_B = brain content of bicarbonate ions, $m^3\ CO_2/m^3$ blood

α_{BCO_2} = solubility coefficient for carbon dioxide in the brain, m^2/N

p_BCO_2 = partial pressure for carbon dioxide in the brain, N/m^2

$$c_{vBCO_2} = B_b + 0.375[K_{O_2} - c_{vBHbo_2}]$$

$$- [0.16 + 2.3\,K_{O_2}]\left[\log\left(\frac{c_{vBCO_2} - \alpha_{CO_2}p_BCO_2}{1.33\,p_BCO_2}\right) - 0.14\right] + \alpha_{CO_2}p_BCO_2 \tag{4.5.24}$$

where B_b = blood content of bicarbonate ions, m^3 CO_2/m^3 blood

c_{vBCO_2} = concentration of carbon dioxide as it leaves the brain, m^3 CO_2/m^3 blood

K_{O_2} = blood oxygen capacity, m^3 O_2/m^3 blood

α_{CO_2} = solubility coefficient for carbon dioxide in the blood, m^2/N

Equation 4.5.23 is a modified carbon dioxide buffer relation for the brain with the hemoglobin and oxyhemoglobin effects removed. An oxygen balance gives

$$c_{vBO_2} = (\alpha_{O_2}/\alpha_{BO_2})\, c_{BO_2} + c_{vBHbo_2} \tag{4.5.25}$$

where c_{vBO_2} = oxygen concentration in venous blood leaving the brain, m^3/m^3

α_{O_2} = blood solubility of oxygen, m^2/N

α_{BO_2} = brain solubility of oxygen, m^2/N

c_{BO_2} = brain concentration of oxygen, m^3/m^3

c_{vBHbo_2} = oxyhemoglobin concentration in venous blood leaving brain, m^3/m^3

As before (Equations 4.5.18–4.5.21),

$$c_{vBHbO_2} = K_{O_2}\left[1 - \exp(Sc_{BO_2}/\alpha_{BO_2})\right]^2 \tag{4.5.26}$$

$$c_{BO_2} = \alpha_{BO_2}\, p_B O_2 \tag{4.5.27}$$

$$S = 0.0033694(\mathrm{pH}_{vB}) - 0.00075743(\mathrm{pH}_{vB})^2 + 0.000050116(\mathrm{pH}_{vB})^3 + 0.00341 \tag{4.5.28}$$

where pH_{vB} = acidity of blood leaving the brain compartment, dimensionless

$$\mathrm{pH}_{vB} = 9 - \log c_{vBH^+} \tag{4.5.29}$$

where c_{vBH^+} = concentration of hydrogen ions in the blood leaving the brain, μmol/m^3

The Henderson–Hasselbach equation describes the equilibrium between hydrogen ion concentration, bicarbonate concentration, and dissolved carbon dioxide. Assuming equal dissolved carbon dioxide concentrations on either side of the blood–brain barrier but unequal bicarbonate and hydrogen ion concentrations gives

$$c_{vBH^+} = K_{H^+}\left[\frac{\alpha_{CO_2}\, p_B CO_2}{c_{vBCO_2} - \alpha_{CO_2}\, p_B CO_2}\right] \tag{4.5.30}$$

$$\mathrm{pH}_B = 9 - \log c_{BH^+} \tag{4.5.31}$$

$$c_{BH^+} = K_{H^+}\left[\frac{\alpha_{CO_2}\, p_B CO_2}{c_{BCO_2} - \alpha_{CO_2}\, p_B CO_2}\right] \tag{4.5.32}$$

where c_{BH^+} = concentration of hydrogen ions in the brain compartment, μ/m^3

A nitrogen balance gives

$$c_{vBN_2} = (\alpha_{N_2}/\alpha_{BN_2})c_{BN_2} \tag{4.5.33}$$

$$c_{BN_2} = \alpha_{BN_2}\, p_B N_2 \tag{4.5.34}$$

where c_{vBN_2} = nitrogen concentration in venous blood leaving the brain, m^3/m^3

α_{N_2} = solubility of nitrogen in blood, m^2/N

c_{BN_2} = nitrogen concentration in brain compartment, m^3/m^3

α_{BN_2} = solubility of nitrogen in brain, m^2/N

Equations for the tissue compartment are analogous to those for the brain compartment. The carbon dioxide balance is

$$c_{TCO_2} = B_T - 0.62 \left[\log\left(\frac{c_{TCO_2} - \alpha_{TCO_2} p_T CO_2}{1.33 \, p_T CO_2} \right) - 0.14 \right] + \alpha_{TCO_2} p_T CO_2 \qquad (4.5.35)$$

where c_{TCO_2} = tissue concentration of carbon dioxide, m^3/m^3
$\quad B_T$ = tissue content of bicarbonate ions, $m^3 \, CO_2/m^3$ tissue
$\quad \alpha_{TCO_2}$ = solubility coefficient for carbon dioxide in the tissue, m^2/N
$\quad p_T CO_2$ = partial pressure for carbon dioxide in the tissue, N/m^2

$$c_{vTCO_2} = B_b + 0.375 \left[K_{O_2} - c_{vTHbo_2} \right]$$
$$- \left[0.16 + 2.3 K_{O_2} \right] \left[\log\left(\frac{c_{vTCO_2} - \alpha_{CO_2} p_T CO_2}{1.33 \, p_T CO_2} \right) - 0.14 \right] + \alpha_{CO_2} p_T CO_2 \quad (4.5.36)$$

where B_b = blood content of bicarbonate ions, $m^3 \, CO_2/m^3$ blood
$\quad c_{vTCO_2}$ = venous concentration of carbon dioxide as it leaves the tissue, m^3/m^3
$\quad K_{O_2}$ = blood oxygen capacity, m^3/m^3
$\quad \alpha_{CO_2}$ = solubility coefficient for carbon dioxide in the blood, m^2/N
The tissue oxygen balance gives

$$c_{vTO_2} = (\alpha_{O_2}/\alpha_{TO_2}) c_{TO_2} + c_{vTHbo_2} \qquad (4.5.37)$$

where c_{vTO_2} = oxygen concentration in venous blood leaving the tissue, m^3/m^3
$\quad \alpha_{TO_2}$ = blood solubility of oxygen, m^2/N
$\quad c_{TO_2}$ = tissue concentration of oxygen, m^3/m^3
$\quad c_{vTHbo_2}$ = oxyhemoglobin concentration in blood leaving the tissue, m^3/m^3

$$c_{vTHbo_2} = K_{O_2} [1 - \exp(Sc_{TO_2}/\alpha_{TO_2})]^2 \qquad (4.5.38)$$

$$c_{TO_2} = \alpha_{TO_2} p_T O_2 \qquad (4.5.39)$$

$$S = 0.0033694(pH_{vT}) - 0.00075743(pH_{vT})^2 + 0.000050116(pH_{vT})^3 + 0.00341 \quad (4.5.40)$$

where pH_{vT} = acidity of venous blood leaving the tissue compartment, dimensionless

$$pH_{vT} = 9 - \log c_{vTH^+} \qquad (4.5.41)$$

where c_{vTH^+} = concentration of hydrogen ions in the blood leaving the tissue, $\mu mol/m^3$

$$c_{vTH^+} = K_{H^+} \left[\frac{\alpha_{CO_2} p_T CO_2}{c_{vTCO_2} - \alpha_{CO_2} p_T CO_2} \right] \qquad (4.5.42)$$

$$pH_T = 9 - \log c_{TH^+} \qquad (4.5.43)$$

$$c_{TH^+} = K_{H^+} \left[\frac{\alpha_{CO_2} p_T CO_2}{c_{TCO_2} - \alpha_{CO_2} p_T CO_2} \right] \qquad (4.5.44)$$

The tissue nitrogen balance gives

$$c_{vTN_2} = (\alpha_{N_2}/\alpha_{TN_2}) c_{TN_2} \qquad (4.5.45)$$

$$c_{TN_2} = \alpha_{TN_2} p_{TN_2} \qquad (4.5.46)$$

where c_{vTN_2} = nitrogen concentration in blood leaving the tissue, m^3/m^3
$\quad\quad \alpha_{N_2}$ = solubility of nitrogen in blood, m^2/N
$\quad\quad c_{TN_2}$ = nitrogen concentration in the tissue compartment, m^3/m^3
$\quad\quad \alpha_{TN_2}$ = solubility of nitrogen in tissue, m^2/N

Hydrogen ion concentration in the cerebrospinal fluid, used as an input to the controller, is

$$c_{CSFH^+} = K_{H^+} \left[\frac{\alpha_{CSFCO_2} p_{CSF} CO_2}{B_{CSF}} \right] \tag{4.5.47}$$

where c_{CSFH^+} = hydrogen ion concentration in the CSF, $\mu mol/m^3$
$\quad\quad \alpha_{CSFCO_2}$ = solubility of carbon dioxide in the CSF, m^2/N
$\quad\quad p_{CSF}CO_2$ = partial pressure of carbon dioxide in the CSF, N/m^2
$\quad\quad B_{CSF}$ = bicarbonate content in the CSF, $m^3 CO_2/m^3 CSF$

and

$$pH_{CSF} = 9 - \log c_{CSFH^+} \tag{4.5.48}$$

Dependence of cardiac output and brain flood flow on arterial carbon dioxide and oxygen partial pressures is defined from information appearing in the literature. An arbitrary first-order lag is assigned to the responses. Cardiac output is given by

$$\ddot{Q} = \frac{\dot{Q}_N + \Delta\dot{Q}_{O_2} + \Delta\dot{Q}_{CO_2} - \dot{Q}}{\tau_c} \tag{4.5.49}$$

where $\dot{Q}$ = blood flow rate, m^3/sec
$\quad\quad \ddot{Q}$ = rate of change of blood flow rate, m^3/sec^2
$\quad\quad \tau_c$ = cardiac output time constant, sec
$\quad\quad \dot{Q}_N$ = normal (resting) blood flow rate, m^3/sec
$\quad\quad \Delta\dot{Q}_{O_2}$ = change in cardiac output due to oxygen pressure change, m^3/sec
$\quad\quad \Delta\dot{Q}_{CO_2}$ = change in cardiac output due to carbon dioxide pressure, m^3/sec

$$\Delta\dot{Q}_{O_2} = 1.6108 \times 10^{-4} - 3.6066 \times 10^{-8} p_aO_2$$
$$+ 2.7419 \times 10^{-12}(p_aO_2)^2 - 7.0566 \times 10^{-17}(p_aO_2)^3, \quad p_aO_2 < 13.865\,kN/m^2 \tag{4.5.50a}$$

$$\Delta\dot{Q}_{O_2} = 0, \quad p_aO_2 \geqslant 13.865\,kN/m^2 \tag{4.5.50b}$$

where p_aO_2 = partial pressure of oxygen in the blood when leaving the lung, N/m^2
In the lung, there is assumed no alveolar–arterial pressure difference. Thus

$$p_aO_2 = (p_{atm} - pH_2O)F_{AO_2} \tag{4.5.51}$$

$$\Delta\dot{Q}_{CO_2} = (5.0 \times 10^{-6})(p_aCO_2 - 5333), \quad 5333 \leqslant p_aCO_2 \leqslant 7999\,N/m^2 \tag{4.5.52a}$$

$$\Delta\dot{Q}_{CO_2} = 0, \quad \text{all other values of } p_aCO_2 \tag{4.5.52b}$$

where p_aCO_2 = partial pressure of carbon dioxide as it leaves the lung, N/m^2
Again,

$$p_aCO_2 = (p_{atm} - pH_2O)F_{ACO_2} \tag{4.5.53}$$

Brain blood flow is determined from

$$\ddot{Q}_B = \frac{\dot{Q}_{BN} + \Delta\dot{Q}_{BO_2} + \Delta\dot{Q}_{BCO_2} - \dot{Q}_B}{\tau_B} \qquad (4.5.54)$$

where $\dot{Q}_B$ = brain blood flow rate, m^3/sec

$\ddot{Q}_B$ = rate of change of brain blood flow rate, m^3/sec^2

$\dot{Q}_{BN}$ = normal brain blood flow rate, m^3/sec

$\Delta\dot{Q}_{BO_2}$ = change in brain blood flow rate due to oxygen partial pressure, m^3/sec

$\Delta\dot{Q}_{BCO_2}$ = change in brain blood flow rate due to carbon dioxide partial pressure, m^3/sec

τ_B = time constant for brain blood flow rate changes, sec

$$\Delta\dot{Q}_{BO_2} = 4.6417 \times 10^{-5} - 1.6539 \times 10^{-8} p_a O_2$$
$$+ 2.4410 \times 10^{-12} (p_a O_2)^3 - 1.6346 \times 10^{-16} (p_a O_2)^3$$
$$- 4.0389 \times 10^{-21} (p_a O_2)^4, \qquad p_a O_2 < 13.865 \, kN/m^2 \qquad (4.5.55a)$$

$$\Delta\dot{Q}_{BO_2} = 0, \qquad p_a O_2 \geqslant 13.865 \, kN/m^2 \qquad (4.5.55b)$$

$$\Delta\dot{Q}_{BCO_2} = 3.8717 \times 10^{-7} - 3.8845 \times 10^{-7} p_a CO_2$$
$$+ 7.5168 \times 10^{-13} (p_a CO_2)^2, \qquad p_a CO_2 \leqslant 5066 \, N/m^2 \qquad (4.4.56a)$$

$$\Delta\dot{Q}_{BCO_2} = 0, \qquad 5066 \leqslant p_a CO_2 \leqslant 5866 \, N/m^2 \qquad (4.5.56b)$$

$$\Delta\dot{Q}_{BCO_2} = -2.5967 \times 10^{-4} + 9.5097 \times 10^{-8} p_a CO_2$$
$$- 1.2140 \times 10^{-11} (p_a CO_2)^2 + 6.6056 \times 10^{-16} (p_a CO_2)^3$$
$$- 1.1473 \times 10^{-20} (p_a CO_2)^4 \qquad p_a CO_2 > 5866 \, N/m^2 \qquad (4.5.56c)$$

Arterial concentrations of carbon dioxide, oxygen, and nitrogen at the entrance of the brain and tissue reservoirs are determined in terms of their concentrations in pulmonary venous (systemic arterial) blood leaving the lung. Because there is a delay between the time blood leaves the lung and arrival at each compartment, the appropriate gas concentration at the lung appeared at a previous time, prior to its arrival in each compartment:

$$c_{aBCO_2} = c_{aCO_2} \delta(t - \tau_{aB}) \qquad (4.5.57)$$

$$c_{aBO_2} = c_{aO_2} \delta(t - \tau_{aB}) \qquad (4.5.58)$$

$$c_{aBN_2} = c_{aN_2} \delta(t - \tau_{aB}) \qquad (4.5.59)$$

$$c_{aTCO_2} = c_{aCO_2} \delta(t - \tau_{aT}) \qquad (4.5.60)$$

$$c_{aTO_2} = c_{aO_2} \delta(t - \tau_{aT}) \qquad (4.5.61)$$

$$c_{aTN_2} = c_{aN_2} \delta(t - \tau_{aT}) \qquad (4.5.62)$$

where c_{aBi} = concentration of gas i at the entrance to the brain, m^3/m^3

c_{ai} = concentration of gas i leaving the lung, m^3/m^3

c_{aTi} = concentration of gas i at the entrance to the tissue compartment, m^3/m^3

τ_{aB} = time delay between lung and brain, sec

τ_{aT} = time delay between lung and tissue, sec

$$\delta(t - \tau) = 0, \qquad t \neq \tau \tag{4.5.63}$$
$$= 1, \qquad t = \tau$$

Similarly, mixed venous concentrations of the three gases at the lung are determined by mixing brain and tissue blood and including an appropriate time delay:

$$c_{vCO_2} = \frac{\dot{Q}_B c_{vBCO_2} \delta(t - \tau_{vB}) + (\dot{Q} - \dot{Q}_B) c_{vTCO_2} \delta(t - \tau_{vT})}{\dot{Q}} \tag{4.5.64}$$

$$c_{vO_2} = \frac{\dot{Q}_B c_{vBO_2} \delta(t - \tau_{vB}) + (\dot{Q} - \dot{Q}_B) c_{vTO_2} \delta(t - \tau_{vT})}{\dot{Q}} \tag{4.5.65}$$

$$c_{vN_2} = \frac{\dot{Q}_B c_{vBN_2} \delta(t - \tau_{vB}) + (\dot{Q} - \dot{Q}_B) c_{vTN_2} \delta(t - \tau_{vT})}{\dot{Q}} \tag{4.5.66}$$

where c_{vi} = mixed venous concentration of gas i, m^3/m^3
$\quad c_{vBi}$ = concentration of gas i leaving the brain, m^3/m^3
$\quad c_{vTi}$ = concentration of gas i leaving the tissue, m^3/m^3
$\quad \tau_{vB}$ = time delay between brain and lung, sec
$\quad \tau_{vT}$ = time delay between tissue and lung, sec

Transport delays are not constants but vary with blood flow rates. To calculate these delays, the volume of the appropriate vascular segment through which blood flows is divided by the average flow rate during the proper past time interval ($\tau_{ax} - \tau_{ax1}$):

$$\tau_{aB} = [1.062 \times 10^{-3}]\left[\left(\frac{1}{\tau_{aB} - \tau_{aB1}}\right)\int_{t - \tau_{aB}}^{t - \tau_{aB1}} \dot{Q}\, dt\right]^{-1} + [15.0 \times 10^{-6}]\left[\left(\frac{1}{\tau_{aB1}}\right)\int_{t - \tau_{aB1}}^{t} \dot{Q}_B\, dt\right]^{-1} \tag{4.5.67}$$

$$\tau_{aT} = [1.062 \times 10^{-3}]\left[\left(\frac{1}{\tau_{aT} - \tau_{aT1}}\right)\int_{t - \tau_{aT}}^{t - \tau_{aT1}} \dot{Q}\, dt\right]^{-1}$$
$$+ [735.0 \times 10^{-6}]\left[\left(\frac{1}{\tau_{aT1}}\right)\int_{t - \tau_{aT1}}^{t} (\dot{Q} - \dot{Q}_B)\, dt\right]^{-1} \tag{4.5.68}$$

$$\tau_{vB} = [60.0 \times 10^{-6}]\left[\left(\frac{1}{\tau_{vB} - \tau_{vB1}}\right)\int_{t - \tau_{vB}}^{t - \tau_{vB1}} \dot{Q}\, dt\right]^{-1} + [188 \times 10^{-6}]\left[\left(\frac{1}{\tau_{vB1}}\right)\int_{t - \tau_{vB1}}^{t} \dot{Q}\, dt\right]^{-1} \tag{4.5.69}$$

$$\tau_{vT} = [2.94 \times 10^{-3}]\left[\left(\frac{1}{\tau_{vT} - \tau_{vT1}}\right)\int_{t - \tau_{vT}}^{t - \tau_{vT1}} (\dot{Q} - \dot{Q}_B)\, dt\right]^{-1}$$
$$+ [188 \times 10^{-6}]\left[\left(\frac{1}{\tau_{vT1}}\right)\int_{t - \tau_{vT1}}^{t} \dot{Q}\, dt\right]^{-1} \tag{4.5.70}$$

where τ_{ax} = transit time for blood from the lung to reach compartment x, sec

In each of these equations, there is a term similar to τ_{aB1}. The pathway taken by the blood is assumed to consist of segment 1 carrying the total cardiac output ($\dot{Q}$), an attached segment carrying blood to (or from) the brain ($\dot{Q}_B$) in series with the first segment, and a parallel segment carrying blood to (or from) the tissue compartment $(\dot{Q} - \dot{Q}_B)$, also in series with the first segment. If τ_{aB1} is considered to be the time required to pass through the arteries serving only the brain, then $(\tau_{aB} - \tau_{aB1})$ is the time required for blood, which eventually reaches the brain, to pass through the common segment. In the venous direction, τ_{vB1} is considered to be the time spent in the common segment, and $(\tau_{vB} - \tau_{vB1})$ is the time to pass through those veins draining blood exclusively from the brain compartment. Another delay time, τ_{ao}, is the lung to carotid body delay time and is required for use in the controller equations:

$$\tau_{ao} = [1.062 \times 10^{-3}] \left[\left(\frac{1}{\tau_{ao} - \tau_{ao1}} \right) \int_{t-\tau_{ao}}^{t-\tau_{ao1}} \dot{Q} \, dt \right]^{-1} + [8.0 \times 10^{-6}] \left[\left(\frac{1}{\tau_{ao1}} \right) \int_{t-\tau_{ao1}}^{t} \dot{Q}_B \, dt \right]^{-1} \tag{4.5.71}$$

where τ_{ao} = lung to carotid body delay time, sec

$\quad\quad \tau_{ao1}$ = time for blood to pass through the arteries carrying only brain compartment blood, sec

Two controller equations were tested with the previous mathematical description of the controlled system. The first is the simpler:

$$\dot{V}_i = 1.1c_{BH^+} + 0.00983p_BCO_2 + \Omega - \dot{V}_n \tag{4.5.72}$$

$$\Omega = [7.87 \times 10^{-5}][231 - (p_{atm} - pH_2O)F_{AO_2}(t - \tau_{ao})]^{4.9},$$

$$(p_{atm} - pH_2O)F_{AO_2}(t - \tau_{ao}) < 231 \tag{4.5.73a}$$

$$\Omega = 0, \quad (p_{atm} - pH_2O)F_{AO_2}(t - t_{ao}) \geqslant 231 \tag{4.5.73b}$$

where $\dot{V}_i$ = inhalation flow rate, m^3/sec

$\quad\quad \dot{V}_n$ = a constant adjusted so that $p_ACO_2 \cong 5333 \, N/m^2$ (40.0 mm Hg) at rest, breathing air at sea level, m^3/sec

The second equation is

$$\dot{V}_i = 1.138c_{CSFH^+} + 0.01923c_{aH^+}(t - \tau_{ao}) + \Omega - \dot{V}_n \tag{4.5.74}$$

and includes newer information about the roles of the cerebrospinal fluid and peripheral receptors.

Grodins et al. (1967) rearranged the preceding equations and solved the resulting equations on a digital computer. Solution of these equations was not entirely straightforward because there are variable time lags in each of these.

Several versions of the model were described by Grodins et al. (1967). The final version includes the CSF compartment and delay time values calculated from past-average blood flows. These inclusions are presented in equations previously given.

The authors subjected their model to normal conditions as well as hypoxia at sea level, hypoxia at altitude, inhalation of carbon dioxide, and metabolic acidosis. The hyperpnea of exercise could not be reproduced.

Normal values of constants not already included in the equations are given in Table 4.5.1. In Figure 4.5.2 is shown the response of the model to a 5% CO_2 pulse. The model gives an initial rapid rise in ventilation followed by a slower rise toward a steady-state value, similar to experimental results.

Since the formulation of the model by Grodins et al. (1967), other attempts have been made to provide more satisfying solutions to the problem of identification of respiratory control mechanisms. The problem was stated succinctly by Grodins (1981). If arterial partial pressure (p_aCO_2) is considered to be the stimulus to alveolar ventilation rates, then an increase in carbon

TABLE 4.5.1 Normal Parameter Values Used in the Respiratory Model[a]

Parameter	Value	
α_{CO_2}	$5.05 \times 10^{-6}\,\mathrm{m^2/N}$	$(6.73 \times 10^{-4}\,1/\mathrm{mm\,Hg})$
α_{O_2}	$2.38 \times 10^{-8}\,\mathrm{m^2/N}$	$(3.17 \times 10^{-5}\,1/\mathrm{mm\,Hg})$
α_{N_2}	$1.29 \times 10^{-7}\,\mathrm{m^2/N}$	$(1.72 \times 10^{-5}\,1/\mathrm{mm\,Hg})$
K_{H^+}	$795\,\mu\mathrm{mol/m^3}$	$(795\,\mathrm{nmol/L})$
V_B	$0.001\,\mathrm{m^3}$	$(1.000\,\mathrm{L})$
V_T	$0.039\,\mathrm{m^3}$	$(39.00\,\mathrm{L})$
V_L	$0.003\,\mathrm{m^3}$	$(3.00\,\mathrm{L})$
V_{CSF}	$0.0001\,\mathrm{m^3}$	$(0.100\,\mathrm{L})$
p_{atm}	$101.3\,\mathrm{kN/m^2}$	$(760\,\mathrm{mm\,Hg})$
B_b	$0.5470\,\mathrm{m^3/m^3}$	$(0.5470\,\mathrm{L\,CO_2(STPD)/L\ blood\ at\ 37°C})$
B_B	$0.5850\,\mathrm{m^3/m^3}$	$(0.5850\,\mathrm{L\,CO_2\ (STPD)/L\ brain\ at\ 37°C})$
B_T	$0.5850\,\mathrm{m^3/m^3}$	$(0.5850\,\mathrm{L\,CO_2\ (STPD)/L\ tissue\ at\ 37°C})$
B_{CSF}	$0.5850\,\mathrm{m^3/m^3}$	$(0.5850\,\mathrm{L\,CO_2\ (STPD)/L\ CSF\ at\ 37°C})$
D_{CO_2}	$1.025 \times 10^{-12}\,\mathrm{m^5/N\cdot sec}$	$(81.99 \times 10^{-7}\,\mathrm{L\ (STPD)/min/mm\,Hg})$
D_{O_2}	$5.452 \times 10^{-14}\,\mathrm{m^5/N\cdot sec}$	$(4.361 \times 10^{-7}\,\mathrm{L\ (STPD)/min/mm\,Hg})$
D_{N_2}	$3.155 \times 10^{-14}\,\mathrm{m^5/N\cdot sec}$	$(2.524 \times 10^{-7}\,\mathrm{L\ (STPD)/min/mm\,Hg})$
F_{iCO_2}	0.0000	(0.0000)
F_{iO^2}	0.2100	(0.2100)
F_{iN_2}	0.7900	(0.7900)
K_{O_2}	0.2000	$(0.2000\,\mathrm{L\ (STPD)/L\ blood})$
$\dot{M}_{BCO_2}$	$8.33 \times 10^{-7}\,\mathrm{m^3/sec}$	$(0.050\,\mathrm{L\ (STPD)/min})$
$\dot{M}_{BO_2}$	$8.33 \times 10^{-7}\,\mathrm{m^3/sec}$	$(0.050\,\mathrm{L\ (STPD)/min})$
$\dot{M}_{TCO_2}$	$3.03 \times 10^{-6}\,\mathrm{m^3/sec}$	$(0.182\,\mathrm{L\ (STPD)/min})$
$\dot{M}_{TO_2}$	$3.58 \times 10^{-6}\,\mathrm{m^3/sec}$	$(0.215\,\mathrm{L\ (STPD)/min})$
$\dot{Q}_N$	$1.000 \times 10^{-4}\,\mathrm{m^3/sec}$	$(6.000\,\mathrm{L/min})$
$\dot{Q}_{BN}$	$1.250 \times 10^{-5}\,\mathrm{m^3/sec}$	$(0.750\,\mathrm{L/min})$
τ_C	$1.67 \times 10^{-3}\,\mathrm{sec}$	$(0.100\,\mathrm{min})$
τ_B	$1.67 \times 10^{-3}\,\mathrm{sec}$	$(0.100\,\mathrm{min})$

[a]Compiled from Gradins et al., 1967.

dioxide production during exercise ($\dot{V}_{CO_2}$) or an increase in inhaled carbon dioxide (F_{iCO_2}) will increase p_aCO_2, and alveolar ventilation would be stimulated. Because this is assumed to be a proportional controller, there would be some steady-state error remaining after the increase, and the error would be inversely related to controlled gain. This is a very attractive explanation for exercise hyperpnea.

Unfortunately, if the controller gain is estimated from its response to carbon dioxide inhalation at rest, the error observed in moderate exercise is not nearly enough to account for the ventilation. A method of circumventing this problem is to add a term to the controller equation which is proportional to $\dot{V}_{CO_2}$. Now, alveolar ventilation rate will increase and p_aCO_2 will remain at its resting level. Nevertheless, this mathematical solution may have no basis in physiological reality.

Saunders Modification of Grodins Model. Saunders et al. (1980) went in a different direction. They modified the Grodins et al. (1967) model to include cyclic ventilation, respiratory dead volume, variable lung volume, blood shunting past the lung, a separate muscle compartment, and a different controller equation (Figure 4.5.3). They deleted the separate CSF compartment of Grodins et al. (1967).

Lung volume was assumed to comprise alveolar volume and dead volume. In turn, dead

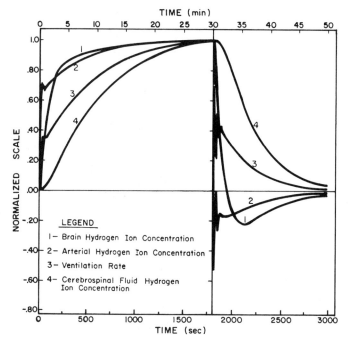

Figure 4.5.2 Computer-generated plot of Grodins model response to a 5% CO_2 pulse. The pulse was applied at zero time and terminated at 1800 sec (30 min). The ordinate scale is nondimensional. (Adapted and used with permission from Grodins et al., 1967.)

volume consisted of an alveolar component and an anatomical (nonalveolar) dead volume:

$$V_L = V_A + V_D \tag{4.5.75}$$

$$V_D = V_{Dalv} + V_{Danat} \tag{4.5.76}$$

where V_{Danat} = anatomical dead volume, m³, considered to be a constant Saunders et al. set

$$V_D = V_{Danat} = 1.75 \times 10^{-4} \, \text{m}^3, \qquad V_T \leqslant 8.75 \times 10^{-4} \, \text{m}^3 \tag{4.5.77a}$$

$$V_D = 0.2 \, V_T, \qquad V_T > 8.75 \times 10^{-4} \, \text{m}^3 \tag{4.5.77b}$$

$$V_{Dalv} = V_D - 1.75 \times 10^{-4} \, \text{m}^3, \qquad V_T > 8.75 \times 10^{-4} \, \text{m}^3 \tag{4.5.77c}$$

$$V_{Dalv} = 0.01, \qquad V_T < 8.75 \times 10^{-4} \, \text{m}^3 \tag{4.5.77d}$$

After some manipulation, they obtained, for inhalation in the alveolar space,

$$\dot{F}_{AX} = \frac{(F_{DX} - F_{AX})(\dot{V}_L - \dot{V}_{Dalv}) + \dot{T}_X}{V_L - V_{Dalv}} \tag{4.5.78}$$

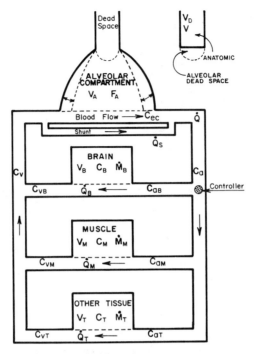

Figure 4.5.3 The controlled system for the Saunders et al. (1980) model. Lung structure is different from the Grodins model, and muscle tissue is given its own compartment. (Used with permission from Saunders et al., 1980.)

where F_{AX} = fractional concentration of gas X in the alveolar space, m^3/m^3

$\quad F_{DX}$ = fractional concentration of gas X in the dead space, m^3/m^3

$\quad \dot{F}_{AX}$ = rate of change of fractional concentration in alveolar space, $m^3/m^3 \cdot sec$

$\quad V_L$ = lung volume, m^3

$\quad V_{D\text{alv}}$ = alveolar dead volume, m^3

$\quad \dot{V}_L$ = rate of change of lung volume, m^3/sec

$\quad \dot{V}_{D\text{alv}}$ = rate of change of alveolar dead volume, m^3/sec

$\quad T_X$ = instantaneous rate of gas transfer of gas X to/from the alveolar compartment, m^3/sec

Unlike the Grodins et al. (1967) equations, Saunders et al. (1980) considered only oxygen and carbon dioxide gases.

During exhalation, they obtained

$$\dot{F}_{AX} = \frac{\dot{T}_X}{V_L - V_{D\text{alv}}} \tag{4.5.79}$$

In the dead volume, during inhalation,

$$\dot{F}_{DX} = \frac{\dot{V}_L(F_{iX} - F_{DX})}{V_D} \tag{4.5.80}$$

where F_{DX} = fractional concentration of gas X in the dead volume, m^3/m^3

$\quad F_{iX}$ = fractional concentration of gas X in the inspired gas, m^3/m^3

$\quad \dot{F}_{DX}$ = rate of change of fractional concentration in the dead volume, $m^3/m^3 \cdot sec$

During exhalation,

$$\dot{F}_{DX} = \frac{(\dot{V}_L - \dot{V}_{Dalv})(F_{DX} - F_{AX})}{V_D} \tag{4.5.81}$$

These equations complicate the original Grodins et al. (1967) equations by the inclusion of an alveolar gas-exchanging volume and a dead volume, both of which vary in size.

Saunders et al. (1980) described other slight modifications to the Grodins et al. (1967) oxygen and carbon dioxide dissociation equations in blood and tissue. In the muscle compartment an equation was included to account for muscle myoglobin[92] dissociation.

$$V_{mO_2} = 3.38 \times 10^{-6} p_m O_2, \qquad\qquad 0 < p_m O_2 \leqslant 924 \, \text{N/m}^2 \tag{4.5.82a}$$

$$V_{mO_2} = 3.126 \times 10^{-8} p_m O_2 + 2.8302 \times 10^{-4}, \qquad 924 < p_m O_2 \leqslant 4528 \, \text{N/m}^2 \tag{4.5.82b}$$

$$V_{mO_2} = 4.167 \times 10^{-9} p_m O_2 + 4.05662 \times 10^{-4}, \qquad 4528 \, \text{N/m}^2 < p_m O_2 \tag{4.5.82c}$$

where V_{mO_2} = volume of oxygen carried on myoglobin in the muscle compartment, m^3
$\quad\; p_m O_2$ = partial pressure of oxygen in the muscle, N/m^2
Then

$$c_{mO_2} = \frac{(p_m O_2 \alpha_{O_2})/p_{atm} + V_{mO_2}}{V_m} \tag{4.5.83}$$

where c_{mO_2} = muscle oxygen concentration, m^3/m^3
$\quad\; \alpha_{O_2}$ = oxygen solubility coefficient, m^2/N
$\quad\; p_{atm}$ = atmospheric pressure, N/m^2
$\quad\; V_m$ = volume of muscle compartment, m^3
Saunders et al. substituted

$$\text{pH}_a = 8.76 - 0.64 \log_{10}(p_a CO_2 - 5333) \tag{4.5.84}$$

where pH_a = arterial blood acidity level, dimensionless
$\quad\; p_a CO_2$ = arterial partial pressure for carbon dioxide, N/m^2
for the Grodins et al. equations (4.5.20 and 4.5.21). The level of pH, or hydrogen ion concentration, was not calculated for tissues.

Ventilation was modeled as a sine wave with

$$f = \dot{V}/V_T \tag{4.5.85}$$

$$V_T = 1.48 \times 10^{-3} \dot{V}, \qquad 0 < \dot{V} \leqslant 1.745 \times 10^{-4} \, \text{m}^3/\text{sec} \tag{4.5.86}$$

$$V_T = 4.80 \times 10^{-3} \dot{V}, \qquad 1.745 \times 10^{-4} < \dot{V} \tag{4.5.87}$$

---

[92]Myoglobin is an iron-containing pigment in red muscles which resembles hemoglobin but binds one, rather than four, moles of O_2 per mole of myoglobin. Its dissociation curve is a rectangular hyperbolic shape rather than the sigmoid shape of hemoglobin. Since the myoglobin dissociation curve is placed to the left of the hemoglobin dissociation curve, myoglobin absorbs oxygen from hemoglobin. Myoglobin content is greatest in muscles specialized for sustained contraction, and its purpose seems to be a small reservoir of oxygen to be used when external oxygen supply through the blood is severely limited (Ganong, 1963).

where f = breathing rate, breaths/sec

$\dot{V}$ = average ventilation rate, m³/sec

V_T = tidal volume, m³

Functional residual capacity (FRC) was calculated to approach residual volume (RV) linearly as tidal volume approached vital capacity (VC):

$$FRC = 2.9 \times 10^{-3} - 0.312 V_T \qquad (4.5.88)$$

Values of 1.5×10^{-3} m³ for RV and 4.5×10^{-3} m³ for VC were used. The mean ventilation volume includes the initial volume (FRC) and the average integral of the sinusoidal flow rate:

$$\bar{V} = FRC + V_T/2 \qquad (4.5.89)$$

Therefore,

$$V_L = FRC + (V_T/2)[1 - \cos(2\pi f t + \phi)] \qquad (4.5.90)$$

and

$$\dot{V}'_L = \pi f V_T \sin(2\pi f t + \phi) \qquad (4.5.91)$$

where t = time, sec

ϕ = phase angle, rad

$\dot{V}'_L$ = flow rate into the lung uncorrected for respiratory quotient, m³/sec

Actual flow rate is

$$\dot{V}_L = \dot{V}'_L + (\dot{T}_{O_2} - \dot{T}_{CO_2}) \qquad (4.5.92)$$

where $\dot{T}_X$ = transfer rate of gas X to/from the alveolar compartment, m³/sec

$$\dot{T}_{CO_2}/\dot{T}_{O_2} = RQ \qquad (4.5.93)$$

where RQ = respiratory quotient, dimensionless

$$\dot{T}_{O_2} = \dot{Q}(c_{aO_2} - c_{vO_2})\frac{\kappa_s}{[p_{atm} - pH_2O]} \qquad (4.5.94)$$

$$\dot{T}_{CO_2} = \dot{Q}(c_{vCO_2} - c_{aCO_2})\frac{\kappa_s}{[p_{atm} - pH_2O]} \qquad (4.5.95)$$

where $\dot{Q}$ = total cardiac output, m³/sec

c_{aX} = arterial concentration of gas X, m³/m³

c_{vX} = mixed venous concentration of gas X, m³/m³

κ_s = conversion factor from STPD to BTPS conditions

= 115.03 kN/m²

p_{atm} = atmospheric pressure = 101.3 kN/m²

pH_2O = partial pressure of water vapor at body temperature

= 6.28 kN/m²

Blood shunting around the lung influenced gas concentrations. A mass balance gives

$$c_{aX} = c_{ecX}[1 - (\dot{Q}_s/\dot{Q})] + c_{vX}(\dot{Q}_s/\dot{Q}) \qquad (4.5.96)$$

where c_{aX} = arterial concentration of gas X, m^2/m^3

c_{vX} = mixed venous concentration of gas X, m^3/m^3

c_{ecX} = pulmonary end-capillary concentration of gas X, m^3/m^3

$(\dot{Q}_s/\dot{Q})$ = shunt fraction, dimensionless

The controller equations used were based on those by Jukes and Cunningham (Cunningham, 1974) and include interaction between hypoxia and hypercapnia (see Equation 4.3.7). Saunders et al. placed the controller so as to sample arterial blood delayed by the lung-to-brain transport time. The controller responded to changes in the arterial partial pressures of oxygen and carbon dioxide. Average partial pressures were used after filtering with a second-order digital filter.

$$\dot{V} = (2.75 \times 10^{-7})[\bar{p}_a CO_2 - 5066] \left[\frac{1 + 2133}{\bar{p}_a O_2 - 4000} \right], \qquad \bar{p}_a CO_2 \geqslant 5333 \, N/m^2 \qquad (4.5.97a)$$

$$\dot{V} = (1.25 \times 10^{-8})[\bar{p}_a CO_2 - 2666] \left[2.2 \left(1 + \frac{2133}{\bar{p}_a O_2 - 4000} \right) - 2.0 \right] + 2.33 \times 10^{-7},$$
$$2666 \leqslant \bar{p}_a CO_2 \, 5333 \, N/m^2 \qquad (4.5.97b)$$

$$\dot{V} = 6.667 \times 10^{-5}, \qquad 0.0 < \bar{p}_a CO_2 < 2666 \, N/m^2 \qquad (4.5.97c)$$

where $\dot{V}$ = average ventilation rate, m^3/sec

$\bar{p}_a CO_2$ = average arterial CO_2 partial pressure, N/m^2

$\bar{p}_a O_2$ = average arterial O_2 partial pressure, N/m^2

Saunders et al. (1980) tested their model with several different situations, including increased inspired CO_2 fraction, step increase in mixed venous blood CO_2 concentration, hypoxic gas mixtures, CO_2 rebreathing, exercise, and breath-holding during exercise. Mixed results were obtained, with the worst results for exercise simulation.

Exercise was simulated by an abrupt increase in oxygen uptake and carbon dioxide production in the muscle compartment together with an appropriate increase in cardiac output. To maintain numerical stability, the muscle myoglobin oxygen storage reservoir had to be maintained at $4 \times 10^{-4} \, m^3$ (400 mL). At a simulation level of $100 \, N \cdot m/sec$, the model again failed with a negative muscle pO_2. The main responsible factor proved to be that ventilation increased too slowly to maintain sufficient oxygen supply in arterial blood during the transient period following the onset of exercise. To restore numerical stability, the controller gain dealing with carbon dioxide had to be increased fivefold, the blood shunt fraction had to be reduced from 5% to 1%, and blood had to be diverted from the other tissue to the muscle compartment if muscle pO_2 fell to $0.667 \, N/m^2$ (5 mm Hg).

Even with numerical stability achieved, the resulting transients for $p_a CO_2$ and ventilation were far from realistic (Figure 4.5.4), showing a lag of about 6 sec with a marked overshoot in ventilation and oscillation in $p_a CO_2$.

Saunders (1980) used the previous model to propose and test a simple, elegant, and apparently successful explanation for the hyperpnea of exercise and elevated carbon dioxide breathing. As previously mentioned, Yamamoto (1960) had drawn attention to the amplitude of oscillations of arterial CO_2 partial pressure ($p_a CO_2$). Because $p_a CO_2$ can decrease only during inspiration, there is a recurring oscillation of $p_a CO_2$ which has a period dependent on the respiration rate. The amplitude of this oscillation increases during exercise (CO_2 loading via the mixed venous blood) and decreases during CO_2 inhalation (CO_2 loading via the lungs). That there is a large difference in respiratory response to these two sources of CO_2 loading, with exercise provoking a rapid increase in ventilation followed by a slower rise toward the steady state (see Section 4.3.4), and CO_2 inhalation provoking a much slower rise in ventilation, has stimulated thought that the amplitude of oscillations could provide information to the controller beyond that provided by the mean $p_a CO_2$ alone.

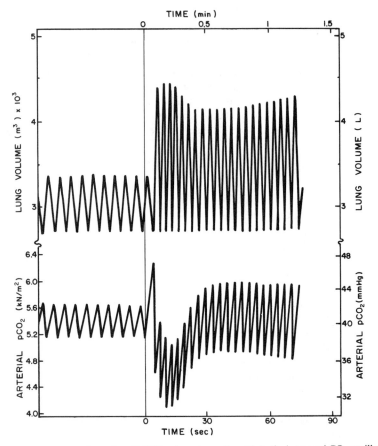

Figure 4.5.4 Sudden onset of exercise of 100 N·m/sec at zero time. Note the increased CO_2 oscillations after the transient, due to the increased CO_2 inflow in venous blood. (Adapted and used with permission from Saunders et. al., 1980.)

Saunders (1980) demonstrated that it is not the amplitude of the oscillations but rather the rate of rise of p_aCO_2 with time that could provide the necessary controller information. The general shape of p_aCO_2 oscillations is seen in Figure 4.5.5. The rising limb of the CO_2 oscillation occupies more than half the cycle because of dead volume and respiratory waveshape. The rate of rise is almost constant during the rising limb. The magnitude of the rate of rise depends on the size of the dead volume, breathing waveshape, and the respiration rate. These effects have been seen experimentally as well as analytically (Saunders, 1980).

Saunders (1980) proposed that the rate of rise[93] of p_aCO_2, (dp_aCO_2/dt), be considered the important controller signal. In view of the many neural receptors which are sensitive to both a stimulus level and a rate of rise of the stimulus, this hypothesis appears to be physiologically sound.

[93]Saunders actually considers the *maximum* rate of rise of arterial CO_2 partial pressure to be the controller stimulus. Since the rate of rise is nearly constant, there will be little difference between maximum and instantaneous rates.

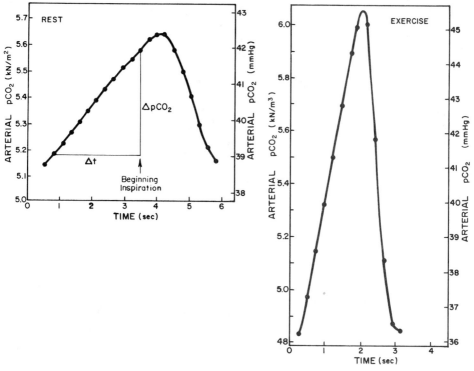

Figure 4.5.5 The general shape of pCO_2 oscillations obtained at rest (*left*) and at 100 N·m/sec (*right*). The ascending limb with slope $\Delta pCO_2/\Delta t$ occupies two-thirds of the cycle in both cases. From left to right, tidal volumes are 63×10^{-5} m^3 (0.63 L) and 170×10^{-5} m^3 (1.7 L) and respiration rates are 0.187/sec (11.2/min) and 0.343/sec (20.6/min). (Adapted and used with permission from Saunders, 1980.)

Saunders then proposed that this stimulus be incorporated within a feedforward[94] loop not so much to maintain mean arterial pCO_2 at a constant level of 5333 N/m^2 (40 mm Hg) seen during exercise as to remove excess metabolic CO_2. The ventilation required to maintain p_aCO_2 at a level of 5333 N/m^2 is related to the rate of rise of p_aCO_2 during the oscillation by the feedforward controller equation:

$$\dot{V} = 7.00 \times 10^{-7}(dp_aCO_2/dt) \tag{4.5.98}$$

where $\dot{V}$ = average ventilation rate, m^3/sec
(dp_aCO_2/dt) = rate of rise of arterial CO_2 partial pressure, N/(m^2·sec)
which is a simple linear relationship.

Using only the feedforward equation (4.5.98) and the controlled system described in Saunders

---

[94]Saunders (1980) gave a clear explanation for the difference between feedforward and feedback control: "If we start with the purpose of maintaining isocapnia, it is natural to start thinking in terms of negative feedback. If however we start with the purpose of eliminating a CO_2 load with maximal efficiency, we may think of a different approach. Thus, an engineering plant controller, faced with a sudden increase in raw material to process, recruits extra staff and mobilises spare machinery. If done well, supplies of rate-limiting components and energy sources will remain constant, and the output of processed material will match the input. In the respiratory system also, faced with a sudden need to process CO_2, the effective mechanism is a direct coupling to the elimination rate." A feedback plant controller would have reduced the CO_2 load which the plant processes by accumulating CO_2 somewhere near the input.

et al. (1980), and with no feedback whatsoever, the system remained stable, mean p_aCO_2 remained at $5426\ N/m^2$ with a somewhat irregular tidal volume showing an occasional deep breath (Figure 4.5.6). Such irregularity in tidal volume is a characteristic of natural breathing.

Circulation time delays can be calculated by the simple process of dividing the volume of the relevant circulation segment by the instantaneous flow rate. However, for rapid changes in flow rate, such as those which accompany the onset of exercise, this approach is incorrect, and the procedure described by Grodins et al. (1967) had to be used.

Using this approach, the delay time between lung and controller (assumed to be in the proximity of the carotid body) has been calculated. The effect of doubling cardiac output on p_aCO_2 oscillations is shown in Figure 4.5.7. It can be seen that even before the blood reaches the controller site, the rate of rise of p_aCO_2 increases. The chemical signal can travel faster than the blood flow!

Saunders (1980) modified the feedforward equation (4.5.98) somewhat to match real data better, which resulted in

$$\dot{V} = 7.69 \times 10^{-7}(dp_aCO_2/dt) - 1.67 \times 10^{-5} \tag{4.5.99}$$

The resulting simulated exercise ventilation at $100\ N\cdot m/sec$ is shown in Figure 4.5.8. It can be seen that the abrupt increase in breathing, followed by the slow rise to steady state, is simulated well even without explicit neural input.

Finally, a controller to simulate both exercise and CO_2 breathing incorporated the resting controller Equations (4.5.97a–4.5.97c) and the feedforward Equation (4.5.99):

$$\dot{V} = \text{Equation } 4.5.97 + \text{Equation } 4.5.99 - 1.23 \times 10^{-4} \tag{4.5.100}$$

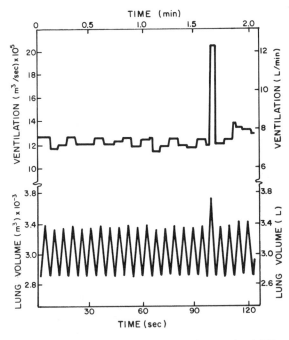

Figure 4.5.6 Ventilation demanded by feedforward control as in Equation 4.5.98 at rest (upper plot), and resulting tidal breathing volume trace. (Adapted and used with permission from Saunders, 1980.)

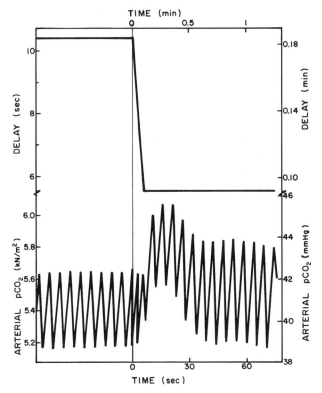

Figure 4.5.7 Delay between lung and controller (upper plot) and arterial pCO_2 delayed as seen by the controller (lower plot), when blood flow is suddenly doubled at zero time. (Adapted and used with permission from Saunders, 1980.)

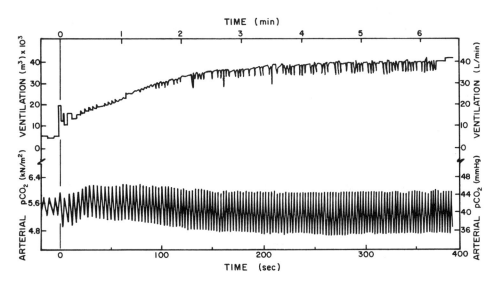

Figure 4.5.8 Demanded ventilation and arterial pCO_2 oscillations in simulated exercise at 100 N·m/sec. Feedforward controller as in Equation 4.5.99. (Adapted and used with permission from Saunders, 1980.)

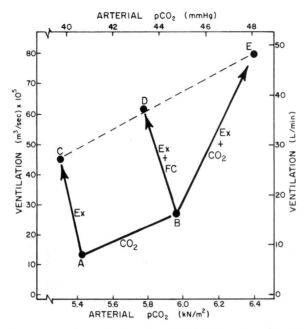

Figure 4.5.9   Steady-state results for ventilation and arterial pCO_2 from the model with controller equation (4.5.100). A = resting point: AB = 4% CO_2 breathing; AC = 50 N·m/sec exercise; BD = 4% CO_2 breathing with superimposed 50 N·m/sec exercise and inspired CO_2 inflow rate constant; BE = 4% CO_2 breathing with superimposed exercise at 50 N·m/sec. (Adapted and used with permission from Saunders, 1980.)

The resulting controller performance is seen in Figure 4.5.9. Resting response to increased inspired CO_2 is given by AB. The transition between rest and exercise is given by AC and is isocapnic within 133 N/m². Exercise plus inhaled CO_2 gives the response represented by CE. Notice that exercise response to inhaled CO_2 occurs at the same slope as resting CO_2 response, with an apparent shift in intercept. Indeed, this hypothesized respiratory controller is consistent with many of the experimental observations that have been so difficult to reproduce in other models (Allen and Jones, 1984).

Yamamoto CO₂ Model.   This model was formulated explicitly to reproduce classic experiments in respiratory control: those by Kao (1963), Yamamoto and Edwards (1960), Greco et al. (1978), and Ponte and Purves (1978). The model is somewhat simpler than the model of Grodins et al. (1967) because the only gas considered was carbon dioxide (oxygen was ignored and hydrogen ions were replaced by CO_2), and there is no explicit cerebrospinal fluid compartment. This model (Yamamoto, 1978, 1981) does, however, show a steady-state hyperpnea to CO_2 introduced at the tissues, with no concomitant rise in mean arterial carbon dioxide partial pressure, and it shows a steady-state hyperpnea to inhaled carbon dioxide which involves a proportionate increase in mean p_aCO_2.

The basic model, formulated for a normal man, includes the two large components of a controlled system and a controlling system (Figure 4.5.10). The controlled system includes lung, brain, and peripheral tissues. Each of these, in turn, consists of a cellular space, an extracellular space, and a capillary blood volume. For the lung, however, the alveolar space is equivalent to the cellular space of tissue. Lung tissue is treated as a single compartment interposed between capillary and gas. The lung gas space consists of alveolar and dead spaces. Respiratory drive is

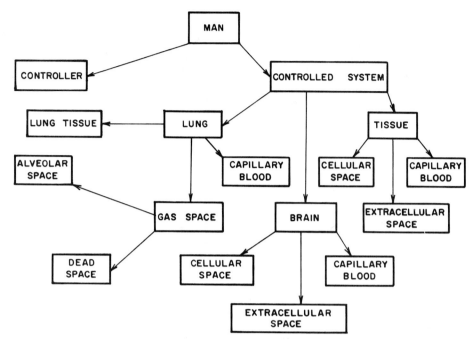

Figure 4.5.10 Organization of the Yamamoto CO_2 model.

computed as a hypothetical muscle pressure which must overcome thoracic and airway impedances to expand or contract alveolar volume.

Components of the controlled system are connected by a branched first-in–first-out file representing the circulating blood. It is in this manner that circulatory delays are incorporated within the model (Figure 4.5.11). There are 100 elements to this file, with each element representing $60 \times 10^{-6}\,\text{m}^3$ of blood (and total systemic blood volume of $6 \times 10^{-3}\,\text{m}^3$ blood). Blood gas values are contained in these elements, and they slowly and sequentially make their ways from one point in the system to another. As cardiac output increases, the volume of blood in each element remains constant, but the transit time decreases. Shifts in blood volume are thus not included. At rest the total transit time is 0.6 sec (cardiac output = $1.0 \times 10^{-4}\,\text{m}^3/\text{sec}$), but at an elevated cardiac output of $3.3 \times 10^{-4}\,\text{m}^3/\text{sec}$, transit time decreases to 0.18 sec. In all cases, total transit time is represented by 100 cycles of computation ($100T_b$).

The site of the respiratory controller is assumed to be the brain. The circulatory branch to the respiratory controller is a sequential subfile whose origin is determined by the volumetric distance of the brain from the heart. Mixed venous blood is produced by the merger of brain and peripheral tissue blood flows.

Table 4.5.2 lists dimensions and typical resting conditions for the simulated man. Basic equations of the model follow below.

Carbon dioxide material balances for the brain compartment are formulated for intracellular fluid:

$$V_{Bi}\,\alpha_{Bi}\,\frac{dp_{Bi}}{dt} = \dot{M}_B - K_{Bi}(p_{Bi} - p_{Be}) \tag{4.5.101}$$

where V_{Bi} = brain intracellular volume, m^3

α_{Bi} = solubility of CO_2 in intracellular volume, m^2/N (or $\text{m}^3\,CO_2\cdot\text{m}^2/(\text{m}^3\text{ tissue}\cdot\text{N})$)

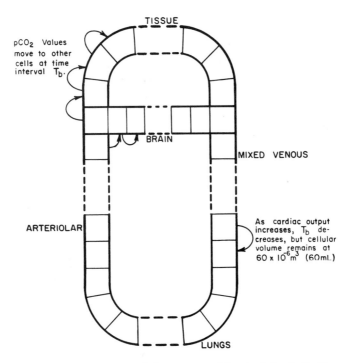

TISSUE

pCO₂ Values
move to other
cells at time
interval T_b.

BRAIN

MIXED VENOUS

ARTERIOLAR

As cardiac output
increases, T_b de-
creases, but cellular
volume remains at
60 x 10⁻⁶ m³ (60mL)

LUNGS

Figure 4.5.11 First-in–first-out (FIFO) cellular structure of the circulation in the Yamamoto model.

p_{Bi} = partial pressure of CO_2 in brain intracellular space, N/m^2
t = time, sec
$\dot{M}_B$ = brain metabolic rate, $m^3\,CO_2$ STPD/sec
K_{Bi} = proportionality constant, $m^5/(N \cdot sec)$
p_{Be} = partial pressure of CO_2 in brain extracellular space, N/m^2
For the extracellular fluid:

$$V_{Be}\alpha_{Be}\frac{dp_{Be}}{dt} = K_{Bev}(p_{Bc} - p_{Be}) - K_{Be}(p_{Be} - p_{Bi})$$ (4.5.102)

where V_{Be} = brain extracellular volume, m^3
α_{Be} = solubility of CO_2 in extracellular fluid, m^2/N
p_{Be} = CO_2 partial pressure in extracellular space, N/m^2
K_{Bev}, K_{Be} = proportionality constants, $m^5/(N \cdot sec)$
p_{Bc} = CO_2 partial pressure in brain capillary blood, N/m^2
and for the brain capillary blood:

$$V_{Bc}\alpha_{Bc}\frac{dp_{Bc}}{dt} = \dot{Q}_B\alpha_{Bc}(p_a - p_{Bc}) + K_{Bc}(p_{Be} - p_{Bc})$$ (4.5.103)

where V_{Bc} = brain capillary volume, m^3
α_{Bc} = solubility of CO_2 in blood, m^2/N
$\dot{Q}_B$ = brain blood flow, m^3/sec
p_a = arterial CO_2 partial pressure, N/m^2
K_{Bc} = constant, $m^5/(N \cdot sec)$

TABLE 4.5.2 Dimensions and Typical Resting Conditions of the Simulated Man

	Blood Volumes, m³		
	Intracellular	Interstitial	Capillary
Tissues, including brain	50×10^{-3}	8×10^{-3}	360×10^{-6}
Brain, including respiratory controller	1.2×10^{-3}	200×10^{-6}	70×10^{-6}
Respiratory controller	60×10^{-6}	10×10^{-6}	3.5×10^{-6}
Lung		1.0×10^{-3}	180×10^{-6}
Blood (total)		6.0×10^{-3} (6.0 L)	

Pulmonary properties
  FRC $2.5 \times 10^{-3} \, m^3$
    (2.5 L)
  Compliance $1.02 \times 10^{-6} \, m^5/N$
    (0.1 L/cm H_2O)
  Tidal volume $500 \times 10^{-6} \, m^3$
    (0.5 L)
  Minute volume $1.375 \times 10^{-4} \, m^3/sec$
    (8.25 L/min)
  Anatomic dead space $150 \times 10^{-6} \, m^3$
    (150 mL)
  Resistance $706 \, kN \cdot sec/m^5$
    (0.12 cm $H_2O \cdot min/L$)
  Respiration rate 0.28/sec
    (16.5/min)
  Alveolar ventilation rate $9.67 \times 10^{-5} \, m^3/sec$
    (5.8 L/min)

Circulatory properties
  Cardiac output $1.0 \times 10^{-4} \, m^3/sec$
    (6.0 L/min)
  Cerebral blood flow $12.5 \times 10^{-6} \, m^3/sec$
    (750 mL/min)
  Mean arterial pressure $13.3 \, kN/m^2$
    (100 Torr)
  Solubility of CO_2 in blood $5.36 \times 10^{-5} \, m^3 \, CO_2 \cdot m^2/(m^3 \, blood \cdot N)$
    (0.00714 mL CO_2/(mL blood·Torr))
  Solubility of CO_2 in body water $5.25 \times 10^{-6} \, m^3 \, CO_2 \cdot m^2/(m^3 \, tissue \cdot N)$
    (70×10^{-5} mL CO_2/(mL·Torr))

Resting metabolism
  CO_2 production rate (total) $4.17 \, m^3$ STPD/sec
    (250 mL STPD/min)
  Cerebral CO_2 production rate $5.5 \times 10^{-7} \, m^3 \, CO_2$ STPD/(kg·sec)
    (3.3 mL CO_2 STPD/(100 g·min))

Other
  Mean arterial CO_2 partial pressure $5357 \, N/m^2$
    (40.18 Torr)
    min $5269 \, N/m^2$
    (39.52 Torr)
    max $5498 \, N/m^2$
    (41.24 Torr)
  Systemic venous CO_2 partial pressure $6171 \, N/m^2$
    (46.29 Torr)
  Cerebral venous CO_2 partial pressure $6485 \, N/m^2$
    (48.64 Torr)
  Alveolar–arterial CO_2 gradient $67 \, N/m^2$
    (0.5 Torr)
  Neural membrane CO_2 gradient $69 \, N/m^2$
    (0.52 Torr)

Source: Adapted and used with permission from Yamamoto, 1978.

Carbon dioxide material balances for the lung compartments begin with the alveolar space:

$$\frac{dp_A}{dt} = \left[\frac{dV_A}{dt}(p_D - p_A) + K_{Ap}RT_A(p_p - p_A)\right][V_L - V_D]^{-1} \qquad (4.5.104)$$

where p_A = alveolar partial pressure of CO_2, N/m^2
V_A = alveolar volume, m^3
p_D = dead volume CO_2 partial pressure, N/m^2
K_{Ap} = constant, $m^2 \cdot mol/(N \cdot sec)$
p_p = pulmonary tissue CO_2 partial pressure, N/m^2
V_L = total lung volume, m^3
V_D = dead volume, m^3
R = gas constant, $N \cdot m/(mol \cdot °K)$
T_A = absolute temperature of alveolar gas, $°K$
For lung tissue:

$$V_p \alpha_p \frac{dp_p}{dt} = K_{pA}(p_A - p_p) + K_{pc}(p_c - p_p) \qquad (4.5.105)$$

where V_p = volume of pulmonary tissue, m^3
α_p = solubility of CO_2 in pulmonary tissue, m^2/N
p_p = CO_2 partial pressure in pulmonary tissue, N/m^2
K_{pA}, K_{pc} = constants, $m^5/(N \cdot sec)$
p_c = CO_2 partial pressure in capillary blood, N/m^2
and for pulmonary blood:

$$V_c \alpha_c \frac{dp_a}{dt} = \alpha_c \dot{Q}(p_v - p_A) + K_{pc}(p_p - p_a) \qquad (4.5.106)$$

where V_c = volume of pulmonary capillary blood, m^3
α_c = solubility of CO_2 in pulmonary blood, m^2/N, $= \alpha_{Bc}$
$\dot{Q}$ = cardiac output, m^3/sec
p_v = mixed venous blood CO_2 partial pressure, N/m^2
In the dead space (inspiration):

$$V_D \frac{dp_D}{dt} = (\kappa_s p_i - p_D)\frac{dV_A}{dt}, \qquad \frac{dV_A}{dt} \geqslant 0 \qquad (4.5.107)$$

where κ_s = conversion of STPD to BTPS, dimensionless
p_i = CO_2 partial pressure in inhaled air, N/m^2
In the dead space (expiration):

$$V_D \frac{dp_D}{dt} = (p_D - p_A)\frac{dV_A}{dt}, \qquad \frac{dV_A}{dt} < 0 \qquad (4.5.108)$$

Carbon dioxide material balances for other tissues are, for intracellular space:

$$V_{Ti}\alpha_{Ti} \frac{dp_{Ti}}{dt} = \dot{M}_{Ti} - K_{Ti}(p_{Ti} - p_{Te}) \qquad (4.5.109)$$

where V_{Ti} = volume of tissue intracellular space, m^3
$\quad\quad \alpha_{Ti}$ = solubility of CO_2 in tissue intracellular space, m^2/N
$\quad\quad p_{Ti}$ = CO_2 partial pressure in tissue intracellular space, N/m^2
$\quad\quad \dot{M}_{Ti}$ = rate of CO_2 production in tissue intracellular space, $m^3 CO_2$ STPD/sec
$\quad\quad K_{Ti}$ = constant, $m^5/(N \cdot sec)$
$\quad\quad p_{Te}$ = CO_2 partial pressure in extracellular fluid, N/m^2
For extracellular space:

$$V_{Te}\alpha_{Te}\frac{dp_{Te}}{dt} = K_{Tc}(p_{Tc} - p_{Tc}) - K_{Te}(p_{Te} - p_{Ti}) \quad\quad (4.5.110)$$

where V_{Te} = tissue extracellular volume, m^3
$\quad\quad \alpha_{Te}$ = CO_2 solubility in tissue extracellular volume, m^2/N
$\quad K_{Tc}, K_{Te}$ = constants, $m^5/(N \cdot sec)$
$\quad\quad p_{Tc}$ = CO_2 partial pressure in tissue blood, N/m^2
And for tissue capillary blood:

$$V_{Tc}\alpha_{Tc}\frac{dp_{Tc}}{dt} = K_{Tc}(p_{Te} - p_{Tc}) + \dot{Q}_T(p_{Ta} - p_{Tc}) \quad\quad (4.5.111)$$

where V_{Tc} = volume of tissue capillary blood, m^3
$\quad\quad \alpha_{Tc}$ = solubility of CO_2 in tissue capillary blood, m^2/N, $= \alpha_{Bc}$
$\quad\quad \dot{Q}_T$ = tissue blood flow, m^3/sec
$\quad\quad p_{Ta}$ = CO_2 partial pressure at the entrance to the tissue capillaries, N/m^2
Cardiac output, as given by Yamamoto (1978), does not depend on blood gases, as given by Grodins et al. (1967), but instead depends on metabolic rate:

$$\dot{Q} = 7.542 \times 10^{-5} + 5.9\dot{M} \quad\quad (4.5.112)$$

where $\dot{Q}$ = cardiac output, m^3/sec
$\quad\quad \dot{M}$ = total body metabolic rate, $m^3 CO_2/sec$
Circulatory resistance is given by

$$R_v = \frac{2.22 \times 10^{-4}}{\dot{Q}} \quad\quad (4.5.113)$$

where R_v = total vascular resistance, $N \cdot sec/m^5$
Cerebral blood flow is given by

$$\dot{Q}_B = \frac{R_v}{R_b}\dot{Q} \quad\quad (4.5.114)$$

The cerebral blood volume aliquot, taken to be the basic unit of blood flow to the brain, is

$$V_{BB} = \dot{Q}_B \Delta t \quad\quad (4.5.115)$$

where V_{BB} = brain blood volume aliquot, m^3
$\quad\quad \Delta t$ = circulation time for each aliquot, sec
and

$$\Delta t = Q_H/\dot{Q}_B \quad\quad (4.5.116)$$

where Q_H = unit blood volume, m^3

Q_H is $60 + 10^{-6}$ when calculation time H is 0.60 sec. For mixed venous blood,

$$p_v = \frac{[p_{Tc}(t - N_1 \Delta t)] V_{Tc} + [p_{Bc}(t - N_2 \Delta t)] V_c}{V_c + V_{Tc}} \qquad (4.5.117)$$

where $V_c + V_{Tc} = 60 \times 10^{-6} \, m^3$

N_1, N_2 = circulatory lags, dimensionless

Pulmonary mechanics are described by

$$\dot{V}_A = \frac{K_R R(nT_b) - (V_L - \text{FRC})/C}{R} \qquad (4.5.118)$$

where K_R = constant, dimensionless

$R(nT_b)$ = computed respiratory drive, N/m^2

C = respiratory compliance, m^5/N

R = respiratory resistance, $N \cdot \text{sec}/m^5$

T_b = circulatory computation time, sec

$\dot{V}_A$ = alveolar ventilation rate, m^3/sec

Respiratory drive represents the envelope of neural impulses in the motor nerves of respiration. It is chosen to be a trapezoidal waveshape that switches from inhalation to exhalation at 0.45 times the respiratory period. Magnitude and frequency of this signal are computed from the CO_2 level of the blood. The frequency drive is calculated from the amplitude by[95]

$$F(nT_b) = \left\{ \sum_0^n (0.09)[A(nT_b) + 12] T_b \right\} \text{MOD} \, 1.0 \qquad (4.5.119)$$

where $F(nT_b)$ = frequency signal for the respiratory drive, dimensionless

$A(nT_b)$ = amplitude signal for the respiratory drive, dimensionless

n = number of breaths, dimensionless

Since A and F are functions of nT_b, time has been assumed to advance in quanta. That is, the amplitude and frequency drives do not change during the circulatory time but only between computation times (at time = nT_b). Also, since the amplitude signal $A(nT_b)$ is summed in Equation 4.5.119, the frequency drive has memory: frequency depends somewhat on previous values of amplitude.

The respiratory drive during inspiratory effort is

$$R(nT_b) = 0.7 A(nT_b) + 0.6 F(nT_b) A(nT_b), \qquad 0 < F(nT_b) \leqslant 0.45 \qquad (4.5.120)$$

where $R(nT_b)$ = computed respiratory drive, N/m^2

During expiration it is

$$R(nT_b) = A(nT_b)[0.5 - 0.8 F(nT_b)] \qquad (4.5.121)$$

Expiration required active muscular effort at all levels of CO_2 excitation. Forcing expiration to be passive was found to change the model behavior only a little.

The equation describing $A(nT_b)$ is the controller equation, and it was this relationship that was the object of study for Yamamoto (1978). The controlling system was assumed to be that part

---

[95]The form $X \text{MOD} Y$ is abbreviated notation for modulo arithmetic. The value for $X \text{MOD} Y$ is the remainder after X is divided evenly by Y. Thus $8.25 \text{MOD} 4 = 0.25$, and $9.0 \text{MOD} 1.0 = 0.0$. Equation 4.5.119 always returns the fractional part of the quantity inside the braces.

of the brain which was concerned with respiration. For an assumed brain mass of 1.4 kg, only 5% (70 g) was assumed to participate in the controller. This brain tissue itself required description by tissue material balance equations (4.5.101–4.5.103). For this portion of the brain, resting blood flow and metabolism were scaled to 5% of those appearing in Table 4.5.2.

Yamamoto (1978) assumed that increased neural output from the brain controller region was accompanied by an increase in local metabolism, with a concomitant increase in carbon dioxide production. An increase in respiratory center activity did not result in a general increase in CO_2 production of the whole brain. The relation between neural activity and CO_2 production is given by

$$\frac{d\dot{M}_B}{dt} = 9.73 \times 10^{-5} - (5.83 \times 10^{-3})\dot{M}_B + 5.00 \times 10^{-6} A(nT_b) \qquad (4.5.122)$$

where $\dot{M}_B$ = brain CO_2 production rate, m^3/sec

Carbon dioxide production was calculated to be $3.85 \times 10^{-5}\, m^3$ STPD/sec. Yamamoto (1978) discusses in greater detail the origin of the coefficient values.

Respiratory controller blood flow was assumed to exhibit the same dependence on arterial carbon dioxide partial pressure as does the entire brain. Rather than use the equations (4.5.50a and b) by Grodins et al. (1967), Yamamoto chose to fit experimental data quatratically. These equations were then scaled to 70 g of brain tissue.

$$\dot{Q}_B(nT_b) = 6.25 \times 10^{-7}, \qquad 5013 < p_aCO_2 < 5866\, N/m^2 \qquad (4.5.123a)$$

$$\dot{Q}_B(nT_b) = 6.2047 \times 10^{-7} - (1.3777 \times 10^{-8})\sqrt{455.71 - (9.0744 \times 10^{-2})p(nT_b)},$$
$$p_aCO_2 < 5013\, N/m^2 \qquad (4.5.123b)$$

$$\dot{Q}_B(nT_b) = 1.6655 \times 10^{-7} + (4.7102 \times 10^{-4})\sqrt{(2.6540 \times 10^{-3})p(nT_b) - 14.606},$$
$$5866\, N/m^2 < p_aCO_2 \qquad (4.5.123c)$$

where $\dot{Q}_B$ = blood flow through respiratory controller, m^3/sec

$p(nT_b)$ = arterial carbon dioxide partial pressure evaluated in discrete time, N/m^2

This computation occurs in discrete, or quantized, time, and spaced one circulatory computation time (T_b) apart.

To introduce a first-order temporal response into vascular changes, Yamamoto (1978) computed blood flow with a first-order difference equation:

$$\dot{Q}'_B(nT_b) = 0.85\dot{Q}_B[(n-1)] + 0.15\dot{Q}_B(nT_b) \qquad (4.5.124)$$

where $\dot{Q}'_B(nT_b)$ = actual blood flow at time = nT_b, m^3/sec

Under resting conditions this is approximately equivalent to a first-order differential equation with a time constant of 4.2 sec.

The nature of the control mechanism was postulated by Yamamoto (1978) as consisting of three contributing components:

1. A term linearly proportional to brain extracellular carbon dioxide partial pressure.
2. A term linearly related to the transmembrane gradient of CO_2 in the neuron.
3. A term linearly related to the difference between the present value of p_aCO_2 and the average value of p_aCO_2 some time ago.

The first term represents the generally accepted view that cerebrospinal fluid is important in respiratory control; the second term gives a gradient detector without a fixed set point, which

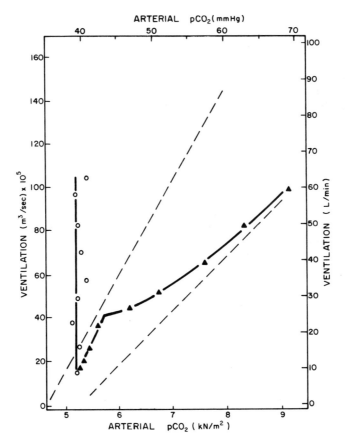

Figure 4.5.12 Ventilation as a function of arterial partial pressure of carbon dioxide for the Yamamoto model. Two responses are clearly obtained dependng on the means of CO_2 introduction. Metabolically produced CO_2 elicits an isocapnic response with almost infinite sensitivity. Inhaled CO_2 elicits ventilation proportional to pCO_2 within an experimentally determined high- and low-sensitivity range. (Adapted and used with permission from Yamamoto, 1978.)

accentuates transient response; and the third term incorporates a time-variant signal into the controller.

$$A(nT_b) = 3.2(p_{Be} - 6079) + 51.0(p_{Bi} - p_{Be}) + 2.0[R_{aa}(0) - R_{aa}(H)] \qquad (4.5.125)$$

where p_{Be} = brain extracellular CO_2 partial pressure, N/m^2
$\quad p_{Bi}$ = brain intracellular CO_2 partial pressure, N/m^2
$\quad R_{aa}(t)$ = autocovariance function evaluated at time lag t, dimensionless[96]
$\quad H$ = delay constant in equivalent file locations, dimensionless

[96]The autocovariance function determines the variation of a signal with itself when delayed by some time interval. A periodic signal will display a periodic autocovariance function. A nonperiodic signal will usually display some monotonically decreasing autocovariance function with maximum value (of 1.0) appearing at a time delay of 0.0. The autocovariance term was used here to give a moving difference value and was calculated from

$$2.0\{p_aCO_2(nT_b) - p_aCO_2[(n - H)T_b]\}^2$$

Values of p_aCO_2 used were in the current cerebral arteriolar position and the one in the cerebral artery H computational cycles earlier in the first-in–first-out file.

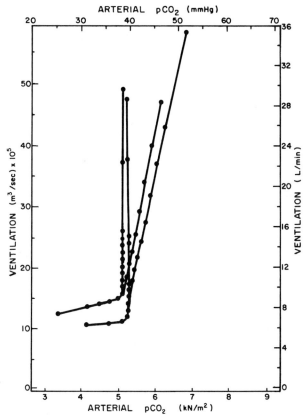

Figure 4.5.13 Model responses over an extended range of arterial pCO_2. Both metabolic CO_2 (vertical lines) and inhaled CO_2 (inclined lines) produce a dog-leg characteristic. (Adapted and used with permission from Yamamoto, 1978.)

Yamamoto used delay values of 1.26 and 1.19 sec, which gave different file location sequences.

Results from the model are seen in Figure 4.5.12. Response to metabolic CO_2 production is isocapnic, whereas response to CO_2 inhalation falls within the range of experimental observations which are described as proportional. The cusp in the model results for CO_2 inhalation is ascribed to the inability of the circulatory file to produce a constant value of the delay constant H. More circulatory segments would presumably alleviate the problem. From the standpoint that the model met the judgement criteria for metabolic and inhaled CO_2, it appears to be successful.

Yamamoto (1981) modified this model in order to reproduce some experimental observations that show that an isocapnic response is not always solicited in response to intravenous CO_2 loading. He was able to demonstrate, with the modified model, a CO_2 response that includes the dog-leg, or hockey-stick, characteristic previously described (see Section 4.3.4). These model results are shown in Figure 4.5.13.

With similar objectives, Swanson and Robbins (1986) investigated two optimal controller structures which also predict isocapnic response to metabolic CO_2 load and nonisocapnic response to inspired CO_2 load. In these structures, cost functionals with two terms (one involving the cost associated with maintaining an arterial carbon dioxide partial pressure at a set point and the other involving the excess cost of breathing) were minimized for controller operation. Direct comparison to the Yamamoto model has not been made, but it is clear that all three of these models are at least partially successful in reproducing exercise ventilatory effects.

4.5.2 Fujihara Control Model

Fujihara et al. (1973a, b) experimentally applied a series of impulse, step, and ramp work loads to subjects pedaling a bicycle ergometer. Work rates were changed silently, and without warning. The range of work loads studied was 33–360 N·m/sec.

By changing work rates with impulse inputs, especially, Fujihara et al. were able to distinguish between a set of competing models to describe respiratory transient responses. The model that best described their experimental data is

$$\Delta \dot{V}_E(S) = \frac{AE^{-st_{D1}}}{(1 + s\tau_1)} + \frac{Be^{-st_{D2}}}{(1 + s\tau_2)(1 + s\tau_3)} \tag{4.5.126}$$

where $\Delta \dot{V}_E(S) =$ change in minute ventilation, m³/sec
  $A, B =$ constants, m³/sec
  $t_{D1}, t_{D2} =$ time delays, sec
  $\tau_1, \tau_2, \tau_3 =$ time constants, sec
  $s =$ complex Laplace transform parameter,[97] sec⁻¹

This transfer function has a time response to an impulse work load as in Figure 4.5.14 (left) and to a step input work load as in Figure 4.5.14 (right). This function provides for the rapid and slower ventilatory responses to abrupt exercise described earlier (see Section 4.3.4), but it also exhibits no identifiable fast response to high levels of exercise when made abruptly higher (Bennett et al., 1981).

Estimates of parameters appearing in Equation 4.5.126 are listed in Table 4.5.3. Fujihara et al. used mainly unsophisticated graphical techniques for determining these values.

Bennett et al. (1981) confirmed the form of Equation 4.5.126 as the correct description of the response of the respiratory system to abrupt changes in ventilatory demand. However, their findings came as a result of the application of a pseudorandom binary sequence of work rates between the limites of 25 and 100 N·m/sec to subjects exercising on a bicycle ergometer. Bennett et al. obtained their parameter estimates (Table 4.5.4) by using autocorrelation and cross-correlation techniques. Values for t_{D1} could not be estimated except for subject BB. A comparison of values between Tables 4.5.3 and 5.5.4 shows a somewhat larger variability in the values of Bennett et al., but an overall similarity of estimates.

4.5.3 Optimization Models

A fairly complete historical discussion of optimization models in respiration was given in Section 4.3.4, and the reader is urged to review that discussion before continuing here. Many

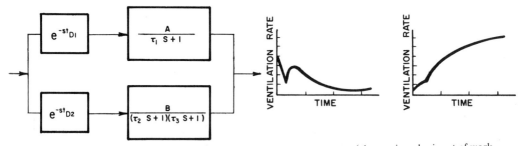

Figure 4.5.14 Time responses of the Fujihara et al. (1973) respiratory model to an impulse input of work (*left*) and step work input (*right*). (Used with permission from Bennett et al., 1981.)

---

[97]See Appendix 3.3 and the description of the Fujihara et al. model in Section 3.4.5 for further explanation of equivalence of time-domain differential equations and s-domain transfer functions.

TABLE 4.5.3   Best Fit Parameters of the Transfer Function for Minute Ventilation (Equation 4.5.126) for the Change in Workload from 32.7 to 400 N·m/sec

Subject	A, m³/sec (L/min)		B, m³/sec (L/min)		t_{D1}, sec	t_{D2}, sec	τ_1, sec	τ_2, sec	τ_3, sec
RA	3.67×10^{-5}	(2.2)	2.42×10^{-4}	(14.5)	5	15	8	50	25
YF	2.33×10^{-5}	(1.4)	2.00×10^{-4}	(12.0)	6	18	6	45	25
JH	3.33×10^{-5}	(2.0)	1.50×10^{-4}	(9.0)	1	20	8	40	12
JRH	5.00×10^{-5}	(3.0)	2.08×10^{-4}	(12.5)	3	20	8	40	8
RW	3.67×10^{-5}	(2.2)	1.60×10^{-4}	(9.6)	1	21	7	40	10
Avg	3.67×10^{-5}	(2.2)	1.92×10^{-4}	(11.3)	3.2	18.8	7.4	43.0	16.0

Source: Adapted and used with permission from Fujihara et al., 1973a.

TABLE 4.5.4   Parameter Estimates of the Transfer Function for Minute Ventilation (Equation 4.5.126) for a Pseudorandom Binary Sequence of Workloads Between 25 and 100 N·m/sec

Subject	A, m³/sec (L/min)		B, m³/sec (L/min)		t_{D1}, sec	t_{D2}, sec	τ_1, sec	τ_2, sec	τ_3, sec
FB	2.07×10^{-5}	(1.24)	2.63×10^{-4}	(15.77)	—	20.2	3.8	12.4	100.0
PR	4.87×10^{-5}	(2.92)	1.50×10^{-4}	(8.99)	—	22.0	17.9	7.3	52.7
PI	2.13×10^{-5}	(1.28)	2.70×10^{-4}	(16.20)	—	0.0	2.1	49.8	49.9
WF	3.13×10^{-5}	(1.88)	1.54×10^{-4}	(9.21)	—	14.6	7.4	7.5	48.8
BB	6.85×10^{-5}	(4.11)	2.24×10^{-4}	(13.14)	6.4	17.0	7.4	16.7	100.7
Avg	3.82×10^{-5}	(2.29)	2.11×10^{-4}	(12.66)	—	14.8	7.7	18.7	70.4

Source: Adapted and used with permission from Bennett et al., 1981.

optimization models have been proposed but none have yet been integrated within comprehensive system models such as the Grodins model or the Yamamoto model. Most of these models, based on respiratory system mechanics, incorporate only the simplest respiratory mechanical descriptions. Some, such as the models by Johnson and Masaitis (1976) and Johnson and McCuen (1980), are special-purpose models directed to explanation of responses while wearing respiratory protective masks. Others, such as the Yamashiro and Grodins series (1971, 1973; Yamashiro et al., 1975) and the Hämäläinen series (1973; Hämäläinen and Sipilä, 1980; Hämäläinen et al., 1978a, c), form connected sets of evolving complexity. In this section two models are highlighted; the first gives insight into the differences between breathing at rest and exercise, and the second reestablishes the connection between rest and exercise.

Yamashiro and Grodins Model. The purpose of the Yamashiro and Grodins (1971) model was to determine if airflow shape is regulated in an optimal manner. To show this, they assumed a simple respiratory mechanical system composed of a single constant compliance and single constant resistance. Expiration was assumed to be passive and contributed nothing to the calculation of respiratory work.

Yamashiro and Grodins assumed that airflow rate can be described by an infinite Fourier series:

$$\dot{V} = \sum_{i=1}^{\infty} a_i \sin(i\omega t) \qquad (4.5.127)$$

where $\dot{V}$ = airflow, m³/sec
   a_i = Fourier coefficients, m³/sec
   ω = radial frequency, rad/sec

t = time, sec
i = index, dimensionless

and

$$\omega = 2\pi f \tag{4.5.128}$$

where f = respiration rate, sec^{-1}
Tidal volume is given by the integral of the flow rate:

$$V_T = \int_0^{t_i} \dot{V} dt \tag{4.5.129}$$

where V_T = tidal volume, m^3
t_i = inhalation time, sec

$$t_i = \pi/\omega \tag{4.5.130}$$

Therefore,

$$V_T = \sum_{i=1}^{\infty} \frac{2a_{2i-1}}{(2i-1)\omega} \tag{4.5.131}$$

Total breathing pressure[98] is

$$p = V/C + R\dot{V} \tag{4.5.132}$$

Total respiratory work becomes

$$W = \int_0^{V_T} p\,dV = \frac{V_T^2}{2C} + R \int_0^{\pi/\omega} \sum_{i=1}^{\infty} \sum_{j=1}^{\infty} a_i a_j \sin(i\omega t)\sin(j\omega t)\,dt$$

$$= \frac{V_T^2}{2C} + \frac{R\pi}{2\omega} \sum_{i=1}^{\infty} a_i^2 \tag{4.5.133}$$

where W = respiratory work, N·m
and the average work rate is

$$\bar{\dot{W}} = Wf = \frac{V_T^2 f}{2C} + \frac{R}{4} \sum_{i=1}^{\infty} a_i^2 \tag{4.5.134}$$

The respiratory system problem is subject to the constraint that tidal volume must satisfy the alveolar ventilation and dead space ventilation requirements:

$$V_T = V_D + \dot{V}_A/f \tag{4.5.135}$$

where V_D = dead volume, m^3
$\dot{V}_A$ = alveolar ventilation rate, m^3/sec
To find the optimal airflow waveshape, the rate of work (Equation 4.5.134) must be minimized

---

[98]Yamashiro and Grodins did not include the second Rohrer coefficient for resistance (Equation 4.2.70). Johnson and Masaitis (1976) showed that the same optimal airflow waveform obtained by Yamashiro and Grodins can result from inclusion of the second Rohrer coefficient.

subject to the constraint of Equation 4.5.135. Rewritten, these equations become

$$\bar{W} = \frac{f}{2C}(V_D + \dot{V}_A/f)^2 + \frac{R}{4}\sum_{i=1}^{\infty} a_i^2 \tag{4.5.134a}$$

$$V_D f + \dot{V}_A - \frac{i}{\pi}\sum_{i=1}^{\infty}\frac{a_{2i-1}}{(2i-1)} = 0 \tag{4.5.135a}$$

Yamashiro and Grodins used the Lagrange multiplier method[99] to solve this problem of constrained optimization. Let

$$F^* = \frac{1}{2fC}(V_D f + \dot{V}_A)^2 + \frac{R}{4}\sum_{i=1}^{\infty} a_i^2 + \lambda\left[V_D f + \dot{V}_A - \frac{1}{\pi}\sum_{i=1}^{\infty}\right] \tag{4.5.136}$$

where F^* = Lagrange function, N·m/sec
λ = Lagrange multiplier, N/m²
The extreme was found by simultaneously solving for all i:

$$\frac{\partial F}{\partial f} = \frac{V_D}{fC}(V_D f + \dot{V}_A) - \frac{1}{2f^2 C}(V_D f + \dot{V}_A)^2 + \lambda V_D = 0 \tag{4.5.137}$$

$$\frac{\partial F}{\partial a_i} = \frac{R a_i}{2} = 0, \qquad i \neq 2j - 1 \tag{4.5.138a}$$

$$\frac{\partial F}{\partial a_i} = \frac{R a_i}{2} - \frac{\lambda}{\pi i} = 0, \qquad i = 2j - 1 \tag{4.5.138b}$$

Therefore,

$$\lambda = \frac{\pi(2i-1)R a_{2i-1}}{2} = \frac{(V_D f + \dot{V}_A)\pi^2 R}{2\sum_{i=1}^{\infty}[1/(2i-1)^2]} \tag{4.5.139}$$

And since

$$\frac{\pi^2}{8} = \sum_{i=1}^{\infty}\frac{1}{(2i-1)^2} \tag{4.5.140}$$

then

$$\lambda = 4R(V_D f + \dot{V}_A) \tag{4.5.141}$$

From Equation 4.5.139,

$$f = \frac{1}{16RC}\sqrt{1 + 32RC V_A/V_D - 1} \tag{4.5.142}$$

Substituting Equation 4.5.141 into Equation 4.5.139 yields

$$a_{2i-1} = \frac{8}{\pi(2i-1)}(V_D f + \dot{V}_A) \tag{4.5.143}$$

---

[99]The Lagrange multiplier method is used for solving constrained optimization problems. See Appendix 4.1 for an explanation of the method.

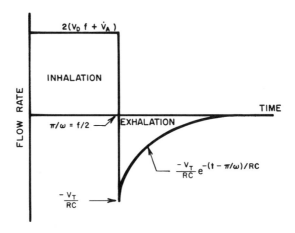

Figure 4.5.15 Optimal respiratory airflow waveshapes generated by the model of Yamashiro and Grodins (1971).

And these Fourier coefficients correspond to a rectangular airflow wave of amplitude $2(V_D f + \dot{V}_A)$ and duration $f/2$.

The expiratory waveshape for passive exhalation was found by setting respiratory pressure to zero in Equation 4.5.132. The solution is

$$\dot{V} = -[V_T/RC] \exp[-(t - \pi/\omega)/RC] \qquad (4.5.144)$$

These optimal waveshapes appear in Figure 4.5.15. There is a great deal of similarity between these waveshapes and inhalation during exercise and exhalation at rest. Later work (Johnson and Masaitis, 1976; Ruttimann and Yamamoto, 1972; Yamashiro and Grodins, 1973; Yamashiro et al., 1975) confirms the rectangular waveshape which minimizes respiratory work rate. The same waveshape can be obtained for both inhalation and exhalation when exhalation is no longer considered to be passive. These waveshapes are characteristic of exercise (see Figure 4.3.35).

Resting inspiratory waveforms do not appear to be rectangular in shape but are much more akin to sinusoids. Yamashiro and Grodins (1971) investigated this condition as well. They noted that the inspiratory muscles continue to contract well into expiration, performing negative work and adding considerably to respiratory inefficiency. Why this should be so is open to speculation, but Yamashiro and Grodins noted that by slowing the transition to exhalation, rapid changes in airflow are avoided, and this may have some utility for improved gas transport in the lungs.

One measure that heavily penalizes high-frequency respiratory components is the mean-squared acceleration (MSA). Yamashiro and Grodins obtained the respiratory waveform which minimized MSA. Acceleration is found by differentiating Equation 4.5.127 with respect to time:

$$\ddot{V} = \sum_{i=1}^{\infty} \pi i a_i f \cos(2\pi i f t) \qquad (4.5.145)$$

and

$$\text{MSA} = \frac{1}{T} \int_0^T \ddot{V}^2 dt = \frac{2\pi^2}{T^2} \sum_{i=1}^{\infty} a_i^2 i^2 \qquad (4.5.146)$$

where $T = 1/f$

Including the constraint on alveolar ventilation and dead volume, as before, gives the Lagrange equation:

$$F^* = 2\pi^2 f^2 \sum_{i=1}^{\infty} a_i^2 i^2 + \lambda \left[V_D f + \dot{V}_A - \frac{1}{\pi} \sum_{i=1}^{\infty} \frac{a_{2i-1}}{2i-1} \right] \qquad (4.5.147)$$

The extremum is found by solving for all i:

$$\frac{\partial F}{\partial a_i} = 0 = 4\pi^2 f^2 i^2 a_i, \qquad\qquad i \neq 2j-1 \qquad (4.5.148a)$$

$$\frac{\partial F}{\partial i} = 0 = 4\pi^2 f^2 (2j-1)^2 a_{2j-1} - \frac{\lambda}{\pi(2j-1)}, \quad i = 2j-1 \qquad (4.5.148b)$$

Solving,

$$a_{2i-1} = \frac{\lambda}{4\pi^3 f^2 (2i-1)^3} \qquad (4.5.149)$$

which, when substituted into the constraint of Equation 4.5.135, gives

$$V_D f + \dot{V}_A = \frac{\lambda}{4\pi^2 f^2} \sum_{i=1}^{\infty} \frac{1}{(2i-1)^4} \qquad (4.5.150)$$

Since

$$\frac{1}{30} = \frac{16}{5\pi^4} \sum_{i=1}^{\infty} \frac{1}{(2i-1)^4} \qquad (4.5.151)$$

then

$$\lambda = 384 f^2 (V_D f + \dot{V}_A) \qquad (4.5.152)$$

and

$$a_{2i-1} = \frac{384(V_D f + \dot{V}_A)}{4\pi^2 (2i-1)^3} \qquad (4.5.153)$$

The first seven harmonics were added together and plotted in Figure 4.5.16. The waveshape is very nearly a sinusoid,[100] and it appears to be similar to resting inspiratory waveshape.

What the Yamashiro and Grodins model has shown is the different natures of respiratory optimization during rest and exercise. For rest, the inspiratory waveshape generated by minimizing the mean-squared acceleration appears to be realistic; during exercise, the inspiratory waveshape generated by minimizing the average respiratory power appears to be close to reality.

Hämäläinen Model. Although there have been more recent improvements to the optimization models developed by Hämäläinen (Hämäläinen and Spililä, 1980, 1984), the model described in

[100]The waveshape, as generated by Yamashiro and Grodins, was somewhat asymmetrical, with the rise in inspiration faster than the fall. It was less peaked than a sinusoid. Hämäläinen and Viljanen (1978b) pointed out that the asymmetry was due to the awkward Fourier series method of solution. For a linear second-order system model, the closed form result is a parabolic arch for both inspiration and expiration.

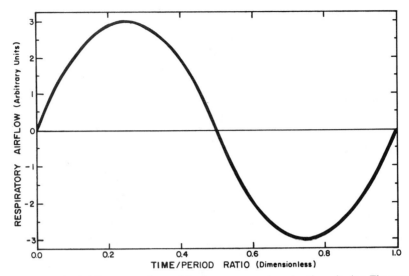

Figure 4.5.16 Optimal airflow pattern for a minimal mean-squared acceleration criterion. The waveform is a symmetrical parabolic arch for both inhalation and exhalation (Hämäläinen and Viljanen, 1978a). Comparing this waveshape with those in Figure 4.3.35a shows similarity with the inhalation airflow form. (Adapted and used with permission from Yamashiro and Grodins, 1971.)

Hämäläinen and Viljanen (1978b) is still noteworthy. It is the first published model that linked the respiratory waveshapes of exercise with those at rest and indicated how the range of respiratory waveshapes could be predicted using but one unified cost functional.[101]

Hämäläinen and colleagues began with a very simple mechanical model of the human respiratory system, which included one constant resistance and one constant compliance term:

$$p = V/C + R\dot{V} \tag{4.5.154}$$

where p = total driving pressure produced by the respiratory muscles, N/m^2
$\quad V$ = change in lung volume from resting conditions, m^3
$\quad C$ = total respiratory compliance, m^5/N
$\quad R$ = total respiratory resistance, $N \cdot sec/m^5$
$\quad \dot{V}$ = airflow rate, m^3/sec

Hämäläinen and Viljanen proposed two different cost functionals for inhalation and exhalation. These were proposed because, they argued, the inspiratory muscles continue their inspiratory action during the initial stages of exhalation. Inspiratory muscles thus perform negative work during this time. Oxygen consumption of muscles during negative work is unlike that during positive work, and the direct additional of physical work done by inspiratory and expiratory muscles therefore is not a satisfactory analog to total oxygen consumption. They proposed instead that the integral square of the driving pressure should correlate with the oxygen consumption of exercise. Presumably, there is no expiratory muscle negative work included in inhalation.

The cost functional for inhalation is

$$J_i = \int_0^{t_i} (\ddot{V}_i^2 + \alpha_i p \dot{V}) \, dt \tag{4.5.155}$$

---

[101]The cost functional is the penalty function that must be minimized to solve the problem. In the previously described Yamashiro and Grodins model, the cost functionals were average work rate and mean-squared acceleration (see Section 4.3.4).

where J_i = symbolic notation for inspiratory cost functional, m^6/sec^3
$\quad\ddot{V}$ = rate of change of inspiratory airflow rate, m^3/sec^2
$\quad\alpha_i$ = inspiratory weighting parameter, $m^5/(N\cdot sec^3)$
$\quad t_i$ = inhalation time, sec
and the cost functional for exhalation is

$$J_e = \int_{t_i}^{t_i+t_e} (\ddot{V}_e^2 + \alpha_e p^2)\, dt \qquad (4.5.156)$$

where J_e = symbolic notation for expiratory cost functional, m^6/sec^3
$\quad\ddot{V}_e$ = rate of change of expiratory airflow rate, m^3/sec^2
$\quad\alpha_e$ = expiratory weighting parameter, $m^{10}/(N^2\cdot sec^4)$

In their model, Hämäläinen and Viljanen minimized the value of each of these cost functionals to determine the time course of respiratory airflow. Other possible sources of variation, such as durations of inspiration and expiration, are presumed known. There are other optimization models which predict these values (Johnson and Masaitis, 1976; Johnson and McCuen, 1980; Yamashiro and Grodins, 1973; Yamashiro et al., 1975).

Each of these cost functionals supposedly represents the oxygen consumption of the respiratory muscles. The second term in J_i includes the product $p\dot{V}_i$, or the respiratory muscle power. The first term in both J_i and J_e describes the reduction in muscular efficiency that accompanies rapid changes in muscular contraction.

Constraints and boundary conditions of this model are

$$V(0) = V_r \qquad (4.5.157a)$$

$$V(t_i) = V_r + V_T \qquad (4.5.157b)$$

$$V(t_i + t_e) = V(T) = V_r \qquad (4.5.157c)$$

$$\dot{V}(0) = 0 \qquad (4.5.157d)$$

$$\dot{V}(t_i) = 0 \qquad (4.5.157e)$$

$$\dot{V}(t_i + t_e) = \dot{V}(T) = 0 \qquad (4.5.157f)$$

where V_r = lung resting volume, m^3
$\quad T$ = respiratory period, sec
The parameters α_i and α_e are to be considered as individual parameters, which vary from person to person.

To solve this system of equations, Hämäläinen obtained the following integrand for J_i:

$$L_i(V, \dot{V}, \ddot{V}) = \dot{V}^2 + \alpha_i(R\dot{V}^2 + V/C) \qquad (4.5.158)$$

Using the Euler–Lagrange equation,[102] the following fourth-order differential equation is obtained:

$$V'''' - \alpha_1 RV'' = 0 \qquad (4.5.159)$$

---

[102]The method of calculus of variations is often used to find the function which, over its entire range, minimizes some cost functional. If there are constraints on the problem, the method of Lagrange multipliers is combined with calculus of variations to give a set of conditions that must be met by the solution, and from which the solution can be obtained. The problem eventually reduces to an algebraic problem of solution of the Euler–Lagrange equation. See Appendix 4.2 for further details.

where primes indicate derivatives. Equation 4.5.159 has a solution:

$$\dot{V}(t) = g_{i1} + g_{i2}\exp(t\sqrt{R\alpha_i}) + g_{i3}\exp(-t\sqrt{R\alpha_i}), \qquad \alpha_i > 0 \qquad (4.5.160)$$

where g_{i1}, g_{i2}, g_{i3} = lengthy, complicated functions of equation parameters, $m^3/\sec$
In the case of exhalation,

$$L_e(V, \dot{V}, \ddot{V}) = \ddot{V}^2 + \alpha_e[R^2\dot{V}^2 + 2R\dot{V}V/C + V^2/C^2] \qquad (4.5.161)$$

gives the following differential equation:

$$V'''' - \alpha_2 R^2 V'' + \alpha_e V/C^2 = 0 \qquad (4.5.162)$$

Solutions for this equation are

$$
\begin{aligned}
\dot{V}(t) = {} & \omega_2[\exp(\omega_1 t)][-d_1\sin(\omega_2 t) + d_2\cos(\omega_2 t)] \\
& + \omega_1[\exp(\omega_1 t)][d_1\cos(\omega_2 t) + d_2\sin(\omega_2 t)] \\
& + \omega_2[\exp(-\omega_1 t)][-d_3\sin(\omega_2 t) + d_4\cos(\omega_2 t)] \\
& - \omega_1[\exp(-\omega_1 t)][d_3\cos(\omega_2 t) + d_4\sin(\omega_2 t)], \qquad 0 < \alpha_e < 4/C^2 R^4
\end{aligned} \qquad (4.5.163)
$$

$$\omega_1 = 0.5[2\alpha_e^{0.5}/C - \alpha_e R^2]^{0.5} \qquad (4.5.164)$$

$$\omega_2 = \frac{[4\alpha_e/C - \alpha_e^2 R^4]^{0.5}}{4} \qquad (4.5.165)$$

where d_1–d_4 = complicated integration constants, m^3
and

$$
\begin{aligned}
\dot{V}(t) = {} & d_1\omega_3[\exp(\omega_3 t)] - d_2\omega_3[\exp(-\omega_3 t)] \\
& + d_3\omega_4[\exp(\omega_4 t)] - d_4\omega_4[\exp(-\omega_4 t)], \qquad \alpha_e > 4/C^2 R^4
\end{aligned} \qquad (4.5.166)
$$

$$\omega_3 = \{0.5[\alpha_e R^2 + (\alpha_e^2 R^4 - 4\alpha_e/C^2)^{0.5}]\}^{0.5} \qquad (4.5.167)$$

$$\omega_4 = \{0.5[\alpha_e R^2 - (\alpha_e^2 R^4 - 4\alpha_e/C^2)^{0.5}]\}^{0.5} \qquad (4.5.168)$$

These equations were numerically evaluated by computer, and the results appear in Figures 4.5.17–4.5.19. In Figure 4.5.17 the airflow pattern for different values of the constants α_i

TABLE 4.5.5 Standard Conditions Used by Hämäläinen in Generating Figures 4.5.17–4.5.19[a]

Condition	Value	
Tidal volume (V_T)	$5 \times 10^{-4}\,m^3$	(0.5 L)
Inhalation time (t_i)	2.0 sec	
Exhalation time (t_e)	2.5 sec	
Compliance (C)	$1.22 \times 10^{-6}\,m^5/N$	(0.120 L/cm H_2O)
Resistance (R)	$3.92 \times 10^5\,N\cdot\sec/m^5$	(4.0 cm $H_2O\cdot\sec$/L)
Inspiratory weighting parameter (α_i)	$2.04 \times 10^{-5}\,m^5/N\cdot\sec^3$	(2.0 L/$\sec^3\cdot$cm H_2O)
Expiratory weighting parameter (α_e)	$1.04 \times 10^{-11}\,m^{10}/N^2\cdot\sec^4$	(0.1 $L^2/\sec^4\cdot cm^2 H_2O$)

[a]Compiled from Hämäläinen and Viljanen, 1978c.

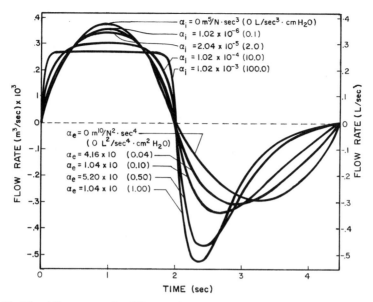

Figure 4.5.17 The airflow pattern for different values of the weighting parameters α_i and α_e for a set of standard conditions (Table 4.5.5). (Adapted and used with permission from Hämäläinen and Viljanen, 1978a).)

and α_e is seen. Other parameters appear in Table 4.5.5. As α_i increases, inhalation waveshape tends to rectangular, and as α_e increases, exhalation waveshape tends to exponential.

Figure 4.5.18 shows the effect of respiratory resistance on breathing waveshape. As resistance increases, both inhalation and exhalation become more nearly rectangular.

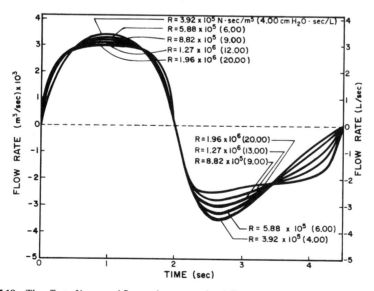

Figure 4.5.18 The effect of increased flow resistance on the airflow pattern. As resistance increases, the flow waveshape flattens, also seen experimentally. (Adapted and used with permission from Hämäläinen and Viljanen, 1978a.)

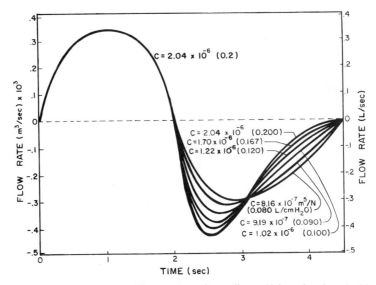

Figure 4.5.19 The airflow pattern for different values of compliance. (Adapted and used with permission from Hämäläinen and Viljanen, 1978a.)

Compliance is seen, in Figure 4.5.19, to affect only exhalation. The greater the compliance, the more nearly exponential is the waveshape.

Adding resistance to the respiratory system affects the breathing waveshape similarly to increasing flow rate (Silverman et al., 1951). Thus we would expect that the increased hyperpnea of exercise would result in a progression of waveshapes beginning with the nearly sinusoidal at rest and ending with the nearly rectangular during heavy exercise. This progression can be seen in the Hämäläinen model as resistance is increased. In this way, the model has united the waveshapes seen during rest and exercise and has provided indication of a common explanation for both.

4.5.4 Brief Discussion of Respiratory Control Models

The control models chosen for inclusion illustrate some very interesting, and contrasting, aspects of respiratory control. The model of Grodins et al. (1967) is not so much a control model as a system model, and the model did little to elucidate respiratory control mechanisms. It was left to Saunders (1980) to extend the model to produce reasonable qualitative responses to exercise, and Saunders did this by describing a respiratory controller located within the carotid bodies. He postulated a simple feedforward mechanism based on rate of change of arterial pCO_2, and he discovered the amazing result that a humoral signal could travel faster than the blood it was flowing in. Yamamoto (1978), on the other hand, produced the essentials of a model which should give reasonable exercise response, but, unlike Saunders' model, required a respiratory controller within the brain. Models of both Saunders and Yamamoto were found to be very sensitive to circulatory delays. Because experimental results have shown that respiratory control actually emanates from at least the two sites of carotid bodies and brain respiratory center, it is encouraging that both Saunders and Yamamoto did so well with their models, but it should also be clear that each is probably considering only one side of the control issue.

The Fujihara model was included because it used experimental results to answer a specific question about respiratory control. It is very interesting that Bennett et al., coming from a different direction, converged on the same results. However, these models do not have the global character of the Saunders and Yamamoto models.

The optimization models are very interesting and seem to be headed in the direction of explaining respiratory phenomena at a very low level. However, they still have the shortcoming that they are not global in nature, and they have not been assimilated within overall respiratory control models. The challenge is to incorporate these models within the upper level models to provide the details of respiratory responses.

APPENDIX 4.1
LAGRANGE MULTIPLIERS

In determining the optimum value of some function $F(x, y, \ldots, z)$, there may arise the situation where some other constraints $G_i(x, y, \ldots, z) = C_i$ must be satisfied by the solution. Here we consider the optimum of $F(x, y, \ldots, z)$ to be found as an extremum with respect to the variables $x, y, \ldots, z$. Any number of constraints $G_i(x, y, \ldots, z) = C_i$ may be imposed, so long as C_i are constants. A necessary condition for the required extremum is

$$\frac{\partial F^*}{\partial x} = \frac{\partial F^*}{\partial y} = \cdots = \frac{\partial F^*}{\partial z} = 0 \tag{A4.1.1}$$

where $F^* = F + \sum_{i=1}^{n} \lambda_i G_i$. The constants λ_i are called undetermined Lagrange multipliers. Upon forming F^* and taking the derivatives in Equation A4.1.1, a system of equations is obtained involving $x, y, \ldots, z$ and λ_i. These are then solved simultaneously with the equations $G_i(x, y, \ldots, z) = C_i$ to obtain values of λ_i. Finally, the same set of equations is solved for the required values of $x, y, \ldots, z$. This method is valid only when the Jacobian matrix is not zero (Sokolnikoff and Redheffer, 1958):

$$J(z_1, z_2, \ldots, z_j) = \begin{vmatrix} \dfrac{\partial G_1}{\partial z_1} & \dfrac{\partial G_1}{\partial z_2} & \cdots & \dfrac{\partial G_1}{\partial z_j} \\[2ex] \dfrac{\partial G_2}{\partial z_1} & \dfrac{\partial G_2}{\partial z_2} & \cdots & \dfrac{\partial G_2}{\partial z_j} \\[2ex] \vdots & \vdots & & \\[2ex] \dfrac{\partial G_i}{\partial z_1} & \dfrac{\partial G_i}{\partial z_2} & \cdots & \dfrac{\partial G_i}{\partial z_j} \end{vmatrix} \neq 0 \tag{A4.1.2}$$

Lagrange multipliers are useful in optimization problems whenever constraints must be introduced. An example of the use of Lagrange multipliers can be found in Equations 4.5.134–4.5.141 in Section 4.5.3. Here the function F is represented by the average rate of work $\bar{W}$ in Equation 4.5.134. The constraint G is given by the tidal volume relationship in Equation 4.5.135. By combining these to form F^*, Equation 4.5.136 is obtained. The various derivatives required for solution are obtained in Equations 4.5.137 and 4.5.138, and the value of the unknown Lagrange multiplier is found in Equation 4.5.141. One derivative Equation 4.5.138 was used to obtain the value for λ, and the other derivative Equation 4.5.137 was used to find the value of the parameter of interest, f, once λ was known. This f then satisfies both the original minimization of work rate criterion and the constraint that tidal volume must remain at a fixed value.

APPENDIX 4.2
METHOD OF CALCULUS OF VARIATIONS

When extreme values of integrals subject to certain constraints are to be found, the method of calculus of variations is often used. Consider the integral

$$I_1 = \int_{x_2}^{x_1} F(x, y, y')\, dx \tag{A4.2.1}$$

where $y' \equiv dy/dx$ and $F(x, y, y')$ is assumed to be known. $F(x, y, y')$ also has continuous second-order partial derivatives with respect to the arguments x, y, and y'. We desire to find the unknown function $y = y(x)$ for which the integral I_1 is a minimum. The function $y = y(x)$ is found with the help of the Euler equation (Sokolnikoff and Redheffer, 1958):

$$\frac{\partial F}{\partial y} - \frac{d}{dx}\left(\frac{\partial F}{\partial y'}\right) = 0 \tag{A4.2.2}$$

On completing the differentiation indicated in Equation A4.2.2, we obtain the second-order ordinary differential equation

$$\frac{\partial F}{\partial y} - \frac{\partial^2 F}{\partial x\, \partial y'} - \frac{\partial^2 F}{\partial y\, \partial y'} y' - \frac{\partial^2 F}{\partial y'^2} y'' = 0 \tag{A4.2.3}$$

The general solution of this equation contains two arbitrary constants that must be chosen so that the curve $y = y(x)$ passes through the boundary points (x_0, y_0) and (x_1, y_1). If the integral (A4.2.1) had been

$$I_2 = \int_{x_0}^{x_1} F(x, y, y', y'', \ldots, y^{(n)})\, dx \tag{A4.2.4}$$

then the Euler equation would be

$$\frac{\partial F}{\partial y} - \frac{d}{dx}\left(\frac{\partial F}{\partial y'}\right) + \frac{d^2}{dx^2}\left(\frac{\partial F}{\partial y''}\right) - \cdots - (-1)^n \frac{d^n}{dx^n}\left(\frac{\partial F}{\partial y^{(n)}}\right) = 0 \tag{A4.2.5}$$

with several dependent variables,

$$I_3 = \int_{x_0}^{x_1} F(x, y, \ldots, z, y', \ldots, z')\, dx \tag{A4.2.6}$$

several simultaneous Euler equations

$$\frac{\partial F}{\partial y} - \frac{d}{dx}\left(\frac{\partial F}{\partial y'}\right) = 0$$

$$\vdots \tag{A4.2.7}$$

$$\frac{\partial F}{\partial z} - \frac{d}{dx}\left(\frac{\partial F}{\partial z'}\right) = 0$$

must be satisfied (Weinstock, 1952). Euler equations are also possible for double integral problems (Sokolnikoff and Redheffer, 1958).

If the integral I_1 was subject to an integral constraint,

$$J = \int_{x_0}^{x_1} G(x, y, y')\, dx \tag{A4.2.8}$$

where J has some known constant value, the method of Lagrange multipliers is used to form another functional,

$$F^* = F + \lambda G \tag{A4.2.9}$$

and the Euler–Lagrange equation

$$\frac{\partial F^*}{\partial y} - \frac{d}{dx}\left(\frac{\partial F^*}{\partial y'}\right) = 0 \tag{A4.2.10}$$

must be satisfied (Weinstock, 1952, p. 20). In this case, once the form for λ is found from Equation A4.2.10, its value is obtained by substitution into the constraint J.

As an example of this technique, we find the inhalation flow rate required to minimize inspiratory work, assuming $p_i = K_1 \dot{V} + K_2 \dot{V}^2$:

$$W_i = \int_0^{t_i} p_i dV = \int_0^{t_i} p_i \frac{dV}{dt} dt = \int_0^{t_i} p_i \dot{V}_i dt$$

$$= \int_0^{t_i} (K_1 \dot{V}_i^2 + K_2 \dot{V}_i^3)\, dt \tag{A4.2.11}$$

Ordinarily, a minimum value for W_i could be obtained by setting $\dot{V}_i = 0$. So we add the constraint that the tidal volume must be maintained:

$$V_T = \int_0^{t_i} \dot{V}_i dt \tag{A4.2.12}$$

The Lagrange function F^* becomes

$$F^* = K_1 \dot{V}_i^2 + K_2 \dot{V}_i^3 + \lambda \dot{V}_i \tag{A4.2.13}$$

and the Euler–Lagrange equation

$$\frac{\partial F^*}{\partial \dot{V}_i} - \frac{d}{dt}\left(\frac{\partial F^*}{\partial \dot{V}_i}\right) = 0 \tag{A4.2.14}$$

becomes

$$3K_2 \dot{V}_i^2 + 2K_1 \dot{V}_i + \lambda = 0 \tag{A4.2.15}$$

since

$$\frac{d}{dt}\left(\frac{\partial F^*}{\partial \dot{V}_i}\right) = 0 \tag{A4.2.16}$$

Solving the quadratic Equation A4.2.15 for $\dot{V}_i$ gives

$$\dot{V}_i = \frac{-K_1 \pm \sqrt{K_1^2 - 3\lambda K_2}}{3K_2} \tag{A4.2.17}$$

which is substituted into the constraint Equation A4.2.12 to give

$$V_T = t_i \left\{\frac{-K_1 \pm \sqrt{K_1^2 - 3\lambda K_2}}{3K_2}\right\} \tag{A4.2.18}$$

The Lagrange multiplier value is

$$\lambda = \frac{-1}{3K_2}\left[\left(\frac{3K_2 V_T}{t_i} + K_1\right)^2 - K_1^2\right] \tag{A4.2.19}$$

Substituting this value into Equation A4.2.17 and taking the positive square root because $\dot{V}_i$ must be positive, we have

$$\dot{V}_i = V_T/t_i \tag{A4.2.20}$$

Thus the airflow waveshape to minimize inspiratory work is a constant flow rate. Further uses of this technique can be found in Johnson and Masaitis (1976).

SYMBOLS

A	area, m^2
$A(nT_b)$	amplitude signal for the respiratory drive, dimensionless
A_m	maximum total cross-sectional generational airway area, m^2
$A_n(0)$	total cross-sectional area at beginning of nth generational airways, m^2
$A_{n+1}(L)$	total cross-sectional area at end of $(n+1)$th generation of airways, m^2
B	bulk modulus of air, N/m^2
B_B	brain bicarbonate content, $m^3 CO_2/m^3$ brain
B_b	blood bicarbonate content, $m^3 CO_2/m^3$ blood
B_{CSF}	bicarbonate content of cerebrospinal fluid, $m^3 CO_2/m^3$ CSF
B_T	tissues bicarbonate content, $m^3 CO_2/m^3$ tissue
b	coefficient, dimensionless
C	compliance, m^5/N
CO	cardiac output, m^3/sec
C_{cw}	chest wall compliance, m^5/N
C_{dyn}	dynamic compliance, m^5/N
C_i	compliance of compartment i, m^5/N
C_{lt}	lung tissue compliance, m^5/N
C_{pl}	pleural compliance, m^5/N
C_{stat}	static compliance, m^5/N
c	coefficient, m^2/N
c_0	initial concentration, m^3/m^3
c_a	concentration of gas in systemic arterial blood, m^3 gas$/m^3$ blood
c_{aB}	brain arterial concentration, m^3/m^3
c_{aHbo_2}	arterial concentration of oxyhemoglobin, m^3/m^3
c_{ao}	concentration at airway opening, m^3/m^3
c_B	brain concentration, m^3/m^3
c_{CO_2}	concentration of carbon dioxide, $m^3 CO_2/m^3$ blood
c_{CSF}	concentration in cerebrospinal fluid, $\mu mol/m^3$
c_{effCO_2}	carbon dioxide concentration of effective blood compartment, $m^3 CO_2/m^3$ blood
c_H	hemoglobin concentration, kg hemoglobin$/m^3$ blood
$c_{HCO_3^-}$	bicarbonate concentration, kg/m^3
c_i	concentration of constituent i, mol/m^3
c_{i0}	initial concentration of surfactant macromolecule, mol/m^3
$c_{i\infty}$	equilibrium concentration of surfactant macromolecule constituent i, mol/m^3
c_{im}	gas concentration entering mixing point from dead volume, m^3/m^3

c_{in}	input concentration, m^3/m^3
c_m	concentration at mixing point, m^3/m^3
c_{mO_2}	muscle oxygen concentration, m^3/m^3
c_{O_2}	concentration of oxygen, $m^3\ O_2/m^3$ blood
c_T	tissue concentration, m^3/m^3
c_v	mixed venous concentration of gas, m^3 gas/m^3 blood
c_{vB}	brain venous concentration, m^3/m^3
c_{vT}	concentration in tissue venous blood, m^3/m^3
$\dot{c}_B$	rate of change of concentration in brain, $m^3/(m^3{\cdot}\text{sec})$
$\dot{c}_T$	rate of change of concentration in tissue, $m^3/(m^3{\cdot}\text{sec})$
D_i	diffusion coefficient of constituent i in a multicomponent system, m^2/sec
D_{ij}	diffusion constant of constituent i through medium j, m^2/sec
D_L	lung diffusing capacity, $m^5/(N{\cdot}\text{sec})$
D_{LCO}	lung diffusing capacity for carbon monoxide, $m^5/(N{\cdot}\text{sec})$
D_x	diffusion coefficient for constituent x, $m^5/(N{\cdot}\text{sec})$
$\mathscr{D}_{ij}$	longitudinal dispersion coefficient, m^2/sec
d	diameter, m
d	integration constant, m^3
ERV	expiratory reserve volume, m^3
$F(nT_b)$	frequency signal for respiratory drive, dimensionless
FRC	functional residual capacity, m^3
F_A	fractional concentration in alveolar air, m^3/m^3
F_{AeCO_2}	fractional concentration of CO_2 from alveolar volume in exhaled gas, m^3/m^3
F_{AiCO_2}	fractional concentration of CO_2 in inhaled air to alveolar volume, m^3/m^3
F_D	fractional concentration in dead space, m^3/m^3
F_{DeCO_2}	fractional concentration of CO_2 from dead volume in exhaled gas, m^3/m^3
F_{eCO_2}	fractional concentration of carbon dioxide in exhaled dry gas, m^3/m^3
F_{eN_2}	fractional concentration of nitrogen in exhaled dry gas, m^3/m^3
F_{eO_2}	fractional concentration of oxygen in exhaled dry gas, m^3/m^3
F_i	fractional concentration of constituent i, m^3/m^3
F_{iN_2}	fractional concentration of nitrogen in inhaled dry gas, m^3/m^3
F_{iO_2}	fractional concentration of oxygen in inhaled dry gas, m^3/m^3
F^*	Lagrange function, various units
$\dot{F}_A$	rate of change of fractional concentration in alveolar space, sec^{-1}
$\dot{F}_D$	rate of change of fractional concentration in dead space, sec^{-1}
f	friction pressure loss per unit distance, N/m^3
f	respiratory frequency, breaths/sec
G_1	constant, m^3
G_2	constant, dimensionless
G_3	constant, $(N{\cdot}\text{sec}/m^2)^{1/2}$
g	acceleration due to gravity, m/sec^2
g_{ij}	equation parameters, m^3/sec
H	delay constant, sec
H	hemoglobin concentration, kg hemoglobin/m^3 blood
HCO_3^-	bicarbonate ion concentration, kg/m^3
Ht	fractional hematocrit, dimensionless
H^+	hydrogen ion concentration, kg/m^3
H_a^+	arterial hydrogen ion concentration, kg/m^3
H_{a0}^+	arterial threshold hydrogen ion concentration, kg/m^3
H_{c0}^+	central hydrogen ion concentration, kg/m^3
H_{c0}^+	central threshold hydrogen ion concentration, kg/m^3
h_f	friction loss, m

h_i	pressure coefficient, N/m^2	
I	inertance, $N \cdot sec^2/m^5$	
IRV	inspiratory reserve volume, m^3	
I_D	collision integral for diffusion, dimensionless	
I_{law}	lower airway inertance, $N \cdot sec^2/m^5$	
I_m	mouthpiece inertance, $N \cdot sec^2/m^5$	
I_{uaw}	upper airway inertance, $N \cdot sec^2/m^5$	
J_e	expiratory cost functional, m^6/sec^3	
J_i	inspiratory cost functional, m^6/sec^3	
J_i	molar flux of constituent i, $mol/(m^2 \cdot sec)$	
J_i'	modified inspiratory cost functional, m^6/sec^3	
j	imaginary operator, denoting a phase angle	
K	coefficient, $N \cdot sec^n/m^{(2+n)}$	
K_1	first Rohrer coefficient, $N \cdot sec/m^5$	
K_2	second Rohrer coefficient, $N \cdot sec^2/m^8$	
K_3	third resistance coefficient, $N \cdot sec/m^2$	
K_4	exhalation resistance coefficient, N/m^2	
K_5	exhalation resistance coefficient, sec^{-1}	
K_{Ap}	constant, $m^2 \cdot mol/(N \cdot sec)$	
K_{Bc}	constant, $m^5/(N \cdot sec)$	
K_{Be}	proportionality constant, $m^5/(N \cdot sec)$	
K_{Bev}	proportionality constant, $m^5/(N \cdot sec)$	
K_{Bi}	proportionality constant, $m^5/(N \cdot sec)$	
K_{H^+}	dissociation constant for carbonic acid, $\mu mol/m^3$	
K_{O_2}	total blood oxygen carrying capacity, m^3/m^3	
K_{pc}	constant, $m^5/(N \cdot sec)$	
K_R	constant, dimensionless	
K_{Tc}	constant, $m^5/(N \cdot sec)$	
K_{Te}	constant, $m^5/(N \cdot sec)$	
K_{Ti}	constant, $m^5/(N \cdot sec)$	
k	Ainsworth coefficient, $N \cdot sec^n/m^{(2+3n)}$	
k	Boltzmann constant	
k	coefficient of proportionality, $m^5/(sec \cdot N)$	
k_1	constant, $N \cdot sec/m^5$	
k_2	constant, $N \cdot sec^2/m^8$	
k_3	constant, dimensionless	
k_4	constant, m^{-3}	
L	inductance, $N \cdot sec^2/m^5$	
L	length, m	
La^-	lactate ion concentration kg/m^3	
L_i	dimensionless constant	
l_e	entrance length, m	
M	proportionality constant, N/m^5	
Mc	Mach number, dimensionless	
M_i	molecular weight of gas i, dimensionless	
$\dot{M}_B$	rate of evolution in brain tissue, m^3/sec	
$\dot{M}_T$	rate of evolution in tissue, m^3/sec	
$\dot{M}_{TI}$	rate of CO_2 production in tissue	
m	body mass, kg	
m	limiting flow rate exponent, dimensionless	
m_{uaw}	mass in upper airway compartment, kg	
N	total number, dimensionless	

Na^+	sodium ion concentration, kg/m^3
N_1, N_2	circulatory lags, dimensionless
N_i	neural discharge, arbitrary units
n	Ainsworth exponent, dimensionless
n	exponent, dimensionless
n	number of breaths, dimensionless
n	number of moles, mol
n_1, n_2	hyperbola parameters, dimensionless
n_i	constituent gas number of moles, mol
P	pressure factor, $N \cdot sec/m^5$
p	pressure, N/m^2
p_1, p_2	vertical asymptotes for hyperbola, N/m^2
$p(nT_b)$	arterial CO_2 partial pressure evaluated in discrete time, N/m^2
p_A	pressure at alveolar level, N/m^2
$p_A CO$	mean alveolar partial pressure for carbon monoxide, N/m^2
p_a	arterial partial pressure, N/m^2
p_{alv}	alveolar pressure, N/m^2
p_{ao}	pressure at airway opening, N/m^2
p_{app}	pressure applied to any element of the respiratory system, N/m^2
p_{atm}	atmospheric pressure, N/m^2
p_{aw}	pressure drop in airway, N/m^2
p_B	partial pressure in brain, N/m^2
p_B	total barometric pressure, N/m^2
p_{Bc}	CO_2 partial pressure in brain capillary blood, N/m^2
p_{Be}	partial pressure of CO_2 in brain extracellular volume, N/m^2
p_{Bi}	partial pressure of CO_2 in brain intracellular space, N/m^2
p_b	pressure at exit from common airway, N/m^2
p_{bs}	pressure at the body surface, N/m^2
pCO_2	partial pressure of carbon dioxide, N/m^2
p_{CSF}	partial pressure in cerebrospinal fluid, N/m^2
p_c	CO_2 partial pressure in capillary blood, N/m^2
p_D	CO_2 partial pressure in lung dead volume, N/m^2
p_e	expiratory pressure developed by the respiratory muscles, N/m^2
P_e	Péchlet number, dimensionless
p_{fric}	friction pressure loss, N/m^2
pH	acidity, dimensionless
pH_2O	vapour pressure of water, N/m^2
p_i	CO_2 partial pressure in inspired air, N/m^2
p_i	constituent gas partial pressure, N/m^2
p_i	inspiratory pressure developed by the respiratory muscles, N/m^2
p_{in}	pressure loss due to inertance, N/m^2
p_{ir}	resistive contribution to inspiratory pressure, N/m^2
pK	logarithm of reaction constant, dimensionless
p_{kin}	kinetic energy component of pressure, N/m^2
p_m	partial pressure in muscle, N/m^2
p_m	pressure at entrance to common airway (mouth), N/m^2
p_{max}	amplitude of muscle pressure, N/m^2
p_{mus}	muscle pressure, N/m^2
p_n	normal, or set-point, partial pressure, N/m^2
pO_2	partial pressure of oxygen, N/m^2
p_o	pressure constant, N/m^2
p_p	CO_2 partial pressure in pulmonary tissue, N/m^2
p_{pl}	intrapleural pressure, N/m^2

$p_{\text{pl}i}$	pleural pressure of compartment i, N/m^2
p_{res}	pressure loss due to resistance, N/m^2
p_s	sinusoidal pressure factor, $N \cdot sec/m^5$
p_{st}	static recoil pressure due to compliance, N/m^2
$(p_{\text{st}})_{\text{sur}}$	surfactant contribution to static pressure, N/m^2
p_T	tissue partial CO_2 pressure, N/m^2
p_{Ta}	CO_2 partial pressure at the entrance to the tissue capillaries, N/m^2
p_{Tc}	CO_2 partial pressure in tissue blood, N/m^2
p_{Te}	CO_2 partial pressure in tissue extracellular fluid, N/m^2
p_{Ti}	CO_2 partial pressure in tissue intracellular space, N/m^2
p_{tm}	transmural pressure, N/m^2
p_{tp}	transpulmonary pressure, N/m^2
p_v	mixed venous blood CO_2 partial pressure, N/m^2
Δp	pressure difference, N/m^2
Δp_{CSF}	rate of change of partial pressure in cerebrospinal fluid, $N/(m^2 \cdot sec)$
Q_H	unit blood volume, m^3
$\dot{Q}$	blood flow rate, m^3/sec
$\dot{Q}$	blood flow through brain, m^3/sec
$\dot{Q}_{\text{eff}}$	effective pulmonary perfusion rate, m^3/sec
$\dot{Q}_N$	normal (resting) blood flow rate, m^3/sec
$\dot{Q}_{\text{pulm}}$	total pulmonary blood flow rate, m^3/sec
$\dot{Q}_s$	pulmonary shunt blood flow rate, m^3/sec
$\dot{Q}_T$	blood flow through tissue, m^3/sec
$\Delta \dot{Q}_{CO_2}$	change in cardiac output due to carbon dioxide pressure, m^3/sec
$\Delta \dot{Q}_{O_2}$	change in cardiac output due to oxygen pressure, m^3/sec
$\ddot{Q}$	rate of change of blood flow rate, m^3/sec
R	gas constant, $N \cdot m/(mol \cdot {}^\circ K)$
R	resistance, $N \cdot sec/m^5$
R	respiratory exchange ratio, m^3/m^3
Re	Reynolds number, $dv\rho/\mu$, dimensionless
$R(nT_b)$	computed respiratory drive, N/m^2
RQ	respiratory quotient, m^3/m^3
RQ_i	respiratory quotient of substance i, m^3/m^3
RV	residual volume, m^3
R_{aa}	autocovariance function, dimensionless
R_{aw}	airway resistance, $N \cdot sec/m^5$
R_B	brain vascular resistance, $N \cdot sec/m^5$
R_C	common airway resistance, $N \cdot sec/m^5$
R_{cw}	chest wall resistance, $N \cdot sec/m^5$
R_i	constituent gas constant, $N \cdot m/(mol \cdot {}^\circ K)$
R_i	inspiratory resistance, $N \cdot sec/m^5$
R_i	resistance of component i, $N \cdot sec/m^5$
R_{law}	lower airway resistance, $N \cdot sec/m^5$
R_{lt}	lung tissue resistance, $N \cdot sec/m^5$
R_m	mouthpiece resistance, $N \cdot sec/m^5$
R_p	pulmonary resistance, $N \cdot sec/m^5$
R_r	respiratory resistance, $N \cdot sec/m^5$
R_{uaw}	upper airway resistance, $N \cdot sec/m^5$
R_v	total vascular resistance, $N \cdot sec/m^5$
r	radius, m
r_i	collision diameter of gas i alone, m

r_i	specific resistance of compartment i, N·sec/m^2
r_{ij}	collision diameter of a pair of gases, m
S	hemoglobin saturation, dimensionless
s	complex Laplace transform parameter, sec^{-1}
T	absolute temperature, °K
T	respiratory period, sec
TLC	total lung capacity, m^3
T_A	absolute temperature of alveolar gas, °K
T_b	circulatory computation time, sec
$\dot{T}_x$	instantaneous rate of gas transfer of gas x to/from the alveolar compartment, m^3/sec
t	time, sec
t_e	exhalation time, sec
t_D	delay time, sec
t_d	dead time, sec
t_i	inspiratory time, sec
U_{O_2}	caloric equivalent of oxygen, N·m/cm^3
$u(x)$	unit step function, dimensionless
V	volume, m^3
VC	vital capacity, m^3
$\dot{V}_0$	limiting flow rate, m^3/sec
V_A	alveolar volume, m^3
$V_{A\infty}$	alveolar volume at thermodynamic equilibrium of surfactant macromolecule diffusion, m^3
V_a	volume of air moving between lower and upper airways, m^3
V_{Ae}	exhaled volume from alveolar space, m^3
V_{Ai}	inhaled volume to alveolar space, m^3
V_{amb}	volume of gas at ambient conditions, m^3
V_B	volume of brain compartment, m^3
V_{BB}	brain blood volume aliquot, m^3
V_{BC}	brain capillary volume, m^3
V_{Be}	brain extracellular volume, m^3
V_{Bi}	brain intracellular volume, m^3
V_C	volume of pulmonary capillary blood, m^3
V_{CSF}	volume of cerebrospinal fluid, m^3
V_D	respiratory dead volume, m^3
$V_{D\,alv}$	alveolar contribution to dead volume, m^3
$V_{D\,anat}$	anatomical dead volume, m^3
V_{De}	exhaled volume from dead space, m^3
V_e	exhaled volume, m^3
V_i	atomic diffusion volume, m^3
V_i	constituent gas volume, m^3
V_i	volume of compartment i, m^3
V_L	lung volume, m^3
V_{law}	lower airway volume, m^3
V_m	volume of muscle compartment, m^3
V_{mO_2}	volume of oxygen carried on myoglobin, m^3
V_p	volume of pulmonary tissue, m^3
V_{pl}	pleural cavity volume, m^3
V_r	lung resting volume, m^3
V_{rc}	rib cage volume, m^3
V_T	tidal volume, m^3

V_T	tissue volume, m^3
V_{TE}	tissue extracellular volume, m^3
V_{TI}	volume of tissue intracellular space, m^3
V_{tg}	thoracic gas volume, m^3
V_{uaw}	upper airway volume, m^3
V^*_{max}	constant, dimensionless
V^*_{min}	constant, dimensionless
$\dot{V}$	flow rate, m^3/sec
$\dot{V}_A$	alveolar ventilation rate, m^3/sec
$\dot{V}_{CO}$	rate of carbon monoxide uptake by the lungs, m^3/sec
$\dot{V}_{CO_2}$	rate of carbon dioxide efflux, m^3/sec
$\dot{V}_D$	dead volume ventilation rate, m^3/sec
$\dot{V}_E$	respiratory minute volume, m^3/min
$\dot{V}_e$	expiratory flow rate, m^3/sec
$\dot{V}_{Ec}$	intracranial receptor contribution to minute volume, m^3/sec
$\dot{V}_i$	inspiratory flow rate, m^3/sec
$\dot{V}_i$	volume flow rate of constituent i, m^3/sec
$\dot{V}_L$	limiting flow rate, m^3/sec
$\dot{V}_L$	rate of change of lung volume, m^3/sec
$\dot{V}_{N_2}$	rate of nitrogen uptake, m^3/sec
$\dot{V}_n$	constant flow rate to adjust pCO_2, m^3/sec
$\dot{V}_{O_2}$	rate of oxygen uptake, m^3/sec
V_{ws}	wave speed flow rate, m^3/sec
$\ddot{V}$	volume acceleration, m^3/sec^2
$\ddot{V}_e$	expiratory volume acceleration of the lung, m^3/sec^2
$\ddot{V}_i$	inspiratory volume acceleration of the lung, m^3/sec^2
v	fluid velocity, m/sec
v_s	speed of sound, m/sec
v_{ws}	wave speed flow rate, m/sec
W	work, $N \cdot m$
W_i	inspiratory work, $N \cdot m$
$\bar{\dot{W}}_i$	average inspiratory power, $N \cdot m/sec$
x	distance, m
X_c	reactance of compliance, $N \cdot sec/m^5$
Z	airway generation, dimensionless
Z_m	amplitude of the mechanical impedance, $N \cdot sec/m^5$
ΔZ	height difference, m
α	airway area normalization, dimensionless
α	CO_2 control constant, N/m^2
α	hypoxic control constant, $m^5/(N \cdot sec)$
α	solubility in the blood, m^2/N
α_0	value of α at $p = 0$, dimensionless
α_B	solubility in the brain, m^2/N
α_{Bc}	solubility of CO_2 in blood, m^2/N
α_{Be}	solubility of CO_2 in brain extracellular fluid, m^2/N
α_{Bi}	solubility of CO_2 in brain intracellular volume, m^2/N
α_C	solubility of CO_2 in pulmonary blood, m^2/N
α_{CO_2}	solubility of CO_2 in plasma, $mol/(N \cdot m)$
α_{CSF}	solubility in cerebrospinal fluid, m^2/N
α_e	expiratory weighting parameter, $m^{10}/(N^2 \cdot sec^4)$
α_i	inspiratory weighting parameter, $m^5/(N \cdot sec^3)$
α_{O_2}	oxygen solubility coefficient, m^2/N

α_T	solubility in tissue, m^2/N
α_{Tc}	solubility of CO_2 in tissue capillary blood, m^2/N
α_{Te}	CO_2 solubility in tissue extracellular volume, m^2/N
α_{Ti}	solubility of CO_2 in tissue intracellular space, m^2/N
α_0'	derivative of α_0 with respect to pressure at $p = 0$, m^2/N
β	CO_2 control constant, N/m^2
β_0	intercept of β sensitivity, N/m^2
β_1	sensitivity of β to $[HCO_3^-]$ changes, $N \cdot m/kg$
β_i	inspiratory coefficient, m^2/N
γ	CO_2 control constant, N/m^2
γ	specific weight, N/m^3
$\delta(t - \tau)$	Dirac delta function, dimensionless
Δ	difference
ε	energy of molecular interaction, $N \cdot m$
ε_i	volume coefficient, m^3
η	neuromuscular gain, N/m^2/neural pulses
θ	phase angle, rad
θ	temperature, $°C$
θ_{crit}	critical phase angle, rad
κ	CO_2 control constant, $m^5/(N \cdot sec)$
κ_s	conversion factor from STPD to BTPS conditions, kN/m^2
λ	Lagrange multiplier, various units
λ_0	hypoxia threshold, $m^5 \cdot sec/N$
λ_1, λ_2	constants, N/m^2
λ_H	hypoxia sensitivity, $m^5 \cdot sec/N$
μ	viscosity, $kg/(m \cdot sec)$
μ_0	central receptor response independent of H^+, m^3/sec
μ_v	central receptor sensitivity to H^+, m^3/sec
ν	muscle force–length effect, N/m^5
ρ	density, kg/m^3
τ	surface tension, N/m
τ	time constant, sec
τ_{aB}	transit time for blood from the lung to reach the brain, sec
τ_{ao}	lung to carotid body delay time, sec
τ_{aT}	transit time for blood from the lung to reach the tissue, sec
τ_B	time constant for brain blood flow, sec
τ_C	cardiac output time constant, sec
τ_D	delay time, sec
τ_i	diffusion time constant of surfactant macromolecule constituent i, sec
τ_{vB}	transit time for blood from the brain to reach the lung, sec
τ_{vT}	transit time for blood from the tissue to reach the lung, sec
ϕ	muscle force–velocity relationship, $N \cdot sec/m^5$
ψ	sense of respiratory effort, dimensionless
ω_n	natural frequency, rad/sec

REFERENCES

Abbrecht, P. H. 1973. Respiration, in class notes for Physiological Systems Analysis for Engineers (Course 7305). University of Michigan, Ann Arbor.

Adams, L., J. Garlick, A. Guz, K. Murphy, and S. J. G. Semple. 1984. Is the Voluntary Control of Exercise in Man Necessary for the Ventilatory Response? *J. Physiol.* **355**: 71–83.

Agostoni, E., and J. Mead. 1964. Statics of the Respiratory System, in *Handbook of Physiology, Volume 1, Section 3*. Respiration W. O. Fenn and H. Rahn, ed. American Physiological Society, Washington, D.C., Chapter 13. pp 387–410.

Ainsworth, M., and J. W. Eveleigh. 1952. A Method of Estimating Lung Resistance in Humans, Technical Paper No. 320, Chemical Experimental Establishment, Ministry of Supply, Porton, Wiltshire, England.

Allen, C. J., and N. L. Jones. 1984. Rate of Change of Alveolar Carbon Dioxide and the Control of Ventilation During Exercise. *J. Physiol.* **355**: 1–9.

Altose, M. S., W. C. McCauley, S. G. Kelsen, and N. S. Cherniack. 1977. Effects of Hypercapnia and Inspiratory Flow-Resistive Loading on Respiratory Activity in Chronic Airways Obstruction. *J. Clin. Invest.* **59**: 500–507.

Anderson, C. B. 1967. Mechanics of Fluids, in *Marks' Standard Handbook for Mechanical Engineers*, 7th ed., T. Baumeister, ed. McGraw-Hill, New York, p. 3-50.

Anthonisen, N. R., and R. M. Cherniak. 1981. Ventilatory Control in Lung Disease, in *Regulation of Breathing*, T. F. Hornbein, ed. Marcel Dekker, New York, pp. 965–987.

Archie, J. P., Jr. 1968. An Analytic Evaluation of a Mathematical Model for the Effect of Pulmonary Surfactant on Respiratory Mechanics. *Dis. Chest* **53**: 759–765.

Astrand, P. O., and K. Rodahl. 1970. *Textbook of Work Physiology*. McGraw-Hill, New York.

Bakker, H. K., R. S. Struikenkamp, and G. A. DeVries. 1980. Dynamics of Ventilation, Heart Rate, and Gas Exchange: Sinusoidal and Impulse Work Loads in Man. *J. Appl. Physiol.* **48**: 289–301.

Barbini, P. 1982. A Non-Linear Model of the Mechanics of Breathing Applied to the Use and Design of Ventilators. *J. Biomed. Eng.* **4**: 294–304.

Bartels, H., and E. Witzleb. 1956. Der Einfluss des arteriellen CO_2—Drucks auf die chemoreceptorischen Aktionspotentiale im Carotissinusnerven. *Arch. ges. Physiol.* **262**: 466–471.

Bartlett, R. G. 1973. Respiratory System, in *Bioastronautics Data Book*, J. F. Parker, Jr., and V. R. West, ed. NASA, Washington, D.C., pp. 489–531.

Bates, J. H. T. 1986. The Minimization of Muscular Energy Expenditure During Inspiration in Linear Models of the Respiratory System. *Biol. Cybern.* **54**: 195–200.

Baumeister, T., ed. 1967. *Marks' Standard Handbook for Mechanical Engineers*, 7th ed. McGraw-Hill, New York, pp. 4-22, 4-32, 11-96.

Bechbache, R. R., H. H. K. Chow, J. Duffin, and E. C. Orsini. 1979. The Effects of Hypercapnia, Hypoxia, Exercise and Anxiety on the Pattern of Breathing in Man. *J. Physiol.* **293**: 285–300.

Ben Jebria, A. 1984. Convective Gas Mixing in the Airways of the Human Lung—Comparison of Laminar and Turbulent Dispersion. *IEEE Trans. Biomed. Eng.* **BME-31**: 498–506.

Ben Jebria, A., and M. Bres. 1982. Computer Simulation of Ternary Diffusion in Distal Airways of the Human Lung. *Int. J. Bio-Med. Comput.* **13**: 403–419.

Bennett, F. M., P. Reischl, F. S. Grodins, S. M. Yamashiro, and W. E. Fordyce. 1981. Dynamics of Ventilatory Response to Exercise in Humans. *J. Appl. Physiol.* **51**: 194–203.

Berger, A. J., R. A. Mitchell, and J. W. Severinghaus. 1977. Regulation of Respiration. *N. Engl. J. Med.* **297**: 92–97.

Berger, A. J., R. A. Mitchell, and J. W. Severinghaus. 1977. Regulation of Respiration. *N. Engl. J. Med.* **297**: 138–143.

Berger, A. J., R. A. Mitchell, and J. W. Severinghaus. 1977. Regulation of Respiration. *N. Engl. J. Med.* **297**: 194–201.

Billings, C. O. 1973. Atmosphere, in *Bioastronautics Data Book*, J. F. Parker, Jr., and V. R. West, ed. NASA, Washington, D.C., pp. 35–63.

Birath, G. J. 1959. Respiratory Dead Space Measurements in a Model Lung and Healthy Human Subjects According to the Single Breath Method. *J. Appl. Physiol.* **14**: 517–520.

Biscoe, T. J., and P. Willshaw. 1981. Stimulus–Response Relationships of the Peripheral Arterial Chemoreceptors, in *Regulation of Breathing*, T. F. Hornbein, ed. Marcel Dekker, New York, pp. 321–345.

Bledsoe, S. W., and T. F. Hornbein. 1981. Central Chemosensors and the Regulation of Their Chemical Environment, in *Regulation of Breathing*, T. F. Hornbein, ed. Marcel Dekker, New York, pp. 347–428.

Blide, R. W., H. D. Kerr, and W. S. Spicer. 1964. Measurement of Upper and Lower Airway Resistance and Conductance in Man. *J. Appl. Physiol.* **19**: 1059–1069.

Bouhuys, A., and B. Jonson. 1967. Alveolar Pressure, Airflow Rate, and Lung Inflation in Man. *J. Appl. Physiol.* **22**: 1086–1100.

Brancatisano, T., D. Dodd, and L. A. Engel. 1983. Factors Influencing Glottic Dimensions During Forced Expiration. *J. Appl. Physiol.* **55**: 1825–1829.

Briscoe, W. A., and A. B. DuBois. 1958. The Relationship Between Airway Resistance, Airway Conductance, and Lung Volume in Subjects of Different Age and Body Size. *J. Clin. Invest.* **37**: 1279–1285.

Brown, A. C., and G. Brengelmann. 1966. Energy Metabolism, in *Physiology and Biophysics*, T. C. Ruch and H. D. Patton, ed. W. B. Saunders, Philadelphia, pp. 1030–1049.

Burki, N. K., K. Mitchell, B. A. Chaudhary, and F. W. Zechman. 1978. The Ability of Asthmatics to Detect Added Resistive Loads. *Am. Rev. Resp. Dis.* **117**: 71–73.

Campbell, E. J. M., and A. Guz. 1981. Breathlessness, in *Regulation of Breathing*, T. F. Hornbein, ed. Marcel Dekker, New York, pp. 1181–1195.

Campbell, E. J., and S. S. Lefrak. 1978. How Aging Affects the Structure and Function of the Respiratory System. *Geriatrics* **33**(6): 68–74.

Casaburi, R., B. J. Whipp, K. Wasserman, W. L. Beaver, and S. N. Koyal. 1977. Ventilatory and Gas Exchange Dynamics in Response to Sinusoidal Work. *J. Appl. Physiol.* **42**: 300–311.

Celli, B. R. 1988. Arm Exercise and Ventilation. *Chest* **93**: 673–674.

Cerny, F. J. 1987. Breathing Pattern During Exercise in Young Black and Caucasian Subjects. *J. Appl. Physiol.* **62**: 2220–2223.

Chang. H. K., and O. A. El Masry. 1982. A Model Study of Flow Dynamics in Human Central Airways. Part I. Axial Velocity Profiles. *Resp. Physiol.* **49**: 75–95.

Cherniack, N. S., and M. D. Altose. 1981. Respiratory Responses to Ventilatory Loading, in *Regulation of Breathing*, T. F. Hornbein, ed. Marcel Dekker, New York, pp. 905–964.

Cherniack, R. M. 1959. The Oxygen Consumption and Efficiency of the Respiratory Muscles in Health and Emphysema. *J. Clin. Invest.* **38**: 494–499.

Christie, R. V. 1953. Dyspnoea in Relation to the Visco-Elastic Properties of the Lung. *Proc. Roy. Soc. Med.* **46**: 381–386.

Cinkotai, F. F., T. C. Sharpe, and A. C. C. Gibbs. 1984. Circadian Rhythms in Peak Expiratory Flow Rate in Workers Exposed to Cotton Dust. *Thorax* **39**: 759–765.

Clément, J., J. Pardaens, H. Bobbaers, and K. P. van de Woestijne. 1981. Estimation of Resistance and Elastance of the Lungs in the Presence of Alinearities. A Model Study. *J. Biomech.* **14**: 111–122.

Cole, P., R. Forsyth, and J. S. J. Haight. 1982. Respiratory Resistance of the Oral Airway. *Am. Rev. Resp. Dis.* **125**: 363–365.

Comroe, J. H. 1965. *Physiology of Respiration.* Year Book Medical Publishers, Chicago.

Cunningham, D. J. C. 1974. Integrative Aspects of the Regulation of Breathing: A Personal View, in *MTP International Review of Science: Physiology Series One, Volume 2, Respiratory Physiology*, J. G. Widdicombe, ed. University Park Press, Baltimore, pp. 303–369.

Cunningham, D. J. C., D. G. Shaw, S. Lahiri, and B. B. Lloyd. 1961. The Effect of Maintained Ammonium Chloride Acidosis on the Relation Between Pulmonary Ventilation and Alveolar Oxygen and Carbon Dioxide in Man *Q. J. Exp. Physiol.* **46**: 322–334.

Dawson, S. V., and E. A. Elliott. 1977. Wave-Speed Limitation on Expiratory Flow—A Unifying Concept. *J. Appl. Physiol.* **43**: 498–515.

Deffebach, M. E., N. B. Charan, S. Lakshminarayan, and J. Butler. 1987. The Bronchial Circulation. *Am. Rev. Resp. Dis.* **135**: 463–481.

Dejours, P. 1963. The Regulation of Breathing During Muscular Exercise in Man: A Neuro-Humoral Theory, in *The Regulation of Human Respiration*, D. J. C. Cunningham and B. B. Lloyd, ed. Oxford University Press/Blackwell Scientific Publications, Oxford, England, pp. 535–547.

De Wilde, R., J. Clément, J. M. Hellemans, M. De Cramer, M. Demedts, R. Boving, and K. P. van de Woestijne. 1981. Model of Elasticity of the Human Lung. *J. Appl. Physiol.* **51**: 254–261.

Dittmer, D. S., and R. M. Grebe, ed. 1958. *Handbook of Respiration.* WADC Technical Report 58-352, Wright Air Development Center, Wright-Patterson Air Force Base, Ohio.

Dorkin, H. L., K. R. Lutchen, and A. C. Jackson. 1988. Human Respiratory Input Impedance from 4 to 200 Hz: Physiological and Modeling Considerations. *J. Appl. Physiol.* **64**: 823–831.

Duron, B. 1981. Intercostal and Diaphragmatic Muscle Endings and Afferents, in *Regulation of Breathing*, T. F. Hornbein, ed. Marcel Dekker, New York, pp. 473–540.

Emmert, R. E., and R. L. Pigford. 1963. Gas Absorption and Solvent Extraction, in *Chemical Engineers' Handbook*, J. H. Perry, ed. McGraw-Hill, New York, pp. 14-1–14-69.

Fencl, V., T. B. Miller, and J. R. Pappenheimer. 1966. Studies on the Respiratory Response to Disturbances of Acid–Base Balance, with Deductions Concerning the Ionic Composition of Cerebral Interstitial Fluid. *Am. J. Physiol.* **210**: 459–472.

Ferris, B. G., J. Mead, and L. H. Opie. 1964. Partitioning of Respiratory Flow Resistance in Man. *J. Appl. Physiol.* **19**: 653–658.

Filley, G. F., R. C. Hale, J. Kratschvil, and E. G. Olson. 1978. The Hyperpnea of Exercise and Chemical Disequilibria. *Chest* **735**: 267S–270S.

Forster, H. V., and J. A. Dempsey. 1981. Ventilatory Adaptations, in *Regulation of Breathing*, T. F. Hornbein, ed. Marcel Dekker, New York, pp. 845–904.

Forster, R. E., A. B. DuBois, W. A. Briscoe, and A. B. Fisher. 1986. *The Lung*. Year Book Medical Publishers, Chicago, pp. 251–252.

Fujihara, Y., J. R. Hildebrandt, and J. Hildebrandt. 1973a. Cardiorespiratory Transients in Exercising Man. I. Tests of Superposition. *J. Appl. Physiol.* **35**: 58–67.

Fujihara, Y., J. Hildebrandt, and J. R. Hildebrandt. 1973b. Cardiorespiratory Transients in Exercising Man. II. Linear Models. *J. Appl. Physiol.* **35**: 68–76.

Fuller, E. N., P. D. Schettler, and J. C. Giddings. 1966. A New Method for Prediction of Binary Gas-Phase Diffusion Coefficients. *Ind. Eng. Chem.* **58**(5): 19–27.

Fung, Y. C., and S. S. Sobin. 1977. Pulmonary Alveolar Blood Flow, in *Bioengineering Aspects of the Lung*, J. B. West, ed. Marcel Dekker, New York, pp. 267–359.

Ganong, W. F. 1963. *Review of Medical Physiology*. Lange Medical Publications, Los Altos, Calif. pp. 198–199, 482–552.

Garrard, C. S., and C. Emmons. 1986. The Reproducibility of the Respiratory Responses to Maximum Exercise. *Respiration* **49**: 94–100.

Geankoplis, C. J. 1978. *Transport Processes and Unit Operations*. Allyn and Bacon, Boston, pp. 263–335.

Gebhart, B. 1971. *Heat Transfer*. McGraw-Hill, New York, p. 581.

Gottfried, S. B., M. D. Altose, S. G. Kelsen, C. M. Fogarty, and N. S. Cherniack. 1978. The Perception of Changes in Airflow Resistance in Normal Subjects and Patients with Chronic Airways Obstruction. *Chest* **73**: 286S–288S.

Gray, J. S., F. S. Grodins, and E. T. Carter. 1956. Alveolar and Total Ventilation and the Dead Space Problem. *J. Appl. Physiol.* **9**: 307–320.

Greco, E. C., W. E. Fordyce, F. Gonzales, P. Reischl, and F. S. Grodins. 1978. Respiratory Responses to Intravenous and Intrapulmonary CO_2 in Awake Dogs. *J. Appl. Physiol.* **45**: 109–114.

Grodins, F. S. 1981. Exercise Hyperpnea. The Ultra Secret. *Adv. Physiol. Sci. (Respiration)* **10**: 243–251.

Grodins, F. S., J. Buell, and A. J. Bart. 1967. Mathematical Analysis and Digital Simulation of the Respiratory Control System. *J. Appl. Physiol.* **23**: 260–276.

Grodins, F. S., and S. M. Yamashiro. 1978. *Respiratory Function of the Lung and Its Control*. Macmillan, New York.

Grunstein, M. M., M. Younes, and J. Milic-Emili. 1973. Control of Tidal Volume and Respiratory Frequency in Anesthetized Cats. *J. Appl. Physiol.* **35**: 463–476.

Hämäläinen, R. P. 1973. Adaptive Control of Respiratory Mechanics. *Trans. ASME J. Dyn. Syst. Meas. Control* **95**:327–331.

Hämäläinen, R. P. 1975. *Optimization Concepts in Models of Physiological Systems*. Report B27, Helsinki University of Technology, Systems Theory Laboratory, Espoo, Finland.

Hämäläinen, R. P., and A. Sipilä. 1980. *Optimal Control of Inspiratory Airflow in Breathing*. PAM-12, Center for Pure and Applied Mathematics, University of California, Berkeley.

Hämäläinen, R. P., and A. Sipilä. 1984. Optimal Control of Inspiratory Airflow in Breathing. *Optim. Control Applic. Meth.* **5**: 177–191.

Hämäläinen, R. P., and A. A. Viljanen. 1978a. Modelling the Respiratory Airflow Pattern by Optimization Criteria. *Biol. Cybern.* **29**: 143–149.

Hämäläinen, R. P., and A. A. Viljanen. 1978b. A Hierarchical Goal-Seeking Model of the Control of Breathing. Part I. Model Description. *Biol. Cybern.* **29**: 151–158.

Hämäläinen, R. P., and A. A. Viljanen. 1978c. A Hierarchical Goal-Seeking Model of the Control of Breathing. Part II. Model Performance. *Biol. Cybern.* **29**: 159–166.

Hardy, H. H., R. E. Collins, and R. E. Calvert. 1982. A Digital Computer Model of the Human Circulatory System. *Med. Biol. Eng. Comput.* **20**: 550–564.

Hawkins, G. A. 1967. Thermal Properties of Substances and Thermodynamics, in *Marks' Standard Handbook for Mechanical Engineers*, 7th ed., T. Baumeister, ed. McGrew-Hill, New York, p. 4–13.

Heijmans, F., J. L. Bert, and K. L. Pinder. 1986. Digital Simulation of Pulmonary Microvascular Exchange. *Comp. Biol. Med.* **16**: 69–90.

Hildebrandt, J., and A. C. Young. 1965. Anatomy and Physics of Respiration, in *Physiology and Biophysics*, T. C. Ruch and H. D. Patton, ed. W. B. Saunders, Philadelphia, pp. 733–760.

Hill, E. P., G. G. Power, and L. D. Longo. 1977. Kinetics of O_2 and CO_2 Exchange, in *Bioengineering Aspects of the Lung*, J. B. West, ed. Marcel Dekker, New York, pp. 459–514.

Holmgren, A., and P.-D. Astrand. 1966. D_L and the Dimensions and Functional Capacities of the O_2 Transport System on Humans. *J. Appl. Physio.* **21**: 1463–1470.

Hornbein, T. F. 1966. The Chemical Regulation of Ventilation, in *Physiology and Biophysics*, T. C. Ruch and H. D. Patton, ed. W. B. Saunders, Philadelphia, pp. 803–819.

Hornbein, T. F., and A. Roos. 1963. Specificity of H Ion Concentration as a Carotid Chemoreceptor Stimulus. *J. Appl. Physiol.* **18**: 580–584.

Hyatt, R. E., T. A. Wilson, and E. Bar-Yishay. 1980. Prediction of Maximal Expiratory Flow in Excised Human Lungs. *J. Appl. Physiol.* **48**: 991–998.

Iravani, J., and G. N. Melville. 1976. Ciliary Movement Following Various Concentrations of Different Anticholinergic and Adrenergic Bronchodilator Solutions in Animals. *Postgrad. Med. J.* **51**: 108–115.

Isabey, D., and H. K. Chang. 1982. A Model Study of Flow Dynamics in Human Central Airways. Part II. Secondary Flow Velocities. *Resp. Physiol.* **49**: 97–113.

Jackson, A. C., and H. T. Milhorn, Jr. 1973. Digital Computer Simulation of Respiratory Mechanics. *Comput. Biomed. Res.* **6**: 27–56.

Jacquez, J. A. 1979. *Respiratory Physiology.* McGraw-Hill/Hemisphere, New York.

Jammes, Y., J. Askanazi, C. Weissman, and J. Milic-Emili. 1984. Ventilatory Effects of Biceps Vibration During Leg Exercise in Healthy Humans. *Clin. Physiol.* **4**: 379–391.

Johnson, A. T. 1976. The Energetics of Mask Wear. *Am. Ind. Hyg. Assoc. J.* **37**: 479–488.

Johnson, A. T. 1980. A Model of Respiratory Mechanics, Control, and Mask Wear. Paper prepared for the International Respiratory Research Symposium, NIOSH, Morgantown, W.V.

Johnson, A.T. 1984. Multidimensional Curve Fitting Program for Biological Data. *Comp. Prog. Biodmed.* **18**: 259–264.

Johnson, A. T. 1986. Conversion Between Plethysmograph and Perturbational Airways Resistance Measurements. *IEEE Trans. Biomed. Eng.* **33**: 803–806.

Johnson, A. T., and G. D. Kirk. 1981. Heat Transfer Study of the WBGT and Botsball Sensors. *Trans. ASAE* **24**: 410–417, 420.

Johnson, A. T., C.-S. Lin, and J. Hochheimer. 1984. Airflow Perturbation Device for Measuring Airways Resistance of Humans and Animals. *IEEE Trans. Biomed. Eng.* **31**: 622–626.

Johnson, A. T., and C. Masaitis. 1976. Prediction of Inhalation Time/Exhalation Time Ratio During Exercise. *IEEE Trans. Biomed. Eng.* **23**: 376.

Johnson, A. T., and R. H. McCuen. 1980. A Comparative Model Study of Respiratory Period Prediction on Men Exercising While Wearing Masks. *IEEE Trans. Biomed. Eng.* **27**: 430–439.

Johnson, A. T., and J. M. Milano. 1987. Relation Between Limiting Exhalation Flow Rate and Lung Volume. *IEEE Trans. Biomed. Eng.* **34**: 257–258.

Jones, A. S., J. M. Lancer, A. A. Moir, and J. C. Stevens. 1985. Effect of Aspirin on Nasal Resistance to Airflow. *Br. Med. J.* **290**: 1171–1173.

Jones, N. L. 1984. Dyspnea in Exercise. *Med. Sci. Sports Med.* **16**: 14–19.

Jones, N. L. 1984. Normal Values for Pulmonary Gas Exchange During Exercise. *Am. Rev. Respir. Dis.* **129**: 544–546.

Kao, F. F. 1963. An Experimental Study of the Pathways Involved in Exercise Hyperpnea Employing Cross Circulation Techniques, in *The Regulation of Human Respiration*, D. J. C. Cunningham and B. B. Lloyd, ed. Davis, Philadelphia, pp. 461–502.

Katz-Salamon, M. 1984. The Ability of Human Subjects to Detect Small Changes in Breathing Volume. *Acta Physiol. Scand.* **120**: 43–51.

Kennard, C. D., and B. J. Martin. 1984. Respiratory Frequency and the Oxygen Cost of Exercise. *Eur. J. Appl. Physiol.* **52**: 320–323.

Khoo, M. C. K., R. E. Kronauer, K. P. Strohl, and A. S. Slutsky. 1982. Factors Inducing Periodic Breathing in Humans: A General Model. *J. Appl. Physiol.* **53**: 644–659.

Kim, C. S., L. K. Brown, G. G. Leuvars, and M. A. Sackner. 1983. Deposition of Aerosol Particles and Flow Resistance in Mathematical and Experimental Airway Models. *J. Appl. Physiol.* **55**: 154–163.

Kotses, H., J. C. Rawson, and J. K. Wigal. 1987. Respiratory Airway changes in Response to Suggestion in Normal Individuals, *Psychosomatic Med.* **49**: 536–541.

Lambert, R. K., T. A. Wilson, R. E. Hyatt, and J. R. Rodarte. 1982. A Computational Model for Expiratory Flow. *J. Appl. Physiol.* **52**: 44–56.

Lambertsen, C. J. 1961. Chemical Factors in Respiratory Control, in *Medical Physiology,* P. Bard, ed. C. V. Mosb, St. Louis, pp. 633–655.

Levison, H., and R. M. Cherniack. 1968. Ventilatory Cost of Exercise in Chronic Obstructive Pulmonary Disease. *J. Appl. Physiol.* **25**: 21–27.

Ligas, J. R. 1984. A Non-Linearly Elastic, Finite Deformation Analysis Applicable to the Static Mechanics of Excised Lungs. *J. Biomech.* **17**: 549–552.

Lightfoot, E. N. 1974. *Transport Phenomena and Living Systems.* John Wiley & Sons, New York, p. 100.

Lind, F. G. 1984. Respiratory Drive and Breathing Pattern During Exercise in Man. *Acta Physiol. Scand.* Suppl. 533.

Linehan, J. H., and C. A. Dawson. 1983. A Three-Compartment Model of the Pulmonary Vasculature: Effects of Vasoconstriction. *J. Appl. Physiol.* **55**: 923–928.

Lloyd, B. B., and D. J. C. Cunningham. 1963. A Quantitative Approach to the Regulation of Human Respiration, in *The Regulation of Human Respiration*, D. J. C. Cunningham and B. B. Lloyd, ed. Oxford University Press/Blackwell Scientific Publications, Oxford, England, pp. 331–349.

Longobardo, G. S., N. S. Cherniack, and A. Damokosh-Giordano. 1980. Possible Optimization of Respiratory Controller Sensitivity. *Ann. Biomed. Eng.* **8**: 143–158.

Loring, S. H., and J. Mead. 1982. Abdominal Muscle Use During Quiet Breathing and Hyperpnea in Uninformed Subjects. *J. Appl. Physiol.* **52**: 700–704.

Lorino, H., A.-M. Lorino, A. Harf, G. Atlan, and D. Laurent. 1982. Linear Modeling of Ventilatory Mechanics During Spontaneous Breathing. *Comput. Biomed. Res.* **15**: 129–144.

Love, R. G. 1983. Lung Function Studies Before and After a Work Shift. *Br. J. Indus. Med.* **40**: 153–159.

Lutchen, K. R., F. P. Primiano, Jr., and G. M. Saidel. 1982. A Nonlinear Model Combining Pulmonary Mechanics and Gas Concentration Dynamics. *IEEE Trans. Biomed. Eng.* **29**: 629–641.

Macklem, P. T. 1980. The Paradoxical Nature of Pulmonary Pressure–Flow Relationships. *Fed. Proc.* **39**: 2755–2758.

Macklem, P. T., D. M. Macklem, and A. DeTroyer. 1983. A Model of Inspiratory Muscle Mechanics. *J. Appl. Physiol.* **55**: 547–557.

Mahler, M. 1979. Neural and Humoral Signals for Pulmonary Ventilation Arising in Exercising Muscle. *Med. Sci. Sports* **1**: 191–197.

Mahutte, C. K., E. J. M. Campbell, and K. J. Killian. 1983. Theory of Resistive Load Detection. *Resp. Physiol.* **51**: 131–139.

Martin, B. J., H.-I. Chen, and M. A. Kolka. 1984. Anaerobic Metabolism of the Respiratory Muscles During Exercise. *Med. Sci. Sports Exerc.* **16**: 82–86.

Martin, B. J., E. J. Morgan, C. W. Zwillich, and J. V. Weil. 1979. Influence of Exercise Hyperthermia on Exercise Breathing Pattern. *J. Appl. Physiol.* **47**: 1039–1042.

Martin, B. J., and J. V. Weil. 1979. CO_2 and Exercise Tidal Volume. *J. Appl. Physiol.* **46**: 322–325.

Martin, B. J., J. V. Weil, K. Sparks, R. McCullough, and R. F. Grover. 1978. Exercise Ventilation Correlates Positively with Ventilatory Chemoresponsiveness. *J. Appl. Physiol.* **45**: 557–564.

Martin, H. B., and D. F. Proctor. 1958. Pressure–Volume Measurements on Dog Bronchi. *J. Appl. Physiol.* **13**: 337–343.

Martin, J., M. Aubier, and L. A. Engel. 1982. Effects of Inspiratory Loading on Respiratory Muscle Activity During Expiration. *Am. Rev. Resp. Dis.* **125**: 352–358.

McDonald, D. M. 1981. Peripheral Chemoreceptors: Structure–Function Relationships of the Carotid Body, in *Regulation of Breathing*, T. F. Hornbein, ed. Marcel Dekker, New York, pp. 105–319.

McIlroy, M. B., D. F. Tierney, and J. A. Nadel. 1963. A New Method for Measurement of Compliance and Resistance of Lungs and Thorax. *J. Appl. Physiol.* **18**: 424–427.

Mead, J. 1960. Control of Respiratory Frequency. *J. Appl. Physiol.* **15**: 325–336.

Mead, J. 1961. Mechanical Properties of Lungs, *Physiol. Rev.* **41**: 281–330.

Mead, J. 1978. Analysis of the Configuration of Maximum Expiratory Flow-Volume Curves. *J. Appl. Physiol.* **44**: 156–165.

Mead, J. 1980. Expiratory Flow Limitation: A Physiologist's Point of View. *Fed. Proc.* **39**: 2771–2775.

Mead, J., J. M. Turner, P. T. Macklem, and J. B. Little. 1967. Significance of the Relationship Between Lung Recoil and Maximum Expiratory Flow. *J. Appl. Physiol.* **22**: 95–108.

Mead, J., and J. L. Whittenberger. 1953. Physical Properties of Human Lungs Measured During Spontaneous Respiration. *J. Appl. Physiol.* **5**: 779–796.

Mines, A. H. 1981. *Respiratory Physiology.* Raven Press, New York, pp. 131–157.

Mitchell, R. A., and A. J. Berger. 1981. Neural Regulation of Respiration, in *Regulation of Breathing*, T. F. Hornbein, ed. Marcel Dekker, New York, pp. 541–620.

Miyamoto, Y., Y. Nakazono, T. Hiura, and Y. Abe. 1983. Cardiorespiratory Dynamics During Sinusoidal and Impulse Exercise in Man. *Jpn. J. Physiol.* **33**: 971–986.

Miyamoto, Y., T. Tamura, T. Takahashi, and T. Mikami. 1981. Transient Changes in Ventilation and Cardiac Output at the Start and End of Exercise. *Jpn. J. Physiol.* **31**: 153–168.

Mohler, J. G. 1982. Quantification of Dyspnea Confirmed by Voice Pitch Analysis. *Bull. Eur. Physiopath. Resp.* **18**: 837–850.

Morehouse, L. E., and A. T. Miller. 1967. *Physiology of Exercise.* C. V. Mosby, St. Louis, pp. 133–164, 185.

Muir, D. C. F. 1966. Bulk Flow and Diffusion in the Airways of the Lung. *Br. J. Dis. Chest* **60**: 169–176.

Nada, M. D., and D. A. Linkens. 1977. Adaptive Technique for Estimating the Parameters of a Nonlinear Mathematical Lung Model. *Med. Biol. Eng. Comput.* **15**: 149–154.

Newstead, C. G., R. V. Nowell, and C. B. Wolff, 1980. The Rate of Rise of Alveolar Carbon Dioxide Tension During Expiration *J. Physiol.* **307**: p42.

Nielsen, M., and H. Smith. 1952. Studies on the Regulation of Respiration in Acute Hypoxia. *Acta Physiol. Scand.* **24**: 293–313.

Notter, R. H., and J. N. Finkelstein. 1984. Pulmonary Surfactant: An Interdisciplinary Approach, *J. Appl. Physiol.* **57**: 1613–1624.

O'Connell, J. M., and A. H. Campbell. 1976. Respiratory Mechanics in Airways Obstruction Associated with Inspiratory Dyspnoea. *Thorax* **31**: 669–677.

Otis, A. B., W. O. Fenn, and H. Rahn. 1950. Mechanics of Breathing in Man. *J. Appl. Physiol.* **2**: 592–607.

Padget, P. 1927. The Respiratory Response to Carbon Dioxide. *Am. J. Physiol.* **83**: 384–393.

Pedley, T. J., R. C. Schroter, and M. F. Sudlow. 1977. Gas Flow and Mixing in the Airways, in *Bioengineering Aspects of the Lung*, J. B. West, ed. Marcel Dekker, New York, pp. 163–265.

Peslin, R., J. Papon, C. Duvivier, and J. Richalet. 1975. Frequency Response of the Chest: Modeling and Parameter Estimation. *J. Appl. Physiol.* **39**: 523–534.

Petrini, M. F. 1986. Distribution of Ventilation and Perfusion: A Teaching Model. *Comput. Biol. Med.* **16**: 431–444.

Ponte, J., and M. J. Purves. 1978. Carbon Dioxide and Venous Return and Their Interaction as Stimuli to Ventilation in the Cat. *J. Physiol. London* **274**: 455–475.

Powers, S. K., S. Dodd, J. Woodyard, and M. Mangum. 1985. Caffeine Alters Ventilatory and Gas Exchange Kinetics During Exercise. *Med. Sci. Sports Exerc.* **18**: 101–106.

Prisk, G. K., and A. E. McKinnon. 1987. A Modeling Approach to the Estimation of CO Diffusing Capacity. *J. Appl. Physiol.* **62**: 373–380.

Provine, R. R., B. C. Tate, and L. L. Geldmacher. 1987. Yawning: No Effect of 3–5% CO_2, 100% O_2, and Exercise. *Behav. Neural Biol.* **48**: 382–393.

Rebuck, A. S., and W. E. Woodley. 1975. Ventilatory Effects of Hypoxia and Their Dependence on pCO_2. *J. Appl. Physiol.* **38**: 16–19.

Riley, R. L. 1965. Gas Exchange and Transportation, in *Physiology and Biophysics*, T. C. Ruch and H. D. Patton, ed. W. B. Saunders, Philadelphia, pp. 761–787.

Rohrer, F. 1915. Flow Resistance in the Human Air Passages and the Effect of Irregular Breathing of the Bronchial System on the Respiratory Process in Various Regions of the Lungs, in *Transitions in Respiratory Physiology*, J. B. West, ed. Dowden, Hutchinson, and Ross, Stroudsburg, P., pp. 3–66.

Roy, A. G., and M. J. Woldenberg. 1982. A Generalization of the Optimal Models of Arterial Branching. *Bull. Math. Biol.* **44**: 349–360.

Rubin, S., M. Tack, and N. S. Cherniack. 1982. Effect of Aging on Respiratory Responses to CO_2 and Inspiratory Resistive Loads. *J. Gerontol.* **37**: 306–312.

Ruttiman, V. E., and W. S. Yamamoto. 1972. Respiratory Airflow Patterns that Satisfy Power and Force Criteria of Optimality. *Ann. Biomed. Eng.* **1**: 146–159.

Sackner, M. A. 1976a, Pulmonary Structure and Pathology, in *Biological Foundations of Biomedical Engineering*. J. Kline, ed. Little, Brown, Boston, pp. 231–241.

Sackner, M. A. 1976b. Pulmonary Circulation, in *Biological Foundations of Biomedical Engineering*, J. Kline, ed. Little, Brown, Boston, pp. 287–313.

Sackner, M. A. 1976c. Mechanics of Breathing, in *Biological Foundations of Biomedical Engineering*, J. Kline, ed. Little, Brown, Boston, pp. 315–339.

Sackner, M. A. 1976d. Distribution, Diffusion, and Gas Exchange, in *Biological Foundations of Biomedical Engineering*, J. Kline, ed. Little, Brown, Boston, pp. 267–285.

Saunders, K. B. 1980. Oscillations of Arterial CO_2 Tension in a Respiratory Model: Some Implications for the Control of Breathing in exercise. *J. Theor. Biol.* **84**: 163–179.

Saunders, K. B., H. N. Bali, and E. R. Carson. 1980. A Breathing Model of the Respiratory System: The Controlled System. *J. Theor. Biol.* **84**: 135–161.

Schorr-Lesnick, B., A. S. Teirstein, L. K. Brown, and A. Miller. 1985. Pulmonary Function in Singers and Wind-Instrument Players. *Chest* **88**: 201–205.

Severinghaus, J. W., R. A. Mitchell, B. W. Richardson, and M. M. Singer. 1963. Respiratory Control at High Altitude Suggesting Active Transport Regulation of CSF pH. *J. Appl. Physiol.* **18**: 1155–1166.

Shahid, S. U., B. A. Goddard, and J. B. L. Howell. 1981. Detection and Interaction of Elastic and Flow-Resistive Respiratory Loads in Man. *Clin. Sci.* **61**: 339–343.

Shykoff, B. E., A. van Grondelle, and H. K. Chang. 1982. Effects of Unequal Pressure Swings and Different Waveforms on Distribution of Ventilation: A Non-Linear Model Simulation. *Resp. Physiol.* **48**: 157–168.

Silverman, L., G. Lee, T. Plotkin, I. A. Sawyers, and A. R. Yancey. 1951. Airflow Measurements on Human Subjects With and Without Respiratory Resistance at Several Work Rates. *Arch. Ind. Hyg. Occup. Med.* **3**: 461–478.

Skelland, A. H. P. 1967. *Non-Newtonian Flow and Heat Transfer*. John Wiley & Sons, New York, p. 125.

Slutsky, A. S., G. G. Berdine, and J. M. Drazen. 1980. Steady Flow in a Model of Human Central Airways. *J. Appl. Physiol.* **49**: 417–423.

Smaldone, G. C., and P. L. Smith. 1985. Location of Flow-Limiting Segments via Airway Catheters Near Residual Volume in Humans. *J. Appl. Physiol.* **59**: 502–508.

Sokolnikoff, I. S., and R. M. Redheffer. 1958. *Mathematics of Physics and Modern Engineering*. McGraw-Hill, New York, pp. 264–281.

Spector, W. S. 1956. *Handbook of Biological Data.* Wright Air Development Center Technical Report 56-273, Wright-Patterson Air Force Base, Ohio.

Spells, K. E. 1969. Comparative Studies on Lung Mechanics Based on a Survey of Literature Data. *Resp. Physiol.* **8**: 37–57.

Stănescu, D. C., B. Nemery, C. Veriter, and C. Maréchal. 1981. Pattern of Breathing and Ventilatory Response to CO_2 in Subjects Practicing Hatha-Yoga. *J. Appl. Physiol.* **51**: 1625–1629.

Staub, N. C. 1963. The Interdependence of Pulmonary Structure and Function. *Anesthesiology* **24**: 831–854.

Sue, D. Y., A. Oren, J. E. Hansen, and K. Wasserman. 1987. Diffusing Capacity for Carbon Monoxide as a Predictor of Gas Exchange During Exercise. *N. Engl. J. Med.* **316**: 1301–1306.

Suzuki, S., H. Sasaki, K. Sekizawa, and T. Takishima. 1982. Isovolume Pressure–Flow Relationships in Intrapulmonary Bronchi of Excised Dog Lungs. *J. Appl. Physiol.* **52**: 295–303.

Swanson, G. D. 1979. Overview of Ventilatory Control During Exercise. *Med. Sci. Sports* **11**: 221–226.

Swanson, G. D., and P. A. Robbins. 1986. Optimal Respiratory Controller Structures. *IEEE Trans. Biomed.* **33**: 677–680.

Swanson, G. D., and D. L. Sherrill. 1983. A Model Evaluation of Estimates of Breath-to-Breath Alveolar Gas Exchange. *J. Appl. Physiol.* **55**: 1936–1941.

Tack, M., M. D. Altose, and N. S. Cherniack. 1983. Effects of Aging on Sensation of Respiratory Force and Displacement. *J. Appl. Physiol.* **55**: 1433–1440.

Tatsis, G., K. Horsfield, and G. Cumming. 1984. Distribution of Dead Space Volume in the Human Lung. *Clin. Sci.* **67**: 493–497.

Taylor, G. I. 1953. Dispersion of Soluble Matter in Solvent Flowing Slowly Through a Tube. *Proc. Roy. Soc. London A* **219**: 186–203.

Taylor, G. I. 1954. The Dispersion of Matter in Turbulent Flow Through a Pipeline. *Proc. Roy. Soc. London A* **223**: 446–466.

Tenney, S. M., and J. E. Remmers. 1963. Comparative Quantitative Morphology of the Mammalian Lung: Diffusing Area. *Nature* **197**: 54–56.

Thiriet, M., and M. Bonis. 1983. Experiments on Flow Limitation During Forced Expiration in a Monoalveolar Lung Model. *Med. Biol. Eng. Comput.* **21**: 681–687.

Tobin, M. J., W. Perez, S. M. Guenther, G. D'Alonzo, and D. D. Dantzker. 1986. Breathing Pattern and Metabolic Behavior During Anticipation of Exercise. *J. Appl. Physiol.* **60**: 1306–1312.

Turney, S. Z. 1983. Personal communication. Maryland Institute for Emergency Medical Services Systems, Baltimore.

Ultman, J. S. 1981. Gas Mixing in the Pulmonary Airways. *Ann. Biomed. Eng.* **9**: 513–527.

Vawter, D. L. 1980. A Finite Element Model for Macroscopic Deformation of the Lung. *J. Biomech. Eng.* **102**: 1–7.

Visser, B. F., and S. C. M. Luijendijk. 1982. Gas Mixing in the Small Airways, Described by Old and New Models. *Eur. J. Respir. Dis.* **63**(Suppl.): 26–35.

Vorosmarti, J. 1979. Influence of Increased Gas Density and External Resistance on Maximum Expiratory Flow. *Undersea Biomed. Res.* **6**: 339–346.

Wasserman, K. and R. Casaburi. 1988. Dyspnea—Physiological and Pathaphysiological Mechanisms, *Ann. Rev. Med.* **39**: 503–515.

Weibel, E. R. 1963. *Morphometry of the Human Lung.* Academic Press, New York.

Weiler-Ravell, D., D. M. Cooper, B. J. Whipp, and K. Wasserman. 1983. Control of Breathing at the Start of Exercise as Influenced by Posture. *J. Appl. Physiol.* **55**: 1460–1466.

Weinstock, R. 1952. *Calculus of Variations.* McGraw-Hill, New York, pp. 4–63.

West, J. 1962. Regional Differences in Gas Exchange in the Lung of Erect Man. *J. Appl. Physiol.* **17**: 893–898.

West, J. B., and P. D. Wagner. 1977. Pulmonary Gas Exchange, in *Bioengineering Aspects of the Lung*, J. B. West, ed. Marcel Dekker, New York, pp. 361–457.

Whipp, B. J. 1981. The Control of Exercise Hyperpnea, in *Regulation of Breathing, Part II*, T. F. Hornbein, ed. Marcel Dekker, New York, pp. 1069–1139.

Whipp, B. J., and S. A. Ward. 1981. Cardiopulmonary Coupling During Exercise. *J. Exp. Biol.* **100**: 175–193.

Whipp, B. J., S. A. Ward, N. Lamarra, J.A. Davis, and K. Wasserman. 1982. Parameters of Ventilatory and Gas Exchange Dynamics During Exercise. *J. Appl. Physiol.* **52**: 1506–1513.

Whitelaw, W. A., L. E. Hajdo, and J. A. Wallace. 1983. Relationships Among Pressure, Tension, and Shape of the Diaphragm. *J. Appl. Physiol.* **55**: 1899–1905.

Widdicombe, J. G. 1981. Nervous Receptors in the Respiratory Tract and Lungs, in *Regulation of Breathing*, T. F. Hornbein, ed. Marcel Dekker, New York, pp. 429–472.

Widdicombe, J. G. 1982. Pulmonary and Respiratory Tract Receptors. *J. Exp. Biol.* **100**: 41–57.

Widdicombe, J. G., and J. A. Nadel. 1963. Airway Volume, Airway Resistance, and Work and Force of Breathing: Theory. *J. Appl. Physiol.* **18**: 863–868.

Witzleb, E., H. Bartels, H. Budde, and M. Mochizuchi. 1955. Der Einfluss des arteriellen O_2 — Drucks auf die chemoreceptorischen Aktionspotentiale im Carotissinusnerven. *Arch. qes. Physiol.* **261**: 211–216.

Yamamoto, W. S. 1960. Mathematical Analysis of the Time Course of Alveolar CO_2. *J. Appl. Physiol.* **15**: 215–219.

Yamamoto, W. S. 1978. A Mathematical Simulation of the Hyperpneas of Metabolic CO_2 Production and Inhalation. *Am. J. Physiol.* **235**: R265–R278.

Yamamoto, W. S. 1981. Computer Simulation of Experiments in Responses to Intravenous and Inhaled CO_2. *J. Appl. Physiol.* **50**: 835–843.

Yamamoto, W. S., and M. W. Edwards. 1960. Homeostasis of Carbon Dioxide During Intravenous Infusion of CO_2. *J. Appl. Physiol.* **15**: 807–818.

Yamashiro, S. M., J. A. Daubenspeck, T. N. Lauritsen, and F. S. Grodins. 1975. Total Work Rate of Breathing Optimization in CO_2 Inhalation and Exercise. *J. Appl. Physiol.* **38**: 702–709.

Yamashiro, S. M., and F. S. Grodins. 1971. Optimal Regulation of Respiratory Airflow. *J. Appl. Physiol.* **30**: 597–602.

Yamashiro, S. M., and F. S. Grodins. 1973. Respiratory Cycle Optimization in Exercise. *J. Appl. Physiol.* **35**: 522–525.

Yeates, D. B., and N. Aspin. 1978. A Mathematical Description of the Airways of the Human Lungs. *Resp. Physiol.* **32**: 91–104.

Younes, M., and J. Burks. 1985. Breathing Pattern During and After Exercise of Different Intensities. *J. Appl. Physiol.* **59**: 898–908.

Younes, M. K., and J E. Remmers. 1981. Control of Volume and Respiratory Frequency, in *Regulation of Breathing*, T. F. Hornbein, ed. Marcel Dekker, New York, pp. 621–671.

Young, A. C. 1966. Neural Control of Respiration, in *Physiology and Biophysics*, T. C. Ruch and H. D. Patton, ed. W. B. Saunders, Philadelphia, pp. 788–802.

Zechman, F. W., R. L. Wiley, and P. W. Davenport. 1981. Ability of Healthy Men to Discriminate Between Added Inspiratory Resistive and Elastic Load. *Resp. Physiol.* **45**: 111–120.

Zin, W. A., A. Rossi, and J. Milic-Emili. 1983. Model Analysis of Respiratory Responses to Inspiratory Resistive Load. *J. Appl. Physiol.* **55**: 1565–1573.

CHAPTER 5

Thermal Responses

Now let us suppose that such a vessel is divided into two portions, *A* and *B*, by a division in which there is a small hole, and that a being, who can see individual molecules, opens and closes this hole, so as to allow only the swifter molecules to pass from *A* to *B*.... He will thus, without expenditure of work, raise the temperature of *B*... in contradiction to the second law of thermodynamics.[1]

—James Clerk Maxwell

5.1 INTRODUCTION

Human responses to the thermal environment are many and varied. Active responses include conscious changes of environment, such as removal of clothing, and unconscious changes, such as sweating. Passive responses include heat lost or gained from the environment solely as a result of temperature differences, much as heat is gained or lost by a house in summer or winter. If heat is not removed as rapidly as it is produced, body temperature will rise, thus aiding passive cooling. If heat is removed more rapidly than it is produced, body temperature falls. High rates of muscular exertion generate large amounts of heart, which must be removed or body temperature will increase to and beyond a point dangerous to life. Responses to this challenge are the subject of this chapter.

5.1.1 Passive Heat Loss

Heat flow in a passive system can be predicted by a means analogous to Ohm's law (Figure 5.1.1):

$$q = \Delta\theta/R_{th} \tag{5.1.1}$$

where q = rate of heat flow, N·m/sec
$\Delta\theta$ = temperature difference between two places exchanging heat, °C
R_{th} = thermal resistance appearing between them, °C·sec/(N·m)

Heat flow in Equation 5.1.1 occurs because a temperature difference exists between the body surface and the environment, and it is greatly reduced for surrounding temperatures approaching skin temperature. When this happens, passive cooling is no longer possible, and active mechanisms must be used to remove heat.

In general, thermal resistance is a complicated assemblage of more elementary resistances in series and parallel with one another. The higher the total thermal resistance, the lower the total heat exchange and the more insulated the system.

Heat exchange can occur by conduction, convection, radiation, or evaporation. For a nude individual resting in a thermoneutral environment, 60% of total heat loss is by radiation, 25% by evaporation, 12% by convection, and 3% by conduction (Nilsson, 1987). Conduction and

---

[1] Maxwell introduced his demon in this way to illustrate the statistical nature of heat. Since then, the demon has been the subject of much discussion.

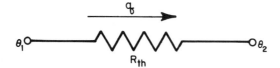

Figure 5.1.1   Diagram of Ohm's law heat exchange. Here the effort variable is temperature and the flow variable is heat.

convection heat losses are normally calculated by means of equations of the form of Equation 5.1.1. Radiation heat losses, although properly proportional to the difference between the fourth powers of the absolute temperatures of the two surfaces exchanging heat, are, for convenience, frequently artifically made to conform to equations of the form of Equation 5.1.1. Evaporation, especially of sweat, must be calculated in a manner different from that given by Equation 5.1.1, although sweat evaporation, if it occurs on the skin surface, directly affects skin temperature and thus $\Delta\theta$.

Passive heat loss from a human occurs not only between the surface and the environment, but also between portions of the body itself. Some thermal models (Brown, 1966) consider the body as a series of shells exchanging heat between them. The simplest is a core-and-shell model (Figure 5.1.2), where the core is taken to represent two-thirds of the body mass and which maintains a nearly constant temperature. The shell, comprising the remaining third of the body mass, is varied in temperature to control the heat loss from the core. Heat exchange between core and shell can be calculated by means of Equation 5.1.1.

Heat loss is only one factor determining the thermal state of the human body. We are also aware that the body generates heat, the amount of which is discussed later. Including this term in a generalized heat balance gives

$$\text{rate of heat gained} - \text{rate of heat lost} + \text{rate of heat generated}$$
$$= \text{rate of change of heat storage} \tag{5.1.2}$$

Since stored heat is manifested as a certain temperature, we see that if the rate of heat lost during exercise is not great enough, deep body temperature will rise, and it may rise to levels dangerous to health.

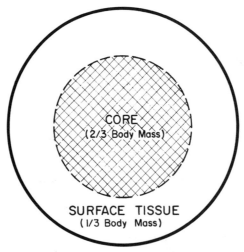

Figure 5.1.2   Simple core and shell model of the human body. This model usually assumes the body shape to be cylindrical, with a cross section appearing as above.

5.1.2 Active Resources

The body is clearly able to actively respond to thermal challenges. Within the thermal comfort zone (or thermoneutral zone), shown in a portion of the psychrometric chart in Figure 5.1.3 (ASHRAE, 1974), vasomotor responses are sufficient to maintain thermal equilibrium. In this region, thermal resistance is actively varied by changing the amount of blood flow to the skin.

In hotter environments, sweating becomes an important active response. Evaporation of sweat absorbs latent heat at the place where evaporation occurs. For nude humans, most of this heat will come from the skin and thus from the interior of the body. For clothed humans where the sweat has soaked through the clothing, evaporation occurs at the surface of the clothes and is not as effective in removing heat as is evaporation from the skin.

In environments colder than thermoneutral, shivering becomes one of the foremost means of producing extra heat. Shivering is the uncoordinated tensing and relaxing of skeletal muscles. This muscular activity generates heat. For an unclothed individual, however, shivering is not an efficient means of heat generation. One of the best insulators is a layer of still air. Shivering under bare skin disrupts this still air layer (Kleiber, 1975) and may also cause greater local surface blood flow. Wearing clothing makes shivering much more effective as a means to generate additional heat because the sill air layer on the outside of the clothing remains relatively undisturbed.

None of the unconscious active mechanisms is as effective as the conscious mechanisms of adding or removing clothing, changing activity level, huddling together, moving to a region of

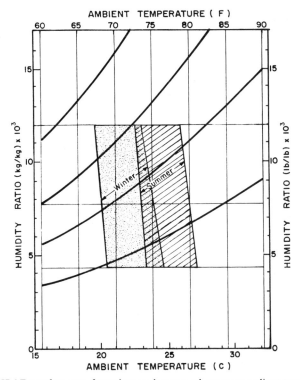

Figure 5.1.3 ASHRAE comfort zone for sedentary humans where mean radiant temperature equals dry bulb temperature and clothing thermal conductance is 10.8 N·m/(m²·°C·sec). The comfort zone is drawn on a standard metric psychrometric chart. (Adapted from ASHRAE, 1981.)

less extreme environment, or modifying the local thermal environment.[2] Indeed, it is the human capacity to accomplish these active responses that has allowed people to exist in harsh environments despite their semitropical nature.

5.2 THERMAL MECHANICS

In this section we deal with specific components of the general heat balance equation (5.1.2). Although heat gained and lost by passive processes can occur by the same mechanisms of conduction, convection, and radiation, we consider them, as appropriate, in the manner in which they normally occur.

Figure 5.2.1 is a schematic representation of the heat loss mechanisms available to the clothed human body. From the core of the body are several parallel pathways for heat loss: (1) evaporation from the respiratory system to the environment, (2) convection from the respiratory system to the environment, and (3) heat transfer through the tissues to the skin surface. This last avenue is accomplished by a combination of conduction and convection, which are difficult to separate. At the skin surface, heat may be removed by conduction through the clothing or by evaporation of sweat. Conducted heat is lost to the environment by convection or radiation, whereas sweat is removed by diffusion through the clothes and by convection at the clothing surface. Each of these processes resists the flow of heat or vapor, as symbolized by the resistances appearing in the diagram. Below each resistance is listed the equation(s) by which it can be calculated.

Body heat is produced by chemical processes needed to maintain the body in proper working order (basal metabolic rate), ingestion of food (specific dynamic action), and muscular contraction. Heat loss occurs by the mechanisms listed in Table 5.2.1. As environmental temperature increases, the role of sweating becomes much greater and that of radiation and convection becomes much less.

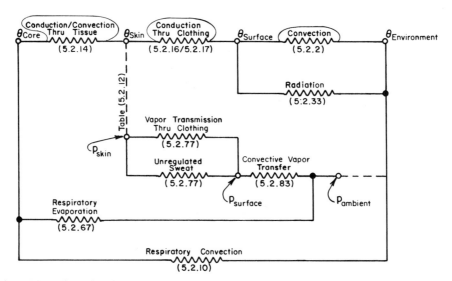

Figure 5.2.1 Thermal resistance representation of the heat loss mechanisms of the clothed human. Numbers in parentheses refer to equation numbers.

[2] Animals such as rats exposed to cold environments can be trained to work for pulses of infrared radiant heat as a physical reward (Refinetti and Carlisle, 1987). This experimental paradigm has been used to study thermoregulatory mechanisms associated with brain thermal stimulation, brain lesions, chemical microinjections, administration of pyrogens, and so on.

TABLE 5.2.1   Percentage Body Heat Loss at 21°C

Body Mechanism	Heat Loss, %
Radiation and convection	70
Sweating	27
Respiration	2
Urination and defecation	1

Source: Used with permission from Ganong, 1963.

TABLE 5.2.2   Variation in Convection Coefficient with Room Air Motion

Air Velocity, m/sec	Convection Coefficient, $N \cdot m/(°C \cdot sec \cdot m^2)$
0.1–0.18	3.1
0.5	6.2
1.0	9.0
2.0	12.6
4.0	17.7

Source: Used with permission from ASHRAE, 1985.

5.2.1   Convection

Heat loss by convection occurs by means of a simultaneous heating and mass movement of a fluid, usually air. To avoid complicated geometrical and boundary layer factors, convection is usually calculated by means of the simplified equation

$$q_c = h_c A(\theta_0 - \theta_a) \tag{5.2.1}$$

where q_c = rate of heat loss[3] by convection, $N \cdot m/sec$
$\quad A$ = surface area, m^2
$\quad \theta_0$ = surface temperature, °C
$\quad \theta_a$ = ambient temperature, °C
$\quad h_c$ = convection coefficient, $N \cdot m/(°C \cdot sec \cdot m^2)$
Relating Equation 5.2.1 to 5.1.1 gives

$$R_{th} = 1/h_c A \tag{5.2.2}$$

Convection that occurs as a result of forced air movement—by means of a fan, or wind, or an exercising subjects, for example—is called forced convection. Convection that occurs because heating of the air surrounding the body expands the air, causing it to rise and establish thermal currents, is called natural convection. During exercise, natural convection is too small in relation to forced convection to be considered.

The convection coefficient h_c is usually a function of air velocity, physical properties of the air, and temperature difference between surface and air (Kreith, 1958).[4] Posture of an individual also

---

[3] Heat loss in newton-meters per second is equivalent to watts or joules per second. In this text conventional units have appeared elsewhere in parentheses next to standard units of measurement. Because of the numerical equivalence of newton-meters per second and watts, thermal values originally in watts do not appear in parentheses.

[4] The convection coefficient for forced convection is usually given as a function of Reynolds number Re, Prandtl number Pr, the thermal conductivity of air k_a, and a significant length L.

$$h_c \propto \frac{k_a}{L} \sqrt{Re} \sqrt[4]{Pr}$$

and thus includes a means to correct as physical properties of air change with temperature, pressure, composition, and so on. The experimental data obtained with humans, however, frequently do not include this generality.

TABLE 5.2.3   Equations Relating Convection Coefficient h_c to Velocity v^a

Equation	Condition	Remarks
$h_c = 8.3v^{0.6}$	Seated	v is room air movement
$h_c = 2.7 + 8.7v^{0.67}$	Reclining	v is lengthwise air movement
$h_c = 8.6v^{0.53}$	Free walking	v is speed of walking
$h_c = 6.5v^{0.39}$	Treadmill	v is speed of treadmill

Source: Used with permission from ASHRAE, 1985.

$^a h_c$ in N·m/(°C·sec·m²), v in m/sec.

TABLE 5.2.4   More Equations Relating Convection Coefficient to Air Velocity

Velocity Range, m/sec	Convection Coefficient, N·m/(°C·sec·m²)
$v < 0.2$	$h_c = 5.4v^{0.466}$
$0.2 < v < 2$	$h_c = 6.8v^{0.618}$
$v > 2$	$h_c = 5.9v^{0.805}$

Source: Used with permission from Nishi and Gagge, 1970.

TABLE 5.2.5   Variation in Convection Coefficient with Activity in Still Air

	Activity Level, N·m/sec (met)	Convection Coefficient, N·m/(°C·sec·m²)
Resting	89 (0.85)	3.1
Sedentary	116 (1.1)	3.3
Light activity	210 (2.0)	6.0
Medium activity	315 (3.0)	7.7

Source: Adapted and used with permission from ASHRAE, 1985.

affects the convection coefficient (ASHRAE, 1985). In general, h_c can be given by a relation of the form (Kleiber, 1975)

$$h_c = k\sqrt{v} \tag{5.2.3}$$

where k = coefficient, (N·sec$^{1/2}$)/(°C·m$^{3/2}$)

v = air velocity surrounding the individual, m/sec

Tables 5.2.2 and 5.2.4 give representative values of the convection coefficient for various room air velocities. Table 5.2.3 gives equations relating the convection coefficient to velocity for several different activities. Because activity is accompanied by relative movement between portions of the body and the surrounding still air, the act of movement itself increases convective heat loss. In Table 5.2.5 is shown the variation between the convection coefficient h_c and activity in still air, originally given in mets.[5] The still air convection coefficient can be calculated (ASHRAE, 1977) from

$$h_c = 5.7(\text{met} - 0.85)^{0.39} = 0.93(M_A - 89)^{0.39} \tag{5.2.4}$$

where M_A = metabolic rate, N·m/sec

[5] A met has been defined as the resting metabolic rate of an average male. As such, its value has been standardized at 58 N/(m·sec), or 105 N·m/sec for a standard man with 1.8 m² surface area. One met is approximately four-thirds of the basal metabolic rate and will maintain comfort of a man with 1 clo of insulation in a room with 0.1 m/sec air velocity, temperature of 21°C, and relative humidity of 50%. (See footnote 8 and accompanying text for a definition of the clo.)

Body Surface Area. Also needed to calculate convective heat loss is the surface area A, By far the most frequently used means of calculation of body surface area of nude humans is from the DuBois formula (Kleiber, 1975):[6]

$$A_{\text{nude}} = 0.07673\,W^{0.425}\,H_t^{0.725} \qquad (5.2.5)$$

where W = body weight, N
$\quad H_t$ = height, m
$\quad A$ = area, m^2

For an average man 1.73 m tall and 685 N (70 kg) weight, a nude surface area of 1.8 m^2 results. Table 5.2.14 gives the distribution of this surface area over parts of the body.

All of this surface area does not contribute to heat loss with the same efficiency. Those areas which are in immediate contact with other parts of the body surface clearly cannot lose heat by convection or radiation. There are other portions of the body surface area that do not feel the full effect of air movement across the body. These, too, are not as efficient in losing heat by convection (and probably not by radiation, as well). Nevertheless, the surface area calculated by means of Equation 5.2.5 gives a reference surface area over which an average heat transfer coefficient may be considered to be effective.

Clothing the human body increases its surface area by a factor of 1.00 to about 1.25. In calculating convection of clothed humans, Equation 5.2.5 must be modified slightly to include this increase in surface area from clothing:

$$A = f_c A_{\text{nude}} \qquad (5.2.6)$$

where f_c = correction factor to account for extra clothing surface area, dimensionless
Values of f_c are given by Equation 5.2.15 or 5.2.16.

Respiratory Convective Heat Loss. A small amount of convective heat loss occurs by respiration. This heat loss is in addition to the heat lost by evaporation (called "latent" heat) from the respiratory system, and this rate of heat loss (called "sensible" heat loss) is determined as the rate of heat transfer required to raise the temperature of the inhaled air to body temperature:

$$q_{c,\text{res}} = \dot{m}_a c_p (\theta_{\text{res}} - \theta_a) = \dot{V} \rho c_p (\theta_{\text{res}} - \theta_a) \qquad (5.2.7)$$

where $q_{c,\text{res}}$ = respiratory convective heat loss N·m/sec
$\quad \dot{m}_a$ = mass rate of flow of air, kg/sec
$\quad c_p$ = specific heat of air, N·m/(kg·°C)
$\quad \theta_a$ = ambient temperature, °C
$\quad \theta_{\text{res}}$ = effective temperature of the respiratory system, °C
$\quad \dot{V}$ = volume flow rate inhaled, m^3/sec
$\quad \rho$ = density of air, kg/m^3

Some difficulty is encountered when applying this equation, however, because $\dot{V}$, ρ, and c_p are all functions of temperature.

Fanger (1967) proposed a simplified form of Equation 5.2.7 using, as an indirect measure of respiratory ventilation rate, the metabolic rate:

$$q_{c,\text{res}} = 0.0014\,M_A(\theta_{\text{res}} - \theta_a) \qquad (5.2.8)$$

where M_A = metabolic rate, N·m/sec

$$\theta_{\text{res}} \simeq 32.6 + 0.066\theta_a + 32\omega_a \simeq 34\,°C \qquad (5.2.9)$$

---

[6]Actually, the DuBois formula is $71.84W^{0.425}H^{0.725}$ where W is measured in kg, H is measured in cm, and A is in cm^2. Jones et al. (1985) give an equation they claim to be more accurate: $A = 0.327 + 0.0071W + 0.0292L_c$, where A is in m^2, W in kg, and L_c is upper half circumference in cm.

TABLE 5.2.6   Values of Parameters for Determination of
Respiratory Convective Heat Loss[a]

Humidity Condition[b]	a, °C	b, dimensionless
Dry (RH < 35%)	24	0.32
Moderate (35% < RH < 65%)	26	0.25
Humid (RH > 65%)	27	0.20

[a] Compiled from Varène, 1986.
[b] Values for normal (10^5 kN/m²) barometric pressure and normal air composition.

where θ_a = ambient temperature, °C

ω_a = ambient humidity ratio, kg H_2O/kg dry air

Thermal resistance of convective losses from the respiratory system is, using the preceding formulation,

$$R_{th} = (714/M_A) \qquad (5.2.10)$$

Varène (1986) proposed a different means to calculate respiratory convective heat loss. He began with Equation 5.2.7, and replaced θ_{res} with a linear function of ambient temperature:

$$\theta_{res} = a + b\theta_a \qquad (5.2.11)$$

where a, b = constants, °C and dimensionless, respectively

Thus

$$q_{c,res} = \dot{V}\rho c_p[a + (b-1)\theta_a] \qquad (5.2.12)$$

In the range $8°C \leqslant \theta_a \leqslant 33°C$ and 10^{-4} m³/sec $\leqslant \dot{V} \leqslant 5.83 \times 10^{-4}$ m³/sec (6–35 L/min), best fit values for a and b were determined by Varène and appear in Table 5.2.6. $\dot{V}$ must be corrected to BTPS conditions (see Section 4.2.2). These parameter values were obtained for normal atmospheric pressure and composition. For nonstandard conditions, the STPD correction of ventilation rate, density values, and specific heat values must be used correctly.

5.2.2 Conduction

Heat is transferred by conduction between parts of the human body and from the body surface through clothing which is worn. Heat loss by conduction may be calculated[7] from

---

[7] Although this form of the conduction equation is often applied to heat transfer in humans, it is absolutely correctly applied only to heat transfer across an area bounded by two flat parallel planes. If thickness is small relative to height and width, Equation 5.2.10 becomes a close approximation to actual heat transfer equation forms. If the conducting medium is too thick, the form of the heat transfer equation must reflect the actual geometrical configuration. While the generalized conduction equation in cartesian coordinates is

$$\frac{\partial^2\theta}{\partial x^2} + \frac{\partial^2\theta}{\partial y^2} + \frac{\partial^2\theta}{\partial z^2} + \frac{q'''}{k} = \frac{1}{\alpha}\frac{\partial\theta}{\partial t}$$

its form in cylindrical coordinates is

$$\frac{\partial^2\theta}{\partial r^2} + \frac{1}{r}\frac{\partial\theta}{\partial r} + \frac{1}{r^2}\frac{\partial^2\theta}{\partial\phi^2} + \frac{\partial^2\theta}{\partial z^2} + \frac{q'''}{k} = \frac{1}{\alpha}\frac{\partial\theta}{\partial t}$$

where q''' = Volume and time rate of internal heat generation, N·m/(sec·m³)

α = thermal diffusivity, m²/sec

TABLE 5.2.7 Thermal Properties of Tissues

Tissue	Thermal Conductivity,[a] N/(°C·sec)	Specific Heat, N·m/(kg·°C)	Density, kg/m³	Reference
Human skin	0.627	3470	1100	Berenson and Robertson, 1973
Muscle	0.498	3470	1080	Pettibone and Scott, 1974
Fat	0.209	1730	850	Pettibone and Scott, 1974
Skin	0.339	3470	1000	Pettibone and Scott, 1974
Blood	—	3470	1050	Pettibone and Scott, 1974
Human surface tissue 2.5 cm deep	0.252	—	—	Kleiber, 1975
Human skin	0.209			Yang, 1980
Subcutaneous tissue	0.419			Yang, 1980

[a]Measured thermal conductivity values can change drastically as temperature changes (Panzner et al., 1986).

$$q_k = \frac{kA}{L}(\theta_i - \theta_o) \qquad (5.2.13)$$

where q_k = heat transfer by conduction, N·m/sec
  k = thermal conductivity, N/(°C·sec)
  A = surface area, m²
  L = thickness of conducting medium, m
  θ_i = temperature of inside surface, °C
  θ_o = temperature of outside surface, °C

The thermal conductivity k is a property of the material through which heat is being conducted. Thermal conductivity is usually somewhat dependent on temperature, but this dependence is largely neglected (Kreith, 1958). Materials having high thermal conductivities (especially metals) are considered to be conductors, whereas materials with low values of thermal conductivity (especially nonmoving gases) are considered to be insulators. In terms of Equation 5.1.1,

$$R_{th} = \frac{L}{kA} \qquad (5.2.14)$$

Different tissues of the human body have different thermal conductivities, as seen in Table 5.2.7 (and Lipkin and Hardy, 1954). These values are necessary to calculate heat conduction from the body core through the peripheral tissues to the body surface, as in a model of the kind illustrated in Figure 5.1.2. When it is necessary to conserve body heat, cutaneous vasoconstriction effectively reduces skin thermal conductivity compared to times when it is necessary to lose body heat (Newman and Lele, 1985).

When calculating heat transfer through the tissues of the skin, muscles, and viscera, a large contribution to heat gain or loss is due to movement of blood flowing through the tissue. Blood heat gain or loss is distributed diffusely throughout the tissue and is considered to be a convective process. However, blood heat transfer is not considered in the same way as the convection just considered. Rather, blood heat transfer is normally considered to be an addition or removal of heat stored in the blood (Hodson et al., 1986), and an additional ($\dot{m}c_p\Delta\theta$) term is added to the generalized conduction equation (see Section 5.2.6).

Clothing. Clothing provides the largest amount of insulation encountered in normal life. The insulation value of clothing is characterized by the accepted, but nonstandard, *clo* unit.[8] A clo is defined as the amount of insulation that would allow 6.45 (N·m)/sec (5.55 kcal/hr) of heat from a 1 m² area of skin of the wearer to transfer to the environment by radiation and convection when a 1°C difference in temperature exists between skin and environment (Goldman, 1967). The higher the clo value of clothing, the less heat will be transferred from the skin. Clo, which contains the insulation of dry clothes plus the underlying still air layer, is usually measured on a manikind with copper skin ("copper man") and heated internally to simulate a human wearer with constant skin temperature (Goldman, 1967). This method allows the normal draping and folding of clothes, which influence measured clo values, to be present.

The combination (k/L) is usually called thermal conductance and will be symbolized here for clothing by C_{cl} with units of N·m/(m²·sec·°C). Thermal conductance is used when material thicknesses are standard (as with bricks or plywood) or, more importantly here, when the thermal conductivity and thickness effects of clothing are not distinct.

Heat conduction through clothing is given by

$$q_k = \frac{6.45A}{\text{clo}}(\theta_{sk} - \theta_0) = C_{cl}A(\theta_{sk} - \theta_0) \tag{5.2.15}$$

where θ_{sk} = mean skin temperature, °C
  θ_0 = temperature at clothing surface, °C

Data for individual pieces of men's and women's clothing appear in Table 5.2.8 (see also Table 5.2.16). In terms of Equation 5.1.1,

$$R_{th} = \frac{\text{clo}}{6.45A} = \frac{1}{C_{cl}A} \tag{5.2.16}$$

Clothing ensembles require combination of conductance values for individual items in Table 5.2.8. By regression this combination has been found to be (ASHRAE, 1985)

$$R_{th} = (0.82 \, \Sigma C_{cl}^{-1})/A \tag{5.2.17}$$

As mentioned earlier, the surface area A can be related to the body surface area as calculated from Equation 5.2.5 by using a factor f_c (Equation 5.2.6). This factor has been found experimentally to be (ASHRAE, 1977)

$$f_c = 1.00 + 1.29/C_{cl} \tag{5.2.18}$$

where f_c = clothing surface area correction factor, dimensionless
for individual clothing items, or

$$f_c = 1.00 + 1.48 \, \Sigma C_{cl}^{-1} \tag{5.2.19}$$

for clothing ensembles.

Mean Skin Temperature. Mean skin temperature must be known to calculate heat loss to the environment by conduction. The preferable means to obtain mean skin temperature is by measurement. However, an estimate can be obtained from the following relationships (ASHRAE, 1977). Each is essentially independent of metabolic rate up to four to five times the

---

[8]The clo unit was defined in 1941 as the insulation of a normal business suit worn comfortably by sedentary workers in an indoor climate of 21°C (70°F).

TABLE 5.2.8 Conductance Values for Individual Items of Clothing

Men Clothing	N·m/(m²·sec·°C)	(clo)	Women Clothing	N·m/(m²·sec·°C)	(clo)
Underwear					
Sleeveless T shirt	110	(0.06)	Bra and panties	130	(0.05)
T shirt	72	(0.09)	Half slip	50	(0.13)
Briefs	129	(0.05)	Full slip	34	(0.19)
Long underwear upper	18	(0.35)	Long underwear upper	18	(0.35)
Long underwear lower	18	(0.35)	Long underwear lower	18	(0.35)
Torso					
Shirt[a]			Blouse		
Light, short sleeve	46	(0.14)	Light	32	(0.20)
Light, long sleeve	29	(0.22)	Heavy	22	(0.29)
Heavy, short sleeve	26	(0.25)			
Heavy, long sleeve	22	(0.29)	Dress		
			Light	29	(0.22)
			Heavy	9.2	(0.70)
Vest			Skirt		
Light	43	(0.15)	Light	65	(0.10)
Heavy	22	(0.29)	Heavy	29	(0.22)
Trousers			Slacks		
Light	25	(0.26)	Light	25	(0.26)
Heavy	20	(0.32)	Heavy	15	(0.44)
Sweater			Sweater		
Light	32	(0.20)	Light	38	(0.17)
Heavy	17	(0.37)	Heavy	17	(0.37)
Jacket			Jacket		
Light	29	(0.22)	Light	38	(0.17)
Heavy	13	(0.49)	Heavy	17	(0.37)
Footwear					
Socks			Stockings		
Ankle length	161	(0.04)	Any length	640	(0.01)
Knee high	65	(0.10)	Panty hose	640	(0.01)
Shoes			Shoes		
Sandals	320	(0.02)	Sandals	320	(0.02)
Oxfords	160	(0.04)	Pumps	160	(0.04)
Boots	81	(0.08)	Boots	81	(0.08)

Source: Adapted and used with permission from ASHRAE, 1985.

[a](5% lower conductance or 5% higher clo for tie or turtleneck)

sitting–resting level [up to 100 (N·m)/sec external work, or 5 mets].[9] For an unclothed subject,

$$\theta_{sk} = 24.85 + 0.332\theta_e - 0.00165\theta_e^2 \qquad (5.2.20)$$

where θ_{sk} = mean skin temperature, °C
θ_e = mean environmental temperature, °C

[9]The efficiency of external work is considered here to be 20%, requiring a metabolic rate five times the external work.

For a clothed subject,

$$\theta_{sk} = 25.8 + 0.267\theta_e \tag{5.2.21}$$

$$\theta_e = (h_c\theta_a + h_r\theta_r)/(h_c + h_r) \tag{5.2.22}$$

where h_c = convection coefficient, N·m/(m²·sec·°C)
$\quad h_r$ = radiation coefficient, N·m/(m²·sec·°C)
$\quad \theta_a$ = ambient temperature, °C
$\quad \theta_r$ = mean radiant temperature, °C

The mean environmental temperature θ_e is essentially a weighted average of mean convective temperature θ_a and mean radiative temperature θ_r.

5.2.3 Radiation

Unlike conduction and convection, which require physical contact between the mass gaining heat and the mass losing heat, radiation heat exchange requires only that there be an unobstructed view from one object to another. Heat is transferred mostly by electromagnetic radiation with a wavelength slightly longer than that of visible light. With a distinctly different modality, radiation heat exchange has been found to depend on the fourth power of the absolute temperature of the body accepting or losing heat:

$$q_{r(1-2)} = \sigma A_1 F_{1-2}(T_1^4 - T_2^4) \tag{5.2.23}$$

where $q_{r(1-2)}$ = heat exchanged by radiation, N·m/sec
$\quad \sigma$ = Stefan–Boltzmann constant
$\quad\quad$ = 5.67×10^{-8} N·m/(m²·sec·°K⁴)
$\quad A_1$ = area of radiating surface, m²
$\quad F_{1-2}$ = shape factor, dimensionless
$\quad T$ = absolute temperature, °K

The rate of heat transfer $q_{r(1-2)}$ is specified between body 1 and body 2. If there are but two objects in the system, heat lost by object 1 equals heat gained by object 2:

$$q_{r(1-2)} = q_{r(2-1)} \tag{5.2.24}$$

With more than two objects, there is no assurance that the rate of heat transferred between each pair of objects will sum to zero.

The shape factor F_{1-2} represents the fraction of total radiant energy leaving body 1 which is intercepted by body 2. The quantity (A_1F_{1-2}) represents the fraction of the surface area of body 1 which could be seen by an observer at various points on body 2 (Figure 5.2.2). Shape factors are

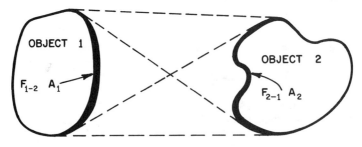

Figure 5.2.2 Two-dimensional representation of line-of-sight areas.

TABLE 5.2.9   Typical Emissivity Values

Substance	Temperature, °C	Emissivity
Water	0	0.95
Water	100	0.96
Ice	0	0.86
Skin	37	0.87
Glass	25	0.93
Plaster	25	0.91
Silver	25	0.02
Black lacquer	25	0.96
White lacquer	25	0.80
Cloth		0.80–0.98
Wood	38	0.93
Skin of white human	35	0.58
Skin of black human	35	0.80

determined solely by geometry. A table of shape factors can be found in Kreith (1958). A reciprocity theorem gives

$$A_i F_{i-j} = A_j F_{j-i} \tag{5.2.25}$$

and because all parts of a surface must be able to be observed by at least some portions of the surrounding surfaces,

$$\sum_{i=1}^{n} F_{i-j} = 1 \tag{5.2.26}$$

Radiation can thus be described as a surface phenomenon that depends on surface characteristics. Equation 5.2.23 describes radiation occurring between perfect radiators and absorbers. To a human observer, a perfect absorber would appear to be totally black, since no incident radiation would be reflected. These are known, therefore, as "black bodies."

Real surfaces are often not totally black. Incident radiation can be reflected and transmitted as well as absorbed. To account for the fraction of radiant energy absorbed and reflected, the absorptivity α and reflectivity ρ are introduced. For opaque surfaces

$$\alpha = 1 - \rho \tag{5.2.27}$$

since transmissivity assumes a value of zero.

In the steady state, where the body is neither gaining nor losing energy, the body emits energy at the same rate as it gains energy. To express the fraction of energy emitted by the body compared to that of a black body, surface emissivity ε is used. Absorptivity and emissivity are nearly identical numerically. If absorptivity and emissivity do not vary with wavelength, the bodies are called "gray bodies,"[10] and the amount of radiation energy transferred between them and their surroundings is a constant fraction of black body radiation. Average emissivities for various substances are given in Table 5.2.9.

[10]For gray bodies, absorptivity α and emissivity ε are the same value if taken at any radiant wavelength. However, it is not uncommon that a body emits the bulk of its radiation at a different temperature than it receives the radiation. Therefore, average values of α and ε are not necessarily the same. Absorptivity α is thus properly evaluated at the temperature corresponding to the emitted radiation striking the body, whereas ε is properly evaluated at the temperature of the body receiving the radiation.

For radiation heat transfer between real surfaces, therefore, Equation 5.2.23 is not adequate. As a matter of fact, the possibility of reflection as well as absorption of incident radiation considerably complicates the calculation of radiation heat exchange. For radiant heat exchange between two bodies,

$$q_{r(1-2)} = \left[\frac{\rho_1}{A_1 \varepsilon_1} + \frac{1}{A_2 F_{2-1}} + \frac{\rho}{A_2 \varepsilon_2} \right]^1 \sigma[T_1^4 - T_2^4] \tag{5.2.28}$$

which accounts for actual surface characteristics. For radiation between more than two bodies, a different scheme must be used for calculation (Kreith, 1958). Fortunately, the case where radiation heat exchange occurs between two bodies, especially where one body, such as a human, is totally enclosed within the other, such as his total environment, is common enough and important enough to minimize the need to consider more complex cases.

For one body completely enclosed within another, when neither body can see any part of itself,

$$F_{ij} = 1 \tag{5.2.29}$$

Furthermore, it is frequently true that the surface area of the enclosing body is much greater than the surface area of the enclosed body ($A_1 \gg A_2$).

Equation 5.2.28 becomes

$$q_{r(1-2)} = \left[\frac{A_2 \rho_2}{A_1 \varepsilon_1} + \frac{1}{F_{2-1}} + \frac{\sigma_2}{\varepsilon_2} \right]^{-1} \tau A_2 [T_1^4 - T_2^4] \tag{5.2.30}$$

Since $A_2 \ll A_1$, and using $F_{2-1} = 1$,

$$q_{r(1-2)} = \left[0 + 1 + \frac{\rho_2}{\varepsilon_2} \right]^{-1} \sigma A_2 [T_1^4 - T_2^4]$$

$$= [\varepsilon_2 + \rho_2]^{-1} \sigma \varepsilon_2 A_2 [T_1^4 - T_2^4]$$

But for an opaque material $\varepsilon_i + \rho_i = 1$,

$$q_{r(1-2)} = \sigma \varepsilon_2 A_2 [T_1^4 - T_2^4] \tag{5.2.31}$$

Radiant Heat Transfer Coefficient. Because it depends on the fourth power of absolute temperature, energy exchange by radiation predominates at large temperature differences between the body losing heat and that gaining heat. Practically speaking, however, conduction and convection cannot be neglected, and heat is transferred by several modes simultaneously. It is thus convenient to define a radiant heat transfer coefficient h_r to be used to calculate radiation energy exchange by a simple temperature difference only:

$$q_r = h_r A (T_0 - T_e) = h_r A(\theta_0 - \theta_e) \tag{5.2.32}$$

and

$$R_{th} = (h_r f_c A_{nude})^{-1} \tag{5.2.33}$$

The similarity of Equations 5.2.32 and 5.2.1 for convection can be immediately seen. Indeed, if, as is often assumed, the mean environmental temperature θ_e equals the temperature of the surrounding air θ_a, an overall heat transfer coefficient h can be used:

$$h = h_r + h_c \tag{5.2.34}$$

and the heat transferred by combined radiation and convection is

$$q = hA(\theta_0 - \theta_a) \tag{5.2.35}$$

The radiant heat transfer coefficient can be related to radiant heat exchange by

$$h_r = \frac{q_r}{A(T_0 - T_e)} = \frac{\sigma\varepsilon[T_0^4 - T_e^4]}{[T_0 - T_e]}$$

$$= \sigma\varepsilon[T_0^3 - T_0^2 T_e + T_0 T_e^2 + T_e^3] \tag{5.2.36}$$

for one body completely enclosed within another. Representative values of h_r for Equation 5.2.32 range from 4.1 to 5.8 N·m/(m²·sec·°C) (Seagrave, 1971) with an average value for normal environments of 4.7 N/(m·sec·°C) (ASHRAE, 1977). Kenney et al. (1987) used a combined coefficient (h) value of 7.5 N·m/(m²·sec·°C) in their work. For a subject wearing shorts and tennis shoes, the radiation coefficient has been estimated at 6.11 N·m/(m²·sec·°C) (Goldman, 1978b). This value is to be reduced to 4.27 N·m/(m²·sec·°C) when the subject wears long-sleeved shirts and trousers.

Similarly, the value of surface area to be used in Equation 5.2.32 can be calculated as a fraction of the total body surface area (Equations 5.2.5 and 5.2.6) available to radiate. This fraction is 0.3 for supine, 0.67 for crouching, 0.70 for sitting, and 0.73 for standing, regardless of sex, weight, height, and body type (Figure 5.2.3).

A 15.4 cm globe with its surface painted flat black has a ratio h_c/h_r of 0.178, which closely approximates the corresponding ratio for an average human body (Goldman, 1978b). Globe temperature, as measured by a thermometer with its bulb at the center of this hollow globe, can be used to estimate mean radiant temperature experienced by a human:

$$\bar{T}_r = (1 + 0.222v^{0.5})(T_g - T_{db}) + T_{db} \tag{5.2.37}$$

where $\bar{T}_r$ = mean radiant temperature, °K
$\quad T_g$ = globe temperature, °K
$\quad T_{db}$ = dry bulb temperature of the air, °K
$\quad v$ = air velocity, m/sec

Solar Heat Load. Human solar heat load can be a very large contributor to heat stress. Roller and Goldman (1968) and Breckenridge and Goldman (1972) presented a means by which this heat load can be analyzed. Referring to Figure 5.2.4, solar heat load in man can be considered to be composed of several components. Sources of radiant energy are (1) direct radiation from the sun, (2) diffuse radiation from dust and water vapor in the sky, and (3) radiation reflected from the terrain. Energy from these three sources impinges on the clothing surface and is reflected, absorbed, or transmitted to the skin [transmittance of light fatigues has been given as 0.02 (Breckenridge and Goldman, 1971), but heavier clothing is assumed to be completely opaque]. Radiant heat absorbed by the clothes is then transmitted by conduction to the skin surface or lost directly from the clothing surface by convection or reradiation. Only that fraction of the total incident radiation that reaches the skin must be considered to be a heat burden to the body. Alternatively, one may consider the solar heat load to be a reduction in possible heat removal from the skin to the clothing surface as a result of the increased surface temperature of the clothes.

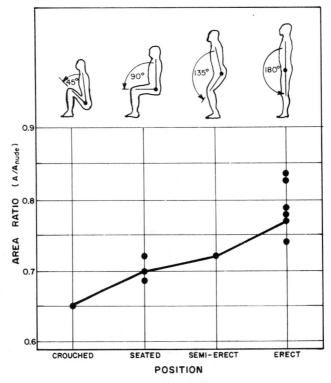

Figure 5.2.3 Ratio of radiation area to nude body surface area as it varies with posture. (Adapted and used with permission from Berenson and Robertson, 1973.)

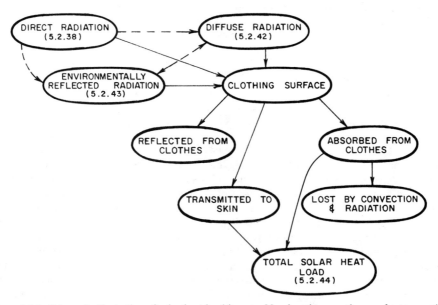

Figure 5.2.4 Schematic illustration of solar heat load in man. Numbers in parentheses refer to equation numbers.

Direct radiant load q_{rdr} is given as

$$q_{rdr} = A_{\text{nude}} f_{cr} \gamma_d I \qquad (5.2.38)$$

where γ_d = fraction of area of nude surface which intercepts direct solar beam (shadow area on a plane normal to the beam), dimensionless

I = intensity of direct sunlight, $N \cdot m/(m^2 \cdot sec)$

f_{cr} = ratio of γ_d for clothed man to γ_d for nude man, dimensionless

For diffuse radiation heat load calculation, Roller and Goldman (1968) proposed a cylindrical model of a man standing in the sun. Direct incident radiation and diffuse radiation impinge directly on the top and sides of the cylinder, but radiation reflected from the terrain hits only the sides. Diffuse radiation on the top plane is simply the area of the top of the cylinder times the diffuse radiation flux.

The top of the cylinder is diagramed in Figure 5.2.5 for incoming rays in one horizontal plane. If uniform radiant flux is assumed, then for any angle ϕ between these rays and a given vertical cross section, the ratio of radiation on the projection of the vertical plane M to the radiation on the entire wall projection N is $\sin \phi$. Integration over the angular span of 0 to π rad gives an average ratio of $2/\pi$.

Rays that are not entirely horizontal will intersect the cylinder wall and the vertical cross section at different heights. Some diffuse rays that would hit the cylinder wall would miss the vertical cross section entirely. Breckenridge and Goldman (1972) assumed their cylinder to have a large enough length-to-diameter ratio to be able to neglect any reduction in intercepted diffuse radiation due to this cause. Thus the total amount of intercepted diffuse radiation on the side of the cylinder is the area of the vertical plane times the diffuse radiation flux on each side times $\pi/2$.

Total diffuse radiation is the sum of radiation on the top and sides of the cylinder:

$$q_{rdf} = \left(\frac{\pi d^2}{4}\right) D + (dL) D \frac{\pi}{2} \qquad (5.2.39)$$

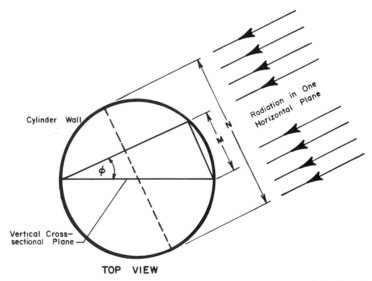

Figure 5.2.5 Geometric model of diffuse radiation on a cylinder. (Used with permission from Breckenridge and Goldman, 1972.)

where q_{rdf} = diffuse radiant heat load, N·m/sec

   d = cylinder diameter, m

   D = intensity of diffuse radiation on a horizontal plane, N/(m·sec)

   L = cylinder length, m

Relating the cylinder dimensions to the nude surface area of a man, which can be calculated from weight and height (Equation 5.2.5), gives

$$d = \sqrt{(4\theta_{\text{nude}}f_c\gamma_z)/\pi} \tag{5.2.40}$$

and

$$L = A_{\text{nude}}f_c\gamma_h/(\pi d) \tag{5.2.41}$$

where γ_z = fraction of the nude area facing the zenith, dimensionless

   γ_h = fraction of the nude area facing horizon, dimensionless

Therefore, Equation 5.2.39 can be rewritten as

$$q_{rdf} = A_{\text{nude}}f_c(\gamma_z + \gamma_h/2)D \tag{5.2.42}$$

Terrain-reflected radiation is assumed to hit only the vertical sides of the cylindrical model. Thus

$$q_{rtr} = A_{\text{nude}}f_c\gamma_h X \tag{5.2.43}$$

where q_{rtr} = terrain reflection heat load, N·m/sec

   X = intensity of terrain-reflected radiation on a vertical plane, N·m/(m²·sec)

Again referring to Figure 5.2.4, of the radiation striking the clothing surface, some is transmitted and some is absorbed. Assuming all the sunlight is absorbed at the clothing surface, and not within the clothing, the resultant heat splits, some flowing through the clothing to the skin surface, and some flowing to the air by convection. Thus

$$q_s = (q_{rdr} + q_{rdf} + q_{rtr})(\tau + \alpha U) \tag{5.2.44}$$

where q_s = solar heat load, N·m/sec

   τ = clothing transmittance, dimensionless

   α = clothing absorptivity, dimensionless

   U = solar heating efficiency factor, dimensionless

and

$$U = \left[f_c\left(\frac{C_a}{C_{cl}}\right) + 1 \right]^{-1} \tag{5.2.45}$$

where C_{cl} = thermal conductance of clothing, N/(m·sec·°C)

   C_a = thermal conductance of the boundary air layer at the nude skin surface, N/(m·sec·°C)

From Figure 5.2.1,

$$C_a = h_r + h_c \tag{5.2.46}$$

Breckenridge and Goldman (1972) use the Winslow equation,

$$C_a = 0.095 + 0.290\sqrt{v} \tag{5.2.47}$$

TABLE 5.2.10   Recommended Values for γ_d, γ_z, γ_h,

Position	γ_d for Solar Angle Of:				γ_z	γ_h
	30°	45°	60°	75°		
Standing						
Facing sun	0.25	0.22	0.18	0.11	0.10	0.60
Profile to sun	0.16	0.14	0.13	0.09	0.10	0.60
Walking	0.27	0.23	0.19	0.13	0.12	0.56
Sitting						
Facing sun	0.22	0.21	0.21	0.18	0.14	0.52
Profile to sun	0.21	0.20	0.19	0.18	0.14	0.52
Prone	0.22	0.24	0.26	0.28	0.30	0.20

Source: Used with permission from Breckenridge and Goldman, 1972.

TABLE 5.2.11   Values of f_{cr} at Four Solar Angles

Position	Light Clothing (such as fagitues)				Heavy Clothing (such as cold-wet uniform)			
	30°	45°	60°	75°	30°	45°	60°	75°
Standing								
Facing sun	1.1	1.1	1.2	1.9	1.3	1.4	1.6	2.2
Profile to sun	1.2	1.2	1.3	1.9	1.5	1.6	1.7	2.2
Walking	1.1	1.1	1.2	1.7	1.3	1.3	1.4	2.0
Sitting								
Facing sun	1.1	1.1	1.1	1.2	1.1	1.1	1.1	1.3
Profile to sun	1.1	1.1	1.1	1.2	1.1	1.1	1.2	1.3
Prone	1.2	1.2	1.1	1.1	1.4	1.4	1.4	1.4

Source: Used with permission from Breckenridge and Goldman, 1972.

and also reduce clothing insulation as wind speed increases:

$$C_{cl}(\text{light clothes}) = \frac{6.45}{0.536 + 0.429e^{-0.422v}} \tag{5.2.48}$$

$$C_{cl}(\text{heavy clothes}) = \frac{6.45}{2.55 - 0.072v} \tag{5.2.49}$$

Clothing transmittance is taken at 0.02 for light clothes and 0.00 for heavy clothes. Clothing absorptivity is 0.8 for army green clothes.

Values for γ_d, γ_z, and γ_h appear in Table 5.2.10, and values for f_{cr} appear in Table 5.2.11. Using measured values of direct, diffuse, and reflected radiation, average predicted solar heat loads were within 4 N·m/sec of actual heat load as measured by a heated copper manikin (Breckenridge and Goldman, 1972).

For the purposes of prediction of solar heat load, it is not always possible to measure each component of solar radiation. Roller and Goldman (1967) tabulated representative values (Table 5.2.12) of solar radiation for nine different geographical areas from meteorological data compiled for summer days at 1400 hours at environmental temperature levels expected to be exceeded in only 5–10% of the days. They adjusted the data to account for conditions of haze, humidity, and cloud cover. Caution should be exercised, however, in using these data, because meteorological conditions are so variable.

TABLE 5.2.12   Summary of Solar Radiant Heat Load Values for Men

| Region | Representative Elevation m | Representative 1400 hr-summer | | | "Hazy" Clear Sky[a] | | Maximum Diffuse Radiation[a] | | Terrestrial Cover[a] | |
| | | Solar Angle, degrees | Temperature C | RH, % | I | D^b | Cloud Type | D^b, N·m/ (m²·sec) | Type | X, N·m/ (m²·sec) |
					N·m/(m²·sec)					
Tropical rain forest	400	60	35	65	845 (725)	180 (155)	Altocumulus	465 (400)	Jungle	45 (40)
Tropical savanna	200	60	39	33	890 (765)	165 (141)	Altocumulus	465 (400)	Lush grass, scattered trees	95 (80)
Tropical–subtropical steppe	1600	60	38	17	1013 (875)	115 (98)	Altocumulus	350 (300)	Grass, bare soil, few trees	105 (90)
Tropical–subtropical desert	1000	60	44	10	1010 (870)	190 (162)	Cirrus	350 (300)	Sand and rocky waste	135 (115)
Humid subtropical	100	60	38	40	850 (732)	180 (155)	Altocumulus	465 (400)	Lush grass and forest	85 (75)
Humid continental	300	52	35	50	835 (720)	185 (159)	Altocumulus	350 (300)	Grass and scattered trees	85 (75)
Subarctic	400	45	27	40	955 (820)	145 (123)	Altostratus	465 (400)	Conifer forest and rocky waste	65 (55)
Tundra	200	38	16	40	985 (847)	130 (111)	Cirrus	350 (300)	Moss, lichens, rocky waste	60 (50)
Ice cap	100	33	−1	30	1095 (940)	265 (227)	Cirrus	580 (500)	Snow	115 (100)

Source: Adapted and used with permission from Roller and Goldman, 1967.

[a]Values in parentheses are original units of kcal/(m²·hr). Unit conversions were rounded to the nearest 5 for N·m/(m²·sec) values.

[b]Values for diffuse radiation D are to be chosen for either clear or cloudy sky not both.

5.2.4 Evaporation

One of the most important modes of heat loss from the body is by means of evaporation of water. This evaporation is composed of three components:

1. Evaporation from the respiratory system.
2. Nonregulated evaporation from the skin.
3. Regulatory sweat evaporation.

Before considering the details of any of these, a general discussion of evaporation must be undertaken.

There is a similarity between convective and evaporative processes because convection involves heat transfer through a thermal boundary layer adjacent to the surface and evaporation involves mass transfer through a concentration boundary layer some fraction of the thickness of the thermal boundary layer (Threlkeld, 1962).[11] Evaporative heat loss from a surface is thus calculated from

$$q_{evap} = h_d A(\omega_{sat} - \omega_a)H \tag{5.2.50}$$

where q_{evap} = evaporative heat loss, N·m/sec
h_d = convection vapor transfer coefficient, kg/(m²·sec)
A = body surface area, m²
ω_{sat} = humidity ratio of air saturated at body temperature, kg H$_2$O/kg dry air
ω_a = humidity ratio of surrounding air, kg H$_2$O/kg dry air
H = latent heat of vaporization of water at body surface temperature, N·m/kg

The similarity between convection and evaporation is embodied by the Lewis number (Threlkeld, 1962)[12]:

$$Le = \frac{h_c}{h_d c} \tag{5.2.51}$$

where Le = Lewis number, dimensionless
c = specific heat capacity of air at constant pressure, N·m/(kg·°C)

The Lewis number can be related to properties of the air, water vapor, and boundary layer dimensions (Johnson and Kirk, 1981); it is illustrated graphically in Figure 5.2.6. The Lewis number can be seen to be slightly dependent on wind velocity and average temperature of body surface and surrounding air.

The specific heat of air c has been measured and can be calculated (Johnson and Kirk, 1981) from

$$c = 1000 + 1880\left(\frac{\omega_{sat} + \omega_a}{2}\right) \tag{5.2.52}$$

---

[11]There are two modes of mass transfer from place to place. The first is molecular diffusion, analogous to heat transfer by conduction. This mode requires a medium through which molecules move that is stationary at least in the direction of molecular movement. The second mode is convection, which occurs when molecules are moved into a volume as bulk movement replaces the mass in that volume. Molecular diffusion is considered later (Equation 5.2.70) and has been discussed as well in Section 4.2.2.

[12]There appears to be some disagreement about the precise definition of the Lewis number. Threlkeld (1962) defines the Lewis number as in Equation 5.2.51 and shows that this is equivalent to $Le = [\alpha/D]^{1-c}$, where α = thermal diffusivity (m²/sec), D = mass diffusivity (m²/sec), and c = dimensionless constant (value generally 0.3–0.4 for turbulent flow). Rohsenow and Choi (1961) define the Lewis number as $Le = (\alpha/D)$. The first definition is the one used for further development in this book. Both show the relationship between mass and thermal diffusivities.

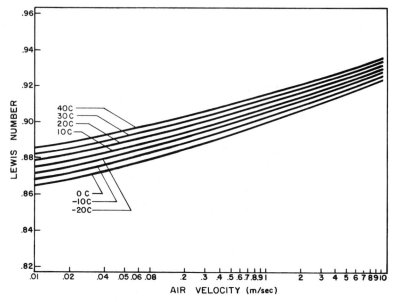

Figure 5.2.6 Lewis number as affected by air velocity and temperature. (Used with permission from Johnson and Kirk, 1981.)

where the specific heat of dry air is 1000 N·m/(kg·°C) and the specific heat of water vapor is 1880 N·m/(kg·°C). Other parameters required in Equation 5.2.50 are the humidity ratio ω_a, which may be obtained most easily from a standard psychrometric chart once two ambient measures are known, and the latent heat of vaporization H, given as (Johnson and Kirk, 1981)

$$H = 2.502 \times 10^6 - 2.376 \times 10^3 \theta, \qquad 0°C < \theta < 50°C \qquad (5.2.53)$$

Frequently, evaporative heat loss is computed from a hybrid equation:

$$q_{\text{evap}} = h_v A(p_{\text{sat}} - p_a) \qquad (5.2.54)$$

where h_v = heat transfer coefficient for evaporation, m/sec
$\quad p_{\text{sat}}$ = partial pressure of water vapor at body surface temperature, N/m²
$\quad p_a$ = partial pressure of water vapor in surrounding air, N/m²
The heat transfer coefficient for evaporation is treated differently by different authors. Seagrave (1971) gives a representative value of h_{va} as

$$h_{va} = 0.104 v^{0.6} \qquad (5.2.55)$$

where h_{va} = heat transfer coefficient for evaporation into air, m/sec
based on reports in the literature (see also Table 5.2.15). Goldman (1967) and ASHRAE (1977) relate h_{va} to the convection coefficient h_c through the Lewis number. Equating Equations 5.2.50 and 5.2.54:

$$h_d A(\omega_{\text{sat}} - \omega_a)H = h_{va} A(p_{\text{sat}} - p_a) \qquad (5.2.56)$$

canceling the area, and making use of Equation 5.2.5.

$$\frac{h_c H(\omega_{sat} - \omega_a)}{Le\, c} = h_{va}(p_{sat} - p_a) \tag{5.2.57}$$

From Lee and Sears (1959), the humidity ratio ω can be related to water vapor partial pressure if the vapor and dry air are assumed to be ideal gases following the ideal gas law:

$$pV = mRT \tag{5.2.58}$$

where p = pressure of gas, N/m^2
$\quad V$ = volume of gas, m^3
$\quad m$ = mass of gas, kg
$\quad R$ = gas constant, N·m/(kg·°K)
$\quad T$ = gas temperature, °K

Since volume and temperature of the mixture are assumed to be the same for both water vapor and dry air,

$$\omega = \frac{m_{H_2O}}{m_{air}} \simeq \frac{R_{air}}{R_{H_2O}} \frac{pH_2O}{p_a} = 0.622 \frac{pH_2O}{p_a} \tag{5.2.59}$$

Thus h_{va} may be obtained from Equation 5.2.57 as

$$h_{va} = \frac{0.622\, h_c H}{Le\, cp_a} \tag{5.2.60}$$

Making some assumptions about skin temperature, humidity ratio of the air, and total atmospheric pressure gives the Lewis relation,

$$h_{va} = 0.0165 h_c \tag{5.2.61}$$

which is used by ASHRAE (1977) to calculate resistance to water vapor heat transfer once

TABLE 5.2.13   **Vapor Pressure Above a Liquid Water Surface at Different Temperature**

Temperature, °C	Vapor Pressure, N/m^2	(mm Hg)
28	3780	(28.4)
29	4005	(30.0)
30	4243	(31.8)
31	4492	(33.7)
32	4760	(35.7)
33	5026	(37.7)
34	5319	(39.9)
35	5626	(42.2)
36	5946	(44.6)
37 (normal body temperature)	6279	(47.1)
38	6626	(49.7)
39	6991	(52.4)
40	7375	(55.3)

convection is known. This similarity among Equation 5.2.61 for evaporation, Equation 5.2.1 for convection, and Equation 5.2.32 for radiation makes calculation of heat loss from these mechanisms simpler than it otherwise would be.

The saturation pressure of water vapor is a function only of temperature. Table 5.2.13 gives this saturated pressure for temperature likely to be encountered at various parts of the body. Some investigators (ASHRAE, 1977; Givoni and Goldman, 1972) have chosen the saturated vapor pressure to be 5866 N/m² (44 mm Hg) and others (Seagrave, 1971) have used 6266 N/m² (47 mm Hg).

Respiratory Evaporation. With this general discussion behind us, we can now turn our attention to the three modes of evaporative heat loss mentioned earlier. First, respired water vapor heat loss[13] can be calculated by means of Equation 5.2.54 with the proper value of h_v. It can also be obtained if respiratory ventilation rate and ambient water vapor conditions are known, since air leaving the respiratory tract can be assumed to be nearly saturated with water vapor at 37°C[14]:

$$q_{evap, res} = \dot{V} \rho H(\omega_{res} - \omega_a) \tag{5.2.62}$$

where $q_{evap,res}$ = respiratory, evaporative heat loss, N·m/sec
ω_{res} = absolute humidity of saturated air at effective respiratory system temperature, kg H$_2$O/kg air
ω_a = absolute humidity of ambient air, kg H$_2$O/kg air
$\dot{V}$ = ventilation rate, BTPS, m³/sec
H = latent heat of vaporization of water, N·m/kg
ρ = density of air, kg/m³

Hanna and Scherer (1986) formulated a model of heat and water vapor transport from the human respiratory tract and found that the two most important parameters governing heat and water transfer are the blood temperature distribution along the airway walls and the total cross-sectional area and perimeter of the nasal cavity. Varène (1986) published a semiempirical equation relating respiratory evaporative heat loss to environmental parameters:

$$q_{evap, res} = 0.001 \dot{V}(59.34 + 0.53 \theta_a - 0.0116 p_a) \tag{5.2.63}$$

where θ_a = ambient temperature, °C
p_a = ambient water vapor pressure, N/m²

Respired heat loss has been empirically found to be proportional to the volume rate of air through the lungs, which in turn is proportional to the metabolic rate. Based on a mean pulmonary ventilation of

$$\dot{m} = 1.67 \times 10^{-6} M_A \tag{5.2.64}$$

where $\dot{m}$ = mass flow of air out of the respiratory system, kg/sec
M_A = metabolic rate per unit area, N·m/(m²·sec)

---

[13]Such heat loss can be a bronchoconstrictive stimulant, resulting in exercise-induced asthma (Sheppard and Eschenbacher, 1984).

[14]Varène et al. (1986) claim that expired air is not water vapor–saturated and they have measured the temperature of expired gas at 31.5°C for mouth breathing and 29.6°C for nose breathing. The reason for temperatures lower than body temperature is that inhaled air cools the respiratory passages and exhaled air subsequently loses heat to them. This countercurrent heat exchange mechanism recovers a great deal of heat that would ordinarily be lost in cold environments. Varène et al. also found about a 7% reduction in convective and evaporative heat loss when breathing through the nose compared to mouth breathing.

and an empirically derived approximation that

$$\omega_{\text{sat}} - \omega_a \simeq 0.029 - 0.80\,\omega_a \qquad \omega_{\text{sat}} - \omega_a > 0 \tag{5.2.65}$$

Fanger (1967) derived an equation for latent heat loss from the respiratory system. In terms of the heat transfer coefficient for evaporation,

$$h_{vr} = 1.725 \times 10^{-5} M_A \tag{5.2.66}$$

where M_A = metabolic rate, N·m/(sec·m^2)
and where p_{sat} is to be taken as 5866 N/m^2 (47 mm Hg) and p_a is 10^5 N/m^2 in Equation 5.2.59.
Thermal resistance of evaporation from the respiratory system is

$$R_{\text{th}} = (h_{vr}\,A_{\text{nude}})^{-1} \tag{5.2.67}$$

where A_{nude} is total body surface area.

Sweating. Evaporative heat loss from sweating skin is both regulatory and nonregulatory. Unstressed skin always sweats about 6% of its maximum capacity. During long exposure to low humidities, dehydration of outer skin layers causes this percentage to drop as low as 2% (ASHRAE, 1977). Each kilogram of sweat requires 2.4×10^6 N·m (670 W·hr) to evaporate (ASHRAE, 1977).[15] The maximum sweating rate for an average man (1.8 m^2 surface area) is about 5×10^{-4} kg/sec. Maximum cooling is about 675 N·m/(m^2·sec) (equivalent to 1200 N·m/sec, or 11.4 mets) for the average man (ASHRAE, 1977). This means that unstressed skin is constantly losing about 40 N·m/(m^2·sec) or 73 N·m/sec total. For relative humidities of 40–60%, ambient temperatures below 20°C, and during rest, evaporative heat loss amounts to 20–25% of the total metabolic rate of the subject (ASHRAE, 1977).

Regulatory sweating comprises the other 94% of maximum capacity, and this 94% is not totally effective. Sweat that rolls off the skin is ineffective; sweat that is absorbed by clothing may evaporate within the clothing or at its surface. Thus a more practical limit to maximum cooling is 350 N·m/m^2 (equivalent to 6 mets). The sweating process involves recruitment of various areas of skin. Sweating does not begin over all areas at the same time or the same temperature. Even in one area, sweating does not reach a maximum value all at once but instead appears to be regulated to lose the required amount of heat. Table 5.2.14 lists preferred temperatures of various regions of the body, along with sweating heat loss from these regions under moderate heat stress. Overall, a skin temperature of 33°C can be assumed to be the most comfortable.

Clothing. Figure 5.2.1 shows two series resistances between the evaporation at the skin and ambient vapor pressure. Clothing presents an impedance to the movement of vapor from the skin and will be considered first.

Nishi and Ibamoto (1969) developed equations for calculation of the heat loss due to evaporation through clothing. They began with the form of heat transfer in Equation 5.2.54,

$$q_{\text{evap}} = h_{vcl} A(p_{\text{sat}} - p_{cl}) \tag{5.2.68}$$

where h_{vcl} = heat transfer coefficient for evaporation from clothing, m/sec
p_{cl} = partial pressure of water vapor at the clothing surface, N/m^2
Evaporative heat loss can also be calculated from the rate of evaporation of water $\dot{m}_v$ multiplied

---

[15]The figure given by ASHRAE is equivalent to the amount of heat required to evaporate an equivalent amount of water. Snellen et al. (1970) measured the heat equivalent of sweat to be 2.6×10^6 N·m/kg (43.3 W·min/g), or about 8% higher than that of water. Their figure was independent of prevailing air temperature or humidity.

TABLE 5.2.14 Thermal Characteristics of Different Parts of the Human Body at Sea Level at Rest

Region	Preferred Temperature, °C	Sweating Heat Loss, N·m/sec (Btu/hr)		Area, m²	Percent Area
Head	34.7	4.7	(15.9)	0.20	11
Chest	34.7	9.6	(32.6)	0.17	9
Abdomen	34.7	5.2	(17.9)	0.12	7
Back	34.7	14.4	(49.3)	0.23	13
Buttocks	34.7	9.7	(33.0)	0.18	10
Thighs	33.0	14.0	(47.7)	0.33	18
Calves	30.8	17.0	(58.0)	0.20	11
Feet	28.6	11.6	(39.7)	0.12	7
Arms	34.7	9.8	(33.4)	0.10	6
Forearms	30.8	10.0	(34.2)	0.08	4
Hands	28.6	18.6	(63.5)	0.07	4
		124.6		1.80	100

Source: Adapted and used with permission from Berenson and Robertson, 1973.

by the latent heat of evaporation of water H:

$$q_{\text{evap}} = \dot{m}_v H \tag{5.2.69}$$

The rate of evaporation of water also equals the rate at which water vapor is transmitted through the clothing by molecular diffusion. Steady-state molecular diffusion is defined by Fick's law (Anderson, 1958; Geankoplis, 1978):

$$\dot{m}_v = DA \frac{dc_v}{dy} \tag{5.2.70}$$

where D = mass diffusivity[16] of water vapor
$\qquad$ = 0.0883 m²/hr
$\qquad A$ = surface area, m²
$\qquad c_v$ = concentration of water vapor, kg/m³
$\qquad y$ = distance along which vapor moves, m
Substituting vapor pressure of water vapor determined from the ideal gas law, Equation 5.2.58 gives

$$\dot{m}_v = \frac{DA}{R_v T} \frac{dp}{dy} \tag{5.2.71}$$

where R_v = gas constant for water vapor
$\qquad$ = 461 N·m/(kg·°K)
$\qquad T$ = absolute temperature, °K
$\qquad p$ = water vapor partial pressure, N/m²
Integrating Equation 5.2.71 from the skin, where $p = p_{\text{sat}}$, to the clothing surface,

---

[16]Nishi and Gagge (1970) give the mass diffusivity of water vapor into air as $D = 0.0784(T/273)^{1.8}$, which means that $D = 0.0883$ m²/hr corresponds to a temperature of 19°C. Yang (1980) gives the mass diffusivity of liquid water through skin as 2.41×10^{-5} m²/hr.

where $p = p_{cl}$,

$$\dot{m}_v = \frac{DA}{R_v T} \frac{(p_{sat} - p_{cl})}{L} \qquad (5.2.72)$$

where p_{cl} = vapor pressure at the clothing surface, N/m^2
$\quad L$ = effective clothing thickness, m
The effective clothing thickness can be approximated by assuming the insulation value of clothing results entirely from dead air trapped in pockets within the fibers:

$$L = k_a/C_{cl} \qquad (5.2.73)$$

where k_a = thermal conductivity[17] of air, $N \cdot m/(m \cdot sec \cdot °C)$
Thus

$$\dot{m}_v = \frac{DA}{R_v T} C_{cl} \frac{(p_{sat} - p_{cl})}{k_a} \qquad (5.2.74)$$

Combining Equation 5.2.68, 5.2.69, and 5.2.74 gives

$$h_{vcl} = \frac{HD}{R_v T} \frac{C_{cl}}{k_a} \qquad (5.2.75)$$

The thickness of the diffusion layer for water vapor has been approximated by the term k_a/C_{cl} based on the assumptions that (1) the physical properties of clothing materials such as thermal conductivity, moisture absorption capacity, porosity, weaving density, thickness, and chemical treatment are ignored; and (2) atmospheric air movement does not break the still air layer in the clothing.

Nishi and Ibamoto (1969) calculated an approximate value of the heat transfer coefficient for evaporation through clothing to be

$$h_{vcl} = 0.0179 \, k_{cl}/L = 0.0179 \, C_{cl} (k_{cl}/k_a) \qquad (5.2.76)$$

With thermal resistance,

$$R_{th} = (h_{vcl} A_{nude})^{-1} \qquad (5.2.77)$$

For perfect vaporproof clothing, $h_{vcl} = 0$, and h_{vcl} is independent of clothing conductance. This restriction, however, applies only to a skin-tight suit completely covering the man (Nishi and Ibamoto, 1969). Other values for h_{vcl} appear in Table 5.2.15.

Nishi and Ibamoto (1969) formed a dimensionless permeation index, P, which they use to help calculate evaporative heat transfer through clothing and the surrounding still air layer:

$$P = \frac{h_{vcl}}{h_{va} + h_{vcl}} = \frac{1}{1 + (h_{va}/h_{vcl})} \qquad (5.2.78)$$

They considered the permeation to be a measure of the cooling efficiency of the evaporative heat loss from the body through the clothing. Actual conditions may cause changes in the permeation as follows:

[17]Johnson and Kirk (1981) give the thermal conductivity of air to be $k_a = 2.416 \times 10^{-2} + 7.764 \times 10^{-5} \theta_a$, $0°C < \theta_a < 50°C$.

TABLE 5.2.15   Heat Transfer Coefficient for Evaporation h_{rcl} and Sweating Efficiency η_{SW} for Four Protective Clothing Ensembles[a]

Clothing	Heat Transfer Coefficient, m/sec	Efficiency
Cotton coveralls	$0.051 v^{0.6}$	0.70
Gore-Tex fabric	$0.051 v^{0.6}$	0.64
Double cotton coveralls	$0.048 v^{0.6}$	0.66
Cotton coveralls and one-piece vapor-barrier suit	$0.034 v^{0.6}$	0.48

[a]Compiled from Kenney et al., 1987. Values were corrected for surface area by assuming body surface area to be $1.8\,m^2$ and clothing surface area correction f_c to be 1.2. Average wind speed was taken to be 0.4 m/sec. Compare these values with that given in Equation 5.2.55, which is for nude or very light clothing, and would be expected to be greater than h_{vcl} for protective clothing.

1. Wind penetration through clothing and ventilation through the neck and sleeves increases P.
2. There is a physiological property that most of the sweat of a clothed man is secreted on exposed parts of the body, which increases P.
3. The interruption of diffusion by the fabric decreases P.

When h_{vcl} is calculated by means of Equation 5.2.76 and h_{va} is calculated from Equation 5.2.61, the resulting permeation agrees well with experimental data presented by Gosselin (1947) and Nagata (1962). This agreement can be seen in Figure 5.2.7 and can be taken as evidence of the validity of Equations 5.2.61 and 5.2.76. Although the permeation index P is used elsewhere in the literature (ASHRAE, 1977), its use here is limited to a role of confirmation of agreement between theory and experiment.

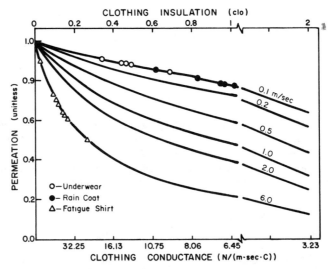

Figure 5.2.7   The relation between the theoretically derived permeation and clothing conductance for different values of air movement. Data were taken from Gosselin (1947) and Nagata (1962). Permeation becomes 1.0 in the unclothed subject at any air movement. (Adapted and used with permission from Nishi and Ibamoto, 1969.)

**TABLE 5.2.16   Heat and Moisture Transfer Characteristics of
Selected Clothing (at 0.3 m/sec effective air motion)**[a]

Uniform	Conductance, N·m/(m²·sec·°C)		im
None (nude)	8.27	(0.78 clo)	0.53
Utility uniform	4.61	(1.40)	0.43
Standard cold-wet	2.02	(3.20)	0.40
Standard cold-dry	1.50	(4.30)	0.43
Nylon twill uncoated coverall	4.78	(1.35)	0.43
Nylon twill coated with urethane	5.08	(1.27)	0.34
Nylon twill coated with butyl	5.24	(1.23)	0.21
Full length plastic raincoat over standard fatigue	3.79	(1.70)	0.25
Coveralls, lightweight, standard cotton	5.00	(1.29)	0.45
Standard fatigues with helmet aviators	4.48	(1.44)	0.42
Combat tropical standard 100% cotton poplin (new)	4.51	(1.43)	0.43
Combat tropical standard 100% cotton poplin (laundered)	4.57	(1.41)	0.41

[a] Selected values from Goldman.

In 1962 Woodcock introduced a dimensionless "impermeability index," im, to be a measure of the resistance of clothing to water vapor. As described by Goldman (1967), the evaporative heat transfer for a nude man or any clothing system could be expressed as the ratio of the actual evaporative heat loss, as hindered by the clothing, to that of a wet bulb with equivalent clothing insulation. This ratio of evaporative loss would vary from 0 for a system with no evaporative vapor transfer to 1 for a system that had no more resistance to evaporative heat transfer than the usual slung wet bulb thermometer. Radiation for men in comparatively still air tends to limit im to 0.5 rather than 1.0 (Table 5.2.16). It is in terms of this index that a model is developed here.

From the definition of the impermeability index, evaporative heat transferred (Goldman, 1967; Nishi and Gaffe, 1970) is

$$q_{\text{evap}} = \frac{\text{im}\,(h_{va}/h_c)(p_{\text{sat}} - p_a)A}{1/(h_r + h_c) + L_{\text{cl}}/k_{\text{cl}}} \tag{5.2.79}$$

Setting this heat loss equal to that treated by Equations 5.2.54 and 5.2.69–5.2.78:

$$q_{\text{evap}} = wPh_{va}(p_{\text{sat}} - p_a)A \tag{5.2.80}$$

where w = fraction of the total surface which is wetted by sweat, dimensionless
The impermeability index is found to be

$$\text{im} = wh_c P\left(\frac{1}{h_r + h_c} + \frac{L_{\text{cl}}}{k_{\text{cl}}}\right) \tag{5.2.81}$$

For completely impermeable clothing, im = 0, $P = 0$, and $h_{vcl} = 0$. For an unclothed subject,

$$\text{im} = \frac{wh_c}{h_r + h_c} \tag{5.2.82}$$

Data obtained from a sweating manikin, where $w = 1$, show almost identical agreement between values of im measured directly and from Equation 5.2.81 when Goldman's fatigue uniform and standard Kansas State University clothing are compared (Nishi and Gaffe, 1970).

As a final consideration under evaporative heat loss through clothing, Nishi and Gaffe (1970) discussed the effect on heat loss of infiltration of sweat into the clothes. If the sweat vaporizes somewhere within the layers of clothing, evaporation is less effective in removing heat from the skin surface. Sweating efficiencies, defined as evaporated sweat to total sweat production, are given in Table 5.2.15.

The water that fills the voids between clothing fibers increases the effective thermal conductance of the clothes and, under some circumstances, tends to compensate for sweating inefficiency. This compensation would be possible only if the surroundings were cooler than the skin surface. Fortunately, this is usually the case during exercise. With high radiant loads, however, sweat infiltration may add to the amount of heat to be removed from the skin surface.

Vapor pressure at the surface of permeable clothing is not the same as ambient vapor pressure. There is an effective resistance between the surface vapor pressure and ambient vapor pressure due to limited movement of water molecules from the clothing surface. A vapor convective process similar to convection of heat removes water vapor from the surface to be added to the ambient air. The similarity between these two convection processes has already been described and developed in Equation 5.2.61. Thus, once the convection coefficient has been determined by one of the equations in Section 5.2.1, vapor convection can be calculated from Equation 5.2.61, and the resistance to water vapor transmission at the clothing surface can be given by

$$R_{th} = (h_{av} f_c A_{nude})^{-1} \qquad (5.2.83)$$

where a correction for surface area has been made.

5.2.5 Rate of Heat Production

In the general heat balance, Equation 5.1.2, the rate of heat generated must be added to the difference between heat gained and lost to obtain the net heat load of an individual. There is, therefore, a qualitative difference between the preceding sections and this, because we are concerned here not with mechanisms of heat transfer but with mechanisms of heat generation.

Heat production in a human is controlled by hormonal secretion, which affects metabolism. Metabolism is composed of the complex, step-wise processes that oxidize food, called catabolism, and formation of energy-rich substances, such as proteins, fats, complex carbohydrates, adenosine triphosphate and adenosine diphosphate, called anabolism. At the cellular level, these processes contribute to the heat generated by the organism.

Basal Metabolic Rate. Heat is produced according to three classifications (Figure 5.2.8): (1) basal metabolic rate, (2) specific dynamic action of food, and (3) skeletal muscular contraction. Basal metabolic rate (BMR) is the summation of heats from all chemical and mechanical processes which must occur to sustain life at a very low level. BMR is usually determined at as complete mental and physical rest as possible, in a comfortable room temperature, and 12–14 hours after the last meal (Ganong, 1963). It includes heat produced by the nervous system, liver, kidneys, and heart muscle. Skeletal muscle tone and gastrointestinal activity should be at a minimum. Actually, metabolic rate during sleep is frequently lower than the BMR measured under standard conditions.

BMR is affected by age, sex, race, emotional state, climate, body temperature, and levels of epinephrine and thyroxine circulating in the blood. Age and sex differences in BMR are illustrated in Table 5.2.17. BMR decreases with age, with a reduction of 2% for each decade increase in years (ASHRAE, 1977). BMR for females at all ages is about 0.9 that of males when

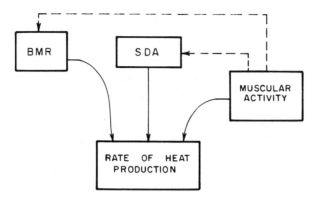

Figure 5.2.8 Factors contributing to the rate of heat production. SDA is specific dynamic action.

TABLE 5.2.17   Age and Sex Differences in BMR

| | Basal Metabolic Rate, | |
| | $N \cdot m/(m^2 \cdot sec)$ | $(kcal/m^2/hr)$ |
Age, Yr	Male	Female
2	66.3 (57.0)	61.0 (52.5)
6	61.6 (53.0)	58.8 (50.6)
8	60.2 (51.8)	54.7 (47.0)
10	56.4 (48.5)	53.4 (45.9)
16	53.1 (45.7)	45.1 (38.8)
20	48.1 (41.4)	42.0 (36.1)
30	45.7 (39.3)	41.5 (35.7)
40	44.2 (38.0)	41.5 (35.7)
50	42.7 (36.7)	39.5 (34.0)
60	41.3 (35.5)	37.9 (32.6)

Source: Adapted and used with permission from Keele and Neil, 1961.

based on body surface area, as in Table 5.2.17. For average sized women with body weights 0.8 those of average men, BMR, not based on area, is about 0.85 that of men.

It has been reported that Chinese and Indians have lower BMRs than Caucasians (Ganong, 1963) and that Eskimos have higher BMRs (Kleiber, 1975). Stress and tension cause increased muscular tensing, which increases the BMR even at rest. An increase in body temperature will raise the BMR as well, due to the increased rate at which chemical activity occurs. For each degree Celsius of fever, the BMR is increased about 9% (Ganong, 1963).[18]

[18]The effect of environmental temperature on the rate of heat production is given by the Van't Hoff equation (Kleiber, 1975):

$$M_\theta = M_0 Q_{10}^{(\theta/10)} \tag{5.2.84}$$

where M_θ = metabolic rate at temperature $\theta°C$, $N \cdot m/sec$

M_0 = metabolic rate at some reference temperature, $N \cdot m/sec$

Q_{10} = Van't Hoff quotient, dimensionless

Typical values of Q_{10} range from 2 to 4. That is, a 10° increase in temperature can cause a twofold to fourfold increase in the metabolic rate. This same effect can be seen in many biological activities and chemical reaction rates.

The Van't Hoff equation is often confused with the Arrhenius equation:

$$M_\theta = M_0^{-\mu/T} \tag{5.2.85}$$

where μ is a constant and T is absolute temperature.

TABLE 5.2.18 Basal Metabolic Rates of Various Animals

Animal	Average Weight, N (kg)		Basal Metabolic Rate			
			Total,		Based on Area,	
	N	(kg)	N·m/sec	(kcal/day)	N·m/(m²·sec)	(kcal/day·m²)
Horse	4325	(441)	241	(4980)	45.9	(948)
Pig	1255	(128)	118	(2440)	52.2	(1078)
Man	631	(64.3)	100	(2060)	50.5	(1042)
Dog	149	(15.2)	37.9	(783)	50.3	(1039)
Rabbit	23	(2.3)	8.4	(173)	37.6	(776)
Goose	34	(3.5)	11.3	(233)	49.3	(1018)
Hen	20	(2.0)	6.9	(142)	48.8	(1008)

Source: Adapted and used with permission from Kleiber, 1975.

BMR for an average man is about 84 N·m/sec or 0.8 met (Seagrave, 1971), which, as can be seen from Table 5.2.21, is due to blood circulation, respiration, digestion, and central nervous system activity.[19] BMR has historically been considered to be proportional to body surface area, since larger body surface areas lose more heat in cool climates and require higher rates of heat production to maintain equilibrium body temperatures. Fasting homeotherms produce about 50 N·m/(sec·m²), or 1000 kcal/(day·m²), based on body surface area (Kleiber, 1975). Table 5.2.18 illustrates this assertion for seven different species.

Another explanation for the variation of BMR with body weight is that BMR should depend on body mass, since it is the body mass that actually produces the heat. This relation is shown somewhat schematically in Figure 5.2.9 in a logarithmic graph (Seagrave, 1971). This explanation is also favored by Kleiber (1975), who argues that, for all species but man, a confusion exists over true surface area. The Dubois area formula (Equation 5.2.5) in man is so widely accepted that the question of surface area in man is not considered serious. Kleiber asserts that BMR should depend on body mass:

$$BMR = 3.39m^{0.75} \tag{5.2.86}$$

where BMR = basal metabolic rate, N·m/sec

m = body mass[20], kg

Body surface area, which has dimensions of length squared, is proportional to mass to the two-thirds power.[21] It is unlikely that a difference in the underlying relationship between BMR and either surface area or body mass could be determined from data which include large amounts of variation. There is not much numerical difference between mass to the two-thirds power and mass to the three-fourths power.

Basal metabolic rate is strongly influenced by environmental temperature, especially cold temperature. Heat-generating mechanisms such as shivering and nonshivering thermogenesis are activated to maintain normal body temperature. When environmental temperature is higher than thermoneutral, metabolic processes are thermally stimulated (Van't Hoff equation), thus raising metabolic rate. Table 5.2.19 shows oxygen consumption indicative of metabolic rate, as it varies with environmental temperature.

Exercise training has been shown to influence resting metabolic rate (Tremblay et al., 1988).

[19]Stolwijk and Hardy (1977) report BMR to be produced by the brain (17% of total), trunk core (60%), skin and musculature (18%), and skeleton and connective tissue (5%).

[20]In standard gravity, this equation becomes $BMR = 0.612W^{0.75}$ where W = body weight in newtons.

[21]As we saw in Chapter 2, area can be expressed in dimensions of L^2. Mass equals density times volume, and density is nearly constant between species. Thus mass is proportional to L^3. Area, expressed in terms of mass, has dimensions $M^{2/3}$.

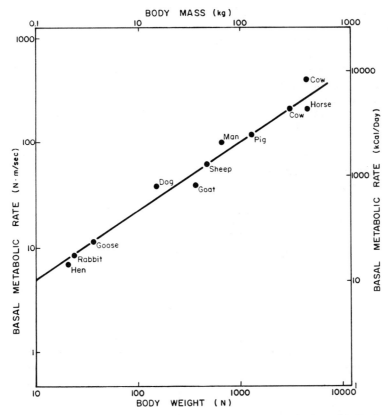

Figure 5.2.9 Logarithmic relation between metabolic rate and body mass. The slope of the line is about 2/3, indicating a relationship between BMR and body mass to the 2/3 power. (Data from Ganong, 1963, and Kleiber, 1975.)

TABLE 5.2.19 **Effect of Environmental Temperature on Resting Oxygen Consumption of Clothed Subjects**

Room Temperature, °C	Oxygen Consumption, m³/sec (mL/min)		Metabolic Rate, N·m/sec
0	5.50×10^{-6}	(330)	115
10	4.83×10^{-6}	(290)	101
20	4.00×10^{-6}	(240)	84
30	4.17×10^{-6}	(250)	87
40	4.25×10^{-6}	(255)	89
45	4.33×10^{-6}	(260)	91

Source: Adapted and used with permission from Grollman, 1930

When exercise-trained subjects were allowed to rest for three days, BMR decreased significantly. Thus comparison of experimental measurements of BMR between different studies should be made cautiously.

Food Ingestion. Recently ingested foods also increase the metabolic rate, and this is known as the specific dynamic action (SDA) of food. The SDA is apparently caused not by digestive action but by catabolism as the food is chemically changed and assimilated into the body.[22] Excess food nutrients, those which are lost to the feces, urine, and gas production, do not result in an SDA (Kleiber, 1975). However, of the catabolized portion, 30% of protein energy is transformed into SDA, 6% of carbohydrate is transformed into SDA, and 4% of fat is transformed into SDA (Ganong, 1963). This means that a portion of food containing 100 N·m (0.024 kcal) of protein, 100 N·m of carbohydrate, and 100 N·m of fat will result in an SDA of 40 N·m. This energy is higher in leaner individuals (Segal et al., 1985) and lower following regular exercise (LeBlanc et al., 1984a; Tremblay et al., 1988). The energy value of the food as it can be utilized by the body is reduced by the amount of the SDA. The SDA may be released over a time period of 6 hours or more.

Muscular Activity. Muscular inefficiency provides the largest component of heat generation. Efficiency is defined as

$$\eta = \frac{\text{external power produced}}{\text{total (heat) power expended}} \qquad (5.2.87\text{a})$$

or

$$\eta = \frac{\text{external work produced}}{\text{chemical energy consumed}} \qquad (5.2.87\text{b})$$

where efficiency defined in Equation 5.2.87a is the instantaneous efficiency, or the efficiency over a period of time characterized by a reasonably constant rate of work.[23] The efficiency defined in Equation 5.2.87b is the efficiency for a particular task. The fact that physical work (force times distance) or power (force times distance divided by time, or force times velocity) appears in the numerator and heat energy or power appears in the denominator recognizes the fact that an equivalence between heat energy and work is demonstrated by the first law of thermodynamics. Food energy, which is the source of muscular energy, is usually measured as heat in a calorimeter; it could just as well be measured as work in a Carnot engine.

The efficiency of muscular activity depends on the muscle used, the nature of the task, and the rate at which the task is performed. In general, the larger muscle groups, such as the gastrocnemius of the lower leg or the triceps extensor cubiti of the upper arm, have higher efficiencies than the smaller muscles such as the opponeus pollicis of the thumb or the levator palpebrae superioris of the eye. The larger muscles perform most external work and have efficiencies of 20–25% (about the same as a gasoline engine); the smaller muscles perform exacting control tasks and have efficiencies of 5% or less. More exacting tasks are usually accomplished with a high degree of antagonistic muscular activity, thus reducing the overall efficiency still further.[24]

Exercise physiologists sometimes define efficiency as (Kleiber, 1975)

$$\eta = \frac{\text{external work}}{\text{total metabolic work} - \text{BMR}} \qquad (5.2.88)$$

With this definition, walking 0.90–1.80 m/sec on a 5% grade, man's mechanical efficiency is

---

[22]LeBlanc et al. (1984) showed that meals identical with regard to composition and caloric content produced four times less heat when the food was placed directly into the stomach by means of a tube (gavage) compared with oral ingestion.
[23]Constant rate of work is the same as constant power.
[24]From the standpoint of thermoregulatory responses, skin temperature, core temperature, and sweating rate appear to be independent of the skeletal muscle mass employed and appear to be dependent only on the absolute metabolic intensity (Sawka et al., 1984b). Thus muscular efficiencies are sufficiently similar to evoke identical responses.

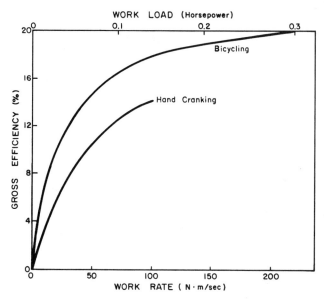

Figure 5.2.10 The gross efficiency for hand cranking or bicycling as a function of the external workload. (Adapted and used with permission from Goldman, 1978a.)

approximately 10%. On a 15–25% grade, it rises to about 20%. Best efficiencies of 20–22% occur with leg exercises that involve lifting body weight. In carpentry and foundry work, where both arms and legs are used, average mechanical efficiency is approximately 10% (ASHRAE, 1977). Gross muscular efficiency varies with the work load, as shown by Figure 5.2.10 (Goldman, 1978a). As the resting metabolic demands of respiration, circulation, central nervous system activity, and digestion become a smaller fraction of overall body oxygen demands, gross efficiency approaches a limiting value of close to 20% for bicycling.

Muscles generally are able to exert the greatest force when the velocity of muscle shortening is zero (isometric exercise).[25] Muscular power must still be expended to maintain this force. Since there can be no external power produced if the velocity is zero, muscular efficiency for isometric exercise is zero.

Exerted muscular force decreases curvilinearly as velocity of shortening increases (Figure 5.2.11).[26] Since power produced equals force times velocity, there is a maximum power condition which occurs at about one-third of maximum speed and one-fourth of maximum force (Milsum, 1966). The rate of energy use by the muscle also varies as rate of shortening increases. Maximum efficiency therefore occurs at a lower speed than maximum power: at about one-quarter of maximum speed and one-half of maximum force (Milsum, 1966). Isotonic exercise, moving a muscle at constant force, will have an efficiency that depends on the rate of shortening and the force applied.

The isometric length–tension relationship of a muscle (Figure 5.2.12) shows that the maximum force developed by a muscle is exerted at its resting length and decreases to zero at twice its resting length and also at its shortest possible length. Resting length is defined as the slightly stretched condition the muscle is in when attached by its tendons to the skeleton (Astrand

[25]Energy consumed as a muscle contracts isometrically is proportional to the area under the curve of muscle force with time (McMahon, 1984).
[26]Hill's analysis showed this curve to be a hyperbola of the form $(F + a)(v + b) = $ constant, where F is the force, v is velocity of shortening, and a and b are parameters. The parameter a is related to the heat liberated by the muscle (Mende and Cuervo, 1976).

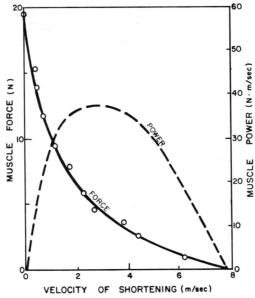

Figure 5.2.11 Force and power output of muscle as a function of velocity. (Adapted and used with permission from Milsum, 1966.)

and Rodahl, 1970). Thus efficiency of muscular contraction depends on the length of the muscle. Since length changes during constant contraction, efficiency is always changing. Figure 5.2.13 shows one aspect of this change in efficiency for stair climbing at different speeds (Morehouse and Miller, 1967).

It is common practice to take the efficiency of muscular exercise as 20%. This means that 80% of the muscular energy expended becomes heat to be removed by the body. Tables 5.2.20–5.2.22 give energy expenditures for various activities performed by men and women.

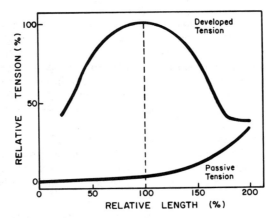

Figure 5.2.12 Length–tension diagram for skeletal muscle. The passive tension curve measures the tension (force/area) exerted by the unstimulated, or relaxed, muscle. The developed tension curve represents the tension developed in a maximally stimulated, isometrically contracting muscle. (Used with permission from Ganong, 1963.)

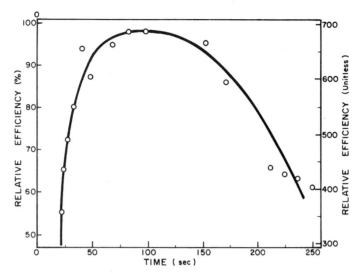

Figure 5.2.13 Mechanical efficiency of the body during stair climbing at different speeds. (Adapted and used with permission from Morehouse and Miller, 1967.)

Specific dynamic action of proteins appears to be unaffected by muscular activity (Kleiber, 1975) and should be added to muscular heat production. Fat and carbohydrate SDA, on the other hand, appears to be abolished by exercise and is not additive (Kleiber, 1975).

Exercise also has a lengthy effect on BMR. Immediately after the termination of nonaerobic exercise, there is an increased metabolic activity to make up the oxygen debt (see Section 1.3). This is immediate and relatively short-lived. Anaerobic work is less efficient than aerobic work, with efficiencies as low as 8% (Morehouse and Miller, 1967). A longer effect is also present. A 10% increase in a man's metabolic rate has been reported for as long as 48 hours after strenuous exercise, and a 25% increase above basal level has been reported 15 hours after work (Kleiber, 1975).

It is the skeletal muscles that produce the extra heat during exercise. Some organs, like the heart, become more active during physical activity. Some, like the brain, do not change. Others, like the kidney and gastrointestinal tract, decrease their activity (Webb, 1973). None of these produces significant heat when compared to skeletal muscle (Table 5.2.23).

Negative work is produced by a muscle when it maintains a force against an external force tending to stretch the muscle. An example of negative work is the action of the leg muscle during a descent on a flight of stairs. The potential energy of the body is decreasing, since the body's mass

TABLE 5.2.20   Classification of Work Intensity

Work	Mets	Oxygen Consumption, m³/sec	(L/min)	Metabolic Rate, N·m/sec	(kcal/min)
Very light work	1–2	$< 0.8 \times 10^{-5}$	(< 0.5)	< 175	(< 2.5)
Light work	2–3	0.8–1.7×10^{-5}	$(0.5$–$1.0)$	175–350	$(2.5$–$5.0)$
Moderate work	3–4	1.7–2.5×10^{-5}	$(1.0$–$1.5)$	$350 - 525]$	$(5.0$–$7.5)$
Heavy work	4–6	$2.5 - 3.3 \times 10^{-5}]$	$(1.5$–$2.0)$	525–700	$(7.5$–$10.0)$
Very heavy work	6–8	$3.3 - 4.2 \times 10^{-5}]$	$(2.0$–$2.5)$	700–875	$(10.0$–$12.5)$
Maximal work	> 8	$> 4.2 \times 10^{-5}$	(> 2.5)	> 875	(> 12.5)

Source: Adapted and used with permission from Morehouse and Miller, 1967.

TABLE 5.2.21 Ergonomic Relationships of Various Activities, Assumed Muscular efficiency = 20%

Task	Physical Work, N·m/sec	Energy Cost, N·m/sec (mets)	Oxygen Consumption, m³/sec (L/min)	Normal Respiratory Minute Volume, m³/sec (L/min)	Normal Heart Rate, beats/sec
Circulation & respiration (rest)	2	10 (0.1)	5.0×10^{-7} (0.03)		
Central nervous system	4	21 (0.2)	1.0×10^{-6} (0.06)		
Circulation & respiration	6	31 (0.3)	1.5×10^{-6} (0.09)		
Gut at rest	10	52 (0.5)	2.5×10^{-6} (0.15)		
Basal (sleep)	17	84 (0.8)	4.0×10^{-6} (0.24)	1.0×10^{-4} (6.0)	1.2
Sit at rest	21	105 (1.0)	5.0×10^{-6} (0.30)		
Very light work	37	183 (1.75)	8.8×10^{-6} (0.53)	1.7×10^{-4} (10)	<1.3
Walk 1.42 m/sec	52	262 (2.5)	1.2×10^{-5} (0.75)		
Light work	68	340 (3.25)	1.6×10^{-5} (0.98)	3.3×10^{-4} (20)	1.3–1.7
Moderate work	105	523 (5.0)	2.5×10^{-5} (1.50)	5.8×10^{-4} (35)	1.7–2.1
Heavy work for 1 hr (50% $\dot{V}_{O_2max}$)	141	707 (6.75)	3.3×10^{-5} (2.03)	8.3×10^{-4} (50)	2.1–2.5
Very Heavy Work	173	864 (8.25)	4.1×10^{-5} (2.48)	1.1×10^{-3} (65)	2.5–2.9
10 min $\dot{V}_{O_2max}$	209	1047 (10.00)	5.0×10^{-5} (3.00)	1.4×10^{-3} (85)	>2.9
Exhausting work	262	1308 (12.50)	6.2×10^{-5} (3.75)		
2-mile record (10 min–anaerobic)	360	1800 (17.2)	8.6×10^{-5} (5.16)		

Source: Adapted and used with permission from Goldman.

TABLE 5.2.22   Energy Expenditure for Various Activities[a]

Activity	Energy Expenditure, N·m/sec	(kcal/min)
Sleeping	49–98	(0.7–1.4)
Personal necessities		
Dressing and undressing	160–272	(2.3–3.9)
Washing, showering, brushing hair	174–195	(2.5–2.8)
Locomotion		
Walking on the level		
0.89 m/sec (2 mph)	133–265	(1.9–3.8)
1.34 m/sec (3 mph)	185–370	(2.8–5.3)
1.79 m/sec (4 mph)	223–488	(3.2–7.0)
Running on the level		
4.47 m/sec (10 mph)	1320–1400	(18.9–20.0)
Recreation		
Lying	91–112	(1.3–1.6)
Sitting	105–140	(1.5–2.0)
Standing	126–174	(1.8–2.5)
Playing with children	237–698	(3.4–10.0)
Driving a car	63–223	(0.9–3.2)
Canoeing 1.79 m/sec (4 mph)	209–488	(3.0–7.0)
Horseback riding (walk–gallop)	209–698	(3.0–10.0)
Cycling 5.81 m/sec (13 mph)	314–774	(4.5–11.1)
Dancing	328–886	(4.7–12.7)
Gardening	300–698	(4.3–10.0)
Gymnastics	174–453	(2.5–6.5)
Volleyball	244–698	(3.5–10.0)
Golf	342–356	(4.9–5.1)
Archery	356–363	(5.1–5.2)
Tennis	495–698	(7.1–10.0)
Football	614–621	(8.8–8.9)
Sculling (1.62 m/sec)	286–781	(4.1–11.2)
Swimming:		
Breast stroke	349–767	(5.0–11.0)
Back stroke	349–767	(5.0–11.0)
Crawl	802–977	(11.5–14.0)
Playing squash	705–1400	(10.1–20.0)
Cross-country running	747–747	(10.5–10.7)
Climbing	698–851	(10.6–12.2)
Skiing	698–1400	(10.0–20.0)
Domestic work		
Sewing, knitting	70–112	(1.0–1.6)
Sweeping floors	112–119	(1.6–1.7)
Cleaning shoes	105–195	(1.5–2.8)
Polishing	167–335	(2.4–4.8)
Scrubbing	202–488	(2.9–7.0)
Cleaning windows	209–251	(3.0–3.6)
Washing clothes	160–349	(2.3–5.0)
Making beds	265–370	(3.8–5.3)
Mopping	293–405	(4.2–5.8)
Ironing	286–293	(4.1–4.2)
Beating carpets and mats	342–544	(4.9–7.8)
Postman climbing stairs	684–963	(9.8–13.8)
Light industry		
Light engineering work (drafting, drilling, watch repair, etc.)	112–167	(1.6–2.4)

TABLE 5.2.22 (*Continued*)

Activity	Energy Expenditure, N·m/sec (kcal/min)	
Medium engineering work (tool room, sheet metal, plastic molding, machinist, etc.)	147–272	(2.1–3.9)
Heavy engineering work (machine idling, loading chemical into mixer, etc.)	251–412	(3.6–5.9)
Printing industry	147–174	(2.1–2.5)
Shoe repair and manufacturing	188–342	(2.7–4.9)
Tailoring		
Sewing	126–188	(1.8–2.7)
Pressing	244–300	(3.5–4.3)
Manual labor		
Shoveling	377–726	(5.4–10.4)
Pushing wheelbarrow	349–488	(5.0–7.0)

[a] Data used with permission from Astrand and Rodahl, 1970.

TABLE 5.2.23 Heat Production of Several Organs in Man

Organ	Heat Production, N·m/sec (kcal/min)		Organ Weight, N	Organ Mass, kg
Skin	11.6	(0.17)	39.23	4.0
Heart	10.5	(0.15)	3.14	0.32
Brain	17.4	(0.25)	13.53	1.38
Kidneys	10.5	(0.15)	2.94	0.30
Muscle				
Rest	16.7	(0.24)	275	28
Exercise	1095	(15.7)	275	28

Source: Adapted and used with permission from Webb, 1973; Berenson and Robertson, 1973.

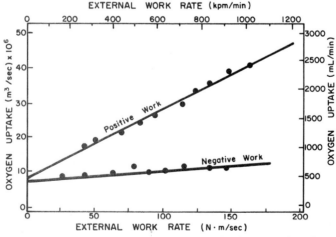

Figure 5.2.14 Oxygen uptake in positive (upper curve) and negative (lower curve) work consisting of riding a bicycle on a motor-driven treadmill, uphill in positive and downhill in negative work (with the movements of the pedals reversed). External work load is shown as positive for both uphill and downhill. The oxygen cost of positive work was nearly six times that for negative work. (Adapted and used with permission from Astrand and Rodahl, 1970.)

is being lowered. If left to itself, this mass would increase its kinetic energy as it accelerated due to gravity. To keep the body's velocity from increasing beyond safe levels, the descent is controlled by the leg muscles. These muscles are using physiological energy and producing negative amounts of mechanical work. It is usually difficult to calculate the actual mechanical efficiency of the muscles while producing negative work (Kleiber, 1975), but negative work generally decreases the overall efficiency of a maneuver (Alexander, 1980). For example, there is a time during walking when both feet are on the ground (see Section 2.4). The trailing foot exerts a force while it shortens and thus is producing positive work; the leading foot, however, exerts a force while it stretches and thus produces negative work. This is the principle of antagonistic muscular activity: the action of the leading foot is required for control of walking (actually, of falling), but the overall mechanical efficiency of walking suffers (Figure 5.2.14).

As shown in Figure 2.4.5, running muscles expend more energy than walking muscles. There is also a minimum energy expenditure for the walking–running composite curve for any given grade of the running surface. As the grade becomes more and more negative (more steeply downhill), this minimum energy expenditure decreases until, at a gradient of about -10%, no further decrease is seen. At slopes more negative than -10%, the energy of walking again increases (McMahon, 1984).

Muscular efficiencies for walking downhill approach -120% (McMahon, 1984). This means that the muscles absorb more energy when walking downhill than they expend during walking. It also means that the heat produced by these muscles is about 220% of their energy expenditure. From Figure 5.2.14, we see that energy expenditure of the muscle undergoing negative work is about one-sixth that of a muscle doing positive work, for the same absolute value of external work load. We might expect, then, a leg muscle going uphill to produce about twice as much heat as a leg muscle going downhill.

Heat production during exercise is thus produced largely by the skeletal muscles. If no better information on metabolic rate is available, then, as long as a significant change in body fat does not occur, the metabolic heat production during a day can be taken as the caloric intake of food during that day. If 145 N·m/sec (3000 kcal/day) of food is eaten, 145 N·m/sec is the average rate of heat production.

5.2.6   Rate of Change of Stored Heat

The last term of the general heat balance Equation (5.1.2) to be defined is the rate of change of heat storage. This term equals the sum of heat gained from the environment, heat lost to the environment, and rate of heat generation. Any imbalance in these quantities will reflect itself in a change of body temperature; during exercise this usually means an increase. This increase of temperature is the manifestation of a rate of change of stored heat, since

$$q_{\text{stored}} = mc\frac{d\theta}{dt} \qquad (5.2.89)$$

where q_{stored} = rate of change of heat storage, N·m/sec
   m = body mass, kg
   c = specific heat of the body, N·m/(kg·°C)
   $d\theta/dt$ = time rate of change of mean body temperature, °C/sec

Physiologists have historically assumed the mass of an average man to be 70 kg (a weight of 686 N). From Tables 5.2.24 and 5.2.25 it can be seen that 70 kg underestimates military personnel body mass but overestimates that for college students. Women's average body mass is about 85% that of comparable men.

The specific heat of the body is taken to be nearly the value for water, since the body is nearly 98% water. This value, which appears in Table 5.2.7, is 3470 N·m/(kg·°C).

The increase in body temperature does not occur as soon as there is a net positive imbalance

TABLE 5.2.24 Body Mass (kg) of Samples of U.S. Males

Group	Number	Percentile 1	5	Mean	95	99	Standard Deviation
Air force flyers (1950)	4,063	56.0	60.3	74.4	94.5	98.1	9.27
Army separatees	24,449	47.1	54.0	70.3	87.0	93.8	9.33
Army pilots	500	56.2	61.8	75.4	89.8	96.6	8.59
Navy pilots (1964)	1,549	58.7	63.7	77.7	92.3	100.2	8.66
FAA tower trainees (21–50 years old)	678	48.5	58.0	73.4	90.3	98.7	10.0
National health survey (18–79 years old)	3,091	50.9	57.3	76.3	98.6	109.5	—

Source: Used with permission fron Van Cott and Kinkade, 1972.

TABLE 5.2.25 Average Body Mass of Samples of U.S. Male Civilians

Group	Maas, kg	(lb)
Railroad travelers	73.0	(167)
Truck and bus drivers	74.4	(164)
Airline pilots	76.2	(168)
Industrial workers	74.4	(170)
College students	64.4	(142)
Eastern, 18 years old	68.0	(150)
Eastern, 19 years old	72.1	(159)
Midwest, 18 years old	67.1	(148)
Midwest, 18–22 years old	70.8	(156)
Draft registrants		
18–19 years old	64.0	(141)
20–24 years old	66.2	(146)
25–29 years old	68.6	(151)
30–34 years old	69.4	(153)
35–37 years old	69.9	(154)
Civilian men	75.3	(166)

Source: Adapted and used with permission from Van Cott and Kinkade, 1972.

in the left-hand side of Equation 5.1.2. Active control mechanisms to be discussed in Section 5.3 attempt to correct the imbalance by causing the body to lose more heat. There appears to be a lag time during which there is no discernible change in deep body temperature (Givoni and Goldman, 1972). The magnitude of this time lag becomes shorter as the metabolic rate becomes higher (see Section 5.5):

$$t_d = \frac{2.1 \times 10^5}{M} \tag{5.2.90}$$

where t_d = delay time, sec

M = metabolic rate, N·m/sec

After the delay time, body temperature still does not increase all at once but instead increases in an exponential manner. The time course of rectal temperature change is discussed in Section 5.5.

A different form of Equation 5.2.89 is used when a convective process is considered, as in heat transfer by the movement of blood or other bodily fluids. In this case, mass moves and (at least in the steady state) temperatures are considered to be static, unlike the condition represented by

Equation 5.2.89, where mass is static and temperatures increase or decrease. The rate of change of heat storage for convective processes is

$$q_{stored} = \dot{m}c\,(\theta_{in} - \theta_{out}) \qquad (5.2.91)$$

where $\dot{m}$ = mass rate of flow, kg/sec
$\quad$ c = specific heat of fluid, N·m/(kg·°C)
$\quad$ θ_{in} = temperature of fluid as it enters the surrounding tissue, °C
$\quad$ θ_{out} = temperature of fluid as it exits the surrounding tissue, °C

The tissue through which the fluid flows is usually assumed to be isothermal, and the convective process is usually assumed to be effective enough that the exiting temperature of the fluid equals the tissue temperature. Depending, then, on blood flow (see Table 5.4.5), a great deal of heat can be delivered to, or removed from, a volume of tissue. While some regions of the body, notably the liver and the brain, produce relatively vast quantities of heat and are thus prone to possess temperatures higher than surrounding tissues and organs, temperature differences are kept small due to the heat removal capacity of the blood flowing through these tissues.

5.3 THERMOREGULATION

Animals that maintain their central body temperatures within relatively narrow limits are termed homeothermic, as compared to poikilothermic animals, which control their body temperatures very imprecisely (Ganong, 1963; Milsum, 1966). Humans are homeotherms and must regulate body temperature within physiologically close limits: enzymatic activity becomes very low below 37°C,[27] and irreversible damage occurs to the central nervous system above 41°C (Milsum, 1966). Very precise thermoregulation occurs only within the thermoneutral zone (see Figure 5.1.3). Outside this zone, thermoregulatory mechanisms are no longer able to maintain body temperature at a constant level, and a rise or fall of deep body temperature occurs in response to the environment.

There are distinct and somewhat independent responses to heat and cold. In exercise it is clear that heat loss mechanisms predominate, but heat maintenance mechanisms can interfere with these and influence thermal response. For this reason, some explanation is given of both responses.

Thermoregulation involves many bodily functions. There appear to be several levels of thermoregulation, with the most precise control occurring with the hypothalamus intact, but with subordinate thermoregulatory structures able to initiate localized and less precise control should hypothalamic direction be lacking (Bahill, 1981; Johnson, 1967; Keller, 1963). Thermoregulation employs feedback of thermal information to the controller, and this thermal information is influenced by various bodily mechanisms intended to lose or maintain heat. We discuss the thermoregulatory structures of sensors, controllers, and activating mechanisms.

5.3.1 Thermoreceptors

Thermoreceptors are small, unencapsulated nerve endings distributed unevenly throughout the body (Hardy, 1961; Hensel, 1963).[28] Thermoreceptors appear to be of two types, warm receptors

---

[27]Because chemical reaction rates are in general higher at higher temperatures, warm-blooded animals are capable of sustained activity levels higher than cold-blooded animals. This has been of consequence in the survival of warm-blooded species because they are capable of seizing prey and escaping capture even at environmental temperatures low enough to immobilize cold-blooded animals (Johnson, 1969).

[28]Several concentrations of skin thermoreceptors are in the palms of the hands and feet, the lips, and the pelvic area. Other concentrations appear to be in the hypothalamus and in the esophagus. Thermoreceptors may also be present in the veins and muscles.

and cold receptors, with the difference being that warm receptors increase discharge frequency[29] with temperature increase in the thermoneutral range, whereas cold receptors decrease discharge frequency with temperature increase in the thermoneutral range (Johnson, 1969). Figure 5.3.1 illustrates the difference between cold and warm receptor outputs. It also shows the paradoxical discharge of cold fibers at high temperatures, which may be responsible for the cold sensation felt when in very hot water (Dodt and Zotterman, 1952b). Somatic cold receptors are much more numerous than warm receptors (Hensel, 1963; Zotterman, 1959) and usually produce an output frequency in the normal range of physiological interest, whereas warm receptors are fairly inactive (Hensel, 1963). Hence it is likely that cold receptors are of primary importance in

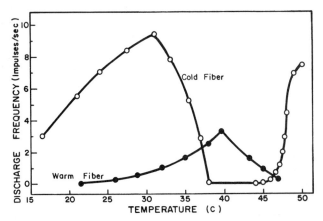

Figure 5.3.1 Graphs showing to the left the steady discharge of a typical single cold fiber (open circles), in the middle a typical single warm fiber (filled circles), and to the right the paradoxical cold fiber discharge (open circles) as a function of temperature. (Used with permission from Dodt and Zotterman, 1952a.)

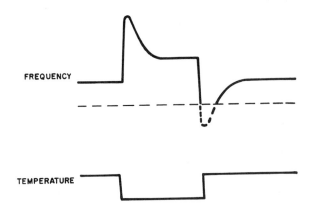

Figure 5.3.2 Cold receptor response. When temperature is lowered, receptor output frequency increases. There is an initial overshoot in frequency, which disappears after a short time. When temperature is increased, steady-state frequency of the cold receptor again decreases. The transient response is negative this time, even causing the receptor to remain silent for a period of time corresponding to the time the frequency would have been negative. Larger temperature steps cause larger transient and steady-state responses.

[29]Neurons appear to carry information encoded as a series of electrical–ionic pulses normally passed from the receptor end to the distal end of the cell. This series of pulses, referred to as the discharge frequency, can carry information related to the frequency of pulse production or related to the temporal pattern of pulse production (Cohen, 1964).

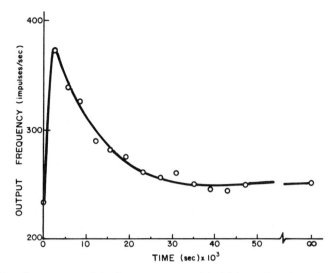

Figure 5.3.3 Transient response of the thermoreceptor model with immediate change in the depolarizing current and exponential change in the Q_{10} term. Simulated is a temperature step decrease of 5°C starting at 25°C. The time constant determining the Q_{10} variation is 10 msec. (Used with permission from Johnson and Scott, 1971.)

thermoregulation while warm receptors perhaps find their main function in conscious temperature sensation (Hardy, 1961; Hensel, 1963; Randall, 1963).

Many different stimuli applied in sufficient magnitudes will cause receptor responses, but the term "adequate stimulus" is applied to the type of stimulus to which the receptor is most sensitive (Patton, 1965). The adequate stimulus for thermoreceptors is temperature level, but strong mechanical stimuli can also cause thermoreceptor outputs (Johnson, 1969). Response thresholds and sensitivities vary depending on location and normal thermal environments. Receptors located in the tongue, for instance, have generally higher threshold temperatures than receptors located in the skin (Hensel et al., 1960; Hensel and Zotterman, 1951). Thermoreceptors appear, as well, to respond to the time rate of change of temperature (Johnson, 1969) and therefore can be termed proportional plus derivative responding (Figure 5.3.2).[30]

Very few models of thermoreceptor action appear in the literature, but the model by Johnson and Scott (1971) is based on the Hodgkin–Huxley equations for neural discharge.[31] Reasonably good agreement was found between model response and thermoreceptor action (Figure 5.3.3). As important as thermoreceptors are to temperature sensation and thermoregulation, they do not usually appear as entities in thermoregulatory models (Hwang and Konz, 1977).

5.3.2 Hypothalamus

At the base of the forebrain (Figure 5.3.4) is a small neural structure called the hypothalamus, which has been found to be the center of thermoregulatory control (Johnson, 1967). The anterior hypothalamus appears to be the site of heat loss control and the posterior hypothalamus the site of control of heat maintenance. The anterior hypothalamus contains temperature-sensitive

[30]Thermal sensations also appear to depend on the total skin area stimulated, known as "spatial summation" (Greenspan and Kenshalo, 1985).
[31]The Hodgkin–Huxley equations describe neural discharge by modeling cell membrane conductances for sodium and potassium. They were first derived to describe the action of the giant squid axon but have since been used as a basis for modeling myocardial activity, skeletal muscle action, and neural receptor mechanisms. For a good motivational background to the Hodgkin–Huxley equations, see Stevens (1966).

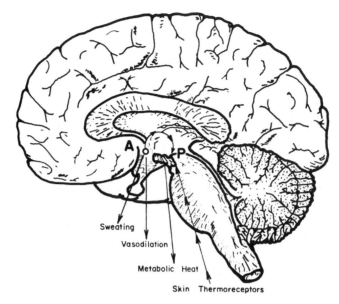

Figure 5.3.4 Thermoregulatory centers and pathways. The posterior hypothalamic "heat maintenance center" (*P*) is synaptic and indifferent to thermal stimulation. The anterior hypothalamic "heat loss center" (*A*) is extremely sensitive to thermal stimulation. Center *A* operates by activating sweat glands and vessels and by depressing the response of metabolizing tissue to cold stimulation of the skin. (Used with permission from Benzinger et al., 1963.)

neurons (Hardy et al., 1962; Nakayama and Eisenman, 1961) but the posterior hypothalamus does not (Benzinger et al., 1963). The anterior hypothalamus has been postulated (Benzinger et al., 1963) as being the terminal sensory organ for warm responses, and it transmits impulses to the sweat glands and vasodilation effectors. The posterior hypothalamus performs not as a terminal sensory organ, but as a relay of impulses from cold skin to the metabolic heat production centers. A connection between these two centers forms a pathway for the warmth receptors in the anterior hypothalamus to inhibit responses to cold from the posterior hypothalamus.

Because Benzinger and colleagues obtained their data from humans on whom hypothalamic temperatures were inaccessible, they measured tympanic membrane temperature (measured in the inner ear at the eardrum) and assumed this to be equivalent to hypothalamic temperature (Benzinger and Taylor, 1963). They discovered that hypothalamic temperature (tympanic temperature) was much more closely related to heat loss and production than was rectal (or deep body) temperature. Drastic changes of metabolic rate elicited by stimuli from the skin due to sudden changes of environmental temperature were transitory, not continuous. Sudden cooling of the body caused the rate of heat production to first rise and then decline to a new, higher level commensurate with the new, lower level of skin temperature. When the skin was suddenly warmed in a water bath, oxygen consumption exhibited a transient depression and then settled at a new, lower, steady rate commensurate with the new, higher level of steady skin temperature. Benzinger et al. (1963) noted the similarity between this type of response and the transient thermoreceptor response seen in Figure 5.3.2 and concluded that skin thermoreceptor outputs, mediated by the posterior hypothalamic heat maintenance center, were the cause of this behavior.

Steady-state responses of humans provide much more evidence for the hypothalamic control centers influenced by cutaneous thermoreceptors. When the skin was cold, and the central (hypothalamic) temperature was below a "set point," heat production increased in an amount related to the difference between the set point and the central temperature level (Figure 5.3.5). A family of curves was obtained, with skin temperature as the third variable. Higher skin temperatures induced lower metabolic rates. No matter what the skin temperature, if the central temperature was above the set point, sweating rates and vasodilation increased rapidly with increased cranial temperature and independently of skin temperature insofar as skin temperature exceeded 33°C. When skin temperature fell below 33°C and central temperature remained above the set point, sweating was inhibited, even to the point of disappearance (Figure 5.3.6). These results indicate that heat loss and heat production can be determined if only the two temperatures, skin and cranial, are known.

This simplified model of the thermoregulatory controller is not universally accepted, however. Most criticism centers about the assumption that hypothalamic temperature can be replaced by tympanic membrane temperature (Randall, 1963). Others note local thermoregulatory responses obtained without hypothalamic intervention (Blair and Keller, 1946; Randall, 1963) or of a smaller magnitude than would be expected from skin and hypothalamic temperatures alone (Hardy, 1961). The first criticism can be settled by experimental measurements, and the second by admitting that there are subordinate thermoregulatory mechanisms involving only local feedback loops which are capable of local thermoregulation of a less precise nature than hypothalamic control (Figure 5.3.7). Perhaps more serious is the fact that hypothalamic temperature has been found to vary greatly within short periods of time. Fusco (1963) found experimentally that when a dog resting in a

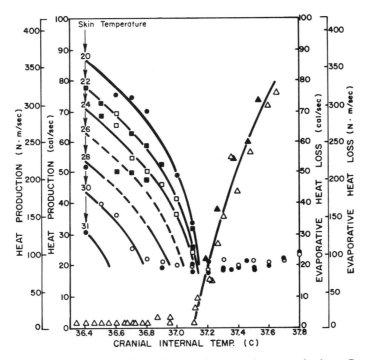

Figure 5.3.5 Experimental determination of human thermoregulatory mechanisms. Cranial internal (presumably hypothalamic) temperature and skin temperature together determine body heat production or loss. At cranial temperatures less than 37.1°C, heat production increases as cranial temperature or skin temperature decreases. Cranial temperatures higher than 37.1°C elicit low, constant heat production rates and evaporative heat loss increases. (Adapted and used with permission from Benzinger et al., 1963.)

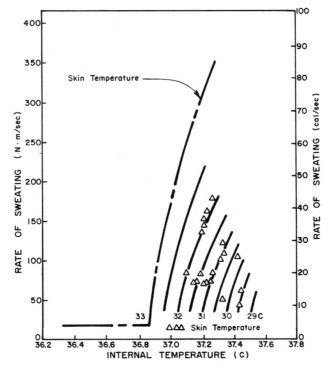

Figure 5.3.6 Intensity of thermoregulatory sweating during cold reception at the skin. At any given cranial internal temperature, sweating rates are seen to be diminished by approximately 170 N·m/sec to every 1°C decrease in level of skin temperature. (Adapted and used with permission from Benzinger et al., 1963.)

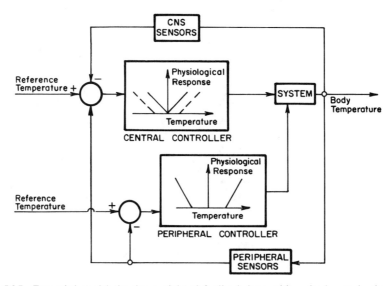

Figure 5.3.7 Expanded model showing peripheral feedback loop with a dead zone in the peripheral controller. This loop would be used only if the CNS controller was damaged or if the pathway back to the CNS was never established. The central controller normally operates without a dead zone (solid lines). Disease or lesions can cause it to operate with a dead zone (dashed lines). (Used with permission from Bahill, 1981.)

thermoneutral environment raised its head, hypothalamic temperature immediately rose.[32] Lowering its head caused hypothalamic temperature to fall. Changes in blood flow were cited to be the cause (Hammel et al., 1963). Pettibone and Scott (1974) showed blood flow to be a major determinant of hypothalamic temperature in poultry, but blood cooling in the neck and heat generation were also found to be important (Morrison et al., 1982). Hypothalamic temperature was also found to be highly variable by Johnson (1967) and to be related to oviposition by Scott et al. (1970) and Hirata et al. (1986). Hammel et al. (1963) note that an animal in a normal thermal environment would exhibit very different responses for the same hypothalamic temperature when exposed to different temperatures or would exhibit the same response at widely different hypothalamic temperatures at different times, depending on whether it was asleep or awake. This brings us to a central issue on thermoregulation: just what is the controlled variable? Is it hypothalamic temperature, deep body temperature, some spatially integrated temperature distribution (Werner, 1986), amount of heat exchanged, or some other, more complex quantity? Different responses to this question form the bases for the thermoregulatory models discussed in Section 5.4

5.3.3 Heat Loss Mechanisms

Heat loss mechanisms are classified in Section 5.1 as active or passive, and passive heat loss was treated completely in Section 5.2. Hypothalamic control facilitates these mechanisms by varying skin temperature and skin wetness, and also by reducing heat production.

Vasodilation. Skin temperature can be controlled by cutaneous vasodilation: arterioles are known to increase their calibers by neural and chemical mechanisms (Ganong, 1963). When the arterioles dilate, warm blood flows in relatively large amounts through vessels close to the skin, thus raising skin temperature. As a consequence, convective and radiative heat loss is facilitated. Vasodilation of the hand begins at an environmental temperature of 22°C, but a general increase in skin heat conductance does not usually occur until an environmental temperature of 28°C has been reached (Robinson, 1963) and may be delayed by nonthermal factors such as motivation and emotion (Brück, 1986; Wenger, 1986).

Hypothalamic control of vasodilation appears to occur directly through efferent nervous pathways and indirectly through circulating hormonal substances which it causes to be released (Ganong, 1963). Local skin effects can sometimes be strong enough to overcome central control.

Innervation of cerebral vessels is scanty and is not of functional importance (Ganong, 1963). This means that temperature of the head is very nearly always high and the head loses a great deal of heat. Heat loss from the head has been estimated as 50% of total body heat loss in the cold, which makes head coverings very effective for maintenance of body heat.

Similarly, head cooling has been suggested as a means to reestablish thermal comfort of humans in hot environments (Brown and Williams, 1982; Nunneley et al., 1982), and many attempts have been made to design cooling helmets. Indeed, any means by which heat can be added to or removed from the head area has almost immediate effects on thermal responses.[33] The magnitude of head cooling that can be accomplished in hyperthermia is limited, however, to about 100 N·m/sec, which limits its use to providing comfort for resting individuals; head cooling cannot be used to significantly reduce the heat burden of heavy exercise in the heat (Nunneley, 1988). Morrison et al. (1982) applied heat to inspired air and found that hyperthermic individuals

---

[32]Although the central nervous system (CNS) weighs only about 2% of total body weight, it accounts for about 20% of total oxygen consumption. The metabolism of the brain is therefore very high. Blood flow through the hypothalamus thus cools rather than heats. When blood flow to the hypothalamus is occluded, hypothalamic temperature rises. Vascularity of the anterior hypothalamus is markedly greater than that of the posterior hypothalamus, and it would be expected to be more sensitive to cooling by the blood (Randall, 1963).

[33]We have shown that a shivering bird can be caused to stop shivering almost immediately by shining a heat lamp on its head. Shining the heat lamp on its body had no noticeable effect on its shivering.

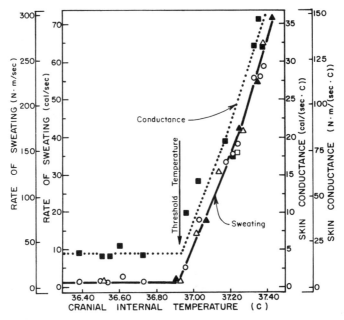

Figure 5.3.8 Combined plot of sweat rates and conductances against cranial internal temperatures from a large number of experiments on one subject. The data show how the thresholds for the onset of sweating (triangles and circles) and vasodilation (squares) coincide at a cranial temperature of 36.9°C. (Adapted and used with permission from Benzinger et al., 1963.)

showed rapid reduction of metabolic heat generation because central heating was accomplished faster in this way than it would have been by heating the entire body.

In Figure 5.3.8 is shown the rate of sweating as well as vasodilation as obtained by Benzinger et al. (1963). Vasodilation is expressed in terms of skin conductance in N·m/(sec·°C) or cal/(sec·°C) and is related to the previous discussion on conduction by being equal to the inverse of thermal resistance defined in Equation 5.2.14.[34] For the subject whose data appears in Figure 5.3.8, there is an apparent increase of skin conductance of 251 N·m/(sec·°C) for each degree Celsius rise in cranial temperature beyond the apparent set point of 36.9°C. This conductance change is due to an increase of 25 cm³/sec blood flow[35] through the skin (for each 1°C rise in cranial temperature) and can drastically increase heat lost to a thermoneutral environment. As an illustration of this point, the thermal resistance diagram of Figure 5.3.9 is considered. Heat flows from the core to the skin surface by conduction and convection, and from the skin surface to the environment by convection and radiation (which may also be included within Benzinger's conductance values). Thermal resistance of surface tissue for this subject is

$$R_{th, sk} = [18.8 + 251 (\theta_r - 36.9)]^{-1} \qquad (5.3.1)$$

where $R_{th, sk}$ = thermal resistance of the skin, °C·sec/(N·m)
θ_r = deep body temperature, °C

[34]There is an unfortunate conflict of definitions here that cannot be easily resolved. The definition of conductance as used in Equation 5.2.16 is the standard definition used by heat transfer engineers. That is, conductance equals thermal conductivity divided by thickness and has units of N·m/(m²·sec·°C). The way the term is used by some physiologists, however, includes skin area as well. Units of N·m/(sec·°C) are associated with this definition. There is no alternative word to use for either of these definitions.

[35]Estimates of overall blood flow to the skin vary from 2.7 cm³/sec per square meter of skin area (160 mL/m²/min) in a nude man resting in the somewhat cool temperature of 28°C to 43 cm³/(sec·m²) (2.6 L/m²/min) in men working in an extremely hot environment (Robinson, 1963).

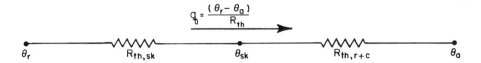

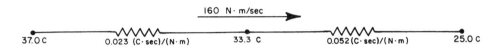

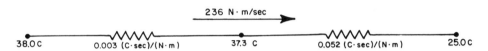

Figure 5.3.9 Decrease in skin thermal resistance and increase of heat flow from the subject whose data appear in Figure 5.3.8, assuming deep body temperature (θ_r) equals cranial (hypothalamic) temperature and that skin conductance is uniform over the body. General case (*top*), internal temperature below threshold (*middle*), internal temperature above threshold (*bottom*).

Assuming a thermoneutral ambient temperature of 25°C (Figure 5.1.3), an average radiation coefficient h_r of 4.7 N/(m·sec·°C) (Section 5.2.3), an average convection coefficient h_c of 6.0 N/(m·sec·°C) (Table 5.2.5), and a surface area of 1.8 m² (Equation 5.2.5), the thermal resistance of radiation and convection acting in parallel is, by Equations 5.2.2 and 5.2.34,

$$R_{\text{th},r+c} = \frac{1}{(h_r + h_c)A} = 0.052°\text{C·sec}/(\text{N·m}) \tag{5.3.2}$$

Skin temperature can be found by realizing that all the heat that flows through the skin through $R_{\text{th,sk}}$ also flows to the environment through $R_{\text{th},r+c}$. Thus

$$\theta_{\text{sk}} = \theta_a + (\theta_r - \theta_a)\left(\frac{R_{\text{th},r+c}}{R_{\text{th},r+c} + R_{\text{th,sk}}}\right) \tag{5.3.3}$$

and total heat flow is

$$q = \frac{\theta_r - \theta_a}{R_{\text{th,sk}} + R_{\text{th},r+c}} \tag{5.3.4}$$

Results are summarized in Figure 5.3.9.

For any given total body heat load, a significantly greater skin conductance was observed by Robinson (1963) during work than at rest. This stimulating effect of neuromuscular work has been likened to the reflex manner of respiratory stimulation during work (see Section 4.3.4). Benzinger et al. (1963), however, reported a decrease in skin conductance during work which they attributed to effects of local skin cooling.

The initial reaction to heat stress is diversion of blood from the splanchnic bed, kidneys, fat, and muscle to the skin to promote heat loss. There will also be an increase in cardiac output (see

Section 3.2.3). When the thermal challenge cannot be met, however, heat stroke ensues. The onset of heat stroke may involve a decrease in central venous pressure and consequent reduction of cardiac output. To compensate, constriction of both arterioles and veins of the skin occurs. The resultant reduced body heat loss and subsequent rise in deep body temperature causes death due to central nervous system damage or the fatal lodging of emboli (blood clots) following intravascular blood coagulation (Hales, 1986). Reduced blood volume due to dehydration while exercising may exacerbate the effect of central venous pressure on cardiac output (Kirsch et al., 1986).

Sweating. Sweating appears to be controlled by local events more than does cutaneous vasodilation (Figure 5.3.6). Very cool skin temperatures can extinguish sweating response despite very high hypothalamic temperatures. Because of this, it is frequently seen that deep body temperature increases rapidly after sudden cessation of exercise (see Section 5.5.2). Apparently the skin cools rapidly because of evaporation of accumulated sweat, causing local vasoconstriction and a sudden decrease of sweating.

Different areas of the body appear to have different preferred temperatures (Table 5.2.14) and therefore begin sweating at different times. As more sweating is required, the surface area engaged in sweating increases up to the maximum, and the rate of sweating in any area also increases (Randall, 1963). The progression of area recruitment is generally from the extremities toward the central regions of the body and headward (Tables 5.3.1 and 5.3.2), thus giving evidence of some

TABLE 5.3.1 **Recruitment of Sweating**

	Usual Order of Recruitment
Dorsum foot	1
Lateral calf	2
Medial calf	3
Laterial thigh	4
Medial thigh	5
Abdomen	6
Dorsum hand	7 or 8
Chest	3 or 7
Ulnar forearm	9
Radial forearm	10
Medial arm	11
Laterial arm	12

Source: Used with permission from Berenson and Robertson, 1973.

TABLE 5.3.2 **Regional Fractions of Total Cutaneous Evaporation, Percentage of Total**

Region	Air Temperature, °C							
	24	26	28	30	32	34	36	37
Head	11.8	12.1	11.9	9.7	8.0	7.0	8.5	8.4
Arm	4.6	4.4	4.2	3.4	2.6	2.2	3.1	3.3
Forearm	8.2	7.2	6.0	4.3	3.2	3.1	4.4	4.3
Trunk	22.8	23.0	22.2	22.2	30.0	33.0	43.0	38.2
Thigh	13.6	13.1	17.1	20.2	22.6	23.8	25.5	22.3
Calf	8.5	9.0	11.9	16.0	20.3	22.8	24.1	19.8
Palm	15.6	15.3	13.1	9.6	6.8	4.6	3.5	2.5
Sole	14.7	15.1	13.5	9.9	6.4	3.7	2.3	1.5

Source: Used with permission from Berenson and Robertson, 1973.

TABLE 5.3.3   Evaluation of the Human Thermostat Set Point from Sweating and Vasodilation

Subject[a]	Sweating Set Point, °C	Vasodilation Set Point, °C	Difference, °C
DS	36.48	36.40	+0.08
JG	—	36.45	—
VG	36.52	36.60	−0.08
MC	36.60	—	—
WD	36.76	36.70	+0.06
MS	36.77	36.80	−0.03
GC	36.80	36.93	−0.13
AS	36.85	36.80	+0.05
Average	36.69	36.67	+0.02

Source: Used with permission from Benzinger et al., 1963.

[a]From these initials, it appears that the subjects may have included the original seven astronauts: Deke Slayton, John Glenn, Virgil (Gus) Grissom, Malcolm (Scott) Carpenter, (W.D. is unknown), Walter (Wally) Marty Schirra Jr., Gordon Cooper, and Alan Sheppard.

local control. Sweating is not a continuous but a cyclic process, marked by alternating periods of high and low sweating activity (Randall, 1963). With full sweating, the trunk and lower limbs provide 70–80% of the total moisture perspired (Berenson and Robertson, 1973).

At maximum sweat cooling capacities of about 1200 N·m/sec (1030 kcal/hr), the sweating mechanism fatigues in 3–4 h, or sooner if adequate water and electrolyte replenishment is not practiced. Sweat rates lower than the maximum, or a high degree of heat acclimatization, will tend to lengthen the time until sweating becomes fatigued.

Benzinger et al. (1963) present evidence that the central (hypothalamic) temperature set point for sweating is the same for vasodilation (Table 5.3.3). Although there is no particular reason why these two mechanisms must have the same set-point temperature, the set-point differences presented by Benzinger et al. (1963) are very small considering the questions that have been raised concerning the equivalence between cranial temperature and hypothalamic temperature.

Grucza et al. (1985) investigated sexual differences in delay of onset and time constant of sweating and their relation to thermoregulation in dry, hot environments. They found no significant differences in time constant between men and women (about 8 min), but a longer delay in onset of sweating was found in women (18.1 vs. 7.8 min). There appeared to be no differences in body temperature responses to the hot environment, so they concluded that whereas both sexes tolerate dry heat exposure equally well, sweating seems to be a more important mechanism for heat loss in men than it is in women. Frye and Kamon (1983) showed that in hot, humid environments, women had higher sweating efficiencies (lower sweating rates compared to required heat removal) but men had higher sweating reserves (higher possible sweating rates).

5.3.4   Heat Maintenance and Generation

In response to cold environments, several effector mechanisms are available to the hypothalamic controller to maintain body warmth. These include vascular, muscular, and hormonal responses.

Vascular Responses. Vasoconstriction occurs in response to cold environments in order to reduce the difference between skin and ambient temperatures. Vasoconstriction is not necessarily the absence of vasodilation; Robinson (1963) states that blood flow to hands and feet is normally maximized by muscle fibers, which must receive constant nervous impulses to produce vasoconstriction. Cutaneous blood flow to the forearms and legs requires increased neural input in order to vasodilate.

What this vasoconstriction accomplishes is a shunting of returning blood from surface veins to veins deep within tissue. Deep veins in limbs normally are located close to arteries (Figure 5.3.10), allowing a large measure of countercurrent heat exchange to take place (Jiji et al., 1984; Weinbaum and Jiji, 1985; Weinbaum et al., 1984). That is, returning venous blood is always colder than entering arterial blood. The close proximity of arteries and venae comitantes allows a strong flow of heat from artery to vein all along the parallel vessels (Figure 5.3.11). Therefore, blood which eventually reaches the limb is precooled and peripheral heat loss is reduced; returning venous blood is heated almost to body temperature and does not significantly cool the

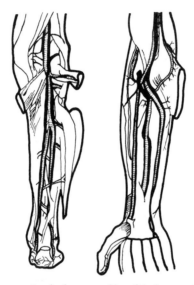

Figure 5.3.10   The heat exchange system in the arm and leg of the human. Arteries (dark) and veins (shaded) are parallel and in intimate contact. (Used with permission from Carlson, 1963.)

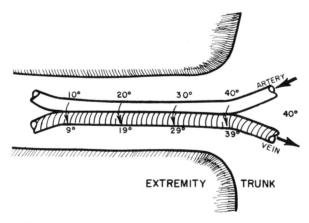

Figure 5.3.11   Schematic presentation of arteriovenous countercurrent heat exchange in an extremity resulting in a steep linear temperature gradient and a consequent reduced peripheral heat loss. (Used with permission from Carlson, 1963.)

main body mass. This mechanism has been highly exploited by vascular structures called "retes," which efficiently transfer large amounts of heat in arctic animals (Carlson, 1963). The effect of vasoconstriction is to increase effective thermal resistance of the tissues, especially of the skin. Haymes et al. (1982) reported on a study of exercise at $-20°C$ in regulation cross-country ski uniforms.[36] Addition of vests to the ski uniforms resulted in a significant rise in skin temperature in the area of the vest and also a significant decrease (about 33%) in tissue resistance. These results would indicate that vasoconstriction, reacting to local warming of the skin, becomes relaxed and allows more heat to pass from the interior of the body.

When local vasoconstriction occurs, subcutaneous fat becomes the cheif insulative layer. A linear relationship has been found between tissue insulation and percentage of body fat (Haymes et al., 1982). However, the insulative shell for the body includes more than just subcutaneous fat. Chilled muscles may also contribute to body insulation.

Shivering. Shivering has been already considered somewhat in Section 5.1, where it was mentioned that shivering in a naked human can interrupt the insulating dead air layer surrounding the skin and thus result in larger amounts of heat loss. Shivering, however, can increase metabolic rate (as measured by total oxygen consumption) by approximately three times (Hemingway and Stuart, 1963).

Shivering is absent in muscles below spinal cord transection, and a major neural pathway from the brain is therefore necessary for shivering to occur. Integrity of the posterior hypothalamus has experimentally been found necessary for shievering to occur (Hemingway and Stuart, 1963).

Nonshivering Thermogenesis. There is a component of cold-induced heat production which is hormonally controlled—nonshivering thermogenesis (Janský, 1971). The two hormones most closely associated with this general increase in BMR are catecholamines (adrenaline, or epinephrine, and noradrenaline, or norepinephrine) produced by the sympathetic nervous system and adrenal glands, and thyroxin, produced by the thyroid gland (Hart, 1963). Among other effects of catecholamines, heat production is very important in cold environments. Catecholamines can be released very shortly after cold challenge. Thyroxin requires somewhat longer time, but it is more important in the long run (Figure 5.3.12). Both of these require the integrity of the hypothalamus (Hart, 1963).

Two thyroid derivatives have been found to be calorigenically potent. Triiodothyronine has been found to be eight times as potent as thyroxin (Figure 5.3.12) in raising the BMR (Ganong, 1963).

The SDA effect does not appear to reduce nonshivering thermogenesis but instead adds to the body's heat production (Hart, 1963). Muscular exercise, like the SDA, also seems to have no direct effect on nonshivering thermogenesis.

To sustain this increased metabolic rate requires a large intake of food. Appetite and hunger, also under hypothalamic control, usually increase in coordinated fashion with metabolic responses to cold (Ganong, 1963).

Age and sex are two factors influencing cold response in humans (Stevens et al., 1987). Wagner and Horvath (1985) found that exposure to cold temperatures resulted in a body temperature maintenance for young men; young women exhibited a maintenance of body temperature at 20°C and a body temperature decline at lower environmental temperatures; older women showed maintenance of body temperature at all environmental temperatures; steady declines in body temperatures were seen for older men. Body fat percentages were found to be important

---

[36]Among their interesting results was that an exercise intensity of at least 1050 N·m/sec (10 mets) had to be attained before the body could maintain thermal equilibrium with the environment in a 4.1 m/sec wind. During the downhill portion of a cross-country ski run, velocities exceed 4.1 m/sec with little muscular activity. Core temperatures have been observed to drop during the downhill portion of the course.

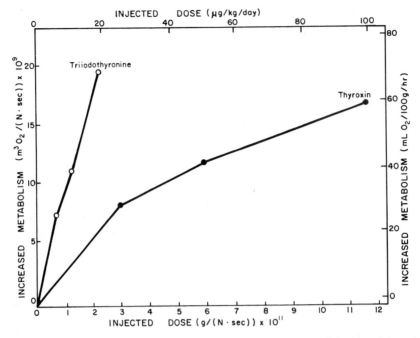

Figure 5.3.12   Calorigenic responses of thyroidectomized rat to subcutaneous injections of thyroxin and 3,5,3-triiodothyronine. Response to the triiodothyronine is much greater. (Adapted and used with permission from Barker, 1962.)

indicators of these results, and the distribution of body fat was also very important (fat beneath the skin acted as an insulating layer).

5.3.5   Acclimatization

Cold acclimatization is generally a coordinated increase in nonshivering thermogenesis and food intake (Hart, 1963). Peripheral vascular readjustments (vasodilation) lead to higher temperatures in limbs and appendages. In general, peripheral vasodilation results in higher amounts of heat lost to the environment by acclimatized individuals. Figure 5.3.13 shows the rapid increase in adrenal cortex activity—releasing norepinephrine—followed by a gradual decline as the exposure to cold continues. Thyroid activity requires a longer time to mobilize but is maintained indefinitely in the cold. Heat production shifts from shivering to nonshivering thermogenesis.

Acclimatization to heat also is acquired as time of exposure to a stressful environment increases; it begins with the first exposure and is well developed in four to seven days (Bass, 1963; Libert et al., 1988). Acclimatization is facilitated by activity in the heat, and it occurs more rapidly to subjects in good physical condition (Bass, 1963). Acclimatization is accompanied by an increase in blood volume (presumably to satisfy competing demands on the blood for heat loss and oxygen transport) of up to 25%, an increased tendency toward earlier vasodilation during exercise, salt conservation, and an increase in sweat production capacity (Bass, 1963; Robinson, 1963). Heat-acclimatized individuals also appear to reduce metabolic heat generation elicited by muscular exercise (Sawka et al., 1983). As acclimatization progresses, increased sweating appears to assume the main heat loss function, and vasodilation and blood volume return to normal (Robinson, 1963). Colin and Houdas (1965) concluded that for nonadapted subjects the mechanism of sweating is activated by centrally located receptors, but that in adapted subjects

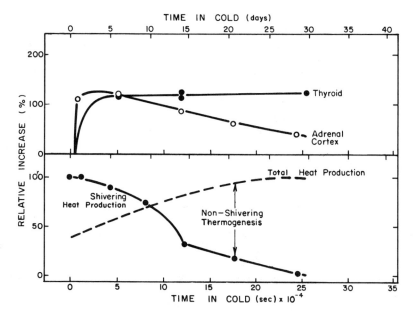

Figure 5.3.13 Summary of endocrinological changes during acclimatization for rats exposed to cold. (Adapted and used with permission from Hart, 1963.)

skin receptors are able to activate sweating before central receptors feed their impulses to the heat loss center. Libert et al. (1988) reported that sweat rates increased for successive exposures of subjects undergoing heat stress, but that sweat rates began declining after three days. No changes in body temperature were noted, but there was an apparent decrease in circulatory strain. Pandolf et al. (1988) reported that age and sex differences in thermoregulatory responses to heat disappeared when body weight, surface area, percentage of body fat, and maximal aerobic capacity were no different between groups. Therefore, regular exercise was found to lessen the effects of thermal stress; young and old men were found to acclimate to the heat in the same way.

Contrary to belief, cold acclimatization does not affect heat acclimatization per se, and heat acclimatization is unable to affect cold acclimatization. Both acclimatizations can coexist in an individual; loss of one or the other results from the absence of an adequate stimulus (Davis, 1963).

5.3.6 Circadian Rhythm

A repeating pattern of temperatures and thermoregulatory responses related to the timing of external events is referred to as a circadian, or biologic, rhythm. The most completely studied of these is the diurnal variation of body temperature. Resting minimum deep body temperature normally occurs during the early morning hours, just before arousal begins (Sawka et al., 1984a; Scott et al., 1970). Resting maximum deep body temperature usually occurs during early evening hours (Sawka et al., 1984a). Deep body temperature differences are accompanied by changes in hypothalamic temperature (Scott et al., 1970); therefore, there are also diurnal variations in the thermoregulatory responses. Peripheral blood flow and sweating rate change diurnally (Sawka et al., 1984a).

Sleep deprivation interferes with normal diurnal thermoregulatory patterns. As sleep deprivation progresses, changes in deep body temperature become less pronounced. Panferova (1964) reported that people with relaxed muscles who were placed in special chairs and water baths for several days began to lose the characteristic body temperature cycle beginning with the second day. Almost a complete loss in the cyclic pattern was seen in some subjects.[37] Activity appears to be a prime stimulant for diurnal rhythms.

Strogatz (1987) reports that subjects who live in isolation chambers without time clues often establish 24–25 hour activity cycles during which their wake–sleep cycles (controlled by the central nervous system) and body temperature cycles (controlled by the neuroendocrine system) are synchronized. Spontaneous desynchronization also occurs, during which time the body temperature cycle remains as before, but the wake–sleep cycle lengthens to 30–50 hours. Entrainment of the two cycles is eventually restored. Strogatz modeled these rhythms as two coupled oscillators that sometimes become unlinked. The application of this model to the disruption caused by jet lag or rotating-shift work schedules has yet to be made.

5.3.7   Exercise and Thermoregulation

The demands of exercise clearly strain thermoregulatory capacity, and thermoregulatory responses interfere with exercise performance. Aside from the obvious increase in heat production as a result of muscular inefficiency (see Section 5.2.5), there are other interferences between exercise performance and thermoregulation. Most importantly, cutaneous vasodilation shunts blood from the muscles to the skin to facilitate heat loss (Roberts and Wenger, 1979). Not only do the muscles then lose a large part of their oxygen supply, but pooling of the blood in the vascular bed makes that much less blood available to support muscular activity. Acclimatization helps to restore the required balance between muscular capacity and thermal normalcy.

There is evidence that exercise lowers the thermoregulatory set point for sweating (Tam et al., 1978), because exercise sweating has been observed to begin at lower mean skin temperatures than does sweating at rest. Exercise also appears to interfere with shivering through some central mechanism (Hong and Nadel, 1979). Nonexercising muscles appear to be inhibited from shivering when other muscle groups are used to perform exercise.

Shivering clearly interferes with muscular work, since the same muscles cannot be used for both. Since shivering muscles are 100% efficient for heat production, but working muscles are only 80–85% efficient for heat production, it can sometimes be difficult to control the muscles to perform external physical work. Muscular heat production can actually decrease in work performance compared to shivering.

Hormonal changes can have subtle effects on exercise performance. Increased levels of catecholamines and thyroxin in the cold, or adrenocorticotropic hormone (ACTH) and adrenal cortical steroids in the heat (Bass, 1963), will likely have effects, sometimes facilitating and sometimes debilitating, on exercise capacity. Injected atropine reduces sweating during exercise, and this effect can be partially overcome by heat acclimatization.

Nicotine is a mild vasoconstrictive agent (Saumet et al., 1986), whereas carbon dioxide and lactic acid produced during exercise are vasodilators (Ganong, 1963), which can lead to increased heat loss. These substances usually improve blood flow through the muscles, but their action may also interfere with proper thermoregulatory adjustments.

Sleep deprivation appears to interfere with thermoregulatory responses during exercise. Sawka et al. (1984a) report that 33 hours of wakefulness followed by moderate intensity cycle ergometer exercise in a temperate environment resulted in a decrease in evaporative (sweating) and dry heat loss (vasodilation) compared to the well-rested condition. The result was an increased rate of rise of deep body temperature in the sleep-deprived state.

Usually, thermoregulatory responses do not significantly interfere with physical work capacity. This is more true of acclimated individuals, who also tend to be in better physical condition.

---

[37]Also affected were normal diurnal cycles in pulse rate, blood pressure, and respiration.

5.4 THERMOREGULATORY MODELS

Models to describe human response to environmental thermal challenges have been proposed by many authors.[38] Good reviews of these appear in articles by Hwang and Konz (1977) and Werner (1986). Some of these have been implemented on analog computers (Brown, 1966; Cornew et al., 1967; Crosbie et al., 1963; Wyndham and Atkins, 1968), others on the digital computer (Gagge, 1973; Stolwijk, 1970). Most are constantly undergoing changes (Charny et al., 1987; Charny and Levin, 1988), which makes constant monitoring of the literature very important.

For the most part, these models incorporate various concepts of human thermoregulation, as well as thermal mechanics, to predict a more or less thorough set of corporal parameters—including central, or deep body, temperature, skin temperature, blood flow, sweat rate, and sometimes much more. Most models do not incorporate long-term changes in thermoregulatory responses (acclimatization), have not been adequately compared with similar or identical sets of data, and cannot deal directly with thermal responses to exercise. For these shortcomings, one must look to the deep body temperature model of Section 5.5, which does not incorporate active thermoregulation and which does not pretend to predict an exhaustive set of physiological parameters.

The models considered in this section are meant to illustrate several different techniques: (1) modeling the human body as a circular cylinder with various distinct layers, (2) modeling the human body as composed of many segments, and (3) modeling thermoregulation to construct a surrogate thermoregulator external to the human body.

5.4.1 Cylindrical Models

Two models are described, both based on replacing the complex geometry of the human body with a simple cylinder composed of distinct layers. It is obvious that the only part of the human body that resembles a cylinder is the trunk, and perhaps the head. Legs (if they remain together), and arms (if they remain close to the torso) can be reasonably included under nonexercise conditions. The cylinder has the advantage of relatively simple heat transfer equations, one-dimensional heat conduction (neglecting end effects), and no thermal concentration points, as exist in a body of rectangular cross section. Other simple geometrical shapes, such as prolate spheroids and oblate spheroids (Moon and Spencer, 1961), which better match actual geometries, also possess the property that their differential equations governing heat conduction are separable (i.e., temporal effects can be treated separately from spatial effects).

Gagge Model. The Gagge (1973) model is a simplified version of that presented by Gagge et al. (1971) and is intended to compare expected physiological heat stress caused by clothing, radiant heat, and air movement. It includes elements of exercise adjustments.

The human body is considered to be a single cylinder with two concentric layers, similar to that diagramed in Figure 5.1.2. The inner layer is the central core and the outer layer is the skin. Thermoregulation is considered to be accomplished by a combination of skin and core temperatures.

Central to the model is a heat balance, similar to that given as Equation 5.1.2. Rate of heat generated M is actually measured. For most tasks, muscular efficiency is taken to be 0%, for bicycle pedaling it is assumed to be 20%. The system of equations used by Gagge to describe the heat balance is

$$q_{stored} = q_{stored, core} + q_{stored, sk} \tag{5.4.1}$$

---

[38]There also appear in the literature many thermal models dealing with animals. As examples of these, see Birkebak et al. (1966) for whole-body models of geese and cardinals.

$$q_{\text{stored, core}} = m_{\text{core}} c \frac{d\theta_r}{dt} = m(1 - \beta) c \frac{d\theta_r}{dt} \tag{5.4.2}$$

$$q_{\text{stored, sk}} = m_{\text{sk}} c \frac{d\theta_{\text{sk}}}{dt} = m \beta c \frac{d\theta_{\text{sk}}}{dt} \tag{5.4.3}$$

$$q_{\text{stored, sk}} = (C_{\text{sk}} + c_{\text{bl}} \dot{V}_{\text{bl}})(\theta_r - \theta_{\text{sk}}) - (q_r + q_c) - (q_{\text{evap}} - q_{\text{evap, res}}) \tag{5.4.4}$$

$$q_{\text{stored, core}} = M - q_{\text{evap, res}} - q_{c, \text{res}} - (C_{\text{sk}} + c_{\text{bl}} \dot{V}_{\text{bl}})(\theta_r - \theta_{\text{sk}}) \tag{5.4.5}$$

$$q_r + q_c = \frac{(h_r + h_c) A (\theta_{\text{sk}} - \theta_e)}{1 + (h_r + h_c)/C_{\text{cl}}} \tag{5.4.6}$$

$$h_r = 4 F_A \sigma (0.5\theta_0 + 0.5\theta_e + 273)^3 [1 + (h_r + h_c)/C_{\text{cl}}] \tag{5.4.7}$$

$$h_c = 5.4 \qquad \text{(bicycle ergometer at 50 rpm)} \tag{5.4.8a}$$

$$= 6.0 \qquad \text{(bicycle ergometer at 60 rpm)} \tag{5.4.8b}$$

$$= 6.51 s^{0.391} \qquad \text{(treadmill walking, still air)} \tag{5.4.8c}$$

$$= 8.60 s^{0.531} \qquad \text{(free walking, still air)} \tag{5.4.8d}$$

$$= 8.60 s^{0.531} + 1.96 v^{0.86} \qquad \text{(free walking in head wind)} \tag{5.4.8e}$$

$$\theta_0 = \theta_e + \frac{\theta_{\text{sk}} - \theta_e}{1 + (h_c + h_r)/C_{\text{cl}}} \tag{5.4.9}$$

$$\theta_e = \frac{h_r \theta_{\text{rad}} + h_c \theta_e}{h_r + h_c} \tag{5.4.10}$$

$$q_{\text{evap, res}} = 1.725 \times 10^{-5} M_{\text{tot}} (p_{\text{sat}} - p_a) \tag{5.4.11}$$

$$q_{c, \text{res}} = 0.0012 M_{\text{tot}} (34 - \theta_a) \tag{5.4.12}$$

$$\theta_r = 37 + \int_0^t \left(\frac{d\theta_r}{dt} \right) dt \tag{5.4.13}$$

$$\theta_{\text{sk}} = 34 + \int_0^t \left(\frac{d\theta_{\text{sk}}}{dt} \right) dt \tag{5.4.14}$$

where A = body surface area, m^2

C_{sk} = skin conductance, $\dfrac{\text{N} \cdot \text{m}}{\text{m}^2 \cdot \text{sec} \cdot {}^\circ \text{C}}$

C_{cl} = clothing conductance, $\text{N}/(\text{m} \cdot \text{sec} \cdot {}^\circ \text{C})$

c = specific heat of body and skin tissue, $\text{N} \cdot \text{m}/(\text{kg}. {}^\circ \text{C})$

c_{bl} = specific heat of blood, $\text{N} \cdot \text{m}/(\text{m}^3 \cdot {}^\circ \text{C})$

F_A = ratio of body radiating area to total surface area, dimensionless

h_c = convection coefficient, $\text{N} \cdot \text{m}/(\text{m}^2 \cdot \text{sec} \cdot {}^\circ \text{C})$

h_r = radiation coefficient, $\text{N} \cdot \text{m}/(\text{m}^2 \cdot \text{sec} \cdot {}^\circ \text{C})$

M_{tot} = total heat generation, including external work, $\text{N} \cdot \text{m}/\text{sec}$

M = net heat generation, total metabolism minus external work, $\text{N} \cdot \text{m}/\text{sec}$

m = total body mass, kg

m_{core} = mass of the core, kg

q_c = convective heat loss, N·m/sec

$q_{c,res}$ = convective heat loss from the respiratory system, N·m/sec

q_{evap} = total evaporative heat loss, N·m/sec

$q_{evap,res}$ = respiratory system evaporative heat loss, N·m/sec

q_r = radiation heat loss, N·m/sec

$q_{stored,core}$ = rate of heat stored in the body core, N·m/sec

$q_{stored,sk}$ = rate of heat stored in the skin shell, N·m/sec

s = walking speed, m/sec

$\dot{V}_{bl}$ = volume rate of blood flow, m³/sec

v = wind speed, m/sec

β = ratio of skin shell mass to total body mass, dimensionless

θ_a = air temperature, °C

θ_e = mean environmental temperature, °C

θ_0 = clothing surface temperature, °C

θ_r = core temperature, °C

θ_{rad} = mean radiant temperature, °C

θ_{sk} = skin temperature, °C

Initial parameter values are given in Table 5.4.1.

The following system of equations was used by Gagge to describe thermoregulation.

1. To account for vasodilation (numerator term) and vasoconstriction (denominator term):

$$\dot{V}_{bl} = \frac{A[0.00175 + 0.0417(\theta_r - 37)]}{[1000 - 500(\theta_{sk} - 34)]}, \qquad \theta_{sk} \leqslant 34, \quad \theta_r > 37 \qquad (5.4.15)$$

TABLE 5.4.1   Parameter Values Used in the Gagge Thermoregulatory Model[a]

Characteristics of average man	
Body mass (m)	70 kg
Body surface area (A)	1.8 m²
Ratio of body's radiating area to total surface area (F_A)	0.72
Minimum skin conductance (C_{sk}/A)	5.28 N·m/(m²·sec·°C)
Normal skin blood flow ($\dot{V}_{bl}/A$)	1.75 × 10⁻⁶ m³/(m²·sec)
Assigned coefficients	
Specific heat of blood (C_{bl})	4.187 N·m/(m³·°C)
Specific heat of body (c)	3.5 N·m/(kg·°C)
Latent heat of water (H)	2.4 N·m/kg
Lewis relation at sea level	0.0165 °C·m²/N
Sea-level barometric pressure	10⁵ N/m²
Stefan–Boltzmann constant (σ)	5.67 × 10⁻⁸ N·m/(m²·sec·°K⁴)
Skin water vapor diffusion fraction (ρ_d)	0.06
Initial conditions	
Skin temperature (θ_{sk})	34°C
Core temperature	
Rectal (θ_r)	37°C
Esophageal	36.6°C
Radiation coefficient (h_r)	5.0 N·m/(m²·sec·°C)
Ratio of skin shell mass to total body mass (β)	0.1
Total evaporative heat loss (q_{evap}/A)	5.0 N·m/m²
Resting metabolic rate (M_r)	58.2 N·m/m²
Convective heat transfer coefficient (h_c) at rest	2.9 N·m/(m²sec·°C)
Convective heat transfer coefficient (h_c) during exercise	5.4 N·m/(m²·sec·°C)

[a]Compiled from Gagge, 1973.

if $\theta_{sk} \leqslant 34$, $(\theta_{sk} - 34)$ becomes 0 and if $\theta_r \leqslant 37$, $(\theta_r - 37)$ becomes 0.

2. To account for evaporative heat loss, the contributing terms of respiratory evaporation, sweating, and skin diffusion are summed. Respiratory evaporation was given previously as Equation 5.4.11. Sweating is controlled by both mean body temperature and peripheral skin temperature:

$$\dot{m}_{sw} = 250\,A\,[\beta(\theta_{sk} - 34) + (1 - \beta)(\theta_r - 37)\exp\,[(\theta_{sk} - 34)/10.7] \tag{5.4.16}$$

where $\dot{m}_{sw}$ = mass of sweat, kg/sec
Passive skin diffusion of water vapor is assumed to be 6% of total sweat capacity:

$$\dot{m}_v = \rho_d \dot{m}_{sw,max} + \dot{m}_{sw} \tag{5.4.17}$$

where ρ_d = fraction of maximum sweating capacity diffused ($\rho_d = 0.06$), dimensionless
$\dot{m}_v$ = total mass of skin water vapor, kg/sec
$\dot{m}_{sw,max}$ = maximum sweating rate, kg/sec
When clothing resistance to water vapor movement (Equation 5.2.77), the relationship between thermal convection coefficient and vapor coefficient (Equation 5.2.60), and latent heat are accounted for, we obtain

$$q_{evap} = q_{evap,res} + 250\,H\,A\beta(1 - \rho_d)(\theta_{sk} - 34) + (1 - \beta)(\theta_r - 37)\exp\,[\theta_{sk} - 34)/10.7]$$
$$+ 0.0165\rho_d h_c A(p_{sat} - p_a)/(1 + 0.922h_c/C_{cl}) \tag{5.4.18}$$

where H = latent heat of water vapor, N·m/kg
p_a = ambient water vapor pressure, N/m^2
p_{sat} = saturated water vapor pressure at skin temperature, N/m^2
and where the second term must be greater than or equal to zero and total calculated evaporative heat loss cannot exceed the maximum value.

3. To account for the change in effective skin thickness which occurs because of active vascular changes,

$$\beta = 0.0442 + 97{\cdot}47 \Bigg/ \left[10^6\!\left(\frac{\dot{V}_{bl}}{A}\right) - 3.85 \right] \tag{5.4.19}$$

4. To account for shivering,

$$M = M_r + 19.4A(34 - \theta_{sk})(37 - \theta_r), \qquad \theta_{sk} \leqslant 34, \quad \theta_r \leqslant 37 \tag{5.4.20}$$

if $\theta_{sk} > 34$, $(\theta_{sk} - 34)$ becomes 0, if $\theta_r > 37$, $(\theta_r - 37)$ becomes 0, and M_r = resting metabolic heat generation, N·m/sec.

Gagge's model can be used to describe thermoregulatory responses to various environmental and exercise conditions, but accuracy of transient predictions depends almost entirely on time steps used for integration.

Wyndham–Atkins Model. Wyndham and Atkins (1968) proposed an analog computer model which is summarized by Hwang and Konz (1977). This is a cylindrical model with four layers (Figure 5.4.1): (1) a central core composed of skeleton and viscera, (2) muscles, (3) deep skin and fatty tissue, and (4) outer skin. Muscular heat generated during exercise is transferred to the deep skin by conduction and vascular convection. Heat flow through the outer skin is assumed to be entirely by conduction, since this layer is assumed to be extremely thin with negligible blood flow.

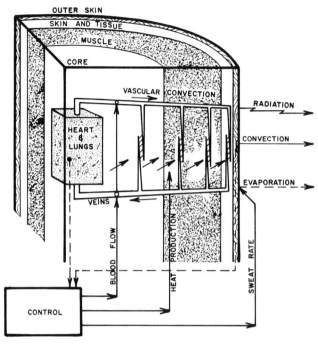

Figure 5.4.1 A simple physical model of heat flow and control in the human body. (Used with permission from Hwang and Konz, 1977. © 1977 IEEE.)

All layers are assumed to be homogeneous with uniform thermal conductivity, metabolic heat production rate, and heat exchange with the blood.

Heat exchange is by conduction, assumed to occur only radially, and by vascular convection, from capillaries only. That is, all arterial blood has the same temperature, no matter which layer it enters. Capillary blood enters at the arterial blood temperature and leaves through the veins at the local tissue temperature.

A control center has temperature receptors near the skin surface, within the spinal cord, and within the hypothalamus. Hypothalamic temperature is nearly equal to arterial blood temperature, and arterial blood temperature is assumed to be the internal reference temperature that controls blood flow, heat production rate, and sweat rate.

The system of equations for heat transfer begins with the generalized heat balance equation (5.1.2) for radial conduction. Rate of change of heat is set equal to radially conducted heat plus heat supplied by the blood:

$$\frac{\partial \theta}{\partial t} = \frac{k}{\rho c r}\frac{\partial}{\partial r}\left(r\frac{\partial \theta}{\partial r}\right) + \frac{1}{c\rho}\left(\frac{M}{V} + \frac{\dot{V}_{bl}}{V}c_{bl}\rho_{bl}[\theta_r - \theta]\right) \tag{5.4.21}$$

where θ = local tissue temperature, °C
  r = radial coordinate, m
  c = specific heat of local tissue, N·m/(kg·°C)
  k = thermal conductivity, $\dfrac{N\cdot m}{m\cdot sec\cdot °C}$
  ρ = density, kg/m³
  M = local tissue metabolic heat generation, N·m/sec

$\dot{V}_{bl}$ = volume of blood flow in a tissue segment, m³/sec
V = volume of local tissue, m³
θ_r = core temperature, °C
c_{bl} = specific heat of blood, N·m/(kg·°C)

$$\sum q_{bl}''' = c_{bl}\frac{\partial \theta_r}{\partial t} \tag{5.4.22}$$

where q_{bl}''' = volume rate of heat exchange with the blood, in each component, N·m/(sec·m³)

$$\sum q_{bl}''' = \frac{\dot{V}_{bl}}{V}c_{bl}\rho_{bl}[\theta_r - \theta]$$

$$q_r = 6.49 A_r(\theta_{sk} - \theta_{rad}) \tag{5.4.23}$$

$$q_c = 7.24(10^{-5}p)^{0.6}v^{0.6}A_c(\theta_{sk} - \theta_a) \tag{5.4.24}$$

$$q_{evap} = 0.0161 A v^{0.37}(p_{sk}K_e - p_a) \tag{5.4.25}$$

where p = atmospheric pressure, N/m²
p_{sk} = saturated vapor pressure of water at skin temperature, N/m²
p_a = partial pressure of water vapor in air, N/m²
v = wind speed, m/sec
K_e = control constant varying between 0 and 1, dimensionless
A = body surface area, m²
A_r = radiation area, m²
A_c = convection area, m²
Heat loss by respiration is neglected.

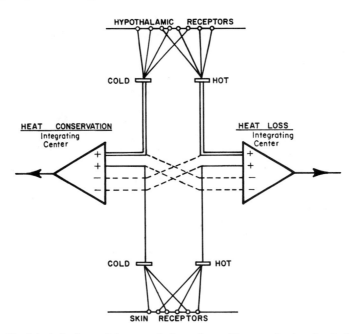

Figure 5.4.2 Physiological scheme of the control of sweating and heat conductance by the hypothalamus and the skin. Cold and hot skin and hypothalamic sensors feed information to hypothalamic control centers for heat maintenance and heat loss. Cross-coupling between the centers coordinates actions. (From Wyndham and Atkins, 1968. Used with permission from Hwang and Konz, 1977. ©1977 IEEE.)

Thermoregulatory equations are based on experimental findings from four highly acclimatized subjects under steady-state conditions (Wyndham and Atkins, 1968) and are therefore limited in range of applicability. To form prediction equations from their data, Wyndham and Atkins assumed a hypothalamic model as in Figure 5.4.2, where facilitation of the effector neurons in the heat loss center by incoming impulses from hypothalamic thermoreceptors and cutaneous thermoreceptors results in sweating and increased thermal conductance. Facilitation of effector neurons in the heat maintenance center results in cutaneous vasoconstriction and shivering. Facilitation of one center inhibits the other.

The equations for sweating are developed only for skin temperatures less than or equal to 33°C, which Wyndham and Atkins termed the "cold zone":

$$q_{evap} = [H/3600][0.55(\theta_r - 36.5) - 0.455(\theta_r - 36.35)(1 - e^{-2.7}[33 - \theta_{sk}])], \qquad \theta_{sk} \geqslant 33°C$$
$$(5.4.26)$$

This equation fits their data only approximately; other equations for evaporative heat loss, as well as other thermoregulatory processes, were not presented. Notice that Wyndham and Atkins assumed temperature set points of 36.5 and 33°C in deep body and skin temperatures. Gagge used temperatures of 37 and 34°C for the same variables.

5.4.2 Multicompartment Model

The Stolwijk (1970) model, which is really an extension of models by Crosbie et al. (1963), their colleagues J. D. Hardy and H. T. Hammel, and others at the John B. Pierce Foundation in New Haven, Connecticut, uses a multicompartment model similar to that presented by Wissler (1963). The body is divided into six segments (head, trunk, arms, legs, hands, and feet) linked together via blood flow to and from a central blood compartment (Figure 5.4.3). Each segment is composed of four layers of core, muscle, fat, and skin. There are thus 24 compartments plus the central blood compartment for a total of 25, each requiring heat balance equations similar to Equation 5.1.2.

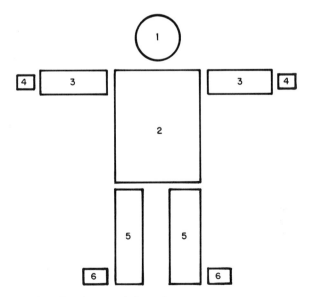

Figure 5.4.3 Representation of passive model of six different segments indicating method of identification: 1 = head; 2 = trunk; 3 = arms; 4 = hands; 5 = legs; 6 = feet. Each segment is composed of four layers: core, muscle, fat, and skin. (Used with permission from Stolwijk and Hardy, 1977.)

The head segment is considered to be a sphere, whereas trunk, arms, hands, legs, and feet are considered to be cylinders. Basic body data and segmental areas, volumes, and masses used by Stolwijk and Hardy (1977) appear in Tables 5.4.2–5.4.4. Table 5.4.5 lists assumed dimensions for each of the body compartments. Volumes appearing in the table are inclusive; that is, inner compartment volumes have not been subtracted from outer compartment volumes. Thus the total volume of 0.0744 m³ (74.4 L) is obtained by adding each of the skin compartment volumes and neglecting the blood compartment volume (which, in reality, appears within the other compartmental volumes).

The heat generation term is composed of basal metabolism (Table 5.4.5) plus activity metabolism. For the three interior layers of core, muscle, and fat, heat input and output occur through tissue conduction and blood flow convection (Figure 5.4.4). Thermal conductances between segments are calculated and appear in Table 5.4.5.

The outer layer of skin exchanges heat with the environment through evaporation, convection, and radiation. Heat transfer coefficient values which appear in Table 5.4.3 are for the natural convection condition and must be modified by Equation 5.4.27 to account for external relative air movement:

$$h = h_r + 3.16 h_c v^{0.5} \tag{5.4.27}$$

where h = combined convection and radiation coefficient, $N \cdot m/(m^2 \cdot sec \cdot {}^\circ C)$ (Table 5.4.3)

h_r = radiation coefficient, $N \cdot m/(m^2 \cdot sec \cdot {}^\circ C)$ (Table 5.4.3)

h_c = convection coefficient, $N \cdot m/(m^2 \cdot sec \cdot {}^\circ C)$ (Table 5.4.3)

v = relative wind speed, m/sec

Because there are 25 compartments, there are many redundant equations in the Stolwijk and Hardy model. The following heat exchange equations are to be applied to each compartment:

1. For heat exchange between each compartment and the blood:

$$q_{c,bl} = 3600 \dot{V}_{bl}(\theta_i - \theta_{bl}) \tag{5.4.28}$$

2. For conduction between segments:

$$q_k = C(\theta_i - \theta_j) \tag{5.4.29}$$

3. For net heat transfer from each compartment:

$$q = M_i - q_{evap} - q_{c,bl} - q_k \tag{5.4.30}$$

TABLE 5.4.2 Basic Data for Stolwijk and Hardy (1977) Average Man

Body mass (m)	74.4 kg
Body surface area (A)	1.89 m²
Height (H_t)	1.72 m
Specific heat (c)	
Skeleton	2.09 N·m/(g·°C)
Fat	2.52 N·m/(g·°C)
Blood	3.74 N·m/(g·°C)
Other tissues	3.78 N·m/(g·°C)
Blood capacity of heart and great vessels	0.0025 m³ (2.5 L)

TABLE 5.4.3 Values for Surface Areas, Volumes, and Heat Transfer Coefficients for the Stolwyk and Hardy Model

Segment	Surface Area		Volume			Heat Transfer Coefficients, N·m/(sec·m²·°C)		
	m²	% of total	m³	(L)	% of total	Radiant (h_r)	Convective (h_c)	Combined ($h_r + h_c$)
Head	0.1326	7.0	0.00402	(4.02)	5.4	4.8	3.0	7.8
Trunk	0.6804	36.0	0.04100	(41.00)	55.1	4.8	2.1	6.9
Arms	0.2536	13.4	0.00706	(7.06)	9.5	4.2	2.1	6.3
Hands	0.0946	5.0	0.00067	(0.67)	0.9	3.6	4.0	7.6
Legs	0.5966	31.7	0.02068	(20.68)	27.8	4.2	2.1	6.3
Feet	0.1299	6.9	0.00097	(0.97)	1.3	4.0	4.0	8.0
Total	1.8877	100.0	0.07440	(74.40)	100.0			

Source: Adapted and used with permission from Stolwijk and Hardy, 1977.

TABLE 5.4.4 Mass (Kg) of the Four Layers in Each Segment of the Stolwijk and Hardy Model

Segment	Total Mass	Core Skeleton	Viscera	Muscle	Fat	Skin
Head	4.02	1.22	1.79	0.37	0.37	0.27
Trunk	38.50	2.83	9.35	17.90	7.07	1.35
Arms	7.06	1.51	0.74	3.37	0.97	0.48
Hands	0.67	0.23	0.03	0.07	0.15	0.19
Legs	20.68	5.02	1.92	10.19	2.38	1.20
Feet	0.97	0.37	0.06	0.07	0.22	0.24
Central blood	2.50	0.00	2.50	0.00	0.00	0.00
Total	74.40	11.18	16.39	31.97	11.16	3.73

Source: Used with permission from Stolwijk and Hardy, 1977.

4. For net heat transfer from skin compartments:

$$q_{sk} = M_i - q_{evap} - q_{c,bl} + q_k - hA(\theta_{sk} - \theta_a) \qquad (5.4.31)$$

5. For local temperature in each compartment:

$$\theta_i = \int d\theta_i = \int \left(\frac{q}{cm}\right) dt \qquad (5.4.32)$$

6. For blood temperature:

$$\theta_{bl} = \int d\theta_{bl} = \int \left(\frac{q_{c,bl}}{c_{bl} m_{bl}}\right) dt \qquad (5.4.33)$$

where θ_i = local temperature in each compartment, °C

θ_{bl} = blood compartment temperature, °C

θ_i, θ_j = adjacent compartment temperatures, °C

θ_{sk} = skin surface temperature, °C

θ_a = ambient temperature, °C

$q_{c,bl}$ = convective heat exchange from local compartment to blood, N·m/sec

q_k = intersegment conduction heat transfer, N·m/sec

q = total heat exchange of each compartment, N·m/sec

q_{sk} = total heat exchange of skin compartment, N·m/sec

q_{evap} = evaporative heat loss, from skin or trunk core, N·m/sec

V_{bl} = local blood flow, m³/sec

C = intersegment conductance, N·m/(sec·°C) (Table 5.4.5)

c = specific heat of local compartment, N·m/(kg.·°C) (Table 5.4.2)

m = mass of local compartment, kg (Table 5.4.4)

M_i = metabolic rate in each compartment, N·m/sec (Table 5.4.5)

t = time, sec

h = combined convection and radiation coefficient, N·m/(m²·sec·°C) (Table 5.4.3)

A = surface area of each segment, m² (Table 5.4.3)

Thermoregulation is accomplished by means of several control signals, each based on the difference between the local compartment temperature θ_i and a local compartment set-point temperature θ_{sp} (Table 5.4.6). If this difference is positive, it indicates warm thermal conditions and a need to remove excess heat. If this difference is negative, heat maintenance measures are

TABLE 5.4.5 Estimated Basal Heat Production, Blood Flow, and Thermal Conductance for Each Compartment

Segment	Compartment	Inclusive Volume, $m^3 \times 10^3$ (L)	Length, cm	Outer Radius, cm	Thermal Conductivity, N/(sec·°C)	Intersegment Conductance, N·m/(sec·°C)	Basal Heat Production, N·m/sec	Basal Blood Flow, m^3/sec $\times 10^6$ (L/sec)
Head	Core	3.01 (3.01)		8.98	0.418		14.95	750.0 (0.7500)
	Muscle	3.38 (3.38)		9.32	0.418	1.61	0.12	2.0 (0.0020)
	Fat	3.75 (3.75)		9.65	0.334	13.25	0.13	2.2 (0.0022)
	Skin	4.02 (4.02)		9.88	0.334	16.10	0.10	24.0 (0.0240)
Trunk	Core	14.68 (14.68)	60	8.75	0.418		52.63	3500.0 (3.5000)
	Muscle	32.58 (32.58)	60	13.15	0.418	1.59	5.81	100.0 (0.1000)
	Fat	39.65 (39.65)	60	14.40	0.334	5.53	2.49	42.7 (0.0427)
	Skin	41.00 (41.00)	60	14.70	0.334	23.08	0.47	35.0 (0.0350)
Arms	Core	2.24 (2.24)	112	2.83	0.418		0.82	14.0 (0.0140)
	Muscle	5.61 (5.61)	112	4.48	0.418	1.40	1.11	19.0 (0.0190)
	Fat	6.58 (6.58)	112	4.85	0.334	8.9	0.21	3.3 (0.0033)
	Skin	7.06 (7.06)	112	5.02	0.334	30.50	0.15	8.3 (0.0083)
Hands	Core	0.26 (0.26)	96	0.93	0.418		0.09	1.7 (0.0017)
	Muscle	0.33 (0.33)	96	1.04	0.418	6.40	0.23	4.0 (0.0040)
	Fat	0.48 (0.48)	96	1.27	0.334	11.20	0.04	0.7 (0.0007)
	Skin	0.67 (0.67)	96	1.49	0.334	11.50	0.06	33.3 (0.0333)
Legs	Core	6.91 (6.91)	160	3.71	0.418		2.59	44.8 (0.0448)
	Muscle	17.10 (17.10)	160	5.85	0.418	10.50	3.32	57.2 (0.0572)
	Fat	19.48 (19.48)	160	6.23	0.334	14.40	0.50	8.7 (0.0087)
	Skin	20.68 (20.68)	160	6.42	0.334	74.50	0.37	47.5 (0.0475)
Feet	Core	0.43 (0.43)	125	1.06	0.418		0.15	2.7 (0.0027)
	Muscle	0.51 (0.51)	125	1.14	0.418	16.13	0.02	0.3 (0.0003)
	Fat	0.73 (0.73)	125	1.36	0.334	20.60	0.05	0.8 (0.0008)
	Skin	0.97 (0.97)	125	1.57	0.334	16.40	0.08	50.0 (0.0500)
Central blood		2.50 (2.50)						
Total		74.4 (74.4)					86.44	4752.2 (4.7522)

Source: Adapted and used with permission from Stolwijk and Hardy, 1977.

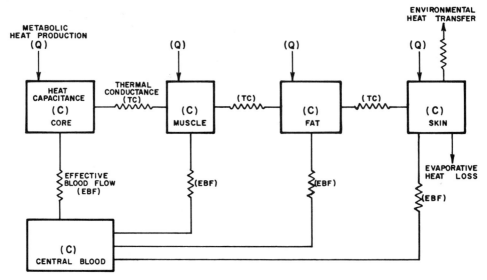

Figure 5.4.4 Schematic representation of heat exchange for the four compartments of Segment I. (Used with permission from Stolwijk, 1971.)

TABLE 5.4.6 Set-Point Temperature Values[a] for the Stolwijk and Hardy Model

Segment	Compartment	Set-Point Temperature, °C
Head	Core	36.96
	Muscle	35.07
	Fat	34.81
	Skin	34.58
Trunk	Core	36.89
	Muscle	36.28
	Fat	34.53
	Skin	33.62
Arms	Core	35.53
	Muscle	34.12
	Fat	33.59
	Skin	33.25
Hands	Core	35.41
	Muscle	35.38
	Fat	35.30
	Skin	35.22
Legs	Core	35.81
	Muscle	35.30
	Fat	35.31
	Skin	34.10
Feet	Core	35.14
	Muscle	35.03
	Fat	35.11
	Skin	35.04
Central blood		36.71

Source: Used with permission from Stolwijk and Hardy, 1977.

[a] Also used as initial condition values.

required. The total control signal is considered to be composed of the error signal in the compartment corresponding to the brain (head core) and error signals from the skin areas of each segment. Weighting is applied to these skin signals in an attempt to account for different thermoreceptor concentrations in different skin areas. Applicable weighting factors for thermosensory inputs appear in Table 5.4.7.

Output signals are required for sweating, vasodilation, shivering, and vasoconstriction. These are then used to vary blood flow, metabolic rate, and skin evaporation heat loss. These four signals are calculated by

$$SW = 372(\theta_{br} - \theta_{spbr}) + 33.7\left(\sum [\theta_{sk} - \theta_{spsk}]F_{th}\right) \tag{5.4.34}$$

$$VD = 489,600(\theta_{br} - \theta_{spbr}) + 61,200\left(\sum [\theta_{sk} - \theta_{spsk}]F_{th}\right) \tag{5.4.35}$$

$$SH = 13.0(\theta_{br} - \theta_{spbr}) + 0.40\left(\sum [\theta_{sk} - \theta_{spsk}]F_{th}\right)\left(\sum [\theta_{sk} - \theta_{spsk}]F_{th}\right) \tag{5.4.36}$$

$$VC = 10.8(\theta_{br} - \theta_{spbr}) - 10.8\left(\sum [\theta_{sk} - \theta_{spsk}]F_{th}\right) \tag{5.4.37}$$

where SW = total efferent sweating command, N·m/sec
VD = total efferent skin vasodilation command, m³/sec
SH = total efferent shivering command, N·m/sec
VC = total efferent skin vasoconstriction command, dimensionless
θ_{br} = brain temperature, °C
θ_{spbr} = brain set-point temperature, °C (Table 5.4.9)
θ_{spsk} = skin set-point temperature, °C (Table 5.4.6)
F_{th} = skin thermosensory fractional weighting factor, dimensionless (Table 5.4.7)
and the summation of differences between local skin temperature and skin set-point temperature is to be performed for all six skin areas.

Heat production is assumed to begin at the basal state and increase in the muscles only during exercise and/or shivering. Basal metabolic rates are assumed constant over a short time span for which this model is to be used. Therefore, acclimatization and other changes in BMR are not

TABLE 5.4.7 Estimates of Distribution of Sensory Input and Effector Output over Various Skin Areas for Stolwijk and Hardy Model

Segment	Surface Area	Thermosensory Input (F_{th})	Applicable Fraction Of:		
			Sweating Command (F_{sw})	Vasodilation Command (F_{vd})	Vasoconstriction Command (F_{vc})
Head	0.1326	0.21	0.081	0.132	0.05
Trunk	0.6804	0.42	0.481	0.322	0.15
Arms	0.2536	0.10	0.154	0.095	0.05
Hands	0.0946	0.04	0.031	0.121	0.35
Legs	0.5966	0.20	0.218	0.230	0.05
Feet	0.1299	0.03	0.035	0.100	0.35

Source: Used with permission from Stolwijk and Hardy, 1977.

considered:

$$M_{mus} = BMR_{mus} + W_{mus}F_{mus} + (SH)F_{sh} \qquad (5.4.38)$$

$$M_{all\ others} = BMR \qquad (5.4.39)$$

where BMR = basal metabolic rate, N·m/sec

M = metabolic rate in each compartment, N·m/sec

W_{mus} = total muscular work rate, N·m/sec

F_{mus} = fraction of work done by each muscle compartment, dimensionless (Table 5.4.8)

F_{sh} = fraction of total shivering done by each muscle compartment, dimensionless (Table 5.4.8)

Evaporative heat loss from the respiratory system is

$$q_{evap,res} = (86.4 + M)(1.725 \times 10^{-4})(5866 - p_{air}) \qquad (5.4.40)$$

and evaporation from the skin is

$$q_{evap,sk} = (q_{evap,b} + [F_{sw}][SW])2^{(\theta_{sk} - \theta_{spsk})/4} \qquad (5.4.41)$$

For all other compartments,

$$q_{evap} = 0$$

where $q_{evap,res}$ = evaporative heat loss from the respiratory system, N·m/sec

$q_{evap,sk}$ = evaporative heat loss from the skin, N·m/sec

$q_{evap,b}$ = basal evaporative heat loss from the skin, N·m/sec (Table 5.4.9)

F_{sw} = fraction of sweating command applicable to each skin compartment, dimensionless (Table 5.4.7)

M = metabolic equivalent of muscular work, N·m/sec

p_a = ambient vapor pressure, N/m²

The fraction F_{sw} accounts for the fact that there is an uneven distribution of sweat gland concentration and skin area in different skin segments. Thus sweating heat loss from each skin segment is different from the others. The term $2^{(\theta_{sk} - \theta_{spsk})/4}$ accounts for a local skin temperature effect on the skin sweating heat loss. Stolwijk and Hardy (1977) indicate that the denominator of the exponent should be 10, but their program shows it as 4.

TABLE 5.4.8 Estimates of Distribution of Heat Production in Muscle Compartments for the Stolwijk and Hardy Model

Segment	Percent of Total Muscle Mass	Fraction of Total Bicycling or Walking Work Done by Muscles (F_{mus})	Fraction of Total Shivering Done by Muscles (F_{sh})
Head	2.323	0.00	0.02
Trunk	54.790	0.30	0.85
Arms	10.525	0.08	0.05
Hands	0.233	0.01	0.00
Legs	31.897	0.60	0.07
Feet	0.233	0.01	0.00

Source: Used with permission from Stolwijk and Hardy, 1977.

TABLE 5.4.9 Basal Evaporative Heat Loss Rate for Each Segment of the Stolwijk and Hardy (1977) Model

Segment	Heat Loss, N·m/sec
Head (skin)	0.81
Trunk (core, respiratory)	10.45
Trunk (skin)	3.78
Arm (skin)	1.40
Hand (skin)	0.52
Leg (skin)	3.32
Feet (skin)	0.72

Total evaporative heat loss cannot exceed the maximum obtained when the skin is totally wet. Maximum evaporative heat loss is checked using the Lewis relationship presented in Equation 5.2.61:

$$q_{\text{evap, max}} = 0.0165 h_c A (p_{\text{sat}} - p_a) \geqslant q_{\text{evap, sk}} \tag{5.4.42}$$

where $q_{\text{evap, max}}$ = maximum evaporative heat loss from the skin, N·m/sec
h_c = convection coefficient, N·m/(m^2·sec·°C) (Table 5.4.3)
A = area of each skin segment, m^2 (Table 5.4.3)
p_{sat} = partial pressure of water vapor at the temperature of the evaporation surface, N/m^2 (Table 5.2.12)

Blood flow to each compartment is also computed. The core and fat compartments are assumed to maintain blood flow at their basal levels (Table 5.4.5). Muscle blood flow is calculated from

$$\dot{V}_{\text{bl}} = \dot{V}_{\text{bl}, b} + 3.60(M - \text{BMR}) \tag{5.4.43}$$

and skin from

$$\dot{V}_{\text{bl}} = \left(\frac{\dot{V}_{\text{bl}, b} + F_{\text{vd}} \text{VD}}{1 + F_{\text{vc}} \text{VC}} \right) 2^{(\theta_{\text{sk}} - \theta_{\text{spsk}})/10} \tag{5.4.44}$$

where $\dot{V}_{\text{bl}, b}$ = basal blood flow, m^3/sec (Table 5.4.5)
F_{vd} = fraction of vasodilation command applicable to each skin area, dimensionless (Table 5.4.7)
F_{vc} = fraction of vasoconstriction command applicable to each skin area, dimensionless (Table 5.4.7)

The term $2^{(\theta_{\text{sk}} - \theta_{\text{spsk}})/10}$ accounts for local temperature effects on skin blood flow.

Model and experimental results are compared in Figure 5.4.5 (Stolwijk and Hardy, 1977). The model gives a reasonably close fit. Another comparison by Hancock (1981) indicates that the model does not always closely predict mean body temperature during exercise. The value of this model, however, goes beyond the comparison with experimental values, because the amount of research that was necessary to estimate parameter values was tremendous. These values, which appear in Tables 5.4.2–5.4.9, can be useful in other anthropometric studies not necessarily related to thermoregulation or exercise.

5.4.3 External Thermoregulation

An external thermoregulatory system has many advantages for the design of space suits or other impermeable clothing where accumulation of sweat poses an extreme design difficulty. Since

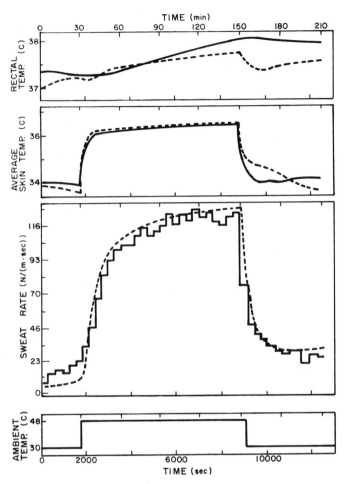

Figure 5.4.5 Comparison of physiological data with theoretical values derived from the model. A subject clad in shorts sat for 1800 sec (30 min) in a neutral environment, 30°C, and transferred quickly to a room at 48°C for 7200 sec (2 hr). A final hour was spent at 30°C. Solid lines denote experimental data; dashed lines denote computed values. (Adapted and used with permission from Stolwijk and Hardy, 1977.)

working subjects are often poor judges of their own thermal states, they cannot be relied upon to adequately control external cooling. Automatic control is thus offered as a reasonable design alternative. This control must be both accurate and timely despite changing activity levels.

Webb et al. (1968, 1970) successfully operated external cooling devices with closed-loop controllers utilizing physiological input feedback. Figure 5.4.6 is the basic diagram of these systems.

Cooling water is circulated by a pump from inside the suit, where it absorbs heat, to an external thermoelectric cooler, where it is cooled. Webb et al. (1968) chose a constant water flow of $2.5 \times 10^{-5} \, m^3/sec$ (1.5 L/min), which would keep a resting subject comfortable at a temperature of 26–32°C yet could remove all metabolic heat a man brought to his surface during hard work.

Two water temperature controller principles were successfully used. The first uses human oxygen consumption as a measure of metabolic heat production. The difficulty with this method is that oxygen consumption can change rapidly, but water inlet temperature requires a longer time to change. There is human body thermal mass, which slows the rate of change of body

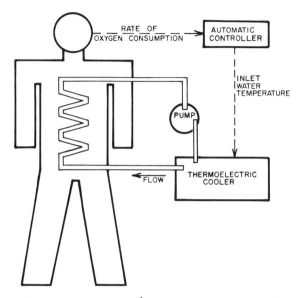

Figure 5.4.6 Diagram of the water loop with the $\dot{V}_{o_2}$ controller and a thermoelectric cooler, a recirculating pump, and a man in the insulated water-cooled clothing assembly. (Used with permission from Hwang and Konz, 1977. © 1977 IEEE.)

temperature upon initiation of activity (see Section 5.5.2). Human and mechanical cooling systems must be matched. Webb et al. (1968) give an equation from which the controller may operate:

$$\tau_c \dot{\theta}_{wi} = -\theta_{wi} + B(M_0 - M) \tag{5.4.45}$$

where τ_c = controller time constant, sec
$\dot{\theta}_{wi}$ = rate of change of inlet water temperature, °C/sec
θ_{wi} = inlet water temperature, °C
B = gain of the system, °C·sec/(N·m)
M = metabolic rate measured from oxygen consumption, N·m/sec
M_0 = reference metabolic rate, N·m/sec

A second controller principle operates by matching heat removed by the cooling water to maintain thermal equilibrium from the skin. This is a much more direct feedback control principle than the controller using oxygen consumption (which is nearly open loop).

Temperature of the inlet and outlet manifolds of the water-cooled suit are used to obtain total amount of heat removed. Average skin temperature is derived from four thermistors placed inside the suit over the thigh muscle, the biceps, the lower abdomen, and the kidney. When this average temperature increases, inlet water temperature decreases to increase heat removal:

$$\dot{m}c(\theta_{wo} - \theta_{wi}) - q_0 = \frac{\theta_{sk} - \theta_{sk0}}{B} \tag{5.4.46}$$

where $\dot{m}$ = mass rate of water flow, kg/sec
c = specific heat of cooling water, N·m/(kg °C)
θ_{wo} = outlet water temperature, °C
q_0 = resting cooling rate, N·m/sec
θ_{sk} = skin temperature, °C
θ_{sk0} = resting skin temperature, °C
B = system gain, °C·sec/(N·m)

5.5 BODY TEMPERATURE RESPONSE

Although the hypothalamic area is the site of precise thermoregulation, human hypothalamic temperature itself is an inaccessible index of thermal stress. Furthermore, the environmental range where thermoregulation finely adjusts bodily responses is fairly narrow. At high levels of exercise, or in very hot environments, the body reacts grossly, not entirely able to maintain a constant body temperature but instead attempting to constrain body temperature rises to those not damaging to itself.

Rectal temperature, as measured 8 cm beyond the sphincter, is an easily obtained index of heat loss, and when rectal temperature approaches 40°C in normal men, heat exhaustion is imminent. Thermoregulatory mechanisms have been known to lose control, with resulting rapid increases in body temperature and probable death.

The major impetus for development of models to predict deep body temperature during exercise has come from two sources: the military and industry. In the military, heat stress can be a significant influence on the capabilities of fighting men (Belyavin et al., 1979), and by knowing probable responses to work, environment, and clothing, suitable adjustments can be made.

Heat stress is also important in industries such as foundries and steel mills, and recent attention has been focussed on better protection of workers (Kamon, 1984). Of these two motivators, work has progressed furthest on the military models (Pandolf et al., 1986). Therefore, most of the following discussion applies mainly to average responses of young, healthy, reasonably fit, heat-acclimatized men. Even among this group, individual differences may be significant and cannot be totally corrected.

5.5.1 Equilibrium Temperature

As long as exercise occurs at or below the comfort zone (the zone of thermoregulation in Figure 5.1.3), rectal temperature depends only on the metabolic level and is independent of climatic conditions (Lind, 1963; Nielsen and Nielsen, 1962). When immediate thermoregulatory mechanisms have reached their limits and can provide no more active control, rectal temperature seems to respond to variations of clothing, work, and environmental conditions (Givoni and Goldman, 1972).

Equilibrium temperature is defined as the temperature reached by the body after all changes have been completed. Equilibrium temperature may require body temperature to move to lethal levels. In such a case, thermal responses of the body will drive body temperature toward the equilibrium temperature, and death will result, unless changes are made in work, environment, or clothing. Equilibrium temperature is assumed to be prescribed by factors in the basic heat balance Equation (5.1.2). These factors are (Givoni and Goldman, 1972) (1) metabolic heat load, (2) radiation and convection heat gain or loss, and (3) the difference between required sweating rate and evaporative capacity of the air. Each is discussed in turn.

Metabolic Heat Load. Metabolic heat load was discussed in Section 5.2.5. Muscular metabolic heat load is the difference between energy required by the muscles and the energy equivalent of external work. Givoni and Goldman (1972) have given an empirical equation for heat production for men walking on any terrain at any speed at any grade:

$$M = 0.10\zeta W\{(2.7 + 3.2(s - 0.7)^{1.65} + 100G[0.23 + 0.29(s - 0.7)]\} - WsG \qquad (5.5.1)$$

where M = net metabolic heat load for walking, N·m/sec
  ζ = terrain factor, dimensionless
  W = total weight (body + load + clothing), N
  s = speed of walking, m/sec
  G = fractional (not percent) grade, dimensionless

The term WsG represents the rate of external physical work accomplished by the muscles: this muscular power is transferred into increased potential energy and does not constitute a heat burden on the body. This formula has been claimed (Givoni and Goldman, 1972) to be usable for running with energy costs up to 1400 N·m/sec, but it cannot be used for walking speeds below 0.7 m/sec, where it is difficult to maintain a smooth movement pattern. For comfort, M should be maintained in the range of 290–525 N·m/sec for average men (Goldman, 1975). At rest a constant value of 105 N·m/sec can be assumed for M.

For the case of downhill walking, leading to negative work, Goldman (1988) indicated that the grade is taken to be a positive number (see Section 5.2.5 for heat production of a muscle performing negative work) and the physical work rate is added to, rather than subtracted from, the expression for metabolic heat load.

Terrain coefficients ζ are corrections applied to terrain surfaces to correct for the increased metabolic cost of walking on these surfaces compared to walking on the treadmill, where Equation 5.5.1 was developed. Values of terrain coefficients valid for men carrying loads of 100–400 N appear in Table 5.5.1.

The weight W to be used in Equation 5.5.1 is the total weight carried, including nude weight, clothing weight, and load carried. It has been found, however, that placement of the load carried will affect the metabolic cost of the load (Soule and Goldman, 1969). Placing the load on the head did not appreciably affect the metabolic rate over that which it would have been had the weight been body weight; placing the load in the hands increased the metabolic cost somewhat; and placing it on the feet increased it greatly. Givoni and Goldman (1971) suggested a correction factor for Equation 5.5.1 which can be used to account for load placement:

$$M' = M + KW_l^2 s^2 \tag{5.5.2}$$

where M' = heat production with load placement correction, N·m/sec
  M = walking metabolic load from Equation 5.5.1, N·m/sec
  K = proportionality factor, sec/(N·m)
  W_l = weight of load, N
  s = walking speed, m/sec

Givoni and Goldman (1971) use $K = 5.51 \times 10^{-3}$ sec/(N·m) [0.015 hr/(km·kg)] for loads in the hands, and $K = 23.5 \times 10^{-3}$ sec/(N·m) [0.064 hr/(km·kg)] for loads on the feet. In the computation of the correction for loads on the feet, only deviations from the weight of standard

TABLE 5.5.1 Terrain Coefficient Values[a]

Terrain	Coefficient (τ)
Treadmill	1.0
Blacktop surface	1.0
Linoleum flooring	1.0
Dirt road	1.1
Hard-packed snow	1.1
Soft snow	1.1 + 0.1 (cm snow print depth left by foot)
Light brush	1.2
Heavy brush	1.5
Plowed field	1.5
Swampy bog	1.8
Firm sand dunes	1.8
Loose sand	2.1

[a]Compiled from Soule and Goldman, 1972; Goldman, 1975; Givoni and Goldman, 1971; Pandolf et al., 1976.

army service boots (15 N, or 1.5 kg) should be taken into account. They indicate that since usual shoes normally weigh 10 N, this adjustment can be omitted with little error. Extra layers of clothing significantly increase metabolic cost, but the increase cannot be attributed entirely to displacement of the load from the axis of the torso (Teitlebaum and Goldman, 1972). Perhaps this effect is due to friction between clothing layers and increased interference of the clothing with natural movement.

Very heavy loads seem to require a disproportionately high amount of energy to carry (Givoni and Goldman, 1971). When the product of the load carried W_l times the speed of walking s exceeds 270 N·m/sec (100 kg·km/hr), a correction is required. If $W_l s < 270$ N·m/sec, no correction should appear:

$$M'' = M + 0.147(W_l s - 270), \qquad W_l s > 270 \tag{5.5.3}$$

where M'' = heat production with heavy load correction, N·m/sec

Givoni and Goldman (1971) also corrected Equation 5.5.1 for heat production while running. They indicate that below an energy cost (external work plus heat production) of about 1000 N·m/sec (900 kcal/hr) walking is more efficient than running (see Figure 2.4.5). Above 1000 N·m/sec, running is more efficient. They thus propose the required running correction to be

$$M''' = [M + 0.47 (1047 - M)][1 + G] \tag{5.5.4}$$

where M''' = heat production for running, N·m/sec

Pandolf et al. (1977) developed an equation for energy expenditure for the same conditions of Equation 5.5.1, except that it does not suffer from the lower walking speed limit of 0.7 m/sec. This equation has five components: (1) metabolic cost of standing without load (calculated as 0.15 N·m/sec per newton of body weight), (2) metabolic cost of standing with a load, (3) metabolic cost of walking on the level, (4) metabolic cost of climbing a grade, and (5) external work. This formula is

$$M = 0.15 W_b + 0.20(W_b + W_l)(W_l/W_b)^2 \\ + 0.102\zeta(W_b + W_l)(1.5 s^2 + 35 sG) - (W_l + W_b)sG \tag{5.5.5}$$

where W_b = body weight, N
   W_l = load weight, N

Although this equation does predict metabolic cost of walking over a wider range of speeds than does Equation 5.5.1, the corrections represented by Equations 5.5.2–5.5.4 have not been validated for use with Equation 5.5.5.

Equation 5.5.5 predicts equal metabolic costs of certain combinations of carried load and walking speed. That is, heavier loads are accompanied by slower speeds. Myles and Saunders (1979) investigated the implications of this equation by testing men carrying different loads at different speeds. Their results confirm that the metabolic cost of load-carrying can indeed be predicted by the methods of Pandolf et al. (1977), and that walking speeds can be adjusted to give the same metabolic costs for heavier loads as with lighter loads. However, there is an extra cost to the cardiopulmonary system of the heavier loads: heart rates for the heavier loads were higher despite equal metabolic costs with lighter loads and higher speeds; breathing rates and minute volumes were higher as well. Ratings of perceived exertion[39] were higher for heavier loads, again despite an equal metabolic cost.

---

[39]Ratings of perceived exertion (RPE), also called reported perceived exertion, measure the intensity of work as apparent to the worker. This is a mental perception of work instead of a physiological measurement. It is postulated that RPE reflects feelings of strain derived from the two sources of the working muscles and the cardiopulmonary system, but the scale was originally selected to correspond to heart rate divided by 10 (Goldman, 1978a; Myles and Saunders, 1979).

Radiation and Convection Heat Exchange. Radiation and convection were discussed in Sections 5.2.1 and 5.2.2. That information is relevant here. However, Givoni and Goldman (1972) use a different set of clothing thermal conductance (C_{cl}) values which include the thermal resistance of a still air layer. Thus the thermal resistances of conduction through clothing and convection through the boundary layer of air, as diagramed in Figure 5.2.1, are combined in their equations. Because body movement as well as wind reduces the insulation value of the surrounding still air layer, a correction must be applied whenever air movement is present.

Givoni and Goldman also assumed a mean radiant temperature equal to the air temperature, so that radiation and convection can be combined, and a mean skin temperature of clothed men in hot environments to be 36°C. Their basic convective and radiative heat exchange equation is

$$(q_r + q_c) = (C_{cl}A)(\theta_a - 36) \tag{5.5.6}$$

Correction for wind and relative air movement caused by motion of the body and limbs through the air has been estimated by

$$v_{eff} = v + 0.004(M - 105) \tag{5.5.7}$$

where v_{eff} = effective air speed, m/sec
v = wind speed, m/sec
$(M - 105)$ = total metabolic rate above the resting level, N·m/sec
M = total metabolic rate, which may include all corrections M', M'', and M''', N·m/sec
and tabulated clothing thermal conductance values are multiplied by the "pumping coefficient," which takes values between $v^{0.2}$ and $v^{0.3}$. Table 5.5.2 includes several of these effective C_{cl} values.

Sweating. Required evaporative cooling to maintain body temperature equilibrium is just the sum of the physical heat exchange and net metabolic heat load:

$$E_{req} = M + (q_r + q_c) \tag{5.5.8}$$

where E_{req} = required evaporative cooling, N·m/sec
Evaporative capacity of the environment depends on the water vapor pressure of the air [obtainable from a psychrometric chart and Equation 5.2.59 and the ability of water vapor to pass through the clothing (im)]. Making use of the Lewis relation value developed in Section 5.2.4, evaporative capacity is given by (Givoni and Goldman, 1972; Goldman, 1975)

$$E_{max} = 0.0165 A \, im \, C_{cl} (p_{sk} - p_a) \tag{5.5.9}$$

TABLE 5.5.2 **Effective Properties of Clothing Including Surrounding Air Layer**

Clothing Type	Effective Clothing Thermal Conductance (C_{cl}), N/(sec·°C·m)	Effective im,[a] dimensionless
Shorts	$11.3v_{eff}^{0.30}$	$1.20v_{eff}^{0.30}$
Shorts and short-sleeved shirt	$8.7v_{eff}^{0.28}$	$0.94v_{eff}^{0.28}$
Standard fatigues	$6.5v_{eff}^{0.25}$	$0.75v_{eff}^{0.25}$
Standard fatigues and overgarment	$4.3v_{eff}^{0.20}$	$0.51v_{eff}^{0.20}$

Source: Adapted and used with permission from Givoni and Goldman, 1972.

[a] An error in the original Givoni and Goldman (1972) publication mislabeled this column as im/clo instead of im (Goldman, 1988).

where E_{max} = maximum evaporative heat loss, $N \cdot m/sec$

p_{sk} = vapor pressure of water at the average skin temperature; for $\theta_s = 36°C$, $p_{sk} = 5866\,N/m^2$

p_a = vapor pressure of air, N/m^2

A = body surface area, = $1.8\,m^2$

If the vapor pressure of the air is above the vapor pressure of the skin, condensation appears on the skin, and the heat of condensation is added to the entire body heat load. Fortunately, this is a very rare occurrence.

Sweating effectiveness depends on where sweat evaporates. In hot, dry environments, air water vapor pressure will be low, and the maximum evaporative heat loss able to be supported by the environment (E_{max}) will be very high, far exceeding the required level of evaporative heat loss (E_{req}). Under these conditions, sweat will evaporate at the skin surface and the percentage of wetted skin area will be low. High air water vapor pressures, caused either by humid ambient conditions or by water-impermeable clothing, require higher percentages of wetted skin area in order to satisfy E_{req}. This leads to sweat accumulation which drips from the skin.

Shapiro et al. (1982) developed an empirical equation predicting rate of sweating for fully heat-acclimatized men:

$$\dot{m}_{sw} = 7.75 \times 10^{-6} A E_{req} (E_{max})^{-0.455}, \qquad 50 < (E_{req}/A) < 360; \quad 20 < (E_{max}/A) < 525 \tag{5.5.10}$$

where $\dot{m}_{sw}$ = rate of sweat mass production, kg/sec

The authors compared predictions from this equation with those by others (most notably the predicted four-hour sweat rate, or P4SR) and found good agreement. This equation, however, has a wider range of applicability.

Equilibrium Body Temperature. Experimental testing and insertion of empirical data have yielded the following equation for final rectal temperature for resting or working men (Givoni and Goldman, 1972):

$$\theta_{rf} = 36.75 + 0.004\,M + (0.00217 A_{cl})(\theta_a - 36) + 0.8 \exp [0.0047(E_{req} - E_{max})] \tag{5.5.11}$$

where θ_{rf} = final (equilibrium) rectal temperature, $°C$

Here, the 36.75 equals the equilibrium rectal temperature corresponding to the basal metabolic rate and the net metabolic rate M may include all corrections in M', M'', and M'''. For resting men with a metabolic rate of $105\,N \cdot m/sec$ in an ambient environment of $36°C$, rectal temperature becomes $37.15°C$.

Below an ambient temperature of $30°C$, rectal temperature appears to be independent of the temperature of the environment. Thus equilibrium rectal temperature can be predicted from Equation 5.5.11 for any temperature below $30°C$ (at least down to $15°C$) by assuming an ambient temperature value of $30°C$.

For comfort, rectal temperature must be less than $38.2°C$. There is a 25% risk of heat casualties for unacclimatized men at a rectal temperature of $39.2°C$, a 50% risk at $39.5°C$, and nearly 100% risk at $40°C$ (Goldman, 1975).

5.5.2 Variation of Rectal Temperature with Time

An infinite amount of heat would be required to instantly raise deep body temperature. Time changes in body temperature depend on many environmental and metabolic factors and are usually characterized by a period of no observable change, an almost exponential change, and a final period of equilibrium. There are three distinct conditions which have been analyzed by Givoni and Goldman (1972). Each is considered in turn.

Changes at Rest Under Heat Stress. When climatic conditions are changed during rest, there is an appreciable time during which no detectable change in rectal temperature occurs. This is especially true for an increase in heat stress. The rate of change at first is slow, then accelerates, and finally diminishes while approaching the new equilibrium level. This complex pattern can be described by (Givoni and Goldman, 1972)

$$\theta_r = \theta_{r0} + (\theta_{rf} - \theta_{r0})(0.1)^{0.4^{[(t-1800)/3600]}} \tag{5.5.12}$$

where θ_r = predicted rectal temperature at any time, °C
  θ_{r0} = rectal temperature when the change first occurs in environmental heat stress, °C
  θ_{rf} = final rectal temperature, °C
  t = time, sec

The complex exponent $0.4^{[(t-18000)/3600]}$ allows prediction at changing rates and gives about 1800 sec (30 min) for the initial time lag when the change is only 10% complete. Time t begins when resting begins. When t approaches infinity, θ_r approaches θ_{rf}. It is possible to estimate the initial resting temperature of young, healthy, heat-acclimatized men by (Givoni and Goldman, 1972)

$$\theta_{r0} = 36 + 0.0015\,W \tag{5.5.13}$$

where W = body weight, N
This equation will give only an estimate, however; it will not yield normal variations due to season, time of day, activities of the previous day and night, and emotional influences.

Elevation During Work. Experiments have shown that rectal temperature during work again does not change immediately, and, in fact, shows no influence of the increase in metabolic rate for quite some time. This time lag becomes shorter as the metabolic rate becomes higher. This was expressed in the form (Givoni and Goldman, 1972)

$$t_{dw} = 208,800/M \tag{5.5.14}$$

where t_{dw} = delay time in onset of increase of rectal temperature during work, sec
  M = total metabolic rate, including external work, N·m/sec
During this period of time, rectal temperature continues to follow the pattern determined by the previous work condition. For work which begins after rest, rectal temperature during the time lag should be computed as if the man were still resting (Equation 5.5.12).

Following the time delay, rectal temperature begins to increase with a time constant that varies directly as the total expected rectal temperature change: a small total change in rectal temperature will be completed in a shorter length of time than a larger change. For a time constant of fixed value, the time for the change to be complete does not depend on the total expected rectal temperature increase. Therefore, a variable time constant was proposed:

$$\tau_w = \frac{3600}{2 - 0.5\sqrt{\theta_{rf} - \theta_{r0}}} \tag{5.5.15a}$$

where τ_w = time constant of rectal temperature increase during work, sec
Berlin (1975) reported that Goldman has used an alternate form for τ_w:

$$\tau_w = \frac{3600}{0.5 + 1.5e^{-0.3(\theta_{rf} - \theta_{r0})}} \tag{5.5.15b}$$

Givoni and Goldman indicated that to avoid the possibility that τ_w could become negative under extreme conditions, they calculate τ_w by

$$\tau_w = \frac{1800}{e^{-0.17(\theta_{rf} - \theta_{r0})}} \tag{5.5.15c}$$

Goldman (1988) indicated that the time constant currently is simply restrained from assuming negative values.

Rectal temperature during work, after the initial delay time, can be computed from (Givoni and Goldman, 1972)

$$\theta_r = \theta_{r0} + (\theta_{rf} - \theta_{r0})(1 - e^{-(t - t_{dw})/\tau_w}) \tag{5.5.16}$$

where the time t begins when the work is initiated and the new equilibrium rectal temperature θ_{rf} must be computed from Equation 5.5.11 for the conditions of work.

Recovery After Work. During recovery from work, the body temperature at first continues to climb and then falls toward the resting value predicted by Equation 5.5.11 for resting conditions. The initial rate of rise in body temperature is probably due to local cooling of the skin by vasodilation and sweating. Without the benefit of as much warming as during work, evaporation of accumulated sweat cools the skin below a point at which local reflex action reduces sweating and perhaps even causes vasoconstriction. Residual heat from the muscles is therefore restricted from escaping, and body temperature rises. This occurs during a recovery delay time of

$$t_{dr} = 900e^{-0.5CP} \tag{5.5.17}$$

where t_{dr} = delay time in onset of cooling during recovery, sec
　　　CP = effective cooling power of the environment, N·m/sec

$$CP = 0.015[0.7E_{\max} + (q_r + q_c) - 105] \tag{5.5.18}$$

where $E_{\max}$ = evaporative cooling capacity of the environment, N·m/sec
Here, evaporative cooling has been assumed to be an average of 70% of maximum evaporative capacity. The resting metabolic rate of 105 N·m/sec has been subtracted from evaporative, convective, and radiative heat losses. Combining Equation 5.5.18 with Equations 5.5.8 and 5.5.9 gives

$$CP = 1.73 \times 10^{-4} \, \text{im} \, C_{cl} A(p_e - p_a) - 0.0150 A(\theta_a - 36)C_{cl} - 1.57 \tag{5.5.19}$$

During this delay time t_{dr}, rectal temperature is assumed to rise one-half as rapidly as predicted from Equation 5.5.16 during work. Thus Equation 5.5.16 would be used to calculate rectal temperature at the end of the period of work, the same equation would be used to predict a rectal temperature during the recovery delay time as if work had not ceased, and the actual rectal temperature during the recovery delay time would be the calculated temperature at the end of work plus one-half the difference between temperature during recovery and at the end of work:

$$\theta_r = \theta_{rw} + 0.5(\theta_{rww} - \theta_{rw}) \tag{5.5.20}$$

where θ_r = rectal temperature during recovery delay time, °C
　　θ_{rw} = predicted rectal temperature at the end of working period, °C
　　θ_{rww} = rectal temperature during the recovery period delay time predicted as if working were still continuing, °C

After the initial rectal temperature rise during recovery, cooling begins. This cooling also occurs at a variable rate described by a time constant (Givoni and Goldman, 1972):

$$\tau_r = \frac{3600}{1.5(1 - e^{-1.5CP})} \tag{5.5.21}$$

and rectal temperature during recovery is

$$\theta_r = \theta_{r0} - (\theta_{r0} - \theta_{rf})(1 - e^{-(t - t_{dr})/\tau_r}) \tag{5.5.22}$$

where θ_{r0} is the highest temperature obtained during recovery. It is calculated from Equations 5.5.16 and 5.5.20 assuming a total time in Equation 5.5.16 of the entire time of working plus the entire recovery delay time t_{dr}.

Effect of Acclimatization. Predicted final rectal temperature from Equation 5.5.11 is valid only for acclimatized men. Givoni and Goldman (1973) found that resting rectal temperatures are an average of 0.5°C lower for acclimatized men compared to unacclimatized men. Further, rectal temperature in the heat for working acclimatized men is a maximum of 1.2°C lower than for unacclimatized men (Figure 5.5.1). This acclimatization process occurs over a number of days, with the number of consecutive days of work experience being reduced one-half day for each day missed. Givoni and Goldman (1973) present this correction[40] to Equation 5.5.11:

$$\theta_{rf(\text{unacc})} = \theta_{rf(\text{acc})} + [0.5 + 1.2(1 - e^{-0.5(\theta_{rf(\text{acc})} - 37.15)})]e^{-0.3N} \tag{5.5.23}$$

where $\theta_{rf(\text{unacc})}$ = unacclimatized equilibrium rectal temperature, °C
$\theta_{rf(\text{acc})}$ = acclimatized equilibrium rectal temperature calculated from Equation 5.5.11, °C
N = number of consecutive days work in heat minus half the number of days skipped, days

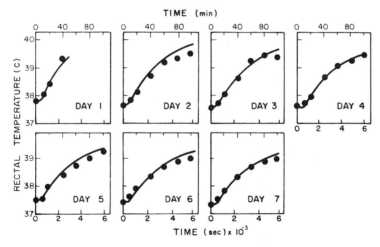

Figure 5.5.1 Acclimatization effects on average rectal temperature response from 24 men walking in 49°C, 20% relative humidity, at 1.6 m/sec. Solid lines are model predictions. Circles are subject data. (Adapted and used with permission from Givoni and Goldman, 1973.)

[40]Givoni and Goldman assumed acclimatization to be complete after 6 days working in the heat. Their equation does not predict acclimatization to be complete until 12–15 days.

Givoni and Goldman (1973) also assumed acclimatization effects to be caused partially by higher circulatory efficiency and partially by a higher sweat production rate. When evaporation is restricted, especially by impermeable clothing, low air movement, or high ambient humidity, sweating acclimatization is of less consequence. To account for this effect,

$$\theta_{rf\,(unacc)} = \theta_{rf\,(acc)} + [0.5 + 1.2(1 - e^{-0.5(\theta_{rf(acc)} - 37.15)})][e^{-0.3N}][1 - e^{-0.005E_{max}}] \quad (5.5.24)$$

where E_{max} is computed according to Equation 5.5.9. With these changes in equilibrium rectal temperature, the time pattern of rectal temperature change occurs in the same manner as before and can be calculated from Equations 5.5.12, 5.5.16, and 5.5.21.

5.5.3 Model Limitations and Performance

This model has been tested by a large number of experiments and found to give good fit (Givoni and Goldman, 1972). In Figure 5.5.2 the agreement between predicted and actual equilibrium rectal temperatures is seen; in the upper left, data produced in studies by Givoni and Goldman (1972) for men resting, walking up a 1% grade, and walking up an 8% grade are compared; in the

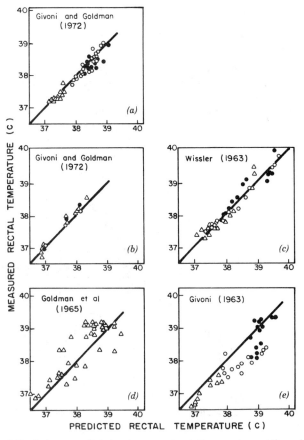

Figure 5.5.2 Correlation between predicted and measured rectal temperatures at the end of work (or resting exposures), from various experimental studies stated in the text. Symbols correspond to different experimental conditions in the original studies. (Used with permission from Givoni and Goldman, 1972.)

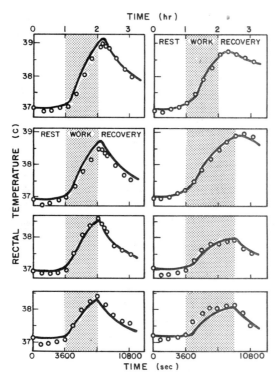

Figure 5.5.3   Comparison of predicted (lines) and measured (circles) patterns of rectal temperature during whole cycles of rest, work, and recovery for a series of tests involving different clothing, ambient temperatures, ambient water vapors, wind speeds, and grades. (Adapted and used with permission from Givoni and Goldman, 1972.)

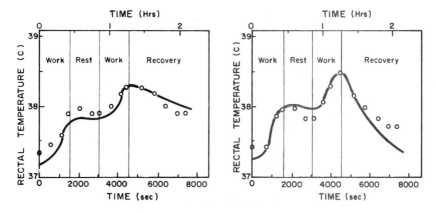

Figure 5.5.4   Comparison between predicted (lines) and measured (circles) patterns of rectal temperature for a whole pattern of work, rest, work, and recovery. The first two work periods and rest periods are identical for the two tests, being conducted at 49°C and ambient water vapor pressure of 2.3 kN/m² (17 mm Hg). The recovery period of the test at the left was conducted at 49°C, whereas the recovery period on the right was at 25°C. (Adapted and used with permission from Givoni and Goldman, 1972.)

middle left, data by Givoni and Goldman (1972) of men in different ambient conditions are compared in the middle right, Figure 5.5.2c is the comparison for data by Wissler (1963) for different rates of step work; in the lower left is the comparison for data by Goldman et al. (1965) for resting men in hot, humid environments; and in the lower right resting and walking data by Givoni (1963) are compared.

The comparison for time patterns of rectal temperature appear in Figure 5.5.3 for a cycle of rest, work, and recovery, and in Figure 5.5.4 for a cycle of work, recovery, work, and recovery. In both figures the period of work is indicated.

The model, however, does have limitations, which are discussed by Goldman (1975). Effects of sex are not known; effects of load carriage are not completely known; sweat inefficiencies due to evaporation inside the clothing and accumulation in some areas have not been incorporated, that is, the model assumes equivalence for all sweating areas, but some areas seem to be more likely to sweat than others; conductance from core to skin has been assumed, but this requires validation; effects of age, physical condition, and motivation have not been adequately studied. This model does not completely describe the physiology of hyperthermia. Nevertheless, for many purposes this model adequately predicts rectal temperature for young, reasonably fit males.

SYMBOLS

A	surface area, m^2
a	constant, °C
B	controller gain for space suit cooling, $°C \cdot sec/(N \cdot m)$
BMR	basal metabolic rate, $N \cdot m/sec$
b	constant, dimensionless
C	thermal conductance, $N \cdot m/(sec \cdot °C)$
CP	cooling power of the environment, $N \cdot m/sec$
C_a	thermal conductance of air layer, $N/(m \cdot sec \cdot °C)$
C_{cl}	thermal conductance of clothing, $N \cdot m/(m^2 \cdot sec \cdot °C)$
C_{sk}	skin conductance, $N \cdot m/(sec \cdot m^2 \cdot °C)$
c	specific heat capacity at constant pressure, $N \cdot m/(kg \cdot °C)$
c_{bl}	specific heat of blood, $\dfrac{N \cdot m}{kg \cdot °C}$
c_v	concentration of water vapor, kg/m^3
D	intensity of diffuse radiation on a horizontal plane, $N \cdot m/(sec \cdot m^2)$
d	diameter, m
E_{max}	maximum evaporative cooling capacity of the environment, $N \cdot m/sec$
E_{req}	required evaporative cooling, $N \cdot m/sec$
F_{1-2}	shape factor from surface 1 to surface, 2, dimensionless
F_{mus}	fraction of work done by muscles, dimensionless
F_{sh}	fraction of total shivering done by muscles, dimensionless
F_{sw}	fraction of sweating command applicable to each skin compartment, dimensionless
F_{th}	skin thermosensory fractional weighting factor, dimensionless
F_{vc}	fraction of vasoconstriction command applicable to each skin area, dimensionless
F_{vd}	fraction of vasodilation command applicable to each skin area, dimensionless
f_c	surface area correction due to clothing, dimensionless
f_{cr}	ratio of γ_d for clothed man to γ_d for nude man, dimensionless
H	latent heat of vaporization of water at body surface temperature, $N \cdot m/kg$
H_t	height, m
h	overall heat transfer coefficient, $N \cdot m/(m^2 \cdot sec \cdot °C)$

h_c	convection coefficient of heat transfer, $\text{N·m/(m}^2\text{·sec·°C)}$
h_d	convection vapor transfer coefficient, $\text{kg/(m}^2\text{·sec)}$
h_r	radiation coefficient of heat transfer, $\text{N·m/(m}^2\text{·sec·°C)}$
h_v	heat transfer coefficient for evaporation, m/sec
h_{va}	heat transfer coefficient for evaporation through air, m/sec
h_{vcl}	heat transfer coefficient for evaporation through clothing, m/sec
h_{vr}	heat transfer coefficient for respiratory evaporation, m/sec
I	intensity of direct sunlight, N/(m·sec)
im	impermeability index of clothing, dimensionless
K_e	Wyndham and Atkins sweating control constant, dimensionless
k	thermal conductivity, N·m/(m·sec·°C)
k_a	thermal conductivity of air, N·m/(m·sec·°C)
k_{cl}	thermal conductivity of clothing, N·m/(m·sec·°C)
L	thickness of conduction layer, m
Le	Lewis number, dimensionless
M	metabolic rate, N·m/sec
M'	metabolic rate corrected for load placement, N·m/sec
M''	metabolic rate corrected for very high loads, N·m/sec
M'''	metabolic rate corrected for running, N·m/sec
M_0	reference, or set point, metabolic rate, N·m/sec
M_A	metabolic rate per unit area, $\text{N·m/(m}^2\text{·sec)}$
M_r	resting metabolic heat load, N·m/sec
M_{tot}	metabolic rate including external work, N·m/sec
m	mass, kg
m_{core}	mass of body core, kg
m_{sk}	mass of skin shell, kg
$\dot{m}$	mass rate of flow, kg/sec
$\dot{m}_{sw}$	mass rate of flow of sweat, kg/sec
$\dot{m}_v$	rate of mass flow of water vapor, kg/sec
N	equivalent number of days of work experience counting toward acclimatization, days
P	permeation index, dimensionless
Pr	prandtl number, $c\mu/k$, dimensionless
p	pressure, N/m^2
p_a	ambient vapor pressure, N/m^2
p_{cl}	vapor pressure at clothing surface, N/m^2
p_{sat}	partial pressure of water vapor, saturated air at the temperature of the evaporation surface, N/m^2
p_{sk}	partial pressure of water vapor, saturated at skin surface temperature, N/m^2
q	rate of heat flow, N·m/sec
q_0	space suit cooling rate at rest, N·m/sec
q_c	convection heat loss, N·m/sec
$q_{c,bl}$	convective heat exchange to blood, N·m/sec
q_{evap}	evaporative heat loss, N·m/sec
$q_{evap,b}$	basal evaporative heat loss from the skin, N·m/sec
$q_{evap,max}$	maximum evaporative heat loss from the skin, N·m/sec
$q_{evap,res}$	evaporative heat loss from the respiratory system, N·m/sec
$q_{evap,sk}$	evaporative heat loss from the skin, N·m/sec
q_k	conduction heat exchange, N·m/sec
q_r	radiation heat transfer, N·m/sec
q_{rdr}	direct radiant heat load, N·m/sec
q_{rdf}	diffuse radiant heat load, N·m/sec

q_{rtr}	terrain reflection heat load, N·m/sec
q_s	solar heat load, N·m/sec
q_{stored}	rate of change of heat storage, N·m/sec
$q_{stored, core}$	rate of heat stored in the body core, N·m/sec
$q_{stored, sk}$	rate of heat stored in the skin shell, N·m/sec
q'''	volume rate of heat generation, N·m/(sec·m^3)
R	gas constant, N·m/(kg·°K)
Re	Reynolds number, $dv\,\rho/\mu$, dimensionless
R_{th}	thermal resistance, °C·sec/(N·m)
R_v	gas constant for water vapor, N·m/(kg·°K)
r	radial coordinate, m
SH	total efferent shivering command, N·m/sec
SW	total efferent sweating command, N·m/sec
s	walking speed, m/sec
T	absolute temperature, °K
t	time, sec
t_{dr}	delay in onset of cooling during recovery, sec
t_{dw}	delay in onset of increase of rectal temperature during work, sec
U	solar heating efficiency factor, dimensionless
V	volume, m^3
VC	total efferent skin vasoconstriction command, dimensionless
VD	total efferent skin vasodilation command, m^3/sec
$\dot{V}$	ventilation rate, BTPS, m^3/sec
$\dot{V}_{bl}$	volume rate of blood flow, m^3/sec
$\dot{V}_{bl,b}$	basal blood flow, m^3/sec
v	air speed, m/sec
v_{eff}	effective air speed, m/sec
W	weight, N
W_{mus}	muscle work rate, N·m/sec
w	fraction of surface wetted by sweat, dimensionless
X	intensity of terrain-reflected radiation on a vertical plane, N·m/(m^2·sec)
y	distance, m
α	thermal diffusivity, m^2/sec
β	ratio of skin shell mass to total body mass, dimensionless
γ_d	fraction of nude subject area which intercepts the direct solar beam, dimensionless
γ_h	fraction of nude surface area facing horizontal, dimensionless
γ_z	fraction of nude surface area facing the zenith, dimensionless
ε	emissivity, dimensionless
η	mechanical efficiency, dimensionless
θ_0	surface temperature, °C
θ_a	air temperature, °C
θ_{bl}	blood temperature, °C
θ_{br}	brain temperature, °C
θ_e	mean environmental temperature, °C
θ_i	temperature at inside surface of conduction layer, °C
θ_{in}	inflow temperature, °C
θ_{out}	outflow temperature, °C
θ_r	predicted rectal temperature at any time, °C
θ_{r0}	initial rectal temperature, °C
θ_{rad}	mean radiant temperature, °C
θ_{res}	effective temperature of the respiratory system, °C

θ_{rf}	final, or equilibrium, rectal temperature, °C
$\theta_{rf(acc)}$	equilibrium rectal temperature for acclimatized men, °C
$\theta_{rf(unacc)}$	equilibrium rectal temperature for unacclimatized men, °C
θ_{rw}	predicted rectal temperature at the end of working period, °C
θ_{rww}	rectal temperature during the recovery delay time predicted as if working were still continuing, °C
θ_{sk}	mean skin temperature, °C
θ_{sk0}	resting skin temperature, °C
θ_{sp}	set-point temperature, °C
θ_{spbr}	brain set-point temperature, °C
θ_{spsk}	skin set-point temperature, °C
θ_{wi}	inlet water temperature for space suit cooling, °C
θ_{wo}	outlet water temperature for space suit cooling, °C
θ_{∞}	bulk fluid temperature, °C
$\dot{\theta}_{wi}$	rate of change of inlet water temperature, °C
$\Delta\theta$	temperature difference, °C
μ	viscosity, kg/(m·sec)
ρ	density, kg/m^3
ρ	reflectivity, dimensionless
ρ_d	water vapor diffusion fraction, dimensionless
σ	Stefan–Boltzmann constant 5.67×10^{-8} N·m/(m^2·sec·°K^4)
τ	clothing transmittance, dimensionless
τ_c	controller time constant, sec
τ_r	time constant for rectal temperature fall during recovery, sec
τ_w	time constant of rectal temperature during work, sec
ϕ	relative humidity as a fraction, dimensionless
ω_a	humidity ratio of surrounding air, kg H$_2$O/kg dry air
ω_{res}	humidity ratio of air saturated at effective respiratory temperature, kg H$_2$O/kg dry air
ω_{sat}	humidity ratio of air saturated at body temperature, kg H$_2$O/kg dry air

REFERENCES

Alexander, R. M. 1980. Mechanics of Walking and Running, in *Perspectives in Biomechanics*, H. Reul, D. N. Ghista, and G. Rau, ed. Harwood, Chur, Switzerland, pp. 355–379.

Anderson, L. B. 1958. Mass Transfer, in *Principles of Heat Transfer*, F. Kreith, ed. International Textbook Co., Scranton, P., pp. 489–519.

Aschoff, J. 1964. Biologishe als Selbsterregte Schwingung [Biological Periodicity as a Self-Stimulated Oscillation]. *Veröff. Arb. Forsch. Landes Nord-Westfallen Natur. Gesellschaftswiss.* **138**: 151–162.

ASHRAE. 1974. Thermal Comfort Conditions, Monograph for Practical Application of ASHRAE Research. *ASHRAE J.* **80**: 90–92.

ASHRAE. 1977. Physiological Principles, Comfort and Health, in *Handbook of Fundamentals*, American Society for Heating, Refrigeration, and Air-Conditioning Engineers, Atlanta, G.A, pp. 8.1–8.36.

ASHRAE. 1981. Thermal Environmental Conditions for Human Occupancy. ANSI/ASHRAE Standard 55-1981.

ASHRAE. 1985. Physiological Principles, Comfort and Health, in *Handbook of Fundamentals*, American Society for Heating, Refrigeration, and Air-Conditioning Engineers, Atlanta, G.A, pp. 8.1–8.32.

Astrand, P. O., and K. Rodahl. 1970. *Textbook of Work Physiology*. McGraw-Hill, New York.

Bahill, A. T. 1981. *Bioengineering: Biomedical, Medical and Clinical Engineering*. Prentice-Hall, Englewood Cliffs, N.J.

Barker, S. B. 1962. Peripheral Actions of Thyroid Hormones. *Fed. Proc.* **21**: 635–641.

Bass, D. E. 1963. Thermoregulatory and Circulatory Adjustments During Acclimatization to Heat in Man, in *Temperature—Its Measurement and Control in Science and Industry*, Part 3, J. D. Hardy, ed. Reinhold, New York, pp. 299–305.

Belyavin, A. J., T. M. Gibson, D. J. Anton, and P. Truswell. 1979. Prediction of Body Temperatures During Exercise in Flying Clothing. *Aviat. Space Environ. Med.* **50**: 911–916.

Benzinger, T. H., C. Kitzinger, and A. W. Pratt. 1963. The Human Thermostat, in *Temperature—Its Measurement and Control in Science and Industry*, Part 3, J. D. Hardy, ed. Reinhold, New York, pp. 637–665.

Benzinger, T. H., and G. W. Taylor. 1963. Cranial Measurements of Internal Temperature in Man, in *Temperature—Its Measurement and Control in Science and Industry*, Part 3, J. D. Hardy, ed. Reinhold, New York, pp. 111–120.

Berenson, P. J., and W. G. Robertson. 1973. Temperature, in *Bioastronautics Data Book*, J. F. Parker, Jr., and V. R. West, ed. NASA, Washington, D.C., pp. 65–148.

Berlin, H. M. 1975. A Computer Program to Predict Heart Rate and Rectal Temperature Response to Work, Environment, and Clothing. Edgewood Arsenal Special Publication ED-SP-75011, Aberdeen Proving Ground, Md.

Birkebak, R. C., C. J. Cremers, and E. A. LeFebrire. 1966. Thermal Modeling Applied to Animal Systems. *J. Heat Transfer* **88**: 125–130.

Blair, J. R., and A. D. Keller. 1946. Complete and Permanent Elimination of Hypothalamic Thermogenic Mechanism Without Affecting the Adequacy of the Heat Loss Mechanism. *J. Neuropath. Exp. Neurol.* **5**: 240–248.

Breckenridge, J. R., and R. F. Goldman. 1971. Solar Heat Load in Man. *J. Appl. Physiol.* **31**: 659–663.

Breckenridge, J. R., and R. F. Goldman. 1972. Human Solar Heat Load. *ASHRAE Trans.* **78**: 110–119.

Brown, A. C. 1966. Further Development of the Biothermal Analog Computer, Aerospace Medical Research Laboratories AMRL-TR-66-197. Wright-Patterson Air Force Base, Ohio.

Brown, G. A., and G. M. Williams. 1982. The Effect of Head Cooling on Deep Body Temperature and Thermal Comfort in Man. *Aviat. Space Environ. Med.* **53**: 583–586.

Brück, K. 1986. Are Non-Thermal Factors Important in the Cutaneous Vascular Response to Exercise? A Proponent's View. *Yale J. Biol. Med.* **59**: 289–297.

Carlson, L. D. 1963. Criteria of Physiological Responses to Cold, in *Temperature—Its Measurement and Control in Science and Industry*, Part 3, J. D. Hardy, ed. Reinhold, New York, pp. 359–362.

Charny, C. K., M. J. Hagmann, and R. L. Levin. 1987. A Whole Body Thermal Model of Man During Hyperthermia. *IEEE Trans. Biomed.* **34**: 375–387.

Charny, C. K., and R. L. Levin. 1988. Simulations of MAPA and APA Heating Using a Whole Body Thermal Model. *IEEE Trans. Biomed.* **35**: 362–371.

Cohen, M. J. 1964. The Peripheral Organization of Sensory Systems, in *Neural Theory and Modelling*, Proceedings of the 1962 Ojai Symposium, R. F. Reiss, ed. Stanford University Press: Stanford, Calif., pp. 273–292.

Colin, J., and Y. Houdas. 1965. Initiation of Sweating in Man After Abrupt Rise in Environmental Temperature. *J. Appl. Physiol.* **20**: 984–989.

Cornew, R. W., J. C. Houk, and L. Stark. 1967. Fine Control in the Human Temperature Regulation System. *J. Theoret. Biol.* **16**: 406–426.

Crosbie, R. J., J. D. Hardy, and E. Fessenden. 1963. Electrical Analog Simulation of Temperature Regulation in Man, in *Temperature—Its Measurement and Control in Science and Industry*, Part 3, J. D. Hardy, ed. Reinhold, New York, pp. 627–635.

Davis, T. R. A. 1963. Acclimatization to Cold in Man, in *Temperature—Its Measurement and Control in Science and Industry*, Part 3, J. D. Hardy, ed. Reinhold, New York, pp. 443–452.

Dodt, E., and Y. Zotterman. 1952a. Mode of Action of Warm Receptors. *Acta Physiol. Scand.* **26**: 345–357.

Dodt, E., and Y. Zotterman. 1952b. The Discharge of Specific Cold Fibres at High Temperatures (The Paradoxical Cold). *Acta Physiol. Scand.* **26**: 358–367.

Fanger, P. O. 1967. Calculation of Thermal Comfort: Introduction of a Basic Comfort Equation. *ASHRAE Trans.* **73**: 111.4.1–111.4.20.

Frye, A. J., and E. Kamon. 1983. Sweating Efficiency in Acclimated Men and Women Exercising in Humid and Dry Heat. *J. Appl. Physiol.* **54**: 972–979.

Fusco, M. M. 1963. Temperature Pattern Throughout the Hypothalamus in the Resting Dog, in *Temperature—Its Measurement and Control in Science and Industry*, Part 3, J. D. Hardy, ed. Reinhold, New York, pp. 585–588.

Gagge, A. P. 1973. A Two-Node Model of Human Temperature Regulation in FORTRAN, in *Bioastronautics Data Book*, J. F. Parker, Jr., and V. R. West, ed., NASA, Washington, D.C., pp. 142–148.

Gagge, A. P., J. A. J. Stolwijk, and Y. Nishi. 1971. An Effective Temperature Scale, Based on a Simple Model of Human Physiological Regulatory Response. *ASHRAE Trans.* **77**: 247–262.

Ganong, W. F. 1963. *Review of Medical Physiology.* (Lange Medical Publications, Los Altos, Calif.

Geankoplos, C. J. 1978. *Transport Processes and Unit Operations.* Allyn and Bacon, Boston, pp. 263–309.

Givoni, B. 1963. Estimation of the Effect of Climate on Man: Development of a New Thermal Index. Building Research Station Research Report to UNESCO, Technion, Haifa, Israel.

Givoni, B. 1969. *Man, Climate and Architecture.* Elsevier, Amsterdam, pp. 42–45.

Givoni, B., and R. F. Goldman. 1971. Predicting Metabolic Energy Cost, *J. Appl. Physiol.* **30**: 429–433.

Givoni, B., and R. F. Goldman. 1972. Predicting Rectal Temperature Response to Work, Environment, and Clothing. *J. Appl. Physiol.* **32**: 812–822.

Givoni, B., and R. F. Goldman. 1973. Predicting Effects of Heat Acclimatization on Heart Rate and Rectal Temperature. *J. Appl. Physiol.* **35**: 875–879.

Givoni, B., and E. Sohar. 1968. Rectal Temperature in the Prediction of Permissible Work Rate in Hot Environments. *Int. J. Biometeorol.* **12**: 41–50.

Goldman, R. F. 1967. Systematic Evaluation of Thermal Aspects of Air Crew Protective Systems, in *Behavioral Problems in Aerospace Medicine*, Conference Proceedings No. 25 of the Advisory Group for Aerospace Research and Development (AGARD), Paris, France.

Goldman, R. F. 1975. Predicting the Effects of Environment, Clothing and Personal Equipment on Military Operations. Paper presented to the Eleventh Commonwealth Defense Conference on Operational Clothing and Combat Equipment, India.

Goldman, R. F. 1978a. Computer Models in Manual Materials Handling, in *Safety in Manual Materials Handling*, C. G. Drury, ed. National Institute of Occupational Safety and Health, Washington, D.C., pp. 110–116.

Goldman, R. F. 1978b. Prediction of Human Heat Tolerance, in *Environmental Stress*, L. J. Folinsbee, J. A. Wagner, J. F. Borgia, B. L. Drinkwater, J. A. Gliner, and J. G. Bedi, ed. Academic Press, New York, pp. 53–69.

Goldman, R. F. 1988. Personal communication.

Goldman, R. F., E. B. Green, and P. F. Iampietro. 1965. Tolerance of Hot, Wet Environments by Resting Men. *J. Appl. Physiol.* **20**: 271–277.

Gosselin, R. E. 1947. Rates of Sweating in the Desert, in *Physiology of Man in the Desert*, E. F. Adolph and associates, ed. Interscience, New York, pp. 44–76.

Greenspan, J. D., and D. R. Kenshalo, Sr. 1985. The Primate as a Model for the Human Temperature-Sensing System. 2. Area of Skin Receiving Thermal Stimulation (Spatial Summation). *Somatosensory Res.* **2**: 315–324.

Grollman, A. 1930. Cardiovascular Reactions to Temperature Changes. *Am. J. Physiol.* **95**: 263–273.

Grucza, R., J.-L. Lecroart, J.-J. Hauser, and Y. Houdas. 1985. Dynamics of Sweating in Men and Women During Passive Heating. *Eur. J. App. Physiol.* **54**: 309–314.

Hales, J. R. S. 1986. A Case Supporting the Proposal that Cardiac Filling Pressure Is the Limiting Factor in Adjusting to Heat Stress. *Yale J. Biol. Med.* **59**: 237–245.

Hammel, H. T., D. C. Jackson, J. A. J. Stolsijk, and J. D. Hardy. 1963. Hypothalamic Temperature in Dog and Monkey and Thermoregulatory Responses to Environmental Factors, Technical Report AMRL-TDE-63-5. Wright-Patterson Air Force Base, Ohio.

Hancock, P. A. 1981. Predictive Validity of a Computer Model of Body Temperature During Exercise. *Med. Sci. Sports Exerc.* **13**: 31–33.

Hanna, L. M., and P. W. Scherer. 1986. A Theoretical Model of Localized Heat and Water Vapor Transport in the Human Respiratory Tract. *J. Biomech. Eng.* **108**: 19–27.

Hardy, J. D. 1961. Physiology of Temperature Regulation. *Physiol. Rev.* **41**: 521–606.

Hardy, J. D., H. T. Hammel, and T. Nakayama. 1962. Observations on the Physiological Thermostat in Homeotherms. *Science* **136**: 636–638.

Hart, J. S. 1963. Physiological Responses to Cold in Nonhibernating Homeotherms, in *Temperature—Its Measurement and Control in Science and Industry*, Part 3, J. D. Hardy, ed. Reinhold, New York, pp. 373–406.

Haymes, E. M., A. L. Dickinson, N. Malville, and R. W. Ross. 1982. Effects of Wind on the Thermal and Metabolic Responses to Exercise in the Cold. *Med. Sci. Sports Exerc.* **14**: 41–45.

Hemingway, A., and D. G. Stuart. 1963. Shivering in Man and Animals, in *Temperature—Its Measurement and Control in Science and Industry*, Part 3, J. D. Hardy, ed. Reinhold, New York, pp. 407–427.

Hensel, H. 1963. Informal Discussion on Thermoreceptors, Symposium on Temperature Acclimation. *Fed. Proc.* **22**: 1156–1166.

Hensel, H., A. Iggo, and I. Witt. 1960. A Quantitative Study of Sensitive Cutaneous Thermoreceptors with C Afferent Fibres. *J. Physiol.* **153**: 113–126.

Hensel, H., and Y. Zotterman. 1951. Quantitative Beziehungen zwischen der Entladung einzelner Kaltefasern und der Temperatur. *Acta Physiol. Scand.* **23**: 291–319.

Hirata, K., T. Nagasaka, A. Hirai, M. Hirashita, T. Takahata, and T. Nunomura. 1986. Effects of Human Menstrual Cycle on Thermoregulatory Vasodilation During Exercise. *Eur. J. Appl. Physiol.* **54**: 559–565.

Hodson, D. A., G. Eason, and J. C. Barbenel. 1986. Modeling Transient Heat Transfer Through the Skin and Superficial Tissue. 1. Surface Insulation. *J. Biomech. Eng.* **108**: 183–188.

Hong, S.-I., and E. R. Nadel. 1979. Thermogenic Control During Exercise in a Cold Environment. *J. Appl. Physiol.* **47**: 1084–1089.

Hwang, C. L., and S. A. Konz. 1977. Engineering Models of the Human Thermoregulatory System—A Review. *IEEE Trans. Biomed. Eng.* **BME-24**: 309–325.

Janský, L., ed. 1971. *Nonshivering Thermogenesis*. Academia, Prague, Czechoslovakia.

Jiji, L. M., S. Weinbaum, and D. E. Lemons. 1984. Theory and Experiment for the Effect of Vascular Microstructure on Surface Tissue Heat Transfer. Part II. Model Formation and Solution. *J. Biomech. Eng.* **106**: 331–341.

Johnson, A. T. 1967. *Measurement and Observations of Hypothalmic Temperature in Poultry*. Unpublished M.S. thesis, Cornell University, Ithaca, N.Y.

Johnson, A. T. 1969. *Thermoreceptor Models*. Unpublished Ph.D. diss., Cornell University, Ithaca, N.Y.

Johnson, A. T., and G. D. Kirk. 1981. Heat Transfer Study of the WBGT and Botsball Sensors. *Trans. ASAE* **24**: 410–417, 420.

Johnson, A. T., and N. R. Scott. 1971. A Computer Model to Analyze and Simulate Thermoreceptor Action. *Trans. ASAE* **14**: 828–836, 840.

Jones, P. R. M., S. Wilkinson, and P. S. W. Davies. 1985. A Revision of Body Surface Area Estimations. *Eur. J. Appl. Physiol.* **53**: 376–379.

Kamon, E. 1984. Advances in Heat Stress Studies, in *Occupational and Industrial Hygiene: Concepts and Methods*, N. A. Esmen and M. A. Mehlman, ed. Princeton Scientific Publishers, Princeton, NJ, pp. 105–122.

Keele, A., and E. Neil. 1961. *Samson Wright's Applied Physiology*. Oxford University Press, London, p. 203.

Keller, A. D. 1963. Temperature Regulation Disturbances in Dogs Following Hypothalamic Ablations, in *Temperature—Its Measurement and Control in Science and Industry*, Part 3, J. L. Hardy, ed. Reinhold, New York, pp. 571–584.

Kenney, W. L., D. A. Lewis, D. E. Hyde, T. S. Dyksterhouse, C. G. Armstrong, S. R. Fowler, and D. A. Williams. 1987. Physiologically Derived Critical Evaporative Coefficients for Protective Clothing Ensembles. *J. Appl. Physiol.* **63**: 1095–1099.

Kirsch, K. A., L. Röcker, H. V. Ameln, and K. Hrynyschyn. 1986. The Cardiac Filling Pressure Following Exercise and Thermal Stress. *Yale J. Biol. Med.* **59**: 257–265.

Kleiber, M. 1975. *The Fire of Life*. Robert E. Krieger Publishing Company, Huntington, N.Y.

Kolka, M. A., W. L. Holden, and R. R. Gonzalez. 1984. Heat Exchange Following Atropine Injection Before and After Heat Acclimation. *J. Appl. Physiol.* **56**: 896–899.

Kreith, F. 1958. *Principles of Heat Transfer*. International Textbook Company, Scranton, Pa.

LeBlanc, J., P. Mercier, and P. Samson. 1984a. Diet-Induced Thermogenesis with Relation to Training State in Female Subjects. *Can. J. Physiol. Pharmacol.* **62**: 334–337.

LeBlanc, J., P. Mercier, and P. Samson. 1984b. Reduced Postprandial Heat Production with Gavage as Compared with Meal Feeding in Human Subjects. *Am. J. Physiol.* **246**: E95–E101.

Lee, J. F., and F. W. Sears, 1959. *Thermodynamics*. Addison-Wesley, London, pp. 317–332.

Libert, J. P., C. Amoros, J. DiNisi, A. Muzet, H. Fukuda, and J. Ehrhart. 1988. Thermoregulatory Adjustments During Continuous Heat Exposure. *Eur. J. Appl. Physiol.* **57**: 499–506.

Lind, A. R. 1963. Tolerable Limits for Prolonged and Intermittent Exposures to Heat, in *Temperature—Its Measurement and Control in Science and Industry*, Part 3, J. D. Hardy, ed. Reinhold, New York, pp. 337–345.

Lipkin, M., and J. D. Hardy. 1954. Measurement of Some Thermal Properties of Human Tissue. *J. Appl. Physiol.* **7**: 212–217.

McMahon, T. A. 1984. *Muscles, Reflexes, and Locomotion*. Princeton University Press, Princeton, N. J., pp. 211–214.

Mende, T. J., and L. Cuervo, 1976. Properties of Excitable and Contractile Tissue, in *Biological Foundations of Biomedical Engineering*, J. Kline, ed. Little, Brown, Boston, pp. 71–99.

Milsum, J. H. 1966. *Biological Control System Analysis*. McGraw-Hill, New York.

Moon, P. H., and D. E. Spencer, 1961. *Field Theory Handbook: Including Coordinate Systems, Differential Equations and Their Solutions*. Springer-Verlag, Berlin.

Morehouse, L. E., and A. T. Miller. 1967. *Physiology of Exercise*. C. V. Mosby, St. Louis.

Morrison, J. B., M. L. Conn, and P. A. Hayes. 1982. Influence of Respiratory Heat Transfer on Thermogenesis and Heat Storage After Cold Immersion. *Clin. Sci.* **63**: 127–135.

Murray, R. W. 1962. Temperature Receptors. *Adv. Comp. Physiol. Biochem.* **1**: 117–175.

Myles, W. S., and P. L. Saunders. 1979. The Physiological Cost of Carrying Light and Heavy Loads. *Eur. J. Appl. Physiol.* **42**: 125–131.

Nagata, H. 1962. Evaporation of Sweat on Clothed Subjects. *Jpn. J. Hyg.* **17**(3): 155–163.

Nakayama, T., and J. S. Eisenman. 1961. Recording of Activity in the Anterior Hypothalamus During Periods of Local Heating. *Fed. Proc.* **20**: 334.

Newman, W. H., and P. P. Lele. 1985. A Transient Heating Technique for the Measurement of Thermal Properties of Perfused Biological Tissue. *J. Biomech. Eng.* **107**: 219–227.

Nielsen, B., and M. Nielsen. 1962. Body Temperature During Work at Different Environmental Temperatures. *Acta Physiol. Scand.* **56**: 120–129.

Nilsson, A. L. 1987. Blood Flow, Temperature, and Heat Loss of Skin Exposed to Local Radiative and Convective Cooling. *J. Invest. Dermatol.* **88**: 586–593.

Nishi, Y., and A. P. Gagge. 1970. Moisture Permeation of Clothing, A Factor Covering Thermal Equilibrium and Comfort. *ASHRAE Trans.* **76**(1): 137–145.

Nishi, Y., and K. Ibamoto. 1969. Model Skin Temperature, An Index of Thermal Sensation in Cold, Warm, and Humid Environments, *ASHRAE Trans.* **75**(2): 94–102.

Nunneley, S. A. 1988. Personal communication.

Nunneley, S. A., D. C. Reader, and R. J. Maldonado. 1982. Head-Temperature Effects on Physiology, Comfort, and Performance During Hyperthermia. *Aviat. Space Environ. Med.* **53**: 623–628.

Pandolf, K. B., B. S. Cadarette, M. N. Sawka, A. J. Young, R. P. Francesconi, and R. R. Gonzalez. 1988. Thermoregulatory Responses of Middle-Aged and Young Men During Dry-Heat Acclimation. *J. Appl. Physiol.* **65**: 65–71.

Pandolf, K. B., B. Givoni, and R. F. Goldman. 1977. Predicting Energy Expenditure with Loads While Standing or Walking Very Slowly. *J. Appl. Physiol.* **43**: 577–581.

Pandolf, K. B., M. F. Haisman, and R. F. Goldman. 1976. Metabolic Energy Expenditure and Terrain Coefficients for Walking on Snow. *Ergonomics* **19**: 683–690.

Pandolf, K. B., L. A. Stroshein, L. L. Drolet, R. B. Gonzalez, and M. N. Sawka. 1986. Prediction Modeling of Physiological Responses and Human Performance in the Heat. *Comput. Biol. Med.* **16**: 319–329.

Panferova, N. E. 1964. O Sutochnom Ritme Funktsii Cheloveka v Usloviyakh Organichennoi Podvizhnosti [The Human Circadian Functional Rhythm Under Conditions of Limited Mobility]. *Fiziol. Zh. SSSR Im. I. M. Sechenova* **50**: 741–746.

Panzner, M., G. Beulich, I. Domschke, H. Hänsgen, and R. Knöner. 1986. Measurements of the Thermal Conductivity of Biological Tissues. *Stud. Biophys.* **113**: 261–266.

Patton, H. D. 1965. Receptor Mechanism, in *Physiology and Biophysics*, T. C. Ruch and H. D. Patton, ed. W. B. Saunders, Philadelphia, pp. 95–112.

Pettibone, C. A., and N. R. Scott. 1974. *Relationship of Temperatures in the Cervical Blood Vessels to Brain Temperatures in Chickens*. ASAE Paper 74-5031, American Society of Agricultural Engineers, St. Joseph, Mich.

Randall, W. C. 1963. Sweating and Its Neural Control, in *Temperature—Its Measurement and Control in Science and Industry*, Part 3, J. D. Hardy, ed. Reinhold, New York, pp. 275–286.

Refinetti, R., and H. J. Carlisle. 1987. A Computational Formula for Heat Influx in Animal Experiments. *J. Therm. Biol.* **12**: 263–266.

Roberts, M. F., and C. B. Wengmr. 1979. Control of Skin Circulation During Exercise and Heat Stress. *Med. Sci. Sports* **11**: 36–41.

Robinson, S. 1963. Circulatory Adjustments of Men in Hot Environments, in *Temperature—Its Measurement and Control in Science and Industry*, Part 3, J. D. Hardy, ed. Reinhold, New York, pp. 287–297.

Rohsenow, W. M., and H. Y. Choi. 1961. *Heat, Mass, and Momentum Transfer*. Prentice-Hall, Englewood Cliffs, N.J., p. 7.

Roller, W. L., and R. F. Goldman. 1967. Estimation of Solar Radiation Environment. *Int. J. Biometeorol.* **11**: 329–336.

Roller, W. L., and R. F. Goldman. 1968. Prediction of Solar Heat Load on Man. *J. Appl. Physiol.* **24**: 717–721.

Saumet, J. L., G. Leftheriotis, A. Dittmar, and G. Delhomme. 1986. Relationship Between Pulse Amplitude and Thermal Exchange in the Finger: The Effect of Smoking. *Clin. Physiol.* **6**: 139–146.

Sawka, M. N., R. R. Gonzalez, and K. B. Pandolf. 1984a. Effects of Sleep Deprivation on Thermoregulation During Exercise. *Am. J. Physiol.* **246**: R72–R77.

Sawka, M. N., K. B. Pandolf, B. A. Avellini, and Y. Shapiro. 1983. Does Heat Acclimation Lower the Rate of Metabolism Elicited by Muscular Exercise? *Aviat. Space Environ. Med.* **34**: 27–31.

Sawka, M. N., N. A. Pimental, and K. B. Pandolf. 1984b. Thermoregulatory Responses to Upper Body Exercise. *Eur. J. Appl. Physiol.* **52**: 230–234.

Scott, N. R., A. T. Johnson, and A. van Tienhoven. 1970. Measurement of Hypothalmic Temperature and Heart Rate of Poultry. *Trans. ASAE* **13**: 342–347.

Seagrave, R. C. 1971. *Biomedical Applications of Heat and Mass Transfer*. Iowa State University Press, Ames.

Segal, K. R., B. Gutin, A. M. Nyman, and F. X. Pi-Sunyer. 1985. Thermic Effect of Food at Rest, During Exercise, and After Exercise in Lean and Obese Men of Similar Body Weight. *J. Clin. Invest.* **76**: 1107–1112.

Shapiro, Y., K. B. Pandolf, and R. F. Goldman. 1982. Predicting Sweat Loss Response to Exercise, Environment, and Clothing. *Eur. J. Appl. Physiol.* **48**: 83–96.

Sheppard, D., and W. L. Eschenbacher. 1984. Respiratory Water Loss as a Stimulus to Exercise-Induced Bronchoconstriction. *J. Allergy Clin. Immun.* **73**: 640–642.

Snellen, J. W., D. Mitchell, and C. H. Wyndham. 1970. Heat of Evaporation of Sweat. *J. Appl. Physiol.* **29**: 40–44.

Soule, R. G., and R. F. Goldman. 1969. Energy Cost of Loads Carried on the Head, Hands, or Feet. *J. Appl. Physiol.* **27**: 687–690.

Soule, R. G., and R. F. Goldman. 1972. Terrain Coefficients for Energy Cost Prediction. *J. Appl. Physiol.* **32**: 706–708.

Stevens, C. F. 1966. *Neurophysiology: A Primer.* John Wiley & Sons, New York.

Stevens, G. L., T. E. Graham, and B. A. Wilson. 1987. Gender Differences in Cardiovascular and Metabolic Responses to Cold and Exercise. *Can. J. Physiol. Pharmacol.* **65**: 165–171.

Stolwijk, J. A. J. 1970. Mathematical Model of Thermoregulation, in *Physiological and Behaviorial Temperature Regulation,* J. D. Hardy, A. P. Gagge, and J. A. J. Stolwijk, ed. Charles C Thomas, Springfield, Ill, pp. 703–721.

Stolwijk, J. A. J. 1971. A Mathematical Model of Physiological Temperature Regulation in Man, NASA Report CR-1855. NASA, Washington, D.C.

Stolwijk, J. A. J., and J. D. Hardy. 1966. Temperature Regulation in Man—A Theoretical Study. *Pflügers Arch.* **291**: 129–162.

Stolwijk, J. A. J., and J. D. Hardy. 1977. Control of Body Temperature, in *Handbook of Physiology, Section 9: Reactions to Environmental Agents,* D. H. K. Lee, ed. Williams & Wilkins, Baltimore, pp. 45–68.

Strogatz, S. H. 1987. Human Sleep and Circadian Rhythms: A Simple Model Based on Two Coupled Oscillators. *J. Math. Biol.* **25**: 327–347.

Tam, H.-S., R. C. Darling, H.-Y. Cheh, and J. A. Downey. 1978. Sweating Response: A Means of Evaluating the Set-Point Theory During Exercise. *J. Appl. Physiol.* **45**: 451–458.

Teitlebaum, A., and R. F. Goldman. 1972. Increased Energy Cost with Multiple Clothing Layers. *J. Appl. Physiol.* **32**: 743–744.

Threlkeld, J. L. 1962. *Thermal Environmental Engineering.* Prentice-Hall, Englewood Cliffs, N.J., pp. 120–209.

Tremblay, A., A. Nadeau, G. Fournier, and C. Bouchard. 1988. Effect of a Three-Day Interruption of Exercise-Training on Resting Metabolic Rate and Glucose-Induced Thermogenesis in Trained Individuals. *Int. J. Obesity* **12**: 163–168.

Van Cott, H. P., and R. G. Kinkade. 1972. *Human Engineering Guide to Equipment Design.* U.S. Government Printing Office, Washington, D.C.

Varène, P. 1986. Computation of Respiratory Heat Exchanges. *J. Appl. Physiol.* **61**: 1586–1589.

Varène, P., L. Ferrus, G. Manier, and J. Give. 1986. Heat and Water Respiratory Exchanges: Comparison Between Mouth and Nose Breathing in Humans. *Clin. Physiol.* **6**: 405–414.

Voit, E. 1901. Über die Grösse des Energiebedarfs der Tiere in Hungerzustande. *Z. Biol.* **41**: 113–154, as cited in Kleiber, 1975.

Wagner, J. A., and S. M. Horvath. 1985. Influences of Age and Gender on Human Thermoregulatory Responses to Cold Exposures. *J. Appl. Physiol.* **58**: 180–186.

Webb, P. 1973. Work, Heat, and Oxygen Cost, in *Bioastronautics Data Book,* J. F. Parker, Jr., and V. R. West, ed. NASA, Washington, D.C., pp. 847–879.

Webb, P., J. F. Annis, and S. J. Troutman. 1968. Automatic Control of Water Cooling in Space Suits, NASA Report CR-1085. NASA, Washington, D.C.

Webb, P., S. J. Troutman, and J. F. Annis. 1970. Automatic Cooling in Water Cooled Space Suits. *Aerosp. Med.* **41**: 269–277.

Weinbaum, S., and L. M. Jiji. 1985. A New Simplified Bioheat Equation for the Effect of Blood Flow on Local Average Tissue Temperature. *J. Biomech. Eng.* **107**: 131–139.

Weinbaum, S., L. M. Jiji, and D. E. Lemons. 1984. Theory and Experiment for the Effect of Vascular Microstructure on Surface Tissue Heat Transfer. Part I. Anatomical Foundation and Model Conceptualization. *J. Biomech. Eng.* **106**: 321–330.

Wenger, C. B. 1986. Non-Thermal Factors Are Important in the Control of Skin Blood Flow During Exercise Only Under High Physiological Strain. *Yale J. Biol. Med.* **59**: 307–319.

Werner, J. 1986. Do Black-Box Models of Thermoregulation Still Have Any Research Value? Contributions of System-Theoretical Models to the Analysis of Thermoregulation. *Yale J. Biol. Med.* **59**: 335–348.

Wissler, E. H. 1963. An Analysis of Factors Affecting Temperature Levels in the Nude Human, in *Temperature—Its Measurement and Control in Science and Industry,* Part 3, J. D. Hardy, ed. Reinhold, New York, pp. 603–612.

Woodcock, A. H. 1962. Moisture Transfer in Textile Systems. *Text. Res. J.* **32**: 628.

Wyndham, C. H., and A. R. Atkins. 1968. A Physiological Scheme and Mathematical Model of Temperature Regulation in Man. *Pflügers Arch.* **303**: 14–30.

Wyndham, C. H., N. B. Strydom, J. F. Morrison, F. D. Dutoit, and J. G. Kraan. 1954. Responses of Unacclimatized Men Under Stress of Heat and Work. *J. Appl. Physiol.* **6**: 681–686.

Yang, W.-J. 1980. Human Micro and Macro Heat Transfer—In Vivo and Clinical Applications, in *Perspectives in Biomechanics*, H. Reul, D. N. Ghista, and G. Rau, ed. Harwood, Chur, Switzerland, pp. 227–311.

Zotterman, Y. 1959. Thermal Sensations. *Handbook of Physiology: Neurophysiology* **1**: 431–458.

Ideas are like rabbits. You get a couple and learn how to handle them, and pretty soon you have a dozen.

—John Steinbeck

Abdomen:
  aorta, 144
  arteries, 131–132, 146
  blood flow, 105, 146
  blood vessel resistance, 105
  capillary resistance, 146
  muscle control, 232
  muscles, 174, 232, 238
  pressure, *see* Intra-abdominal pressure
  skin temperature, 386
  surface area, 386
  sweating, 386
  veins, 144, 146–147
Abdomen–diaphragm, 272
  volume, 279
Abnormal gait, 59
Absolute humidity, 363, 381–383
Absolute temperature and radiation, 362, 372
Absorption of energy, 53
Absorptivity, 373
Acceleration, 31, 53, 56, 61
  and muscle damage, 265
  and muscular efficiency, 265
  and muscular instability, 265
Acclimatization:
  to altitude, 250
  to cold, 416–417
  to cold and heat compared, 417
  to heat, 81, 127, 416, 418, 443
  model of, 127
  period, 131, 416, 443
Acetic acid diffusion constant, 186
Acetoacetate, 9
Acetoacetic acid respiratory quotient, 183
Acetylcholine, *see also* Catecholamines
  during exercise, 24
Achilles tendon, 58
Acidity of blood, 101, 108, 194

Acidosis:
  effect on respiration, 244
  metabolic, 17, 229, 244
ACTH, 10, 24, 418
Actin muscle fibers, 8
Activation factor, *see* Myocardium, activation
  factor
Active optimization process, 268
Active responses to heat, 361, 363
Activity:
  and convection coefficient, 366
  equivalents of foods, 48–49
  level and thermal response, 363
Actomyosin, 8–9
Adaptation to irritants, 238
Adenine, 8
Adenosine, 8
  diphosphate, *see* ADP
  monophosphate, *see* AMP
  triphosphate, *see* ATP
Adenylic acid, *see* AMP
Adequate stimulus, 235, 237, 405
Adiabatic compression of a gas, 278
Adipose tissue, *see* Fatty tissue
Adjoint equations, 152
ADP, 8, 390
Adrenal cortex, 416–417
Adrenal glands, 415
Adrenaline, *see* Epinephrine
Adrenocorticotropic hormone, *see* ACTH
Aerobic capacity, *see* Maximum, oxygen uptake
Aerobic contraction, 8
Aerobic metabolism, 8–9, 24, 183
  contribution to muscle energy demand, 11–12
  efficiency of, 10
  equations, 9
  model of, 21–22
Aerobic threshold, 16–17, 94

Aerosol deposition, 271
Afferent nerves, 231
Afterload, 98
Age, effect on:
  airway resistance, 208, 254
  BMR, 390–391
  blood pressure, 91–92
  body mass, 402
  CO_2 sensitivity, 249
  cold response, 112, 415
  lung volume, 176
  maximum heart rate, 94, 125
  maximum oxygen uptake, 14, 94
  maximum torque, 36
  oxygen response time, 248
  respiratory irritants, 239
  respiratory results, 239
  respiratory sensation, 255
  speed, 5–6, 56
  ventilatory loading, 254
Ainsworth and Eveleigh resistances, 203
Air, 166
  collision diameter, 187
  compliance, *see* Compliance, air
  compression, 212
  conditioning, respiratory, 170
  diffusion volume, 188
  force constant, 187
  gas constant, 180
  as insulator, *see* Insulation, still air
  molecular mass, 180
  movement, respiratory, 174
  physical properties and convection, 365
  resistance during running, 64
  speed and convection coefficient, *see*
    Convection, coefficient and air velocity
  thermal conductivity, *see* Thermal,
    conductivity, of air
Airborne contaminants, 202
Airflow:
  models, 297–298, 771
  pattern, *see* Airflow waveshape
  rate and lung filling, 290
  in respiratory system, 170, 253
Airflow waveshape(s), 166, 175, 219, 232,
    265–266, 280–281, 331
  dimples, 266–267
  optimal, 264, 334–336, 339–340
  and respiratory compliance, 340
  and respiratory flow rate, 338–339
  and respiratory resistance, 339
  rounded corners, 265–266
  sinusoidal, 258, 260, 265–266, 290, 335–336
  square, 290, 333–334
  trapezoidal, 265–266
  triangular, 290
Airplanes, cost of transport, 51–52
Air-supplied masks, 208
Airway(s), *see also* Respiration, airways

angles, 206–207, 283
area, 168, 284–285
area and pressure, 283
branching, 169
cast model, 283
central, 286
collapsible segment, 208
compartments, 275
compliance, *see* Compliance, airway
conductance, 287
contribution to resistance, 208
control, 169, 232
generations, 170
generations and geometric properties, 168, 284
inertance, *see* Inertance, airway
mechanics, 281
muscle control, 232
muscles, 169, 236, 238
narrowing, 209, 230
obstruction, 280
occlusion, 233, 236
opening, 294
peripheral, 286
pressure drop, 282
pressure-flow characteristic, 209–210
resistance, *see* Resistance, airway(s)
segments flow, 207
size and dead volume, 208
transmural pressure, 211
tube characteristic, 212
volume, 279
Alarm, 270
Alcohol:
  diffusion constant, 186
  respiratory quotient, 183
Algebraic equations, 153
Alveolar:
  blood flow, 177
  capillary membrane, 172, 192
  collapse, 171
  compartment, 293–294
  dead volume, 175, 311
  diffusion, 191
  ducts, 168–170, 190
  efficiency, 196
  gas concentration, 191
  hypoxia, 179
  inflation, 171, 175
  membrane, 171–172
  mixing time, 171
  oxygen, 72, 179
  pCO_2 during exercise, 240–241
  pCO_2 and minute volume, 243–245
  pressure, 172, 179, 189, 232
  recruitment, 175
  sacs, 168–169
  size, 170–171
  space, 170, 172, 179, 192, 198, 320–321
  surface area, 169, 192

surface tension, 218, 273
tissue thickness, 171
vasoconstriction, 179
ventilation rate, 177, 229–230, 258, 269, 323, 332
ventilation rate distribution, 178
ventilation volume, 175, 177
volume, 280–281
walls, 169–170
Alveolar air, 72, 189, 197
composition, 181–182, 189, 193
diffusivity, 189
gas pressures, 181–182
Alveolar-arterial CO_2 difference, 193–194, 323
Alveolar-arterial oxygen difference, 193–194
Alveoli, 167–168
Amino acids, 77
oxidation of, 9
Amino acid transport in brain, 228
Ammonia:
collision diameter, 187
diffusion constant, 186
diffusion volume, 188
force constant, 187
gas constant, 180
and hyperventilation, 249
irritation, 239
molecular mass, 180
volume fraction in air, 180
Ammonium chloride acidosis, 244
AMP, 9, 108
Anabolism, 390
Anaerobic contraction, 8
Anaerobic exercise and respiratory quotient, 184
Anaerobic metabolism, 9, 13, 71, 75
and ATP, 9
contribution to muscle energy demand, 11–12, 109
efficiency of, 10
equations, 9
limits to, 10
model of, 22
by respiratory muscles, 26
Anaerobic threshold, 15–17, 94, 229
effect of previous exercise, 16
individual, 17–18
and maximum oxygen uptake, 15
in model, 22
and oxygen uptake, 249
and respiratory exchange ratio, 184
and respiratory response, 241
and training, 15
and ventilation, 250–252
Analog computer, 114
Analog model, 200
Analogy between heat and mass transfer, 381
Anastomoses, *see* Shunts
Anatomic dead volume, 175, 177, 179, 198, 311, 323

Anatomy of respiratory system, *see* Respiration, anatomy
Anesthesia, 230
and occlusion pressure, 233
and respiration, 249
Aneurysm, 112
Anger, 107
Angina pectoris, 98, 112
Angular motion, 43, 47
Aniline diffusion constant, 186
Animal cost of transport, 50–51
Animals:
cardiac output, 96
running speed, 58
walking speed, 46, 58
Ankle, 59
Anoxia, 104, 107, 228
Antagonistic muscles, 394, 401
Antagonistic systems, 101
Antelopes, 52
Anterior hypothalamus, 192, 405. *See also* Hypothalamus, and thermoregulation
Anthropometric studies, 443
Anticipation of work, 128
Anxiety and respiratory responses, 254–255
Aorta, 81, 89, 91, 93, 96, 116
Aortic arch, 100–101, 105, 141, 224, 228
Aortic baroreceptors, 99, 105, 108
Aortic blood flow, 146
Aortic blood volume, 144
Aortic body, 225
Aortic chemoreceptors, 101, 228
Aortic compliance, 144
Aortic inertance, 144
Aortic pressure, 133, 144, 148
Aortic resistance, 144
Aortic valve, 113–115, 122
Apnea, 230, 238
Apneusis, 231
Apneustic center, 231
Apparent viscosity, 86, 88
Appetite, 10, 24, 415
Archimedes, 31
Arctic animals, heat maintenance, 415
Area, of body surface, *see* Body, surface area
Areas of different body parts, 386
Argon:
collision diameter, 187
diffusion volume, 188
force constant, 187
gas constant, 180
molecular mass, 180
volume fraction in air, 180
Arithmetic effect on respiration, 254
Arm(s), 36
arteries, 144
blood flow, 146, 428
capillary resistance, 146
exercise, 93, 109

Arm(s) (*Continued*)
  heat production, 428
  mass, 428
  skin temperature, 386
  surface area, 386, 427
  sweating, 386
  thermal conductivity, 428
  veins, 144, 147
  volume, 427
  weight, 32
Arrhenius equation, 391
Arteries, 81, 93, 131–132
  blood, 96, 143, 198, 224, 267
  blood gas pressures, 181, 228
  blood pressure, 105–107, 114, 122, 144, 323
  blood volume, 81, 144
  carbon dioxide, 193
  chemoreceptor reflex, 107
  chemoreceptors, 107
  compliance, *see* Compliance, arterial
  inertance, *see* Inertance, arterial
  model, 116, 143, 145
  pCO_2, 72, 238–241, 268
  pCO_2 in exercise, 245, 247, 251, 316
  pH, 240, 268, 309, 311
  pO_2, 72
  pO_2 in exercise, 200, 248
  resistance, *see* Resistance, arterial
  weight, 81
Arterial–venous oxygen differences, 77, 97, 103, 109
Arterioconstriction, 104, 409
Arterioles, 74, 81–83, 93, 104, 108, 172, 409
Arteriovenous shunts, *see* Shunts
Artifacts, *see* Noise
Asphalt surface, 66
Aspirin:
  and CO_2 sensitivity, 249
  and nasal resistance, 202
Asthma, 191, 220
Astronauts, 413
Asymptotes, 284
Atelectasis, 253
Athletes:
  heart size, 109
  maximum heart rates, 109
  maximum oxygen uptake, 13
Athletic competition, 2
Athletic records, 2
Atmospheric pressure, 72, 179, 421
ATP, 8–9, 108, 390
  formation:
    aerobic, 9, 11
    equation of, 9
  in liver, 10
  in muscle, 10, 14, 67
  replenishment from creatine phosphate, 9
Atria:
  blood flow, 146
  blood pressure, 144, 147

blood volume, 144
  compliance, 139
  receptors, 100
  systole, 139
  volume, 139
Atrium, 89, 93, 109, 138
Atropine and exercise, 418
Autocorrelation, 330
Autocovariance function, 328
Automobiles, cost of transport, 51–52
Autoregulation of blood flow, *see* Blood, flow, autoregulation
Avogadro's principle, 180
Awareness:
  of metabolic load, 438
  of respiratory loads, 254, 271
Axial streaming of red blood cells, 84

Back:
  bending during walking, 56
  carrying loads, 65–66
  skin temperature, 386
  surface area, 386
  sweating, 386
Backward difference approximation, 149
Banked track, 45
Bantus, 65
Bare skin and shivering, *see* Insulation, still air
Baroreceptor model, 106
Baroreceptors, 100–101, 104–108, 111, 140, 224
Baroreflex, 105
Basal heat production of various segments, 429
Basal metabolic rate, *see* BMR
Basal oxygen consumption, 94
Base excess, 77
Base of support, 32
Bat, 218
Beneken and DeWit cardiovascular model, 131
Benzene diffusion constant, 186
Bernoulli equation, 84, 210
Beta adrenergic receptors, 101
Bicarbonate, *see* Blood, bicarbonate; Brain, bicarbonate
Biceps muscle, 33, 36
Bifurcations, 82, 169, 204, 281
Binary system of gases, 189
Bingham plastic fluids, 78–79
Bioenergetics, 21
Bioengineer, 1, 72, 112, 216, 268
Bioengineering, 1
Biological redundancy, 106, 108
Biological threshold phenomena, *see* Weber-Fechner law
Biomechanics, 53
Birds:
  flying efficiency, 52
  migration, 50
Bison, 52
Black bodies, 373
Bleeding, *see* Hemorrhage

Blood, 72
  acid–base balance, 166
  acidity, 268, 298
  acidity and lactate, 17
  ammonia, 249
  bicarbonate, 17, 73–74, 192, 250, 268, 300
  bicarbonate and metabolic acidosis, 244
  –brain barrier, 228, 251, 304
  buffering, 74, 301
  circulating between compartments, 300, 321
  circulation time, 248
  clots, 412
  coagulation, *see* Blood, clots
  CO_2 concentration, 109
  CO_2 content, 300
  composition, 72, 225
  convection, *see* Convection, blood
  cooling in neck, 409
  density, 369
  dissolved oxygen, 72
  distribution, 81, 103–104
  diversion, 411
  flow:
    autoregulation, 104, 108, 142, 149
    in capillaries, *see* Capillary, blood flow
    control, 82
    distribution, 146, 256
    to head, 81
    in muscles, *see* Muscle, blood flow
    rapid increase, 240
    skin, *see* Cutaneous, blood flow
    after standing, 105
    for various segments, 429, 433
    during work, 13, 81, 145, 410
  gas concentrations, 195, 225, 300
  gases, 73, 192
  glucose, 10, 27, 184
  heat storage, 369
  heat transfer, 369
  hemoglobin oxygen, 72
  inertance, *see* Inertance, blood
  lactate, 11, 13–14, 17, 26, 250
    and aerobic threshold, 17, 250
    and anaerobic threshold, 15–17
    and exercise severity, 250
    model of, 22
  lactic acid, *see* Blood, lactate
  linking compartments, *see* Blood, circulating
    between compartments
  mass, 428
  nitrogen, 73, 300
  O_2 concentration, 109
  one-way conduction, 82
  oxygen-carrying capacity, 17, 72, 300
  pH, 75–76, 108–109, 184
    and anaerobic threshold, 251
    and metabolic acidosis, 244
  plasma, *see* Plasma
  pooling, 105, 147
  pressure, 82, 91–93, 102, 107

  and carotid sinus, 105–106
  and gravity, 107
  and pulmonary capillaries, 172, 177
  pressure control, 24, 83, 99, 104, 111, 140,
    148
  pressure during exercise, 100, 104, 149
  shifting from veins to arteries, 104, 109, 131
  shunts, 82, 173, 179, 193, 198, 310
  sounds, 93
  storage, 82
  thermal properties, 369
  transit time, 74, 173, 194
  venous return, 82
  vessel distention, 84, 112
  vessel resistance, 83, 103
  vessels, 78, 81, 102, 104, 112, 118, 143
  vessel wall effect, 84, 112
  viscosity, 78, 80, 82, 84, 86
  volume, 15, 72, 80–81, 108, 323
  volume in the heat, 416
Blouse thermal conductance, 371
BMR, 366, 390, 421, 440
  contributors to, 390, 392, 398
  depending on body area, 392
  depending on body mass, 392–393
  depending on training, 392
  response to cold, 415
Body:
  acceleration, 38
  a–v oxygen difference, 103
  blood flow, 103
  center of mass, 32, 52–55, 65
    shifting, 33
  core, 369
  fat percentage and cold response, 415
  height, 426
  mass, 103, 362, 401–402, 421, 426, 428
  mass correction to compliance, 217
  mass correction to resistance, 213–214
  oxygen consumption, 103
  parts, weight, 32
  position, *see* Posture
  surface area, 366, 421, 426–427
  surface area correction, *see* Clothing, surface
    area correction factor; Radiation, surface
    area correction
  trunk, weight, 31
  vascular resistance, 103
  velocity, 38
  volume, 427
  water content regulation, 108
  weight, 52, 65
Body temperature:
  effect on BMR, 391
  and gas partial pressures, 180
  and heart rate, 7, 127
  and inhalation, 236
  limit, 26
  and metabolism, 10
  response to heat loss/gain, 361, 436

Body temperature (*Continued*)
  standard pressure, saturated conditions, *see*
    BTPS, conditions
Bohr effect, 75
Bohr equation, 198
Boltzmann constant, 187
Boltzmann radiation constant, *see*
    Stefan-Boltzmann constant
Bone:
  blood flow, 81–82
  blood volume, 81
  elasticity, 42
  energy, 43
  force, 36
  fracture, from jump, 42
  modulus of elasticity, 42
  oxygen consumption, 81
  rupture strength, 42
  weight, 81
Bones and muscles, 33
Boundary layer, surface, 381
Bradycardia, 93, 102, 107–108, 238
Bradykinin, 108
Bradypnea, 230
Brain:
  a–v oxygen difference, 103
  bicarbonate, 229
  body flow, 81–82, 103–105, 225, 246
    and carbon dioxide partial pressure, 307,
      327
    and heat loss, 409
    and oxygen partial pressure, 307
  blood volume, 81, 323
  chemical milieu, 223, 228
  chemoreception, 224, 228
  compartment, 300, 320–321
  contribution to BMR, 392
  environment, 104, 223
  extracellular fluid, 228–229, 232
  heat production, 400, 403, 409
  lesions, 363
  mass, 103, 327, 400
  metabolic rate, 322–323
  motor center, 102
  oxygen consumption, 103–104
  respiratory quotient, 184
  thermal stimulation, 363
  vascular resistance, 103
  weight, 81, 400
Braking a car, 53
Breath-holding, 166, 315
Breathing, *see also* Ventilation
  cycle and gas partial pressures, 193
  and FRC, 175
  synchronized, 166
  waveshape, *see* Airflow waveshape
Breathlessness, *see* Dyspnea
Bricks, 370
Bronchi, 168–170
  air flow, 205

capillary resistance, 146
  entrance length, 205
  mechanical properties, 281, 284
  systemic circulation, 173, 177
Bronchiolar airflow, 205
Bronchiolar entrance length, 205
Bronchiole constriction, 179
Bronchioles, 168–170
Bronchoconstriction:
  and compliance, 216
  from evaporation, 384
  and lung time constant, 220
  and mechanoreceptors, 230
  as resistive loading, 253
  response to chemicals, 239
Bronchodilation and mechanoreceptors, 230
Bronchoreactive drugs, 202
BTPS:
  conditions, 181
  to STPD conversion, 181
Bubble surface tension, 171
Buffer equation:
  for bicarbonate, 74, 229
  for lactate, 250
Buffering of blood, *see* Blood, buffering
Bulk flow of air, *see* Convection, gas flow
Bulk modulus, 277
Bunsen coefficient, 72
Buttocks:
  skin temperature, 386
  surface area, 386
  sweating, 386

Caffeine and respiratory response, 241
Calculus of variations, 337, 341
Caloric equivalent:
  of carbohydrate, 185
  of fat, 185
Caloric value of oxygen consumption, 183, 185,
    222
Calories, in food, 48–49
Calorimeter, 394
Calorimetry, indirect, 185
Calves:
  skin temperature, 386
  surface area, 386
  sweating, 386
Capacitor, 200
Capillary(ies), 15, 74, 81–82, 93, 104
  blood compartment, 320–321
  blood flow, 82, 84, 146, 177
  blood pressures, 91, 93, 146, 177
  blood volumes, 323
  gas partial pressures, 191
  permeability, 82, 108, 147
  resistance, 146
Carbamino hemoglobin CO_2, 73, 77. *See also*
    Carboxyhemoglobin
Carbohydrate, 9–10
  catabolisis and SDA, 393, 397

composition, 183
energy density, 183
metabolism, 183, 247
Carbon dioxide:
  arterial-alveolar difference, 193
  in brain, 228
  capacity of the blood, 73, 195
  cellular, 195
  collision diameter, 187
  concentration in air, 197
  concentration in blood, 109, 173, 195, 199
  concentration and bronchiole constriction, 179
  delivery to lungs, 240, 269
  diffusion, 173, 225
  diffusion constant, 186, 189
  diffusion rate, 192
  diffusion volume, 188
  dissociation curve, 194
  during exercise, 16
  effect(s):
    on heart rate, 223
    on respiration, 232
    on vessel resistance, 149, 418
    on hemoglobin saturation, 74–75
  end-tidal, 240
  fluctuations during breathing cycle, 193
  force constant, 187
  forms in blood, 73–74
  gas constant, 180
  inhalation, 309, 311, 315
  inhaled compared to metabolic, 245–246, 310, 315, 320, 328–329
  irritation, 239
  mass balance, 195, 198–199, 302–303, 305, 321–325
  molecular mass, 180
  oscillations, *see* Oscillations, of pCO_2
  partial pressure in blood, 72–75, 101, 104, 108, 173, 193, 224, 238, 268, 323
  partial pressure chemoreceptors, 224, 226
  partial pressure in lungs, blood, and muscle, 181, 193
  partial pressure and respiratory control, 315
  production, 9, 74, 108, 182, 184, 196, 315
  production rate, 197, 250, 268, 271, 323
    diurnal variation, 202
    during exercise, 240–241
    muscles, compared to mouth, 240
    of neural tissue, 327
  production as respiratory stimulus, 247
  psychophysiological reactions, 222, 224
  reaction constant, 195
  rebreathing, 315
  removal, 71, 74, 190, 196, 298
  respiratory responses, 223–224, 240–245
    equations, 247
  sensitivity, 248–249
  solubility, 195
  storage, 233, 240

  transport, 77
  and vasodilation, 108
  volume fraction in air, 180–182
Carbonic acid, 74, 301
Carbonic anhydrase, 192, 268
Carbon monoxide:
  affinity for hemoglobin, 191
  diffusion volume, 188
  gas constant, 180
  molecular mass, 180
  volume fraction in air, 180
Carboxyhemoglobin, 300
Cardiac blood flow, 121
Cardiac hypertrophy, 91, 109
Cardiac mechanoreceptor reflex, 107
Cardiac output, 27, 77, 82, 94, 103, 148–149, 173, 269, 323
  and carbon dioxide partial pressure, 306
  in cold, 112
  distribution, 146
  in exercise, 96–97, 100, 105, 109
  in heat, 411
  and metabolic rate, 325
  models of, 112, 118
  and norepinephrine, 108
  and oxygen partial pressure, 306
  and oxygen uptake, 195
  and pCO_2 oscillations, 318–319
  while sitting, 94
  after standing, 105
Cardiac power, 98
Cardiopulmonary resuscitation, 230
Cardiovascular system:
  chemical transport, 71
  conflicting demands, 71, 100, 111, 416, 418
  control, 99, 102, 108, 131–132, 148, 223
  dynamics, 109, 111
  fitness, 94
  heat removal, 71
  hypertension, 91
  limits to exercise, 3, 6, 24
  local control, 108
  mechanics, 71, 131
  model, 116, 131
  purpose, 71
  –respiratory interaction, 6, 101, 107–108, 223
  and respiratory similarities, 166, 223, 228
  responses to rapid exercise, 71
Caribou, 52
Carina, 169, 212
Carnot engine, 394
Carotid arteries, 225
Carotid bodies, 7, 99, 224, 268
  blood flow, 225
  and CO_2 removal, 240, 318
  and exhalation, 236
  and hypoxia, 7
Carotid chemoreceptors, 7, 101, 228, 231, 270
Carotid sinus, 100–101, 105, 108

Carotid sinus nerve, 225, 228, 233
  pCO_2 response, 225–226
  pO_2 response, 225–226
Carotid sinus pressure, 105–106, 141, 148
Cartesian coordinates, 84, 368
Cartilage, 168–169
Carts, 66
Casson equation, 79
Cat, 106, 136, 193, 236, 270
Catabolisis, 9, 390, 393
Catecholamines, 24, 107
  effect on blood vessels, 24
  effect on breathing, 24, 254
  effect on carotid chemoreceptors, 108, 228
  effect on exercise, 418
  effect on heat generation, 24, 415
  effect on respiration, 249, 254
Cellular carbon dioxide, 195
Cellular compartment, 320–321
Cellular membrane, 33
Center of mass, body, see Body, center of mass
Central airways, 286
Central blood regulation, 104
Central difference approximation, 149
Central nervous system hyperthermia, 412
Central nervous system metabolism, 409
Central respiratory receptors, see Respiratory,
  chemoreceptors
Central venous pressure, 105, 111, 412
Centrifugal force, 43
Centrifugal separation of blood components, 80
Centripetal force, 43, 55
Cerebellum, 99
Cerebral blood flow, 104–105, 149, 323–325
Cerebral blood vessels, 104, 131–132, 246, 409
Cerebral cortex:
  and cardiovascular control, 101–102
  and respiratory control, 224, 268
Cerebral pCO_2, 246
Cerebral vasoconstriction, see Vasoconstriction,
  cerebral
Cerebrospinal fluid, 228–229, 300–301
  pH, 306, 309, 311
  pH and ventilation, 229–230, 251
Cessation of exercise, 94
  and body temperature, 412
Challenge gas, 191
Check valve, 147
Chemical control of respiration, 224. See also
  Respiration, humoral component
Chemical irritants, 238
Chemical microinjections, 363
Chemical milieu of brain, 223, 228
Chemical responses to exercise, 24
Chemoreceptor(s), 101, 107, 224
  outputs, 238
  sensitivity, see Sensitivity, of chemoreceptors
Chest:
  skin temperature, 386

strapping, 253
surface area, 386
sweating, 386
Chest wall, 167, 173, 253, 271
  compliance, see Compliance, chest wall
  distortion and inspiration, 236
  inertance, see Inertance, chest wall
  resistance, see Resistance, chest wall
  volume–pressure curve, 217
Chicken, 409
  BMR, 392–393
Chilling of face, 107
Chinese lung model, 293
Chloride:
  extracellular, 34
  lost through vomiting, 244
Chronic obstructive pulmonary disease, 191,
  216, 250, 254, 256
Chronotropic effect, 105
Cigarette smoking, 239
Cilia, 168, 239
Cingulate, 102
Circadian rhythm:
  of blood pressure, 418
  of body temperature, 417
  of carbon dioxide production, 202
  of expiratory flow rate, 209
  of hormones, 108
  of lung volume, 202
  of mechanical parameters, 202
  of minute volume, 202
  of respiration, 418
  of respiratory exchange ratio, 202
Circulation:
  pulmonary, see Pulmonary, circulation
  time delay, see Time delay, circulation
Circulatory system model, 116
Clo, 366, 370
Closed loop control, 60, 99, 232, 434
Closing volume, see Residual volume
Cloth emissivity, 373
Clothing, 6, 26–27, 370
  absorbing sweat, 390. See also Sweating,
    ineffective
  adding to metabolic load, 438
  conductance, see Clothing, thermal
    conductance
  effective thickness, 387
  ensemble thermal conductance, 370
  evaporation coefficient, 388
  heat transfer, 364, 422
  permeability, 387
  resistance to water vapor movement, see
    Resistance, of clothing to water vapor
  role in solar heat load, 375–376
  and shivering, see Insulation, still air
  surface area correction factor, 367, 370
  and sweat evaporation, 385
  sweat soaked, 363

thermal conductance, 371, 389
  and absorbed water, 390, 439
  weight, 437
  wetted, 390
Cloud cover, 379–380
Coefficient:
  of determination, 65
  of evaporation, 382, 385, 387–388
  of friction, 43
  of radiation, *see* Radiant heat transfer
    coefficient
  of radiation and convection, *see* Combined
    convection and radiation
Cold-blooded animals, *see* Poikilothermic
  animals
Cold receptors, 403–404. *See also*
  Thermoreceptors
Cold stress, 111. *See also* Thermal, stress
Cold response, 413
Collapse:
  of air passages, 208, 211
  of blood vessels, 147
  of lung, 253
  of respiratory air passages, 147
College students' body mass, 402
Collision diameters, 186
Collision integrals, 188
Combination of mechanical properties, 202
Combinations of components, *see* Mechanical,
  properties combined
Combined convection and radiation, 375,
  410–411, 427, 439
Comfortable metabolic level, 437
Comfort zone, *see* Thermoneutral environment
Common air, 166
Compartments of the lung, *see* Lung,
  compartments
Compass gait during walk, 56
Compensation:
  for partial lung obstruction, 297
  for ventilation/perfusion imbalances, 297
Competition, athletic, *see* Athletic competition
Complementary solution, 241
Compliance, 112, 203, 214
  air, 202
  airway, 201–202, 214
  arterial, 115, 122, 144
  blood vessel, 82
  changes with deep breath, 274
  changes with lung volume, 215
  changes with tidal volume, 274
  chest wall, 201–202, 217
  dynamic, 215–216, 220
  effect on resistance detection, 292
  effect on stretch receptor sensitivity, 230
  exhalation, 215–216
  frequency effect on, 216, 219
  inhalation, 215–216
  loads, 253

lung, 191, 273
lung tissue, 201–202, 212, 216–217, 275, 289
  nonlinear, 273
  parenchymal, 202, 295
  pleural, 275
  reactance of, 219
  respiratory, 202, 215–217, 234, 323, 331, 338
    changes with frequency, 216
    corrected for body mass, 217
    optimal, 267
  specific, 218
  static, 215–216
  venous, 144
  ventricular, 113–115
Compressible gas, 212
Compression, 42
  stress, 42
Concentration boundary layer, 381
Concentric muscular contraction, 53
Condensation, 440
Conductance:
  airway, *see* Airway, conductance
  cell membrane, 405
  definitional conflict, 410
  skin, *see* Thermal, conductance of skin
  thermal, *see* Clothing, conductance;
    Thermal, conductance
Conduction, 361, 364, 368
  analogous to diffusion, 381
  equation, generalized, 368
Conductive zone, respiratory, 169–170
Conductors, 369
Connective tissue:
  blood flow, 81
  contribution to BMR, 392
Conscious awareness:
  of respiration, *see* Awareness, of respiratory
    loads
  of temperature, 405
Conscious responses to heat, 361, 363
Constrained optimization, 333
Conservation:
  of energy, 84, 132, 210
  of mass, 132–133, 196, 269, 298, 301–302, 314,
    321
  of momentum, 84
Conserving energy, 53
Consistency coefficient, 79, 82
Constraints, 61, 63, 337, 341
Contractility, myocardial, *see* Myocardium,
  contractility
Control:
  of airway caliber, 230, 236
  of cardiovascular system, *see* Cardiovascular
    system, control
  closed loop, 60
  criteria for respiration, 270
  of ERV, 236–237
  of exhalation, 236

Control (*Continued*)
  function, 152
  of heart, 99, 102
  of heart rate, *see* Heart rate control
  of heat loss, external, 434
  of inspiration, 231
  loss of, 270
  of nonshivering thermogenesis, 415
  open loop, 60
  optimal, 60
  of pulmonary circulation, *see* Pulmonary,
    circulation, control
  of respiration, 166, 222, 224, 232, 246, 257,
    268, 309
  of respiratory resistance, 236
  of stepping, 60
  of sweating, *see* Sweating, regulatory
  system gain, 106, 310
  of upper airway resistance, 236
Controlled variable:
  cardiovascular, 102
  respiratory, 224
  thermoregulation, 409, 434
Controller:
  equation, *see* Respiration, control equations
  gain, *see* Control, system gain
  stepping, 60
Convection:
  blood, 369, 402
  coefficient, 364–365, 420–421, 427
  coefficient and air velocity, 365–366
  coefficient with activity, 366
  coefficient dependent on other parameters,
    365
  coefficient and metabolic rate, 366
  coefficient and posture, 366
  gas flow, 110, 170, 185, 189
  of mass compared to heat, 370, 390
  respiration, 367–368, 420
  thermal, 361, 364
  water vapor, 370
Convective gas transport, laminar, 190
Convolution integrals, 153
Cooling:
  helmets, 409
  power of the environment, 128, 442
  suit, 434
  water, 434
Coordination of respiratory muscles, 238
Copper, skin manikin, 370, 379, 389
COPD, *see* Chronic obstructive pulmonary
    disease
Core and shell model, 362, 419, 422–423
Coronary blood circulation, 81–82, 84, 103, 112,
    131–132, 142, 146
Coronary capillary resistance, 146
Coronary chemoreceptors, 228
Coronary veins, 146
Cortex, *see* Cerebral cortex

Cost:
  functional, 61, 99, 120, 152, 264, 336
  of transport, 50
Cough, 212, 230, 238
Countercurrent heat exchange, respiratory, 384
Counterflow heat exchange in limbs, 414
Cow BMR, 393
Cranial nerve, *see* Glossopharyngeal nerve
Cranial temperature, *see* Ear drum temperature
Creatine, 9
  from creatine phosphate, 9
  kinase, 9
Creatine phosphate, 9–11, 15, 26
  equation for metabolism, 9
  model of utilization, 21–22
Creep, 79
Critical phase angle for resistance detection,
    291
Cross correlation, 330
Cross-country skiing and thermoregulation, 415
Crouch, 40–41
Crowbar, 34
Cuff, measuring blood pressure, 93
Cushioning of joints, 43
Cutaneous blood flow, 81–82, 103, 410, 421
Cutaneous receptors, 102, 404
Cutaneous vasoconstriction, 111, 149, 413, 421,
    425, 442
  equation, 431
Cutaneous vasodilation, 24, 71, 108, 407, 409,
    421, 442
  equation, 431
Cyclic sweating, 413
Cyclic ventilation in model, 310
Cycling, 2–5, 48–50, 54, 57, 96, 166
  energy by various muscle groups, 431
Cycloid, 61
Cylinder, 91, 426
  coordinates, 368
  model for solar radiation, 377
  thermoregulatory models, 419, 422

Daedalus flight, 27
Dalton's law, 179
Damping ratio, 218
Day/night cycle, *see* Circadian rhythm
Dead volume, *see* Alveolar, dead volume;
    Respiration, dead volume
Dehydration, 27, 412
Delay time, *see* Time delay
Delta function, 125
Density:
  of air in airway, 277, 282
  of blood, 369
  of fat, 369
  of muscle, 369
  of skin, 369
  of tissue, 369
Depolarization, 98

Derivative:
approximation to, 149
of arterial pCO_2, see Oscillations, of pCO_2
response, 100, 227, 230, 269, 341, 404–405
Desert solar load, 380
Detection of resistive loads, see Perception, of
added resistance
Detergent, see Surfactant
Development of vertical force from horizontal,
53
Diabetes, 244
Diaphragm, 147, 167, 173–174, 220, 232–233,
253–254
control, 232
shape, 174
Diastole, 81–83, 89, 92–93, 114
and lung perfusion, 179
Diastolic pressure, 91–93, 108–109, 111
Diatomic oxygen, 72
Dichotomous airway branching, 170
Difference equation, 327
Differential equations, 149, 153, 241, 342, 419
Difficult breathing, see Dyspnea
Diffuse radiation, 375–377, 379–380
Diffusing capacity, see Lung, diffusing capacity
Diffusion, 167, 381
across blood–brain barrier, 302
analogous to conduction, 381
axial and radial, 171
binary mixtures, 186, 279
of carbon dioxide, see Carbon dioxide,
diffusion
coefficient, see Diffusion, constant
constant, 185–186, 381
constants for gases, 186
constant of water, 386
layer thickness, 387
multicomponent mixtures, 189
of oxygen, see Oxygen, diffusion
radial, 190
respiratory, 190
of respiratory gas, 170, 175, 177, 179, 185
of surfactant macromolecules, 273
of water vapor through clothes, 386
Digital computer, 149
Digital filter, 315
Dilatant fluids, 78–79
Dimensional analysis, 46, 95, 278–279, 392
Diode, 119, 131–132, 147
Dipalmitoyl phosphatidyl choline, see
Surfactant
Direct solar radiation, 375–376
Dirt road surface, 66
Discharge frequency, see Neural, firing rate
Discomfort:
and CO_2, 222
during exercise, 26
Disease:
defenses, 71

and pulmonary circulation, 173
and respiratory dead volume, 175
Dispersion coefficient, see Longitudinal
dispersion, coefficient
Dissolved carbon dioxide in blood, 73, 195
Dissolved nitrogen, 73
Dissolved oxygen, 72–73, 195
Dissociation, ionic, see Ionic dissociation
Distance traveled over time, 39
Distensible walls, 147
Distributed parameter model, 112, 117–118
Dithering, 233
Diurnal variations, see Circadian rhythm
Diving, 33
reflex, 101, 107, 230
Dizziness, 242
Dog, 95, 106, 115, 193, 407
BMR, 392–393
Dog-leg of ventilation response, 243–244, 246,
329
Dorsal respiratory neurons, 231–232
DPPC, see Surfactant
Drag, fractional, 4, 52, 64, 84
Drinking water intake, 108
Driving input for respiration, 242
Drugs:
affecting respiration, 249
affecting respiratory mechanical parameters,
202
Dry gas partial pressure, 181
Dry grass surface, 66
DuBois surface area formula, 366–367
Dust irritation, 239
Dynamic compliance, see Compliance, dynamic
Dynamic muscular contraction, 65
Dynamic work, 13, 15, 66
Dyspnea, 230, 254

Ear drum temperature, 406
Eating, 393
Eccentric muscular contraction, 53
ECG, 109
Eddying, 206
Edema, 82, 250
Effective blood perfusion rate of lungs, 199
Effective skin thickness, see Skin, thickness
Effector organs, 104
Efferent fibers, nerve, 102
Efferent nerves, 231, 409
Efficiency:
of aerobic and anaerobic metabolism, 10, 397
of the heart, see Heart, efficiency
of kinetic energy to potential energy
conversion, 41
of muscular exertion, 371
muscle, see Muscle, efficiency
of respiratory muscles, 221–222, 252, 264, 271,
334
of sweating, 388, 413

Effort variable, 113
Egg-laying, *see* Oviposition and hypothalamic
    temperature
E-I transition, *see* Exhalation–inhalation switch
Ejection time, 98
Elastance, 234
Elasticity, 79, 81, 91
    deformation of pulmonary capillaries, 172
    element, muscle, 113
    energy storage, 53, 58, 120, 174
    loading, 253
    load perception, 254
    of lungs, 175, 177
    modulus, 42
    recoil pressure, 214. *See also* Static recoil
        pressure
Elbow, 36
Electrocardiograph (ECG), 109
Electromagnetic radiation, 372
Electromyograph, 59
Electrophrenic stimulation, 234
Elegant experiments, 239
Elephant, 95
Emboli, *see* Blood, clots
Emissivity, 373, 387
    and absorptivity compared, 373
    values, 373
Emotion, 93, 102
    and respiration, 231, 249
    and skin conductance, 409
Emphysema, 191, 220–221
End-diastolic volume, 96
End expiration, 216
End expiratory volume, 232
End inspiration, 216
Endocrine secretions, 101
Endorphins, 24
End-systolic volume, 96, 193
End-tidal air, 175, 197
End-tidal CO_2, 240–241, 251
Endurance, 3–4, 6
    time, *see* Performance, time
    equation, 2
Energy, 9, 17, 21, 38, 53
    absorbed during landing, 42
    absorption, 53
    balance, *see* Conservation, of energy
    chemical, 96
    cost of movement, 47–49
    demands of various activities, 398
    density of fuels, 183
    dissipation, 203
    equivalence of carbohydrate, 185
    equivalence of fat, 185
    equivalence of oxygen utilization, 11, 183,
        185
    expenditure for various activities, 399
    food, 48–49
    of heart beat, 98–99, 118–121

kinetic, 39, 47, 58, 96, 132, 147, 214
    to lift and carry loads, 65
    to maintain transmembrane potential, 33
    of molecular interaction, 187
    optimization, 58–59, 98–99, 118–122, 256–268,
        330–341
    potential, 39, 58, 147, 437
    during running, 57, 64
    sources, 183
    storage, 53, 58, 81, 203, 214
    during walking, 53, 57–59
Engineer, vii
Engineering, vii
Ensemble thermal conductance, 370
Entrance length, 204
Environmental factors, 26, 224
Environmentally reflected radiation, 375–376,
    378–379
Environmental modification, 363
Environmental temperature, mean, *see* Mean,
    environmental temperature
Epicardial receptors, 107
Epiglottis, 175
Epinephrine, *see also* Catecholamines
    and body metabolism, 10, 24
    during exercise, 24
    and glucose regulation, 10
    and vasoconstriction, 108
Epithelial tissue:
    alveolar, 178
    brain, 228
Epithelium, 168
Equilibrium:
    blood oxygen, 74
    cardiovascular, 100
    ionic, 34
    mechanical, 31
    rectal temperature, 436
    thermal, *see* Thermal equilibrium
Equivalent airways resistance, 214
Equivalent dimensions of cylinder, 378
Ergonomics, viii, 65
Errors, *see* Noise
ERV, *see* Expiration reserve volume
Erythrocytes, *see* Red blood cells
Esophageal pressure, 215
Ether diffusion constant, 186
Ethyl alcohol:
    diffusion constant, 186
    respiratory quotient, 183
Ethyl benzene diffusion constant, 186
Ethyl ether diffusion constant, 186
Euler equation, 342
Euler–Lagrange equation, 337, 343
Euphoria and oxygen lack, 242
Eupnea, 230
Evaporation, 361, 364, 381
    coefficient, *see* Coefficient of evaporation
    components, 381

rate for various segments, 430
required, 439
respiratory, 384, 420, 422
site of, 363
skin diffusion, 422
on skin surface, 362–363
of sweat, 362–364, 385, 422, 439. *See also*
    Sweating, regulatory
of sweat by region, 412
Evaporative capacity of environment, 129, 439
Evaporative heat loss, *see* Evaporation,
    respiratory; Evaporation, skin diffusion;
    Evaporation, of sweat
Evolution, 224, 403
Excitement, 107
Exercise:
    airflow waveshape, 265–266, 334
    and airway resistance, 281
    and alveolar air composition, 182, 193
    and alveolar gas fluctuation, 193
    and alveolar inflation, 175
    and ammonia, 249
    and arterial pCO_2, 245–247
    and arterial pO_2, 200
    and blood flow, 82, 96, 109
    and blood lactate, 11
    and blood oxygen content, 199
    and blood oxygen saturation, 194, 200
    blood pressure, 93, 109
    and BMR, 392, 397
    and cerebrospinal pH, 229
    cessation, 240, 250
    and dead volume, 176
    energy sources, 184
    and exhalation time, 236
    and FRC, 175
    gas exchange, 192
    and gas mixing, 184
    heart rate, 94, 107–108, 125
    and heart rate, 240. *See also* Heart rate
    hyperpnea, *see* Hyperpnea
    initial rise in ventilation, *see* Initial rise in
        ventilation
    legs only, 13
    limitation:
        cardiovascular, 3, 6, 13, 71
        long-term, 3, 6. *See also* Sustained work
        respiratory, 3, 6
        thermal, 3, 6
    and lung blood flow, 177, 194
    and lung diffusion capacity, 191–192
    and lung volume, 175–176
    and optimal respiration rate, 260, 264
    and oxygen saturation, 200
    performance, 6
    physiology, vii, 65, 72
    and psychological state, 228
    and pulmonary capillary recruitment, 192, 194
    rate, 26

and respiration, 239, 241
and respiratory dog-leg, 243
and respiratory exchange ratio, 183–184
and respiratory inertial effects, 218
and respiratory muscles, 174
and respiratory ventilation, 224, 239, 241
and SDA, 394
simulation, 315
stimulates diurnal rhythm, 418
stimulation of respiration, 230, 329
stimulation of skin conductance, 411
supine, 13
tests, 109
and thermoregulation, 418
and tidal volume, 175
and ventilation/perfusion, 177, 194
Exercise-induced asthma, 384
Exercising among singers, 176
Exhalation, 107, 147, 174, 231
    active, 175, 326
    affects dead volume, 208
    affects airway resistance, 208
    control, 236
    flow-limiting segment, 287
    limited flow rate, *see* Limiting flow rate
    passive, 175, 214, 219, 258, 331, 334
    resistance, *see* Resistance, exhalation
    Rohrer coefficients, 203
    temperature, 384
    time, 3, 6, 25, 232, 236, 254, 296
    time depending on previous inhalation time,
        236, 254
    time with resistive loading, 254
    unsaturated, 384
    waveshape, 175. *See also* Airflow
        waveshape
Exhalation–inhalation switch, 235, 237
Exhaled carbon dioxide, 197, 242
Exhausting work, 3, 66
Experience, *see* Training
Expiration, *see also* Exhalation
    braking, 236, 238
    center, 231
    flow rate, maximum, 221
    muscles, 232, 253
    pressure, maximum, 221
Expiratory reserve volume, 175–177, 232
    control, 236
    optimal, 267
Expiratory Rohrer coefficients, *see* Rohrer
    coefficients
Expired air:
    composition, 182
    gas pressures, 181
Exponential relationship, 19, 125, 127, 147, 156,
    175, 219, 240–241, 265–266, 295, 306, 334,
    402, 441, 443
External thermoregulation, 433, 435
External work, 52–53, 96, 127, 371, 383

Extracellular compartment, 320–321
Extracellular ions, 33–34, 250
Extravascular fluid, 82

Fahraeus–Lindqvist effect, 84, 88, 112
Familial relationships:
  heart rate, 94
  oxygen uptake, 94
Fasting homeotherms, 392
Fast twitch muscle fibers, 8, 37
Fat:
  catabolisis and SDA, 393, 397
  composition, 183
  metabolism, 183, 247
  tissue blood flow, 411
  tissue mass, 428
  tissue thermal properties, 369
Fatigue, 26
  of sweating, 413
Fatty acids, 244
Fatty tissue:
  blood flow, 81
  blood volume, 81
  energy density, 183
  oxygen consumption, 81
  weight, 81
Fear, 107
Feedback, 60, 99, 232, 236, 246, 317, 403, 407, 434
Feedforward, 60, 246, 310, 317
Feet:
  blood flow, 428
  carrying loads, 65, 437
  heat production, 428
  mass, 428
  during running, 54
  skin temperature, 386
  surface area, 386, 427
  sweating, 386
  thermal conductivity, 428
  volume, 427
  during walking, 54
  weight, 32
Fencing, 33
Fever, 108
  effect on BMR, 391
Fick equation, 185, 386
Fighter planes, 52
Fight or flight reaction, 24
Finite difference techniques, 149
Firing rate, 101, 106
First-in-first-out file, 321
First law of thermodynamics, 394
First-order linear response, 240, 327. *See also*
  Exponential relationship
Fish, 54
Fixed air, 166
Flashner stepping model, 60
Flat black paint, 375
Fliers, 51

Flight, man-powered, 2, 3, 5, 27
Flow:
  behavior index, 79, 82
  rate, *see* Airflow, rate and lung filling; Blood,
    flow
  variable, 113
  velocity, 147
  velocity profile, *see* Velocity, profile
Flow-limiting segment, exhalation, 287
Fluctuations in blood gas pressure, *see*
  Oscillations, of $p\mathrm{CO}_2$
Fluid:
  absorption, 82, 108
  mechanics, 167
  movement through capillary walls, *see*
    Capillary, permeability
  static pressure, 147
Flying, 54
Food, 238, 401
  energy in, 48–49
  ingestion, 393, 415
  metabolism and ventilation, 247
Foot motion, 60
Footwear, thermal conductance, 371
Force:
  amplitude criterion, 262
  balance, 31, 85
  constant, diffusion, 186
  depending on fulcrum, 35
  leg muscles, 40, 46
  source, 113
Force–velocity relationship, 98
Forced convection, 365
Forced exhalation, 211
Forearms:
  skin temperature, 386
  surface area, 386
  sweating, 386
Formation of energy-rich substances, *see*
  Anabolism
Formic acid diffusion constant, 186
Forward difference approximation, 149
Fourier series, 331
Fourier transform, 156
Fox, running speed, 47
Fractional concentration, 196
FRC, *see* Functional residual capacity
Frequency:
  of cilia movement, 239
  effect on compliance, 216, 219
  response, 156
Friction, 43, 44, 50, 84
  between clothing layers, 438
  coefficients for airways, 206
  energy, 43–45
  factor of airways, 283
  pressure loss, 211–212
Fruit puree, 79
Fujihara heart rate model, 125

Fujihara respiratory model, 330
Fulcrum, 31, 34
Fully developed flow, 82–83
Functional residual capacity, 175–177, 202, 215, 233, 297, 314, 323
 change with tidal volume, 314
Functions of respiration, *see* Respiration, functions

Gagge thermal model, 419
Gain, system, *see* Control, system gain
Galloping, 58
Gamma receptors, 101
Gas:
 absorption, 174
 collision diameter, 187
 composition fluctuations, respiration, 182
 concentration in blood, 73
 concentration differences in lungs, 298
 concentration in respiratory system, 296
 constants, 180
 diffusion, 170. *See also* Diffusion
 diffusion constant calculation, 186
 diffusion constants, 186, 189
 diffusion volumes, 188
 distribution in lungs, 286, 293
 exchange through capillaries, 82
 exchange in lungs, 167, 174, 177, 196, 198
 force constants, 187
 fractional concentration, 196
 mixing in airways, 189, 198
 mixing in heart, 193
 mixing in lungs, 176
 movement, *see* Bulk flow of air; Convective gas transport; Gas, transport
 partial pressures:
  in alveolar air, 181
  in arterial blood, 181
  in blood, 73, 104, 181–182
  in expired air, 181
  in inspired air, 181
  in lungs, blood, and muscle, 181
  in mixed venous blood, 181
  in muscle tissue, 181
  in respiration, 179, 181
 transport in conduit, 190
 transport models, 271, 295
 volume fractions in air, 180
Gaseous mixtures, 179–180
Gastric fluid:
 exclusion, 238
 secretion, 184, 244
Gastrocnemius muscle, 394
Gastrointestinal tract:
 blood flow, 81–82, 104
 blood volume, 81
 oxygen consumption, 81
 weight, 81
Gavage, 394

Gender effect:
 on airways resistance, 208
 on blood composition, 72
 on blood gases, 73
 on blood oxygen content, 199
 on blood pressure, 92
 on BMR, 390–391
 on body weight, 391, 401
 on cold response, 112, 415
 on exercise, 4–5
 on heart rate, 94, 109
 on hematocrit, 196
 on hemoglobin mass, 72
 on lifting capacity, 65
 on lung volumes, 176
 on maximum oxygen uptake, 14, 94
 on maximum torque, 37, 39
 on oxygen diffusing capacity, 192
 on respiratory results, 239
 on sweating, 413
 on walking energy, 56
Generalized conduction equation, *see* Conduction, equation, generalized
Generation of heart rhythm, 101
Genetic code, 268
Geometry and conduction equation, 368
Giant squid axon, 405
Givoni and Goldman:
 heart rate model, 127
 rectal temperature model, 437
Glass emissivity, 373
Globe temperature, *see* Mean, radiant temperature
Glomus cells in carotid bodies, 225
Glossopharyngeal nerve, 225, 231–232
Glottis, 169, 175
 air flow, 205, 211
 opening, 236
Glucagon:
 and exercise, 24
 role in glucose regulation, 10
Glucose, 9–10
 in blood, 10
 metabolism, 183
 plasma, 27
 regulation in blood, 10
 released by liver, 10
 transport in brain, 228
Glycerol respiratory quotient, 183
Glycogen, 9–10, 15
 energy density, 183
 metabolism of, equation, 9
 metabolism and metabolic acidosis, 244
 muscle, 26
Glycogenolysis, 24, 184
Glycolysis:
 in muscles, 9, 11
 model of, 21–22
Goat, BMR, 393

Goats, 229–230
Goldman:
  heart rate model, 127
  rectal temperature model, 437
Goose BMR, 392–393
Grams percent units, 245
Graphical determination of minimum, 259
Gravity effect:
  on blood pressure, 105
  on jumping, 41
  on lung volume, 176
  on ventilation/perfusion, 177–178
Gray bodies, 393
Green and Jackman vascular model, 118
Grief, 107
Grodin's respiratory model, 300
Guinea pig, 95
Gut, 256

Haldane effect, 74, 302
Hämäläinen respiratory model, 335
Handcarts, *see* Carts
Hands:
  blood flow, 428
  carrying loads, 65, 437
  heat production, 428
  mass, 428
  skin temperature, 386
  surface area, 386, 427
  sweating, 386
  thermal conductivity, 428
  volume, 427
  weight, 32
Hare, 95
Hats, 409
Haze, 379–380
Head:
  arteries, 144
  blood flow, 81, 131–132, 146, 428
  capillary resistance, 146
  carrying loads, 65, 437
  cooling, 409
  heat loss, 409
  heat production, 428
  mass, 428
  skin temperature, 386
  surface area, 386, 427
  sweating, 386
  thermal conductivity, 428
  veins, 144
  volume, 427
  weight, 32
Health awareness, 176
Heart, 89, 105, 131, 167
  activation oxygen consumption, 98
  a–v oxygen difference, 103
  beginning of life, 71
  beta receptors, 101

blood flow, 81–82, 84, 103. *See also* Coronary,
    blood circulation
blood volume, 81
capillaries, 98
contraction, 89
contraction energy, 124
contraction oxygen consumption, 98
control, 99–102
dilatation, 98
efficiency, 98
energetics, 96
failure, 82
failure simulation, 122, 124
filling, 89–90
gamma receptors, 101
heat production, 402
mass, 103, 400
muscle, *see* Myocardium
oxygen consumption, 81, 98, 103
power output, 98
relaxation oxygen consumption, 98
resting oxygen consumption, 98
stroke volume, 90
vascular resistance, 103
volume, effect of training, 15
weight, 81, 95, 400
Heart rate, 3, 15, 93–94, 107
  acceleration, 94
  and ambient humidity, 128
  and ambient temperature, 127
  athletes, 93
  and body dimensions, 95
  in cold, 112
  control, 101, 105, 140
  during exercise, 6, 14, 16, 24–25, 27, 71, 97,
      100, 105, 108, 111, 125
  effect of CO_2, 223
  effect of temperature, 25, 109, 127
  at exercise onset, 240
  in heat, 108
  increase after standing, 105
  index, 128
  linear with body temperature, 127
  linear with work rate, 94, 109
  and metabolic rate, 128
  and oxygen uptake, 94, 110, 125
  reflex, 107
  resting, 93
  step response, 125
  and temperature, 108, 111
  transient response, 125
  for various activities, 398
Heat:
  accumulation, rate of, 26
  balance, 362, 419, 423, 425. *See also*
      Conservation, of energy
  casualty, 440
  convection analogous to mass convection, 381

dissipation, *see* Heat, removal
effect on heart rate, *see* Heart, rate in heat
energy equivalent to work, *see* First law of
   thermodynamics
exhaustion, 436
generation, 26, 53, 238
loss center, 425. *See also* Anterior
   hypothalamus
loss mechanisms, 236, 364, 409
maintenance, 112
maintenance center, 425. *See also* Posterior
   hypothalamus
production, 363, 390, 392, 396, 415, 436
production of various organs, 400
production of various segments, 429
removal, 53, 71, 111. *See also* Heat, loss
   center, loss mechanisms
storage, 369, 401, 419
storage and blood convection, 403
storage and temperature change, 401
stress, *see* Thermal stress
stroke, 111, 412. *See also* Heat, casualty
Heating air, 170
Heaviside fraction expansion, 155
Heavy work, 3, 189, 265, 397–398
Height of jump, 41
Helicopters, 52
Helium:
   collision diameter, 187
   diffusion volume, 188
   force constant, 187
   gas constant, 180
   molecular mass, 180
   volume fraction in air, 180
Hematocrit, 81, 88, 195–196
   defined, 80
Heme unit, 72
Hemoconcentration, 81
Hemoglobin, 10, 72, 109, 179, 192, 225
   mass in body, 72
   oxygen capacity, 72
   saturation, 73, 75–76, 109, 173, 194, 268
   saturation and respiratory response, 248, 298
   saturation in exercise, 200
   as a weak acid, 74
Hemorrhage, 148
Hen BMR, 392–393
Henderson–Hasselbalch equation, 74, 195, 304
Hepatic vein, 118
Hierarchical control, 60, 267
High blood pressure, *see* Hypertension
High frequency ventilation, 189
High jump, 41
Hill's muscle equation, 136, 395
Hip:
   joint, forces, 36–38
   motion, 60
   during running, 47

during walking, 57
Histamine and vasodilation, 108
Hockey-stick portion of respiratory response,
   see Dog-leg respiratory response
Hodgkin–Huxley equations, 405
Homeostasis, 148, 181, 298
Homeotherms, 392, 403
Horizontal force component, 53
Hormonal control of metabolism, 415
Hormonal response to exercise, 24
Hormones, 107, 390, 409
   and exercise capacity, 418
Horse, 95
   BMR, 392–393
   running speed, 47, 58
Hospital:
   patients, 208
   ventilators, 271
Hot-water faucet, 176
House, 361
Huddling, 363
Human, BMR, 391–393
Humid area solar load, 380
Humidifying air, 170
Humidity ratio, *see* Absolute humidity
Humerus, 36
Humoral agents, 107
Humoral communication, 71
Humoral regulation of respiration, *see*
   Respiration, humoral component
Hunger, 415
Hydraulic analog, of energy processes, 21
Hydrogen:
   collision diameter, 187
   diffusion constant, 186
   diffusion volume, 188
   force constant, 187
   gas constant, 180
   ion concentration, 228, 230
   ions, 74, 250
   ions in brain, 228
   molecular mass, 180
   volume fraction in air, 180
Hydrostatic pressure, 82
Hydroxybutyric acid respiratory quotient, 183
Hyperbolic shape, 284–285, 313, 379, 395
Hypercapnia, 107
   and ERV, 236
   and expiratory braking, 238
   and inhalation, 236
   and occlusion pressure, 233
   and ventilatory load compensation, 254
Hypercapnia–hypoxia interaction, *see*
   Hypoxia–hypercapnia interaction
Hyperpnea, 230, 249, 268, 309, 318, 340
Hypertension, 91, 112, 249
Hyperthermia, 409
Hypertrophy, 91, 109

Hyperventilation, 17, 104, 240
  abolishes initial ventilation rise, 240
Hypocapnia and bronchiole constriction, 179
Hypocapnic vasoconstriction, 104
Hypotension, 107, 238
Hypothalamus:
  and carbohydrate ingestion, 10
  and cardiovascular control, 102, 140
  and hunger, 415
  model, *see* Model, of hypothalamus
  and respiratory control, 224, 231
  and thermoregulation, 403, 405–406, 415
Hypoventilation and second wind, 255
Hypoxia, 98, 112, 172, 179, 224, 309
  and occlusion pressure, 233
  and ventilatory load compensation, 253–254
Hypoxia-hypercapnia interaction, 225, 227,
    243–246, 248, 315
Hypoxic acclimatization, *see* Acclimatization,
    to altitude
Hypoxic respiratory responses, 248
Hysteresis, 218, 274

Ice:
  emissivity, 373
  solar load, 380
Ideal gas law, 179, 202, 383
  and vapors, 179
Illness, 109. *See also* Disease
Impaired breathing, *see* Dyspnea
Impedance, 113
Impermeability index, 389
Impermeable clothing, 389, 434, 440
Impulse work load, 330
Inaccuracy of numerical results, 151
Incompressibility, 134
Incompressible flow, 281
Index of contractility, 120
Indirect calorimetry, 185
Individual anaerobic threshold, 17–18
Inductor, 200
Industrial lifting, 65
Industrial motivation for heat models, 436
Inertance, 112, 203, 218
  abdomen diaphragm, 275
  airway, 201–202, 275
  arterial, 144
  blood, 119, 122, 131, 133, 143
  chest wall, 201–202, 218, 275
  gas, 218, 275
  lower airway, 275–276
  lung tissue, 201–202, 218, 275
  mouthpiece, 275–276
  pressure in lungs, 218
  reactance of, 218
  respiratory, 202, 274
  upper airway, 275–276
  venous, 144

Inert gases, 188, 197
Inertia, 4, 50, 65, 84, 233
  of tissues and air, 258, 261
Inertial pressure, 273
Inert tracer gas, 295
Inferior vena cava, 131–132, 144, 146–147
Inflation receptors, 224
Infrared heat pulses for rats, 363
Ingenious experiments, 239
Inhalation, 93, 107, 174–175, 231
  active component, 234
  affects airway resistance, 208
  affects dead volume, 208
  control, 235
  passive component, 234
  resistance, *see* Resistance, inhalation
  Rohrer coefficients, 203
  time, 232–233, 235, 253, 296
  time/exhalation time ratio, 267
  time with elastic load, 253
  time independent of previous exhalation, 254
  time with resistive load, 254
  waveshape, *see* Airflow waveshape
Inhalation–exhalation switch, 235
Inhaled CO_2:
  and metabolic acidosis, 244
  compared to metabolic CO_2, *see* Carbon
    dioxide, inhaled compared to metabolic
Inhaled gases and respiration, 243
Inhibitory center, 102
Initial rise in ventilation, 230, 239–240,
    318–319, 330
Initial values, 151
Injuries, effects of, 108
Innominate artery, 225
Inotropic effect, 105, 120, 131, 141
Inspiration, *see also* Inhalation
  air heating, 409
  center, 231–232
  control, *see* Control, of inspiration
  duration, *see* Inhalation time
  flow differing from neural signal, 235
  flow rate, 233
    maximum, 221
  muscles, 232, 234, 236, 253, 334, 336
  power criterion, 258
  pressure, 238
    maximum, 221
  reserve volume, 175–177
  Rohrer coefficients, *see* Rohrer coefficients
Inspired air:
  composition, 182
  gas pressures, 181
Instability:
  of muscles, 265
  of numerical solution, 151
Insulation, 361
  of chilled muscles, 415

of clothes, 370
of fat, 415
still air, 363, 369–370, 387, 415, 439
Insulators, 369
Insulin, 10
Integral equations, 150, 153
Interaction:
    between compliance and resistance detection, 292
    between hypercapnia and resistive loads, 254
    of hypoxia and hypercapnia, *see* Hypoxia–hypercapnia interaction
    between hypoxia and resistive loads, 254
    between inspiratioin reflexes, 236
    of pH and pCO$_2$ sensing, *see* pH–pCO$_2$ interaction
    between resistive and elastic loading, 254
    between respiratory and cardiovascular responses, 5, 101, 107, 145, 223, 228
    between respiratory and thermal responses, 6, 236
    between thermoreceptors and mechanical stimuli, 405
Interactions of various stresses, 5
Intercostal muscle(s), 173–174, 220, 232, 236, 238
    control, 232
Intercostal nerves, 236
Intermolecular interactions, 179
Internal work, *see* Physiological work
Interrupter technique, 280
Interstitial fluid, 108–109
    pressure, 82
Interventricular septum, 134
Intestinal arteries, 144, 146, 148
Intestinal blood flow, 146
Intestinal capillary resistance, 146
Intestinal veins, 144, 146
Intra-abdominal pressure, 145, 147, 174
Intracellular ions, 33–34
Intracranial pressure, 104, 107
Intraluminal pressure, 147
Intrapleural space, 167, 174
Intrathoracic pressure, 145, 174
Intraventricular pressure, 98
Intubated animals, 213
Ionic dissociation, 74
Ion permeability, 229
Ions producing transmembrane potential, 33–34
Irritant protection, 230
Irritants, 238
Irritation, 3
    receptors, 224, 230
IRV, *see* Inspiration, reserve volume
Ischemia, 104, 112
Isocapnia, 317, 329
Isometric contraction, 8, 65, 141
Isometric exercise, 98, 109, 395

Isometric pressure:
    of inhalation, 234
    of ventricle, 114
Isopleth, 262
Isothermal compression of gas, 278
Isothermal tissues, 403
Isotonic exercise, 395
Isotropic material, 134
Isotropic response of airways, 284
Isovolume pressure–flow curves, 209–210, 213, 286
IVPF curves, *see* Isovolume pressure–flow curves

Jackson–Milhorn respiratory model, 271
Jacobian matrix, 63, 341
Jet-lag, 418
Jogging, 50
Johnson compliance model, 215
Johnson airways resistance model, 212
Joint cushioning, 43
Joint forces, 36, 37, 43
Joint friction, 43
Joint lubrication, 43
Joint proprioceptors, 230
Jones surface area formula, 367
Jump, vertical, 40, 54
Jumping, 33, 40
    on the moon, 41
Just-noticeable difference, 254, 292
J-valves, 253

Ketone production and metabolic acidosis, 244
Kidney:
    and blood volume control, 108
    a–v oxygen differences, 103
    blood flow, 81–82, 103, 225, 256, 411
    blood volume, 81
    heat production, 400
    mass, 103, 400
    oxygen consumption, 81, 103
    vascular resistance, 103
    weight, 81, 400
Kinematic equations, 61
Kinesiology, 53
Kinetic energy, *see* Energy, kinetic
Knee flexion during walk, 57
Krypton diffusion volume, 188

Lactate:
    muscle, 26
    plasma, 10, 67. *See also* Plasma, lactate
    removal rate, 67, 250
    transport in brain, 228
Lactic acid, 9, 15, 67, 75, 184
    and anaerobic threshold, 17–18
    and metabolic acidosis, 244
    model for formation, 21–22

Lactic acid (*Continued*)
  and oxygen debt, 10, 26
  and vasodilation, 418
Lagrange multipliers, 63, 333, 335, 337, 341, 343
Lagrange's method, *see* Method of Lagrange
Lamb, 193
Lambert flow limitation model, 281
Laminar flow, 82, 203, 210, 283
Laminar resistive pressure loss, 283
Laminar to turbulent transition, 82, 207, 283
Landing phase of walking, 63
Laplace, law of, *see* Law of Laplace
Laplace transform, 154
Larynx, 169, 175, 238, 255
  constriction, 230
  receptors, 230
  resistance, *see* Resistance, larynx
Latent heat, 363, 367
  of vaporization, 381
    of sweat, 385
    of water, 382, 421
Latin, 174
Law of Laplace, 91, 171, 174
Learning stepping motion, 61
Least-squares analysis, 3, 187
LeBas atomic volumes, 187
Leg(s):
  arteries, 131-132, 144, 146
  blood flow, 146, 428
  capillary resistance, 146
  effect on walking efficiency, 54
  exercise, 93, 109
  heat production, 428
  length and walking speed, 46, 56
  mass, 428
  motion, 60
  muscle force, 40
  skin temperature, 386
  surface area, 386, 427
  sweating, 386
  thermal conductivity, 428
  veins, 146-147
  volume, 427
  weight, 32, 45-46
Length-tension:
  inappropriateness, 255, 291
  relationship of muscles, *see* Muscle,
    length-tension relationship
Levator palpebrae superioris muscle, 394
Lever, 31, 34
Levers, classes of, 34, 35
Lewis number, 381
  dependent on air velocity and temperature,
    381-382
Lewis relation between convection and
  evaporation, 383, 421, 439
Lifting:
  body weight, 52, 395

loads, 65
Ligaments, 58
Light activity convection coefficient, 366
Light work, 3, 397-398
Limb(s):
  blood flow, 105
  blood vessel resistance, 105
  movement, 4
  movement and occlusion pressure, 233
  movement stimulates respiration, 230, 240
  weight, 32
Limbic system and respiratory control, 224
Lime, 166
Limiting flow rate, 209-210, 212-213, 265,
  286-287
Limping, 36-38
Lipolysis and metabolic acidosis, 244
Liver, 173
  a-v oxygen differences, 103
  blood flow, 103-104, 108
  heat production, 403
  mass, 103
  oxygen consumption, 103
  synthesis of glycogen from lactic acid, 10
  vascular resistance, 103
Livnat and Yamashiro ventricular model, 118
Load:
  carrying, 32, 65, 437
  heaviness correction, 438
  lifting, *see* Lifting loads
  placement correction, 437
  position, 65, 437
Load-grade-speed trade-off, 438
Lobar bronchi, 168, 170, 212
Lobes of lung, 167, 283, 290, 293
Local cardiovascular control, 108
Local circulation control, 104. *See also* Blood
  flow, autoregulation
Local optimum points, 153
Local tissue oxygen consumption, 104
Logarithmic relationship, 284, 392-393
Log-log plot, 203
Longitudinal dispersion, 190
  coefficient, 190
Long-term effects, 6
Lower airway:
  resistance, *see* Resistance, airway; Resistance,
    lower airway
  volume, 74, 89, 167, 174-175, 276
Lower airways limiting flow, 212
Loss of control, respiratory, *see* Control, loss of
Lumped parameter models, 112, 118,
  200
Lung(s), 74, 89, 167, 174-175, 232
  air distribution, 207
  blood and compliance, 81, 148, 216
  blood volume, 81, 104, 323
  closing volume, *see* Residual volume

compartments, 271, 288, 293–294, 300, 320–321
compliance, *see* Compliance, lung
diffusing capacity, 191, 271
diffusion, 185
filling and emptying, 219–220
fluid, 250
gas distribution, *see* Gas, distribution in lungs
gas mixing, *see* Gas mixing in lungs
inflation receptors, 101, 230
obstruction, 297, 299
perfusion, 175, 177, 239
recoil pressure, 177
resistance, *see* Resistance, lung
resting volume, *see* Resting, volume of lungs
stiffness, 174, 216
stretch receptors, 230
surfactant, *see* Surfactant
time constant, *see* Time constant of the lung
tissue, 167
tissue compliance, *see* Compliance, lung tissue
tissue inertance, *see* Inertance, lung tissue
tissue volume–pressure curve, 217
transfer coefficient, 191
transfer factor, 191
volume, 174, 177, 279, 281, 293
volume diurnal variation, 202
volume effect:
  on airway resistance, 208
  on exhalation, 236–237
  on inhalation, 235
Lutchen gas dynamics model, 293
Lying, blood pressure, 105

Mach number, 212
Magnitude response, 156
Mahutte resistance detection model, 291
Man BMR, 392–393
Margaria bioenergetics model, 21
Mask(s):
  dead volume, 270
  resistance, 270
  respiratory protective, 2, 5, 196, 208, 252–253, 270
Mass:
  balance, *see* Conservation, of mass
  convection analogous to heat convection, 381
  diffusivity, *see* Diffusion constant
  transport, 167
  of various organs, 103
Material balance, *see* Conservation, of mass
Maximum:
  aerobic power, *see* Maximum oxygen uptake
  exercise and respiration, 250
  expiratory flow rate, 221
  expiratory pressure, 220–222
  flow rates, 221
  inspiratory flow rate, 221
  inspiratory pressure, 220–222
  lifting capacity, 65
  minute ventilation, 221
  oxygen uptake, 12, 66, 94, 109
    effect of age, 14
    effect of sex, 14
    effect of training, 14, 26
    and exercise ventilation, 26
    and hemoconcentration, 81
    related to oxygen uptake time constant, 21
    typical, 14
  respiratory power, 221
  respiratory pressures, 221
  sweat cooling, 413
  voluntary contraction, 67
  walking speed, 56
  work, 390
Maxwell's demon, 361
Mean:
  arterial pressure, 323
  blood pressure, 100, 103, 105, 108–109
  blood pressure in cold, 112
  blood pressure set point, 140
  environmental temperature, 371
  radiant temperature, 375, 420, 439
  skin temperature, 370, 420, 439
  squared acceleration, 334
  squared pressure, 265
Measurement artifacts, *see* Measurement, noise
Measurement, noise, 150
Mechanical efficiency, 98
Mechanical equilibrium, 31
Mechanical parameter models, 271
Mechanical properties combine, 202, 217
Mechanical properties of respiratory system, 200, 253
Mechanical stability, 31
Mechanical work, 52–53
Mechanics, definition, 31
Mechanoreceptors, 100, 107, 230, 232, 236, 253
Medium activity convection coefficient, 366
Medulla:
  and cardiovascular control, 99, 101–102, 140
  oblongata chemoreceptors, 224, 228, 231
  and respiratory control, 224, 231–232
Menstrual cycle, 24
Mental activity, strenuous or otherwise, 104
Mesencephalon, 102
Metabolic acidosis, 17, 229, 244, 251, 309
Metabolic CO_2 compared to inhaled, *see* Carbon dioxide, inhaled compared to metabolic
Metabolic cost of air resistance, 64
Metabolic heat production, *see* Heat production
Metabolic rate:
  and cardiac output, 325
  of central nervous system, 409

Metabolic rate (*Continued*)
  and convection coefficient, 366
  and evaporation coefficient, 385
  and heart rate, 438
  and respiratory convection, 367
  and temperature, 392–393
  and temperature time delay, 402
Metabolic state, 196
Metabolism:
  control, 24
  heat effects, 26
  resting, 9, 15
  during walking and running, 58, 66
Metabolite exchange through capillaries, 82
Metabolites, circulating, 107, 184, 240, 268
Met defined, 366
Meteorological data, 379–380
Methanol diffusion constant, 186
Method of Lagrange, 63
Microvessels, 80
Migration of birds and mammals, 50, 52
Military motivation for heat models, 436
Milliequivalence units, 245
Milligrams percent units, 245
Millipedes, 54
Minimization:
  of average muscle pressure, 261
  of energy or power, 58–59
  of inspiratory power, 257–258, 260
  of respiratory power, 265, 271
Minimum cost of transport, 50–51
Minute volume, 175, 177–178, 181
  and CO_2, *see* Carbon dioxide, respiratory
    responses
  during exercise, 239–241, 252
  and O_2, *see* Oxygen, respiratory responses
  with resistive loading, 254
  and respiratory exchange ratio, *see*
    Respiration, exchange ratio and minute
    volume
  response to hemoglobin saturation, 248–249
  of various activities, 398
Mitral valve, 113–114
Mixed venous blood, 96, 194, 198, 321
  gas partial pressures, 181, 193, 315
MOD, *see* Modulo arithmetic
Model(s), 1–2, 59, 112
  of airway dimensions, 283
  airways, 206
  appropriateness, 200
  of baroreceptor action, 106
  of body water content, 108
  cardiovascular, 116
  core and shell, *see* Core and shell model
  expiratory flow limitation, 281
  of gas concentration, 293
  gas transport, 271
  of heart rate thermal response, 127

  of heart rate transient response, 125
  of heart ventricle, 112
  of hypothalamus, 424–425
  lung deformation, 271
  of lung filling, 288
  muscle, 112–113, 136
  muscle mechanics, 113
  of nonNewtonian fluids, 79
  optimization, 118, 257
  power law, 79
  pulmonary vasculature, 271
  of rectal temperature, 437
  of resistance detection, 291
  of respiration, 222
  respiratory, 2, 200
  of respiratory control, 298, 320
  respiratory mechanical, 271, 276
  of respiratory resistance, 213
  solution, 149
  of stepping motion, 59, 62
  of thermal mechanisms, 364, 436
  vascular, *see* Vascular models
  ventricular, *see* Ventricular model
  walking, 54, 59
Moderate work, 3, 265, 397–398
Modulo arithmetic, 326
Modulus of elasticity, 42
Moisture condensation, 170
Molar flux, 186
Molecular diffusion, *see* Diffusion
Moment of inertia, 45, 47
Momentum, 39, 84
Monetary rewards and heart rate, 107
Moody diagram for airways, 206, 283
Moon's gravity, 41
Morphology, 168
Morton bioenergetics model, 21
Motivation and discomfort, 26
Motor cortex, 140
Mouse, 51–52, 95
Mouth:
  breathing, 207
  pressure, 201, 215, 233
  pressure-flow nonlinearity, 203–204
  resistance, *see* Resistance, mouth
Mouthpiece, 275–276
Moving to more benign environment, 363
Mucous, 168, 230, 239
Multicompartment thermoregulation model, 425
Multilevel respiratory control, 267
Muscle(s):
  acceleration, adverse effects of, 265
  aerobic and anaerobic contraction, 9
  anaerobic metabolism, 270
  ATP, 9–10, 15, 26, 67
  blood flow, 24, 74, 81–82, 104, 109, 131
    in exercise, 149
    in heat stress, 411, 418

blood vessels, 105
blood volume, 81
compartment, 310
contraction, 8–9, 34, 37, 65, 82, 90–91, 173, 238
contribution to, 392
depolarization, 34
efficiency, 8, 11, 15, 36, 47, 52, 98, 174, 221, 264, 371, 394, 419
efficiency maximum, 395, 397
efficiency by muscle type, 394
efficiency for negative work, 401
efficiency with work load, 395
elastance, 234
energy consumption, 395
energy expenditure for various body compartments, 431
energy mechanisms, 7–9, 11
energy sources, 183
exertion during walking, 46
fatigue, 26, 37
fibers, 7, 33, 37, 113, 134
force, maximum, 395–396
forces, 36, 41, 46, 52, 60, 114, 136–137, 238, 253, 395
force–velocity relationship, 136, 235, 238, 253, 395
glycogen, 26–27, 184
glycolysis, 9, 26
heart, *see* Myocardium
heat of recovery, 11
heat production, 11, 361, 400, 418
isometric contraction, 8, 65, 141
lactate, 26–27
length–tension relationship, 8, 90, 98, 136, 174, 234, 238, 253, 395–396
mass, 400, 428
maximal voluntary contraction, 67
metabolism, 15, 26, 71
microvasculature, 88
model, *see* Model, muscle
movement and respiration, 240
myoglobin, *see* Myoglobin
negative work, *see* Negative work
nutrient supply, 111
osmotic balance, 9
oxidation processes, 9
oxygen utilization, 73–74, 81, 109, 336
power, maximum, 395–396
pressure, respiratory, 174, 201
production of CO_2, 270
proprioceptors, 230
pumping venous blood, 82, 109
pyruvate, 27
resistance, *see* Resistance, muscle
respiratory, *see* Respiration, muscles
respiratory quotient, 184
resting length, 8, 253, 395
running, 46

shortening rate and tension, *see* Muscle, force–velocity relationship
slow and fast twitch fibers, 8
smooth, 81, 169
sphincter, 82, 436
spindles, 268
stretching, 58
temperature, 26, 109
temperature limiting exercise, 26
tension, 8
thermal properties, 369
tissue gas partial pressures, 181
tone and respiratory compliance, 216
torque, 36, 46, 67
transmembrane potential, 33
in veins, 82
velocity of shortening, *see* Muscle shortening rate
weight, 81, 400
Myocardium, 24, 89, 91, 98, 101, 109, 112–113
activation factor, 136, 142, 148
blood flow in exercise, 149
contractility, 105, 108, 121, 141
contraction force, 136–137, 141
cross-sectional area, 134
energy supply, 142
ischemia, 112, 138
length, 135–136
oxygen consumption, 120, 125
pressures, 114–115
Myoglobin, 10, 15, 74, 313
dissociation, 313
Myosin muscle fibers, 8

Narcotics and occlusion pressure, 233
Nasal air flow, 205
Nasal cavity, 169
Nasal circulatory reflex, 101
Nasal compared to mouth breathing, 384
Nasal to mouth breathing transition, 208, 236
Nasal receptors, 230
Nasal resistance, *see* Resistance, nasal
Natural convection, 365
Natural frequency, 218
Natural frequency of respiratory system, 219
Navier–Stokes equations, 84
Neck blood cooling, 409
Necrosis of tissue, *see* Tissue, necrosis
Negative work, 53, 174, 203, 220, 236, 238, 265, 334, 336, 397, 400, 437
Neocortex, 231
Neon:
    collision diameter, 187
    diffusion volume, 188
    force constant, 187
Nerve(s):
    action potential, 34, 225

Nerve(s) (*Continued*)
  hypothalamic, 425
  transmembrane potential, 34
Nervous impulse, 34, 225
Neural circuits, 231
Neural circuit time, 292
Neural control:
  of heart rate, 101, 109, 131–132
  of inspiration, 235
  of respiration, 224–226, 230, 326. *See also*
    Respiration, neural component
Neural discharge frequency, *see* Neural firing,
  rate
Neural firing:
  rate, 225–226, 233, 404–405
  rate variability, 233
Neural oscillator, 292
Neural output, *see* Neural firing, rate
Neurogenic origin of respiratory response, 240,
  268
Neuromuscular junction, 34
Neuron, *see* Nerve
Neurotic individuals, 254
Newtonian fluids, defined, 79
Newton's Second Law, 39
Nicotine causing vasoconstriction, 418
Night/day cycle, *see* Circadian rhythm
Nitrogen:
  collision diameter, 187
  concentration, 297–299
  diffusion constant, 189
  diffusion volume, 188
  excretion, 183, 185
  force constant, 187
  gas constant, 180
  mass balance, 197, 303–304
  molecular mass, 180
  partial pressure(s), 181
    in blood, 73
    in lungs, blood, and muscle, 181
  role in pulmonary function measurement, 193
  volume fraction in air, 180, 182
  washout maneuver, 297–299
Nitrous oxide:
  collision diameter, 187
  diffusion volume, 188
  force constant, 187
Noise, 150
Nonlinear:
  airway resistance, 213, 289
  compliance, 216, 273, 289
  vascular resistance, *see* Resistance, nonlinear
    vascular
  ventilatory response, 251
Nonlinearities, 112, 153, 187, 203, 218, 226,
  241–242, 248
NonNewtonian fluids, 79, 82, 210
Nonprotein RQ, 184–185

Non-shivering thermogenesis, *see* Heat,
  production
Noradrenaline, *see* Norepinephrine
Norepinephrine, 108. *See also* Catecholamines
  during exercise, 24
Nose breathing, 207–208, 236
No slip condition, 87
Nucleic acid, 8
Nucleus parabrahialis medialis, 236
Nude body heat loss, 361
Nude surface area, *see* Body, surface area
Numerical integration, 151
Numerical solution, 149
Nutrient supply by blood, 111

Objective function, 61
Oblate spheroids, 419
Obstructive pulmonary diseases, 191, 297
Occlusion pressure, 233
  and resistive loading, 254
Ockham's Razor, 1
Ohm's law, 361
Onset of exercise, 230, 240
Open loop control, 60, 106
Opponeus pollicis muscle, 394
Optimal control, 60
Optimal exhalation resistance, 257, 270
Optimal trajectories, 61
Optimization, 151, 299
  of airflow waveshape, 331
  of breathing, 257, 330
  of cardiac power, 99, 118
  cost functionals, *see* Cost, functional
  of power during walking, 58
  of respiratory power, 118, 166, 333
  of respiratory pressure, 260
  of vascular sizes, 118
Oral cavity, 169
Organic acid anions, 33–34
Oscillation(s), 218, 230
  daily, *see* Circadian rhythm
  instability, 151
  of $p\mathrm{CO_2}$, 238, 240, 270, 315, 317, 319
  of pendulum, 45
  of sweating, 413
Osmotic balance, 9
Osmotic pressure, 82
Otis, Fenn, and Rahn respiratory model, 258
Overall heat transfer coefficient, 375
Overdamped system, 218
Overland running, 64
Overshoot, 107, 404
Oviposition and hypothalamic temperature,
  409
Oxygen:
  carrying capacity of blood, 72–73, 109
  collision diameter, 187
  combined with hemoglobin, 72–73

concentration and alveolar vasoconstriction, 179
concentration in blood, 109, 173, 195
consusmption, *see* Oxygen, uptake
content of blood, definition, 72
cost:
    of breathing, 221
    of respiratory muscle work, 264
    of running, 64
debt, 10, 19, 26, 184
    maximum, 15
delivery to tissues, 96, 104, 170
deprivation, 242
diffusion, 173, 192
diffusion constant, 186, 189
diffusion rate, 194
diffusion volume, 188
dissociation curves, 74–76
effect on vessel resistance, 149
–energy production conversion, 11
excess intake due to oxygen debt, 11
fluctuations during breathing cycle, 193
force constant, 187
gas constant, 180
lack, *see* Hypoxia
mass balance, 196, 199, 303–305
molecular mass, 180
partial pressure:
    in blood, 72–73, 75–77, 96, 101, 104, 108
    in the heart, 121
    in lungs, blood, and muscle, 181, 193
    and respiratory control, 315
partial pressure chemoreceptors, 225–226
respiratory responses, 240, 243, 248
saturation, *see* Hemoglobin, saturation
sensitivity, 248, 249
storage, 240, 313
supply, 71, 190, 195
transfer between hemoglobin and myoglobin, 313
transport, 11, 71, 128, 193–194
unavailable to muscles, 166
uptake, 13–14, 81, 103–104, 183, 195, 268
    and alveolar gas composition, 193
    and alveolar size, 170
    and blood oxygen content, 199
    of brain, 104
    and cardiac output, 109, 195
    dead time of, 21, 171
    during exercise, 16, 19, 64–65, 97, 110, 240–241
    dynamics, 19
    energy equivalence, 183, 185
    and heart rate, 94
    kinetics, 19–20
    model of processes, 21–22
    and optimality, 264
    and oxygen diffusing capacity, 192

of respiratory muscles, 256, 264
and STPD conditions, 181
and temperature, 392–393
as thermoregulatory signal, 434
time constant of, 21
of various activities, 398
volume fraction in air, 180, 182
Oxygenated blood, 77
Oxyhemoglobin, 77, 225. *See also* Hemoglobin
Oxymyoglobin, 10

Pacemaker cells, 231
Pain, 107
    and respiration, 231, 255
    suppression, 24
Paint emissivity, 373
Panic, 271
Panting, 236
Pants thermal conductance, 371
Papillary muscle, 136
Parabolic response, 335
Parabolic velocity profile, 83
Paradoxical discharge of cold receptors, 404
Parallel blood vessels, 414
Parallel components, combination of, *see* Mechanical, properties combine
Parasympathetic nervous system, 101, 105
Parenchymal compliance, *see* Compliance, parenchymal
Parrot, 50
Parsimony, principle of, 1
Partial pressure, definition, 72
Partial pressures of blood gases, 73, 75–76, 104
Particular solution of differential equation, 240
Passive exhalation, 174
Passive heat loss, 361
Passive limb movement, 240
Passive responses to heat, 361
Pathogenic causes of metabolic acidosis, 244
Pause, respiratory, 181
pCO_2, *see* Carbon dioxide, partial pressure
Péclet number in respiratory system, 190
Pedaling, 166
Pelvic rotation during walk, 57
Pelvic tilt during walking, 57
Pelvis:
    during walking, 57
    lateral displacement during walking, 57
Pencil, 34
Pendelluft, 290, 293
Pendulum, 45
Perception:
    of added resistance, 254, 291
    of lung volume, 254
    of metabolic loads, 438
Perceptive changes and CO_2, 222
Performance:
    functional, *see* Cost, functional

Performance (*Continued*)
  index, 61
  time, 2–4, 6, 12
    and oxygen uptake, 15, 66
    and physiological limits, 2–3
    and work intensity, 2–3
    type of metabolism, 11
Perfusion, 104, 175. *See also* Ventilatory
    perfusion
Peribronchial pressure, 281
Periodic nervous discharge, 231
Peripheral airways, 286
Peripheral resistance, *see* Vascular resistance
Peripheral respiratory receptors, *see*
    Respiration, chemoreceptors
Permeability of capillaries, 108
Permeation index, 387–388
Persistence, 271
pH, *see* Acidity, of blood; Hydrogen, ion
    concentration; Hydrogen, ions
  of brain, 224
  chemoreceptors, 224
  compared to pCO_2 respiratory contribution,
    244
  definition, 74
  effect on hemoglobin saturation, 74, 76
  effect on ventilation, 229–230, 243–244, 268
  shifts in blood and brain, 229
Pharynx:
  air flow, 205
  muscles, 238
Phase angle, 156, 241, 290
  and resistance detection, 291
Phasic response, *see* Derivative response
Phosphagen, *see* Creatine phosphate
Phosphocreatine, *see* Creatine phosphate
Phosphorylation, 184
pH–pCO_2 interaction, 225, 227–228
Phrenic nerve, 232–233
Physical fitness, seasonal, 109
Physical work, *see* External work
Physics:
  applied to living systems, 31
  of movement, 31
Physiological work, 98
Physiologic dead volume, *see* Respiratory, dead
    volume
Physiologist, 112
Physiology, 268
Pig BMR, 392–393
Pigeon, 54
Pinching of veins, *see* Collapse, of blood vessels
Piston, 173
  pump, 89
Plantar flexion during walking, 57
Plasma, 72, 74, 82, 84
  carbon dioxide, 195, 268
  concentrations, units of, 245

diffusion, 171–172, 179, 192
  glucose, 27
  lactate, 10, 67
  layer, 86
  oxygen, 72, 74, 109, 171, 195
  shift, 80
  volume, 27, 80–81, 111
Plaster emissivity, 373
Platelets, 108
Pleura, 174, 253
Pleural cavity, 293–294
  volume, 229
Pleural membrane, 174
Pleural pressure, 201, 271–272, 281
  and airway opening, 208
  distribution, 207, 286
Plywood, 370
Pneumotaxic center, 231–232, 236
Pneumothorax, 174, 253
pO_2, *see* Oxygen, partial pressure
Poikilothermic animals, 403
Poiseuille flow, 83, 279, 283
Poiseuille pressure compared to real, 283
Poisson probability distribution, 225
Pole vault, 41, 54
Polymerization of glucose, 184
Pons:
  and cardiovascular control, 101–102
  and respiratory control, 224, 231–232, 236
Pontryagin maximum principle, 121, 151
Position of load, *see* Load, position
Positive displacement pump, 84
Positive-pressure masks, 253
Positive-pressure ventilation, 208
Posterior hypothalamus, *see* Hypothalamus,
    and thermoregulation
Postinspiratory braking of diaphragm, 253
Posture:
  and blood pressure, 93, 105
  and cardiac output, 94
  and convection coefficient, 365–366
  and hypothalamic temperature, 409
  and lung blood flow, 177
  and lung volumes, 176
  and proprioceptors, 230
  and pulmonary blood volume, 173
  and radiation surface area, *see* Radiation,
    surface area correction
  and respiratory muscles, 238
  and respiratory work, 220, 253
  and venous return, 91
  and ventilation/perfusion ratio, 177
Potassium, intracellular, 33–34, 405
Potential energy, *see* Energy, potential
Potentiation, 292
Poultry, *see* Chicken; Goose, BMR; Hen, BMR
Power:
  of flight, 50–51

law model, 79
minimization, 58
output of heart, 98
of running, 57-58
of walking, 57
Prandtl number and convection, 365
Precapillary sphincter muscles, 82
Predicted four hour sweat rate (P4SW), 440
Preload, 91, 98, 108, 267
Pressure:
  balance, 113, 116, 118-119, 133, 138, 143, 200,
    232, 272, 275, 281, 288, 291, 294, 332
  demand mask, 253
  elastic, see Elasticity, recoil pressure; Static
    recoil pressure
  energy, 96
  gradient, 282
  intracranial, see Intracranial pressure
  loading, 253
  loss:
    in laminar flow, 82
    at mouth, 214
    due to resistance, 203
    in turbulent flow, 83
  respiratory system, 200-201
  saturation, see Saturation, pressure for water
    vapor
Pressure-flow nonlinearities, 203-204
Pressure-volume curve for respiratory system,
    see Volume-pressure curve, for respiratory
    system
Prolate spheroids, 419
Prolonged exercise, 26
Proprioceptors, 224, 230, 268
Propyl benzene diffusion constant, 186
Prostaglandins, 108
Prostanoids, 24
Protein:
  catabolisis and SDA, 393
  composition, 183
  metabolism, 183, 244
  SDA unaffected by activity, 396
Pseudoplastic fluids, 78-79
Pseudorandom binary sequence, 330
Psychological factors in fatigue, 27, 222
Psychological state, exercise, and respiration,
    228
Psychophysiological effects of CO_2, 224, 242
Psychrometric chart, 363, 382, 439
Puberty, effect on blood pressure, 91-93
Pulmonary:
  arterial blood, 173
  artery, 89, 93
  blood:
    flow, 81, 177
    transit time, 173
    volume, 81, 144, 173, 194
  capillary(ies), 171-172, 192

resistance, 146
volume, 173
chemoreflex, 238
circulation, 81, 89, 93, 131-132, 172. *See also*
    Ventilatory perfusion
  blood pressures, 144, 172, 177
  chemoreceptors, 228
  compliance, 144
  control, 172
  gas exchange, 175
  inertance, 144
  oxygen consumption, 81
  resistance, 144
effective compartment, 198. *See also* Gas,
    exchange in lungs
function tests, 193, 197, 201, 297
  for musicians, 176
gas exchange, *see* Gas, exchange in lungs
hypertension, 230
interstitial edema, 250
perfusion, *see* Ventilatory perfusion
resistance, definition, 203
shunt, 77
system weight, 81
vasculature models, 271
venous blood, 173
venous blood pressure, 93
Pulsatile flow, 83, 90
Pulsatile pressure, 101, 106
Pulse pressure, 141, 238
Pumping coefficient, 439
Pumps, 89
Pyrogens, 363
Pyruvic acid, 9
  respiratory quotient, 183

Q_{10}, *see* Van't Hoff equation
Quadripedal animals, 58
Quanta of time, 326
Quicksand, 79

Rabbit, 95
  BMR, 392-393
Race and BMR, 391
Race-related lung volume differences,
    176
Race walking, 2-5, 54, 56
Radial frequency, 156
Radiant heat transfer coefficient, 374-375,
    420-421, 427
Radiant temperature, mean, *see* Mean, radiant
    temperature
Radiation, 361, 364, 372-373
  between two bodies, 374
  coefficient, *see* Radiant heat transfer
    coefficient
  shape factor, 372
  solar, *see* Solar, heat load

Radiation (*Continued*)
  surface area correction, 375–376, 421
  wavelength, 372
Radius (bone), 36
Rain forest solar load, 380
Ramp work rate, 330
Rat, 95, 363
Rat splat, 54
Rate:
  of change of arterial pCO_2, *see* Oscillations,
    of pCO_2
  of change of pressure, 100
  response, *see* Derivative, response
Ratings of perceived exertion, 438
Ratio of inhalation time to exhalation time,
    see Inhalation, time/exhalation time ratio
Reaction constant for carbon dioxide, *see*
    Carbon dioxide, reaction constant
Reactance, 219
Reclining, 105. *See also* Supine blood pressure
Reclining energy expenditures, 47–49
Recoil pressure, *see* Lung, recoil pressure
Recovery from work, 67, 239, 250
Recruitment of sweating, *see* Sweating,
    recruitment
Rectal temperature, 3, 6, 25, 250, 406, 436. *See
    also* Body temperature; Temperature
  in heat, 441
  limit, 26
  during recovery from work, 442
  during work, 441
Rectangular waveshape, *see* Square-wave
    response
Recumbent cardiac output, 95
Red blood cells, 72, 77, 80, 84, 88, 171–172, 179,
    192, 268
Reduced blood, 77
Reflected solar radiation, 375–376
Reflection of incident radiation, 374
Reflectivity, 373
Reflexes, 102, 105, 238
Regression, statistical, 3, 187
Regulation of blood pressure, *see* Blood,
    pressure control
Regulators, 107
Relaxation pressure, 215
Renal blood flow in exercise, 149
Renal output, 108
Repolarization, 98
Residual volume, 175–177, 208, 215, 278, 314
Resistance, 112, 203
  abdomen–diaphragm, 274–275
  airway(s), 201–202, 207, 211, 278, 320
    affected by cigarette smoking, 239
    affected by exercise, 280
    affected by lung volume, 208, 265, 278, 294
    affected by pleural pressure, 208
    children, 208

  optimal, 267
  upper lung compared to lower lung, 283
  at wave speed, 282
  women, 208
arterial, 144
arteriole, 82
blood vessels, 81–82
capillary, *see* Capillary, resistance
chest wall, 201–202, 204, 207, 275
clothing, 370
of clothing to water vapor, 390, 422
conduction, 369
convection, 365
detection, *see* Perception, of added resistance
evaporation heat loss, 385, 387, 389–390
exhalation, 208, 211, 287
external, 211
glottis, 207
inhalation compared to exhalation, 207
larynx, 204, 207
load detection, *see* Perception, of added
    resistance
loading, 253–254
  effect on CO_2 response, 254
  effect on occlusion pressure, 254
loading during exercise, 254
lower airways, 204, 207, 276, 289
lung tissue, 201–202, 207, 275
mouth, 203–204, 207, 236
mouthpiece, 208, 276
muscle, 115
nasal, 202, 204, 207, 236
nonlinear vascular, 147
perception of, *see* Perception, of added
    resistance
peripheral, *see* Vascular resistance
pharynx, 240
power, 259
pressure, 273
pulmonary, 204, 207
pulmonary and respiratory, defined, 203
radiation, 374
respiratory, 191, 202–203, 207, 234, 323, 331,
    338
  control of, 236
respiratory convection, 368
respiratory corrected for body mass, 213–214
in respiratory disease, 254
and respiratory efficiency, 222
and respiratory work, 221
thermal, 361, 411
thermal and vasoconstriction, 415
thoracic, 320
upper airways, 203–204, 207, 276
upper lung airway, 207, 289, 296
vascular, *see* Vascular resistance
venous, 144
ventricular, 113–115

Resistor, 200
Respiration, 2, 166
  airflow, 170
  airways, 167, 169
  airways volume, 177
  anatomy, 167
  blood gas partial pressures, 193
  bronchioles, 168–169
  center, 231
  chemoreceptors, 224, 231, 238, 246, 248, 251
  compliance, *see* Compliance, respiratory
  control, *see* Control, of respiration
  control center, 140, 231–232, 321
  control equations, 309, 315, 317–318, 326
  controlled variable, 224, 316
  controller, 231, 321
  control signals, 238
  convective heat loss, *see* Convection, respiration
  cycle, 93, 174
  dead volume, 175, 177, 189, 196–198, 253, 259, 275, 311, 320–321, 332
    and airway lumen size, 208
    optimal, 267
    throughout breathing cycle, 208
    and tidal volume, 176, 312
  dead volume air, 197, 246
  dead volume compartment, 293–294, 296
  dead volume determination, 197
  disorders, 201, 250
  dynamics, 221
  effector organs, 238
  efficiency, *see* Efficiency, of respiratory muscles
  elastic power, 257
  end point, 271
  evaporation, *see* Evaporation, respiratory
  exchange of CO_2, 196
  exchange ratio, 183, 240, 247. *See also* Respiratory quotient
    and anaerobic threshold, 15–17
    and minute volume, 247
    during exercise, 16
  functions, 166
  gas exchange, *see* Gas, exchange in lungs
  gas measurements, 196
  heat loss, 364
  humoral component, 224, 268, 318, 340
  impairment and exercise, 26
  inertance, *see* Inertance, respiratory
  limits to exercise, 3, 6, 26, 252
  measurements, 271
  mechanical work, 221
  mechanics, 166
  minute volume, *see* Minute volume
  muscle efficiency, 221
  muscle fatigue, 255
  muscle force criterion, 260
  muscle mechanoreceptors, 230
  muscle oxygen uptake, 264, 336
  muscle pressures, 221, 254–255, 261, 280–281, 291, 295, 320
  muscle use patterns, 286
  muscles, 17, 166, 173, 203, 222, 224, 233, 238, 253
  muscles and dyspnea, 255
  muscles and second wind, 255
  muscular work, 166, 175, 220, 255–256, 258, 332, 334
  neural component, 224, 268
  obstruction, 189, 191. *See also* Chronic obstructive pulmonary disease
  optimization, 257, 260
  period, 175–177, 259
  power, maximum, 221
  power criterion, 258
  pressures on blood vessels, 145
  rate, 166, 250, 252, 323
    and CO_2, *see* Carbon dioxide, respiratory responses
    with elastic loading, 253
    during exercise, 257
    optimal, 259, 267, 333
    with resistive loading, 254
    variability, 262
  receptors, 224
  resistance, definition, 203
  resistive power, 257
  response to hemoglobin saturation, 248–249
  responses to CO_2, *see* Carbon dioxide, respiratory responses
  responses to exercise, 224, 239, 241
  rhythm, 224, 230–231, 238
  sensation quantified, 255
  sinus arrhythmia, 107
  steady-state response, 224
  system diagram, 167, 272
  system effective temperature, 367
  system mechanical properties, 200
  system models, 200–201, 271
  system natural frequency, 219
  system overdamping, 218
  system total gas pressure, 181
  ventilation, *see* Ventilation, rate after exercise, rate during exercise
  water vapor, 72
  work, 175, 218, 220, 252. *See also* Respiration, muscular work; Respiration, power
  work and resistance, 221
  zone, 169
Respiratory-cardiac interaction, 6, 101, 107, 145, 223, 228
Respiratory quotient(s), 183, 251. *See also* Respiration, exchange ratio
  of the brain, 184

Respiratory quotient(s) (*Continued*)
of carbohydrates, 183
diurnal variations, 202
during exercise, 184, 189
of fats, 183
of metabolizable substances, 183
of muscles, 184
of protein, 183
of the stomach, 184
Respiratory-thermal interaction, 6, 232
Response, thermal, vii
Rest:
and BMR, 390
and FRC, 175
after work, 67
Resting, *see also* Supine
airflow waveshapes, 265–266, 335–336
blood pressure, 93
convection coefficient, 366
energy expenditure, 50
heart rate, 93, 95
metabolic rate, *see* BMR
oxygen consumption, 104
rectal temperature, 440
transmembrane potential, 33
volume of lungs, 175, 253, 274
Restrictive pulmonary disease, 191
Retes, 415
Reticular substance, 101–102
Reynolds number, 82, 84, 205–206
and convection, 365
and entrance length, 205
local, 282
tracheal, 283
Rheopectic fluids, 79
Rib cage, 175, 272
volume, 279
Ribose, 8
Ribs, 173, 220
Robinson's ventricle model, 112
Rohrer equation, 203, 283
Rohrer coefficients, 203–204
airway, 204, 275
for exhalation and inhalation, 203, 278
pulmonary, 204
respiratory, 204
variation, 203
Rostral pons area, 236
Rotating shift work, 418
Rough terrain, 66
Round-off error, 150
RQ, *see* Respiratory quotient
Runners, 2, 4, 51
Running, 2–6, 31, 41, 44, 46, 48–57, 166
energy expenditure, 399, 438
load correction, 438
overland, 64
treadmill, 64
uphill, 64
Runny nose, 170
Rupture strength of bone, 42
RV, *see* Residual volume

Salt:
conservation in the heat, 416
loss and fatigue, 27
Sandquist circulatory system model, 116
Saturation:
of oxygen, *see* Hemoglobin, saturation
pressure for water vapor, 383–384
Saunders respiratory control model, 310
Savanna solar load, 380
Scaleni muscles, 174
SDA, 393
depending on body type, 394
depending on exercise, 394
release time, 394
s-domain, 125, 141, 154, 330
Sea level barometric pressure, *see* Atmospheric
pressure
Seasonal variations in physical fitness, 109
Second law of thermodynamics, 361
Second wind, 254–255
Sedentary convection coefficient, 366
Seesaw, 34
Segmental bronchi, 168, 170
Semitropical nature of man, 363
Sensible heat, 367
Sensitivity:
of chemoreceptors, 225, 228
of stretch receptors, 230
of test protocol, 25
Sensor firing rates, 100
Sensors, mechanical, 60, 100
Separable differential equations, 419
Septum, *see* Interventricular septum
Sequential file, 321
Series components, combination of, *see*
Mechanical properties combine
Serotonin, 108
Serum, 82
Sesquipedalian entry, 486
Set-point:
mean blood pressure, 140
pCO_2, 265, 327
temperature, 407–408, 425
for sweating, 413, 418
for various body compartments, 433
for vasodilation, 413
Severe exercise, 104
Sex, *see also* Gender effect
effect on blood composition, 72
effect on exercise, 4–5, 56, 65
effect on maximum torque, 37
Shape factor, *see* Radiation, shape factor

Shear rate, 78–79, 84
Shear stress, 78–79, 90–91
Sheep BMR, 393
Shirt thermal conductance, 371
Shivering, 112, 363, 415, 425
    energy by various muscle groups, 431
    equation, 431
    and heat source, 409
    inhibited during exercise, 418
    requiring neural control, 415
Shoes:
    effect on stepping motion, 60
    thermal conductance, 371
Shortening velocity of muscle, *see* Muscle,
        shortening rate and tension
Shunting:
    of blood from muscles to skin, 418
    of warm blood, 414
Shunts, 82, 173, 179, 193, 198, 414
Shykoff respiratory model, 286
Sigh, 274
Sigma effect, 86, 88
Sigmoid shape, 75–76, 100–101, 313
Silver emissivity, 373
Simpson's rule, 150
Sine-wave response, 107, 240–241
Singers, 176
Sinusoidal waveshape, 258, 260, 295, 313,
        334–336
Sitting heart rate, 129
Skating, 2–5
Skeletal mass, 428
Skeletal muscle, *see also* Muscle
    a–v oxygen difference, 103
    blood flow, 103
    heat production, 397
    mass, 103
    oxygen consumption, 103
    vascular resistance, 103, 108
Skiing, 2–3
    and body temperature, 415
    energy expenditure, 399, 415
Skin:
    a–v oxygen difference, 103
    blood flow, *see* Cutaneous blood flow
    blood volume, 81, 104
    conductance, *see* Thermal conductance, of
        skin
    conductance during work, 411
    contribution to BMR, 392
    dehydration, 385
    diffusion, 170
    emissivity, 373
    heat loss, 411
    heat production, 399
    irritation, 27
    mass, 103, 400, 428
    oxygen consumption, 81, 103

receptors, *see* Cutaneous receptors
surface evaporation, *see* Evaporation, on skin
        surface
temperature:
    mean, *see* Mean, skin temperature
    preferred, 385–386, 412
    from thermal resistance, 411
    and thermoregulation, 406. *See also*
        Hypothalamus; Thermoregulation
    and vasodilation, 409
thermal properties, 369
thickness, 422
vascular resistance, 103
weight, 81, 400
Slacks thermal conductance, 371
Sleep:
    deprivation and thermoregulatory response,
        417–418
    effect on respiration, 249
    and hypothalamic temperature, 409
Slow twitch muscle fibers, 8, 37
Smell, 230, 238
Smoke irritation, 239
Smoking among singers, 176
Smooth muscle fibers, *see* Muscle, smooth
Sneeze, 212, 230, 238
Socks thermal conductance, 371
Sodium:
    extracellular, 33–34, 405
    pump, 34
Solar heat load, 375–376
Solar heat load values, 380
Solar radiation components, 376
Solubility:
    of CO_2 in blood, 323
    of CO_2 in body fluid, 323
    of oxygen, 72
Solution and gas partial pressure, 72
Sonic velocity in tube, 211
Sophistication of subjects, effect on
        experimental results, 239
Sound sensitivity, 292
Sparrow, 51–52
Spatial summation of receptor outputs, 405
Spatial-temporal effects, 112
Specific dynamic action of food, *see* SDA
Specific heat:
    of air, 367, 381
    of blood, 369, 421, 426
    of body, 401, 421
    of bone, 426
    of fat, 369, 426
    of gases, 278
    of muscle, 369
    of skeleton, 426
    of skin, 369
    of tissue, 369, 426
Specific humidity, *see* Absolute humidity

Speed, 39
  and levers, 35–36
  of response, 233
  of sound, 211–212
  of sports competition, 4
  of walking, 46, 56, 58–59
Sphere, 91, 134, 171, 426
Spheroids, 419
Sphincter muscles, *see* Muscles, sphincter
Sphygmomanometer, 93
Spinal cord, 102, 228, 231–232
  transection, 415
Splanchnic bed, 104–105, 118, 411
Splanchnic blood flow in exercise, 149
Spleen blood flow, 104
Spontaneous breathing model results, 280
Spring constant, 42
Sprinting, 2
Squamous epithelium, 169
Square-wave response, 107, 334
Stability:
  mechanical, 31, 33, 172, 238
  numerical, 315, 318
Stair climbing efficiency, 396–397
Standard temperature and pressure, 72, 75, 181.
  See also STPD
Standing:
  blood pressure, 105
  cardiac output, 95
  lung volume, *see* Posture, and lung volumes
Starling's law, 90, 108, 112, 116, 122
State equations, 153
Static compliance, *see* Compliance, static
Static equilibrium, 31
Static pressure in tube, 211
Static recoil pressure, 272–273, 285
Static work, 13, 15, 66, 109
Steady flow, 281
Steady-state:
  error, 268
  respiratory response, 224, 241, 268
Stefan–Boltzmann constant, 372, 421
Stefan–Maxwell hard sphere model, 187
Step:
  change in work rate, 241, 330
  response, heart rate, *see* Heart rate, step
    response
Steppe solar load, 380
Stepping, 54, 60, 166
Sternum astoid muscles, 174
Steroids and exercise, 418
Stiffness, 279
Still air layer, *see* Insulation, still air
Stimulation, 102, 405
  of breathing, 230
Stolwijk and Hardy thermoregulatory model, 425
Stomach respiratory quotient, 184
Stop-flow technique, 274, 280

Storage:
  blood vessels, 82, 100, 104
  of energy, *see* Energy, storage
  of heat, *see* Heat, storage
STPD:
  to BTPS conversion, 181
  conditions, definition, 72, 181
Strain, definition, 42
Stress:
  definition, 42
  effect on BMR, 391
  relaxation, 79
  and respiration, 249
Stress–strain relationship of materials, 42, 134
Stresses:
  independence of various, 6
  interaction of various, 6
Stretching lungs and chest wall, 257
Stretch receptors, 100, 231, 253
Stride, 46
Stringed instrument players, 176
Stroke, 112
  volume, 14, 89, 93–94, 122
    in cold, 112
    in exercise, 97, 100, 105, 108, 110
    after standing, 105
Stupor, 222
Subarctic solar load, 380
Subbronchi, 169
Subclavian artery, 225
Subthreshold stimuli, 236
Sulfur dioxide irritation, 239
Sulfuric acid and metabolic acidosis, 244
Sulfur metabolism, 244
Sun of the microcosm, 71
Superior vena cava, 131–132, 144, 146–147
Supine:
  blood pressure, compared to upright, 105
  exercise, compared to upright, 13
  lung volume, *see* Posture, and lung volumes
  ventilation/perfusion, *see* Posture, and
    ventilation/perfusion
  work:
    compared to upright, 13
    oxygen uptake of, 21
    time constant of oxygen uptake, 21
Surface area:
  body, *see* Body, surface area
  correction for clothing, *see* Clothing, surface
    area correction factor
  correction for radiation, *see* Radiation, surface
    area correction
Surface emissivity, *see* Emissivity
Surfaces, walking, *see* Terrain, coefficients
Surface tension, 273
Surfactant, 171–172, 273, 280
Survival, 224, 403
Suspensions, 79

Sustained work, 66
Swallowing, 175, 230, 238–239
Sweat:
    absorbed by clothing, *see* Sweating, ineffective
    accumulation, 434, 440, 442
    evaporation, *see* Evaporation, of sweat
    glands, 108
    latent heat of vaporization, 385
    rate, 440
    rolling off skin, *see* Sweating, ineffective
Sweater thermal conductance, 371
Sweating, 361, 425, 439
    and acclimatization, 416
    and dehydration, 27, 80
    different areas, 386
    efficiency, 388
    equation, 425, 431
    ineffective, 385, 390
    local control of, 412
    nonregulatory, 385
    nonsteady, *see* Cyclic sweating
    rate, 410
    recruitment, 385, 412
    regulatory, 385, 407–408, 412
    of trunk, 413
Swim bladders, 54
Swimmers, 3–4, 51
Swimming, 2–5, 48–50, 166
    energy expenditure, 399
Swing phase of walking, 63
Sympathetic nerves, 101–105, 109, 140, 415
    and chemoreceptor output, 228
Synchronized body temperature and sleep, 417
Synchronized breathing, 166, 257, 297
Syphon, 91
Systemic:
    arterial baroreceptor reflex, 105
    arteries, 144
    arterioles, 172. *See also* Arterioles
    blood pressure, *see* Blood, pressure
    blood volume, 321
    circulation, 89, 104, 117, 131–132, 143
    circulation gas measurements, 196
    veins, 144
Systole, 81, 83, 89, 92–93, 113
    time difference between atrial and ventricular,
        139
Systolic pressure, 91–93, 98, 108–109, 111
Systolic work, 120

Tachycardia, 93
Tachypnea, 230
Taylor dispersion, 190
Temperature:
    and activity level, 403
    of blood, 194
    and cardiovascular control, 108
    effects:

on enzymatic activity, 391, 403
on heart rate, 111
on hemoglobin saturation, 76
on inhalation, 235–236
on metabolism, 392–393. *See also* Van't
    Hoff equation
on occlusion pressure, 233
on plasma volume, 111
on respiration, 249
on sonic velocity, 212
on tidal volume, 175, 250
regulation, *see* Thermoregulation
and second wind, 255
set-point, *see* Set-point, temperature
skin, *see* Skin, temperature
threshold, 405
tympanic membrane, *see* Ear drum
    temperature
Tendons, 33, 58, 230, 395
Tension-time index of the heart, 98
Terminal bronchioles, 168–169
Termination of inspiration, 236
Terrain:
    coefficients, 437
    coefficients for walking, 66
    reflected heat load, *see* Environmentally
        reflected radiation
Thermal boundary layer, 381
Thermal comfort, 409
Thermal comfort zone, *see* Thermoneutral
    environment
Thermal conductance, 370, 425
    for clothing, 370–371, 389
    and heat loss, 410–411
    of skin, 409–410, 421
    for various segments, 429
Thermal conductivity, 369
    of air, 365, 387
    of fat, 369
    of muscle, 369
    of skin, 369
    of tissue, 369
Thermal currents, 365
Thermal diffusivity, 368, 381
Thermal discomfort limiting exercise, 26
Thermal equilibrium, 166, 363
Thermal limits to exercise, 3, 6, 26
Thermal mechanics, 364
Thermal overload, *see* Heat, stroke
Thermal resistance, *see* Resistance
Thermal–respiratory interaction, *see*
        Respiratory–thermal interaction
Thermal response, *see* Response, thermal
Thermal shells, *see* Core and shell model
Thermal stress, 111, 441
Thermodynamics:
    first law, 394
    second law, 361

Thermoelectric cooler, 434
Thermogenesis, *see* Heat, production
Thermoneutral environment, 361, 363, 403, 436
Thermoreceptor(s), 268, 403, 425. *See also*
    Cold receptors; Warm receptors
  distribution, 403
  inputs by various body segments, 432
  model, 405
Thermoregulation, 24, 223, 363, 403
  different levels, 407–408
  equations, 421, 431, 435
  external, *see* External thermoregulation
Thickness of clothing, *see* Clothing, effective
    thickness
Thick-walled vessel, 134
Thighs:
  skin temperature, 386
  surface area, 386
  sweating, 386
  weight, 32
Thixotropic fluids, 79
Thoracic cage, 175, 238
Thoracic cavity, 147, 173
Thorax:
  aorta, 144
  arteries, 131–132, 146
  blood flow, 146
  blood volume, 177
  compartments, 147
  gas volume, 208
  muscles, 175
  pressure, *see* Intrathoracic pressure
  shape, 173, 220
  stiffness, 216
  veins, 146
  volume, 238
  wall, *see* Chest wall
Threshold:
  detection, *see* Weber–Fechner Law
  level, 225, 405
  loading, 253
  pressure, 100
  stimuli, 235–237, 405
  temperature, 405, 410
Thyroid and carbohydrate ingestion, 10
Thyroid gland, 415–417
Thyroxin:
  and exercise, 24, 418
  and heart rate, 108
  and heat production, 415–416
Tidal volume, 175–177, 189, 233, 259, 323, 332
  with elastic loading, 253
  in exercise, 252
  irregularity, 318
  related to chemoreceptors, 253
  related to mechanoreceptors, 253
Time:
  domain, 154

increment for numerical solution, 151
  sense of, 292
  to exhaustion, *see* Performance, time
Time constant:
  of baroreceptors, 140, 142
  of brain blood flow, 307
  of carbon dioxide production, 240
  of cardiac output change, 306, 310
  of exhalation, 219, 334
  of heart response, 25, 126
  of lung filling, 286
  of the lung, 219
  of lung segments, 191, 219
  of macromolecule diffusion, 274–275
  of oxygen uptake, 20–21, 25, 240
  of rectal temperature change, 441, 443
  of respiratory muscle pressure, 295–296
  of respiratory response, 25, 240, 330–331
  of respiratory system, 219, 261–262
  of respiratory ventilation, 240–242
  of sweating, 413
  of thermal response, 25
  of vascular control, 145
  of vascular segments, 145
Time delay:
  for body temperature change, 402, 441–442
  circulation, 318
  in dead volume gas, 256
  heart rate, 125–126
  between lung and brain, 307, 315
  between lung and tissue, 307
  in oxygen response, 248
  respiratory response, 330–331
  sweating, 413
Tissue:
  blood flow, 104
  compartment, 300, 320–321
  heat transfer, 364
  necrosis, 112
  pH, 108
  thermal properties, 369
  volumes, 323
TLC, *see* Total lung capacity (or Tender loving
    care)
Toluene diffusion constant, 186
Tongue thermoreceptors, 405
Torque:
  balance on body, 31
  on joint, 37, 39, 61, 67
  sign convention, 31
Torso rigidity, 166
Total lung capacity, 175–177
Total respiratory cycle work, 260
Trachea, 168–169, 173, 175, 281
  air composition, 182
  air flow, 181
  mechanics, 281
  Reynolds number, 283

Tracheobronchial receptors, 230
Tracheostomy tube, 236
Track, 45
Training:
    effect:
        on acclimatization, 416
        on BMR, 392
        on heart rate, 95
        on heart size, 109
        on heart weight, 95–96
        on maximal heart rate, 109
        on maximum oxygen uptake, 15, 94
        on metabolism, 392
        on muscle capillary beds, 74
        on respiratory pressure loading, 254
        on stroke volume, 95
        on thermal stress, 417
    and respiratory sensation, 255
Trajectory determination, 60
Transdiaphragmatic pressure, 174
Transient increase:
    in blood lactate, 250
    in ventilation, 240–241
Transient response to blood pH, 244
Transient time, blood circulation, 321
Transition:
    from laminar to turbulent flow, *see* Laminar
        to turbulent transition
    from nose to mouth breathing, *see* Nasal to
        mouth breathing transition
    from rest to exercise, 240, 265
    speed from walking to running, 54, 58
    zone, respiratory, 169–170
    zone in airway cast model, 283
Transit time:
    blood through muscles, 73
    pulmonary blood, 173, 194
Translational motion, 38
Transmembrane potential, 33, 292
Transmission line, 118
Transmissivity, 373
Transmural pressure of blood vessels, 145, 147
Transport time, lung-to-brain, *see* Time, delay
        between lung and brain
Transpulmonary pressure, 295. *See also*
        Respiration, muscle pressures
Trapezoidal integration, 150
Trauma, 82
Treadmill:
    load carrying, 66
    running, 64
    walking, 437
    walking heart rate, 129
Triceps:
    extensor cubiti muscle, 394
    muscle, 33, 36
Trigeminal nerve, 101
Triiodothyronine and heat production, 415–416

Tripalmitin metabolism, 183
Tropical rain forest solar load, 380
Tropical savanna solar load, 380
Trousers thermal conductance, 371
Trucks, cost of transport, 51–52
Truncation error, 150
Trunk:
    blood flow, 428
    contribution to BMR, 392
    heat production, 428
    mass, 428
    surface area, 427
    sweating, 413
    thermal conductivity, 428
    volume, 427
Tube:
    characteristic, 211–212
    narrowing, 211
    resistance, 82–83
    rigidity, 211
Tundra solar load, 380
Turbulence, 206
Turbulent flow, 82, 93, 176, 191, 203–204, 210
Turbulent friction pressure loss, 283
Tympanic membrane temperature, *see* Ear drum
        temperature

Ulna, 36
Unconscious clues to dyspnea, 271
Unconsciousness, 104–105, 222
Unconscious responses to heat, 361
Undamped natural frequency, 219
Underdamped system, 218
Underwear thermal conductance, 371
Unequal lung filling, 286
Universal gas constant, 180
Unsteady flow, 83
Upper airway, 276
    pressure–flow nonlinearities, 203–204
    resistance, *see* Resistance, airway(s);
        Resistance, upper airway
    stiffness, 208
    volume, 278
Upper airways limiting flow, 212
Urinary nitrogen equivalent of protein, 185
Urinary output, 108, 183
Urine concentrations, units of, 245
Useful work, 166

Vagal afferent sources, 101, 233
Vagal tone, 93
Vagus:
    discharge, 236
    effect, 105
    nerve, 101–102, 105, 140, 230, 232
    nerve and respiratory sensation, 255
Valves, 82, 90, 131–132, 144. *See also* Aortic,
    valve; Mitral valve; Veins

Van't Hoff equation, 391
Vapor:
  diffusion constants, 186
  pressure of water, *see* Saturation, pressure for water vapor
  transmission, 364
Vascular innervation, 104
Vascular models, 117–119, 131–132
Vascular pressure, 231
Vascular resistance, 91, 98–100, 103–104, 107, 116, 122, 131–132, 148, 325
  in cold, 112
  control, 145
  and epinephrine, 108
  during exercise, 105, 145
  increase after standing, 105
  nonlinearities, 147
Vasoconstriction, 74, 102, 104
  alveolar, 179
  cerebral, 149, 246
  cutaneous, 369
  and vasodilation compared, 413
Vasodilation, 101, 104, 108, 131
  cerebral, 104, 108
  cutaneous, *see* Cutaneous, vasodilation
Vasomotor:
  center, 99, 101–102, 104, 140
  responses, 363. *See also* Vasoconstriction; Vasodilation
  tone, 101
VC, *see* Vital capacity
Veins, 81–82, 93, 104
Velocity:
  profile, 83, 191, 204–205, 210
  profile in airways, 206
  of shortening, *see* Muscle, shortening rate and tension
Vena cava, 81–82, 89, 91, 93, 131–132
Venae comitantes, 414
Venous blood, 74, 77, 82, 143, 267
  gas partial pressures, 181, 193
  pressure, 82, 105, 111, 144
  return, 82, 90–91, 100
  return in exercise, 109
  volume, 144, 147
Venous collapse, *see* Collapse, of blood vessels
Venous compliance, *see* Compliance, venous
Venous inertance, *see* Inertance, venous
Venous model, 116, 143, 145
Venous pCO_2, 108
Venous pO_2, 109
Venous resistance, *see* Resistance, venous
Venous return path for blood in heat, 414
Venous valves, 82, 131–132, 147
Venous weight, 81
Ventilation:
  and baroreflex, 107
  control, 24, 238
  distribution, 207

during exercise, *see* Hyperpnea
  high frequency, 189
  and inhaled CO_2, 309, 311, 318, 320, 328
  rate after exercise, 250
  rate during exercise, 17, 240–241, 309
  and respiratory exchange ratio, *see* Respiration, exchange ratio, and minute volume
Ventilation/perfusion ratio, 177–178, 194
  distribution, 177
  regulation, 179
Ventilatory compensation, 251, 253
Ventilatory loading, 252
Ventilatory perfusion, 177–178, 196, 239
  rate distribution, 177
Ventilatory response to hemoglobin saturation, 248–249
Ventral respiratory neurons, 232
Ventricle, 89, 93, 96, 112–113, 131
  blood volume, 144
  compliance, *see* Compliance, ventricular
  ejection period, 123
  ejection pressure, 98, 114
  energy and power, 99, 118
  filling, 96
  isovolume contraction, 123
  model, 112, 114, 118–119
  muscle length, *see* Myocardium, length
  pressure, 113, 115, 122–123, 133, 144
  receptors, 107
  resistance, *see* Resistance, ventricular
  volume, 114
  wall, 134
Venule, 81–82, 93, 104
Vertebral extensor muscles, 174
Vertical force component, 54
Vertical jump, 40
Very heavy loads, 438
Very heavy work, 397–398
Very light work, 397–398
Vibration and inhalation, 236
Viscera, 102, 109, 131
  mass, 428
Viscoelastic fluids, 79
Viscosity, blood, *see* Blood, viscosity
Viscous dissipation of energy, 203, 211
Viscous power, *see* Resistance, power
Viscous pressure drop, 84, 203, 282. *See also* Friction
Visible light, 372
Vital capacity, 175–177, 215, 314
  with elastic loading, 254
Vocal cords, 175
Voice:
  box, *see* Larynx
  pitch analysis, 255
Volume:
  fractions of air constituents, 180
  lower airways, 279

lung, *see* Lung volume
receptors, 100
tube, 279
Volume–pressure curve:
  for abdomen–diaphragm, 273–274
  for chest wall, 217, 273–274
  for lung tissue, 217, 274, 276
  for respiratory system, 215
  slope, 215
Voluntary control of respiration, 166, 257
Vomiting and metabolic acidosis, 244

Walking, 2–5, 43, 45, 47–52, 55, 57
  downhill, 437
  efficiency, 52, 401
  energy, 53, 58–59, 66, 399, 401, 436
  energy by various muscle groups, 431
  heart rate, 129
  speed, 46, 54, 58–59
Wall effect in blood vessels, 84
Warm-blooded animals, *see* Homeotherms
Warm receptors, 403–404. *See also*
    Thermoreceptor
Water:
  emissivity, 373
  filtration, 82
  of hydration, 183
  latent heat of vaporization, 382
  mass diffusivity, 386
  vapor, respiratory, 72, 181, 384
  vapor collision diameter, 187
  vapor diffusion constant, 186, 189
  vapor diffusion volume, 188
  vapor force constant, 187
  vapor mass diffusivity, 386
  vapor partial pressure in lungs, blood, and
    muscle, 181
  vapor pressure, 180, 383–384, 390, 440
  vapor saturation pressure, *see* Saturation,
    pressure for water vapor
  vapor transmission through clothes, 385, 439
Waves, 112
Wave-speed formulation, 211, 282
Weather data, 379–380
Weber–Fechner law, 254, 292
Weibel respiratory model, 168–169, 281
Weight-lifting, 33, 65, 166, 395

Weight of various organs, 81
Wetted clothes, 390
Wetted skin area, 440
Whale, 218
Wheel, 54
Wheelbarrow, 34
White blood cells, 72
Wind instrument players, 176
Windkessel vessels, 82
Windpipe, *see* Trachea
Wing, 53–54
Winslow equation for ambient conductance,
    378
Women, speed compared to men, 4–5
Wood emissivity, 373
Work, 3, 52, 218
  of breathing, 220–221
  dynamic, 13, 15
  in energy model, 23
  equivalent to heat energy, *see* First law of
    thermodynamics
  history of subjects, 239
  intensity classification, 3, 397–398
  of posture maintenance, 220
  rate:
    for cardiovascular limited exercise, 24
    during experimental studies, 25
    and heat accumulation, 26
    impulse, 330
    ramp increase, 19, 330
    for respiratory limited exercise, 26
    sinusoidal, 241
    step change, 241, 330
    for thermal limitation to exercise, 26
  and respiration, 240–241
  static, 13, 15
Wrestling, 33
Wyndham–Atkins thermoregulatory model, 422

Yamamoto CO_2 model, 320
Yamashiro and Livnat ventricular model, 118
Yawning, 172
Yield stress, 179
Yoga breathing exercises, 250
Young's modulus, 42
  for biological materials, 42
  for bone, 42